Advances in Plant Alkaloid Research

Advances in Plant Alkaloid Research

Editor

John C. D'Auria

MDPI • Basel • Beijing • Wuhan • Barcelona • Belgrade • Manchester • Tokyo • Cluj • Tianjin

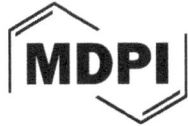

Editor
John C. D'Auria
Research Group
Leader—Metabolic Diversity
Department of Molecular
Genetics Leibniz Institute of
Plant Genetics and Crop Plant
Research (IPK Gatersleben)
Gatersleben
Germany

Editorial Office
MDPI
St. Alban-Anlage 66
4052 Basel, Switzerland

This is a reprint of articles from the Special Issue published online in the open access journal *Molecules* (ISSN 1420-3049) (available at: https://www.mdpi.com/journal/molecules/special_issues/plant_alkaloid).

For citation purposes, cite each article independently as indicated on the article page online and as indicated below:

LastName, A.A.; LastName, B.B.; LastName, C.C. Article Title. *Journal Name* **Year**, *Article Number*, Page Range.

ISBN 978-3-03943-172-4 (Hbk)
ISBN 978-3-03943-173-1 (PDF)

Cover image courtesy of John C. D'Auria.

© 2020 by the authors. Articles in this book are Open Access and distributed under the Creative Commons Attribution (CC BY) license, which allows users to download, copy and build upon published articles, as long as the author and publisher are properly credited, which ensures maximum dissemination and a wider impact of our publications.
The book as a whole is distributed by MDPI under the terms and conditions of the Creative Commons license CC BY-NC-ND.

Contents

About the Editor vii

Preface to "Advances in Plant Alkaloid Research" ix

Ivette M. Menéndez-Perdomo and Peter J. Facchini
Benzylisoquinoline Alkaloids Biosynthesis in Sacred Lotus
Reprinted from: *Molecules* **2018**, *23*, 2899, doi:10.3390/molecules23112899 1

Sebastian Schramm, Nikolai Köhler and Wilfried Rozhon
Pyrrolizidine Alkaloids: Biosynthesis, Biological Activities and Occurrence in Crop Plants
Reprinted from: *Molecules* **2019**, *24*, 498, doi:10.3390/molecules24030498 19

Kathrin Laura Kohnen-Johannsen and Oliver Kayser
Tropane Alkaloids: Chemistry, Pharmacology, Biosynthesis and Production
Reprinted from: *Molecules* **2019**, *24*, 796, doi:10.3390/molecules24040796 63

David A. Restrepo, Ernesto Saenz, Orlando Adolfo Jara-Muñoz, Iván F. Calixto-Botía, Sioly Rodríguez-Suárez, Pablo Zuleta, Benjamin G. Chavez, Juan A. Sanchez and John C. D'Auria
Erythroxylum in Focus: An Interdiciplinary Review of an Overlooked Genus
Reprinted from: *Molecules* **2019**, *24*, 3788, doi:10.3390/molecules24203788 87

López Carlos, Pastrana Manuel, Ríos Alexandra, Cogollo Alvaro and Pabón Adriana
Huberine, a New Canthin-6-One Alkaloid from the Bark of *Picrolemma huberi*
Reprinted from: *Molecules* **2018**, *23*, 934, doi:10.3390/molecules23040934 115

Kang He, Jinxi Wang, Juan Zou, Jichun Wu, Shaojie Huo and Jiang Du
Three New Cytotoxic Steroidal Alkaloids from *Sarcococca hookeriana*
Reprinted from: *Molecules* **2018**, *23*, 1181, doi:10.3390/molecules23051181 121

Luciana R. Tallini, Jaume Bastida, Natalie Cortes, Edison H. Osorio, Cristina Theoduloz and Guillermo Schmeda-Hirschmann
Cholinesterase Inhibition Activity, Alkaloid Profiling and Molecular Docking of Chilean *Rhodophiala* (Amaryllidaceae)
Reprinted from: *Molecules* **2018**, *23*, 1532, doi:10.3390/molecules23071532 129

Mao-Sheng Zhang, Yan Deng, Shao-Bin Fu, Da-Le Guo and Shi-Ji Xiao
Mahimbrine A, a Novel Isoquinoline Alkaloid Bearing a Benzotropolone Moiety from *Mahonia imbricata*
Reprinted from: *Molecules* **2018**, *23*, 1539, doi:10.3390/molecules23071539 157

Matthew W. Turner, Roberto Cruz, Jordan Elwell, John French, Jared Mattos and Owen M. McDougal
Native *V. californicum* Alkaloid Combinations Induce Differential Inhibition of Sonic Hedgehog Signaling
Reprinted from: *Molecules* **2018**, *23*, 2222, doi:10.3390/molecules23092222 163

András Keglevich, Szabolcs Mayer, Réka Pápai, Áron Szigetvári, Zsuzsanna Sánta, Miklós Dékány, Csaba Szántay Jr., Péter Keglevich and László Hazai
Attempted Synthesis of *Vinca* Alkaloids Condensed with Three-Membered Rings
Reprinted from: *Molecules* **2018**, *23*, 2574, doi:10.3390/molecules23102574 173

Olívia Moreira Sampaio, Lucas Campos Curcino Vieira, Barbara Sayuri Bellete, Beatriz King-Diaz, Blas Lotina-Hennsen, Maria Fátima das Graças Fernandes da Silva and Thiago André Moura Veiga
Evaluation of Alkaloids Isolated from *Ruta graveolens* as Photosynthesis Inhibitors
Reprinted from: *Molecules* **2018**, *23*, 2693, doi:10.3390/molecules23102693 195

Fredi Cifuentes, Javier Palacios, Adrián Paredes, Chukwuemeka R. Nwokocha and Cristian Paz
8-Oxo-9-Dihydromakomakine Isolated from *Aristotelia chilensis* Induces Vasodilation in Rat Aorta: Role of the Extracellular Calcium Influx
Reprinted from: *Molecules* **2018**, *23*, 3050, doi:10.3390/molecules23113050 207

Chuxin Liang, Chang Chen, Pengfei Zhou, Lv Xu, Jianhua Zhu, Jincai Liang, Jiachen Zi and Rongmin Yu
Effect of *Aspergillus flavus* Fungal Elicitor on the Production of Terpenoid Indole Alkaloids in *Catharanthus roseus* Cambial Meristematic Cells
Reprinted from: *Molecules* **2018**, *23*, 3276, doi:10.3390/molecules23123276 219

Shaojie Huo, Jichun Wu, Xicheng He, Lutai Pan and Jiang Du
Two New Cytotoxic Steroidal Alkaloids from *Sarcococca Hookeriana*
Reprinted from: *Molecules* **2019**, *24*, 11, doi:10.3390/molecules24010011 235

Folake A. Egbewande, Mark J. Coster, Ian D. Jenkins and Rohan A. Davis
Reaction of Papaverine with Baran Diversinates™
Reprinted from: *Molecules* **2019**, *24*, 3938, doi:10.3390/molecules24213938 243

Ana Calheiros de Carvalho, Luiza De Camillis Rodrigues, Alany Ingrid Ribeiro, Maria Fátima das Graças Fernandes da Silva, Lívia Soman de Medeiros and Thiago André Moura Veiga
Integrated Analytical Tools for Accessing Acridones and Unrelated Phenylacrylamides from *Swinglea glutinosa*
Reprinted from: *Molecules* **2020**, *25*, 153, doi:10.3390/molecules25010153 257

About the Editor

John C. D'Auria Research Group Leader—Metabolic Diversity Department of Molecular Genetics, Leibniz Institute of Plant Genetics and Crop Plant Research (IPK Gatersleben) Gatersleben, Corrensstraße 3, 06466 Seeland, Germany.

Preface to "Advances in Plant Alkaloid Research"

Plant alkaloids are critical components of modern medicine and pharmaceuticals. These compounds are also becoming increasingly important for industrial uses as part of the green chemistry revolution. This Special Issue will focus on the molecular advances being made in understanding how such a large and diverse class of compounds are made by plants and how metabolic engineering advances are increasing the overall yield of crucial precursors.

John C. D'Auria
Editor

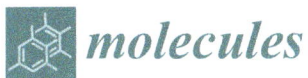

Review

Benzylisoquinoline Alkaloids Biosynthesis in Sacred Lotus

Ivette M. Menéndez-Perdomo and Peter J. Facchini *

Department of Biological Sciences, University of Calgary, Calgary, AB T2N 1N4, Canada; ivette.menendez1@ucalgary.ca
* Correspondence: pfacchin@ucalgary.ca; Tel.: +1-403-220-7651

Received: 24 October 2018; Accepted: 4 November 2018; Published: 6 November 2018

Abstract: Sacred lotus (*Nelumbo nucifera* Gaertn.) is an ancient aquatic plant used throughout Asia for its nutritional and medicinal properties. Benzylisoquinoline alkaloids (BIAs), mostly within the aporphine and bisbenzylisoquinoline structural categories, are among the main bioactive constituents in the plant. The alkaloids of sacred lotus exhibit promising anti-cancer, anti-arrhythmic, anti-HIV, and anti-malarial properties. Despite their pharmacological significance, BIA metabolism in this non-model plant has not been extensively investigated. In this review, we examine the diversity of BIAs in sacred lotus, with an emphasis on the distinctive stereochemistry of alkaloids found in this species. Additionally, we discuss our current understanding of the biosynthetic genes and enzymes involved in the formation of 1-benzylisoquinoline, aporphine, and bisbenzylisoquinoline alkaloids in the plant. We conclude that a comprehensive functional characterization of alkaloid biosynthetic enzymes using both in vitro and in vivo methods is required to advance our limited knowledge of BIA metabolism in the sacred lotus.

Keywords: benzylisoquinoline alkaloids; cytochrome P450 monooxygenase; medicinal properties; methyltransferase; *Nelumbo nucifera*; norcoclaurine synthase; sacred lotus; stereochemistry

1. Introduction

Sacred lotus (*Nelumbo nucifera* Gaertn) is a basal eudicot aquatic plant. It belongs to the small Nelumbonaceae family (order Proteales), which includes only the genus *Nelumbo* and the species *N. lutea* (native to North America) and *N. nucifera* (native to Asia and Australia). Sacred lotus diverged from the core eudicots early in angiosperms evolutionary history, prior to a whole-genome triplication event [1,2]. According to the fossil records, Nelumbonaceae morphology has remained stable since the mid-Cretaceous period, and plastid genome sequencing analysis has established that both *Nelumbo* species, currently found in opposite sides of the Pacific Ocean, diverged relatively recently (~1.5 million years ago) from a common ancestor [3].

For thousands of years lotus has been integrated in traditional medicine, diet, and popular culture, commonly used as an ornamental plant in ponds and designated 'sacred' owing to its religious significance in Buddhism and Hinduism [4]. The plant also displays several outstanding characteristics rarely seen in the angiosperms, such as shoot-before-root emergence, regulated flower thermogenesis, a dim-light photosynthetic plumule, and leaves with wax-covered nanopapillae that create the self-cleaning and water-repellent 'lotus effect' [5–7]. In addition, scared lotus seeds are remarkable for their longevity (radiocarbon dated up to ~1300 years before germination), which is a feature of interest to researchers investigating the molecular mechanisms of aging resistance [8,9].

All parts of sacred lotus are medicinally significant. For example, rhizomes are used in the Chinese traditional medicine for the treatment of liver cirrhosis, dyspepsia, and dysentery; stem preparations are prescribed in Ayurvedic medicine as an anthelmintic and to treat leprosy; leaf extracts possess antiviral, diuretic, and astringent activities and are applied to fever management; flowers are employed to treat cholera and bleeding disorders; and finally seeds and dissected embryos are used as remedies for insomnia, inflammation, cancer, and heart diseases [4,10]. More than 200 secondary metabolites have been isolated from the plant and associated with various pharmacological properties [4]. The isolated compounds comprise different classes of chemicals such as flavonoids, terpenoids, and alkaloids. In particular, benzylisoquinoline alkaloids (BIAs) in the aporphine and bisbenzylisoquinoline structural categories are among the main bioactive constituents of sacred lotus.

Nuciferine, the major aporphine found in *N. nucifera*, has reportedly been effective in the treatment of several types of cancer (e.g., lung, colon, and breast) and neuroblastoma [11–13]. Other bioactive aporphines extracted from sacred lotus are pronuciferine, an alkaloid reported to decrease intracellular triglyceride content in adipocytes, making it a promising metabolite to treat obesity [14]; *N*-nornuciferine, which acts as a melanogenesis inhibitor [15,16]; *O*-nornuciferine (also known as *N*-methylasimilobine) and lysicamine, both possessing potent antioxidant properties; 7-hydroxydehydronuciferine, a metabolite that significantly inhibits the proliferation of melanoma, prostate, and gastric cancer cells [17]; and roemerine, which has been ascribed anti-fungal and anti-malarial properties [18].

Neferine and liensinine are the main bisbenzylisoquinoline components of sacred lotus. The former has been reported to possess anti-arrhythmic effects [19] and to induce apoptosis in human lung cancer [20]; hepatocellular carcinoma [21], and ovarian cancer [22], whereas the latter has been shown to inhibit the growth of breast cancer cells and prevent associated bone destruction [12,23]. In addition, neferine, liensinine, isoliensinine, and nelumboferine exhibit sedative effects in mice models, which could be related to the relaxation properties of tea prepared from sacred lotus embryos [24].

Despite the medicinal importance of BIAs in sacred lotus, relatively little is known about alkaloid metabolic pathways in the plant, or the biosynthetic genes and cognate enzymes. Remarkably, although many BIAs isolated from *N. nucifera* have been detected in the *R*-enantiomer conformation, which contrasts with predominantly *S*-enantiomer conformers found in opium poppy (*Papaver somniferum*) and related plants (order Ranunculales), no studies have yet examined this feature of BIA metabolism in sacred lotus. Such topics are of significance to advance research in the field of plant alkaloid metabolism, particularly in non-model species, and to develop better strategies to bioengineer high-value phytopharmaceuticals in various production systems. Herein, we review the current knowledge of BIAs biosynthesis in sacred lotus.

2. Occurrence of BIAs in Sacred Lotus

Benzylisoquinoline alkaloids (BIAs) constitute a large class of plant specialized metabolites derived from tyrosine [25]. The enantioselective condensation of dopamine (yielding the tetrahydroisoquinoline moiety) and 4-hydroxyphenylacetaldehyde (yielding the benzyl moiety) by norcoclaurine synthase (NCS) generates (*S*)-norcoclaurine, the common precursor to all BIAs [26]. A variety of coupling reactions and functional group modifications establish a large number of structural subcategories and specific compounds with a plethora of pharmacological properties. These include the narcotic analgesics morphine and codeine (morphinans), the muscle relaxant papaverine (1-benzylisoquinoline), the antimicrobial agents sanguinarine (benzophenanthridine) and berberine (protoberberine), the bronchodilator and anti-inflammatory glaucine (aporphine), and the potential anticancer drugs noscapine (phthalideisoquinoline) and dauricine (bisbenzylisoquinoline) [27].

The occurrence of BIAs in nature is restricted to certain plant families, primarily in the order Ranunculales. Consequently, most of the plants that have been investigated with respect to BIA metabolism are members of the Papaveraceae, Ranunculaceae, Berberidaceae, and Menispermaceae families [27–30]. The first and foremost of these is opium poppy (*Papaver somniferum*). However, BIAs also occur sporadically in the orders Piperales and Magnoliales, as well as in the Rutaceae, Lauraceae,

Cornaceae and Nelumbonaceae families [31], but plants belonging to these taxa have received far less attention. Sacred lotus leaves, embryos, and leaf sap are rich in BIAs, although the alkaloid composition and content varies considerably among the nearly 600 known genotypes [32–35]. There are three main subclasses of BIAs in sacred lotus: the 1-benzylisoquinoline, aporphine, and bisbenzylisoquinoline alkaloids (Table 1).

Table 1. Benzylisoquinoline alkaloids (BIAs) detected in different organs of *Nelumbo nucifera*, their chemical formula, and stereochemistry. Alkaloid structures are assigned numbers as shown in Figures 1–4. L: leaf, E: embryo, F: flower, S: seed, R: rhizome, LS: leaf sap, NS: not specified, N/A: not applicable.

No.	Alkaloid	Formula	Enantiomer	Organ	Reference
1-BENZYLISOQUINOLINE					
1	Norcoclaurine	$C_{16}H_{17}NO_3$	(+)-R and (−)-S	L, E	[36–39]
2	Coclaurine	$C_{17}H_{19}NO_3$	(+)-R	L, E, F	[15,37,38]
3	N-Methylcoclaurine	$C_{18}H_{21}NO_3$	(−)-R	L, E, F	[15,37,38]
4	Norarmepavine	$C_{18}H_{21}NO_3$	(+)-R	F	[15,40]
5	N-Methylisococlaurine	$C_{18}H_{21}NO_3$	NS	L, E	[38,41]
6	6-Demethyl-4′-O-methyl-N-methylcoclaurine	$C_{18}H_{21}NO_3$	NS	E	[38]
7	Armepavine	$C_{19}H_{23}NO_3$	(−)-R and (+)-S	L, E, S	[15,38,40,42]
8	4′-O-Methyl-N-methylcoclaurine	$C_{19}H_{23}NO_3$	NS	E	[38]
9	4′-O-Methylarmepavine	$C_{20}H_{25}NO_3$	NS	L	[43]
10	Lotusine	$C_{19}H_{24}NO_3^+$	NS	E	[38]
11	Isolotusine	$C_{19}H_{24}NO_3^+$	NS	E	[38]
APORPHINE					
12	Caaverine	$C_{17}H_{17}NO_2$	(−)-R	L	[17,40]
13	Asimilobine	$C_{17}H_{17}NO_2$	(−)-R	L, F	[15,17,44]
14	Lirinidine	$C_{18}H_{19}NO_2$	(−)-R	L, F	[16]
15	O-Nornuciferine	$C_{18}H_{19}NO_2$	(−)-R	L, F	[16,17,35]
16	N-Nornuciferine	$C_{18}H_{19}NO_2$	(−)-R	L, E, F	[16,17,38]
17	Nuciferine	$C_{19}H_{21}NO_2$	(−)-R	L, E, F	[15,17,35,38]
18	Anonaine	$C_{17}H_{15}NO_2$	(−)-R	L, F	[17,32]
19	Roemerine	$C_{18}H_{17}NO_2$	(−)-R	L, F	[17,18,32,35]
20	Dehydronuciferine	$C_{19}H_{19}NO_2$	N/A	L, R	[16,32,41]
21	Dehydroanonaine	$C_{17}H_{13}NO_2$	N/A	L	[41]
22	Dehydroroemerine	$C_{18}H_{15}NO_2$	N/A	L	[41]
23	Pronuciferine	$C_{19}H_{21}NO_3$	(+)-R and (−)-S	L, E, F	[16,38,40,43]
24	7-Hydroxydehydronuciferine	$C_{19}H_{19}NO_3$	N/A	L	[17]
25	Lysicamine	$C_{18}H_{13}NO_3$	N/A	L, F	[16]
26	Liriodenine	$C_{17}H_9NO_3$	N/A	L	[17]
BISBENZYLISOQUINOLINE					
27	Nelumboferine	$C_{36}H_{40}N_2O_6$	NS	E, LS	[32,45]
28	Liensinine	$C_{37}H_{42}N_2O_6$	1R,1′R	L, E, F, LS	[32,35,44,46]
29	Isoliensinine	$C_{37}H_{42}N_2O_6$	1R,1′S	E	[35,46]
30	Neferine	$C_{38}H_{44}N_2O_6$	1R,1′S	E, LS	[32,35,46]
31	6-Hydroxynorisoliensinine	$C_{36}H_{40}N_2O_6$	NS	E	[38]
32	N-Norisoliensinine	$C_{36}H_{40}N_2O_6$	NS	E	[38]
33	Nelumborine	$C_{36}H_{40}N_2O_6$	NS	E	[45]
TRIBENZYLISOQUINOLINE					
34	Neoliensinine	$C_{63}H_{70}N_3O_{10}$	1R,1′S,1″R	E	[46]

2.1. 1-Benzylisoquinoline Alkaloids

1-Benzylisoquinoline alkaloids occur in trace amounts in several sacred lotus organs (Table 1). Norcoclaurine, also known as higenamine, is the common intermediate for the biosynthesis of all BIAs. It was first reported in sacred lotus embryos a half-century ago [36] and later isolated from *N. nucifera* leaves via anti-HIV bioassay-guided fractionation [37]. Norcoclaurine is notable for its anti-inflammatory, anti-arrhythmic, and anti-thrombotic properties, and is also considered a β-adrenergic receptor agonist [47].

Norcoclaurine subsequently undergoes O- and N-methylation yielding various 1-benzylisoquinoline alkaloid derivatives (Figure 1). Coclaurine (6-O-methylated norcoclaurine), norarmepavine (7-O-methylated coclaurine), N-methylcoclaurine (N-methylated coclaurine), and armepavine (7-O- and N-methylated coclaurine) isolated from sacred lotus flowers have shown melanogenesis inhibition activity, with potential application in the cosmetics industry [15]. Armepavine also exhibited a suppression of T-cell proliferation and an inactivation of NF-kB, among other immunomodulatory effects that could be beneficial for the treatment of autoimmune diseases such as systemic lupus erythematosus and crescentic glomerulonephritis [42,48]. Two quaternary amines, lotusine and isolotusine (most likely derived from N-methylisococlaurine and N-methylcoclaurine, respectively) and three 4′-methoxylated compounds, 6-demethyl-4′-O-methyl-N-methylcoclaurine, 4′-O-methyl-N-methylcoclaurine, and 4′-O-methylarmepavine have also been isolated from the plant [38,43].

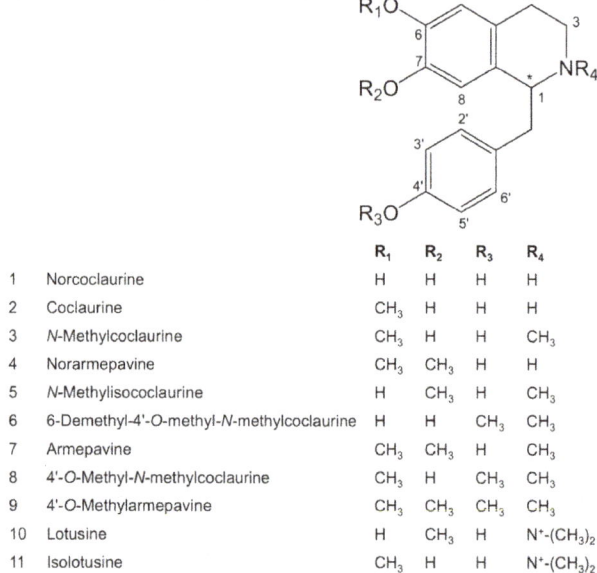

Figure 1. Major 1-benzylisoquinoline alkaloids reported in sacred lotus. Asterisk indicates a chiral center.

2.2. Aporphines

Nelumbo nucifera contains several aporphine alkaloids that accumulate mainly in the leaves (Table 1). Nuciferine is the major alkaloid in this organ, although substantial variation in alkaloid content and composition is found between cultivars [32,33,35,49]. Aporphines in sacred lotus (Figure 2) are presumably derived from 1-benzylisoquinoline intermediates as a result of C8-C2′ coupling reactions, except for pronuciferine, which exhibits C8-C1′ coupling. The C6 and/or C7 positions (Figure 1) are consistently O-methylated, with the only exceptions being anonaine and roemerine (and their dehydro derivatives), in which a methylenedioxy bridge occurs between these carbon atoms. The isoquinoline ring can also be N-methylated, but there are no reports of quaternary (e.g., N,N-dimethylated) amines among sacred lotus aporphines.

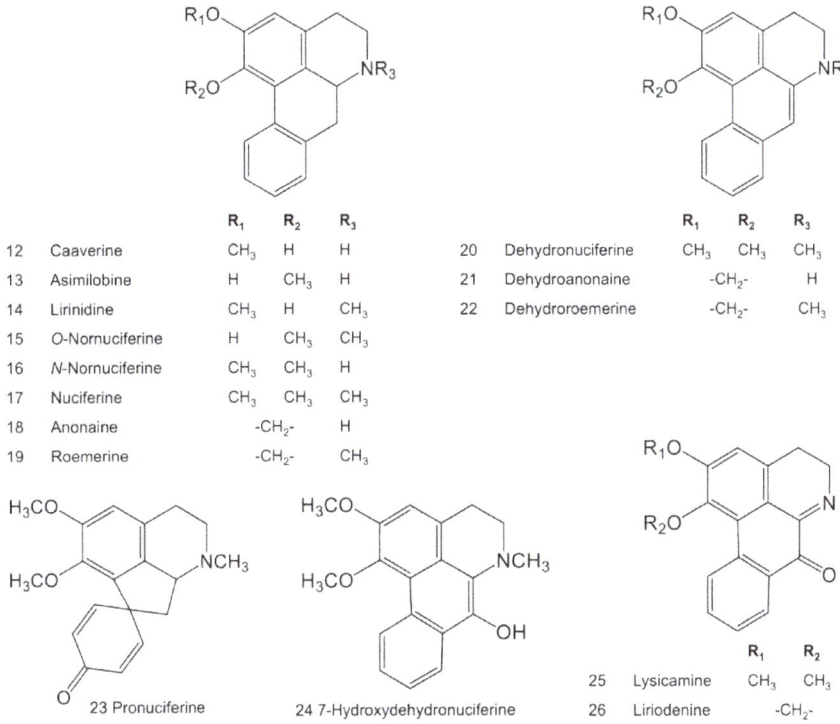

Figure 2. Major aporphine alkaloids reported in sacred lotus.

Curiously, all aporphines reported in *N. nucifera* lack of substitutions in the benzyl moiety presumably derived from 4-hydroxyphenylacetaldehyde. This is a major difference with respect to the aporphines isolated from members of the Ranunculales, such as corytuberine, magnoflorine, isoboldine, and glaucine that are all likely derived via reticuline [50,51]. Reticuline is a 1-benzylisoquinoline alkaloid containing 3'-hydroxyl and a 4'-methoxyl groups and serving as a key branch point intermediate in the biosynthesis of most BIAs in the Ranunculales [27]. However, reticuline has not been reported in sacred lotus, and its absence could indicate the existence of substantial differences in BIA metabolism in this ancient plant. Nevertheless, all 1-benzylisoquinolines isolated from *N. nucifera* so far display a 4'-hydroxyl or 4'-methoxyl moiety, and it remains unclear why aporphines in the plant lack these modifications. Further research on aporphine biosynthesis is required to shed light on this intriguing phenomenon.

2.3. Bisbenzylisoquinolines

Bisbenzylisoquinoline alkaloids accumulate predominantly in the seed embryo of *N. nucifera*. Although it has been suggested that these alkaloids are synthesized in the leaf and then transported in the leaf sap to the embryo [32], the localization of BIA biosynthesis has not been experimentally examined. Neferine and liensinine are the major alkaloid constituents of the embryo, although the bisbenzylisoquinolines profile varies considerably in different genotypes [32,35].

Bisbenzylisoquinoline alkaloids are formed by C6-O-C3' or C8-C3' coupling (or C8-C5' coupling, due to free rotation of the benzyl ring) between two 1-benzylisoquinoline monomers. Different O- and N-methylation patterns create a diverse array of compounds (Figure 3). A more complex structure, the tribenzylisoquinoline alkaloid neoliensinine (Figure 4), has been recently isolated from sacred lotus embryos [46]. As with aporphine biosynthesis, it is not yet known whether the differential O-

and *N*-methylation patterns among bisbenzylisoquinolines and tribenzylisoquinolines are established before or after coupling.

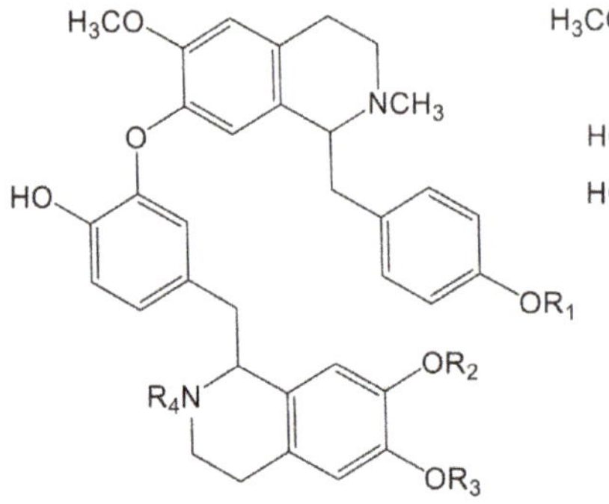

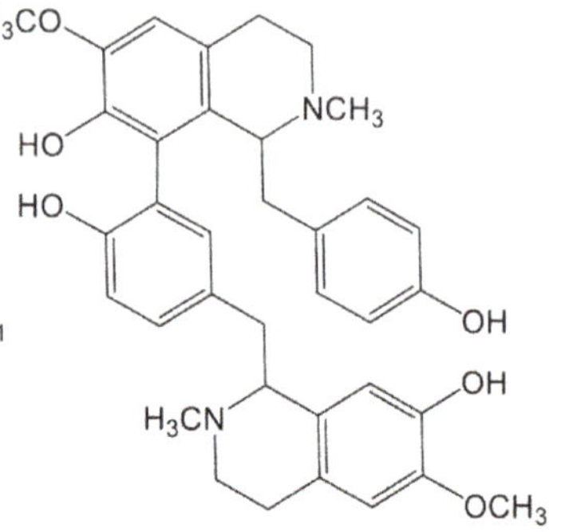

		R₁	R₂	R₃	R₄
27	Nelumboferine	H	H	CH₃	CH₃
28	Liensinine	H	CH₃	CH₃	CH₃
29	Isoliensinine	CH₃	H	CH₃	CH₃
30	Neferine	CH₃	CH₃	CH₃	CH₃
31	6-Hydroxynorisoliensinine	H	CH₃	H	CH₃
32	*N*-Norisoliensinine	H	CH₃	CH₃	H

Figure 3. Major bisbenzylisoquinoline alkaloids reported in sacred lotus.

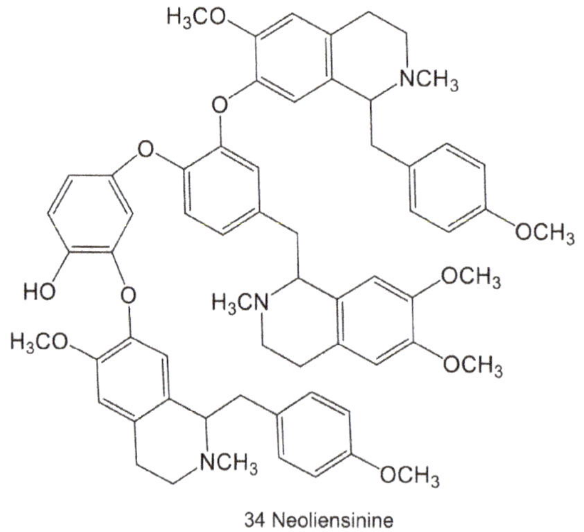

34 Neoliensinine

Figure 4. The tribenzylisoquinoline alkaloid, neoliensinine, reported in sacred lotus.

3. Stereochemistry of BIAs Biosynthesis in *Nelumbo nucifera*

In members of the Ranunculales, BIA stereochemistry is initially introduced by the enantioselective Pictet-Spengler condensation of dopamine and 4-hydroxyphenylacetaldehyde catalyzed by norcoclaurine synthase (NCS) [26]. Norcoclaurine contains a stereogenic atom and can theoretically occur as either the *R* or *S* conformer. To date, all functionally characterized NCS from opium poppy and related members of the Ranunculales yield exclusively (*S*)-norcoclaurine [52–59]. In contrast, norcoclaurine was first reported as an *R*-enantiomer in sacred lotus [36], a result later confirmed by

HPLC coupled with chiral fluorescent detection [39]. The S-enantiomer of norcoclaurine has also been reported from *N. nucifera* leaves [37] (Table 1). In addition, it was recently reported that the embryos contained a racemic mix (59:41) of norcoclaurine-4'-O-β-D-glucoside 1R and 1S diastereomers [60], further supporting the formation of both R and S norcoclaurine conformers.

At least five functional isoforms of norcoclaurine synthase (NnNCS) have been purported in sacred lotus, based on the occurrence of homologs in the genome [34], and in various transcriptomes [34,49,61,62]. These NCS candidates must be functionally characterized to determine which, if any, are responsible for the formation of norcoclaurine and variations in the stereochemistry of BIAs in sacred lotus. Since norcoclaurine has been isolated in both R and S conformations, it is possible that two or more NnNCS isoforms catalyze the Pictet-Spengler condensation with the opposite enantioselectivity. Alternatively, it is also plausible that the diverse BIA stereochemistry in sacred lotus results from a lack of NCS enantioselectivity, leading to the formation of both enantiomers by one enzyme. The unique features of the BIA biosynthetic enzymes from sacred lotus provide exciting targets for advanced structural and biochemical investigations with respect to substrate recognition, product formation and underlying catalytic mechanisms.

Optically active enantiomers or stereoisomers exhibiting similar physicochemical properties might differ in their biological activity. Although the specific physiological role of norcoclaurine is not known, the two enantiomers could be associated with differences in substrate recognition by NCS, and in other biochemical interactions. For example, (S)-norcoclaurine appears superior to (R)-norcoclaurine in suppressing the inducible expression of nitric oxide synthase, a hallmark of septic shock [63].

The majority of BIAs isolated from sacred lotus are R-conformers (Table 1). In contrast, most BIAs in members of the Ranunculales are S-conformers, with the notable exception of the bisbenzylisoquinolines (1R,1'S)-berbamunine, (1R,1'S)-2'-norberbamunine, and (1R,1'R)-guatteguamerine from *Berberis stolonifera* (presumably derived from (R)- and (S)-coclaurine and/or (R)- and (S)-N-methylcoclaurine) [64]. Although aporphines in the S conformation have not been reported in sacred lotus (except for racemic pronuciferine [43], a proaporphine), some 1-benzylisoquinoline alkaloids, such as norcoclaurine and armepavine, have been detected as both R and S enantiomers [16,36,37,39,40,48]. Moreover, the bisbenzylisoquinoline and tribenzylisoquinoline alkaloids have been reported as combinations of various R and S 1-benzylisoquinolines with the exception of (1R,1'R)-liensinine [46].

The stereospecificity (i.e., the ability to distinguish between stereoisomers) of downstream BIA biosynthetic enzymes is not known. For example, norcoclaurine-6-O-methyltransferase from *Thalictrum flavum* accepts both (R)- and (S)-norlaudanosoline (an unnatural analogue of norcoclaurine) [65]. In opium poppy, (S)-reticuline is converted by (i) the berberine bridge enzyme to (S)-scoulerine to form benzophenanthridine, protoberberine, and/or phthalideisoquinoline alkaloids and; (ii) corytuberine synthase to (S)-corytuberine leading to aporphine alkaloids. In contrast, reticuline epimerase is the gateway enzyme in the conversion of (R)-reticuline to morphinan alkaloids since the subsequent enzyme salutaridine synthase (CYP719B1) does not accept (S)-reticuline [30,66]. Enzyme stereospecificity is a critical feature of BIA metabolism in the Ranunculales. The stereospecificity of BIA biosynthetic enzymes in sacred lotus might be considerably different based on the widespread occurrence of R-conformers.

4. BIA biosynthetic Genes and Enzymes in the Sacred Lotus

Analysis of the *Nelumbo nucifera* genome sequence suggest that, after the lineage-specific whole-genome duplication event (approximately 18 to 76 million years ago), several rearrangements (i.e., ancestral chromosome fissions, fusions, and a single inversion) were responsible for the modern diploid karyotype (16 chromosomes) [67,68]. The sacred lotus genome is ~1 Gb in size and encodes approximately 27,000 genes [1,2]. Based on sequence similarity with BIA biosynthetic genes in members of the Ranunculales [30], genes predicted to encode norcoclaurine synthase (NCS), O- and N-methyltransferases (OMT and NMT), and cytochrome P450 (CYP) monooxygenases CYP80A,

CYP80G, and CYP719A (CYP) have been detected in the sacred lotus genome (Figure 5). Although other gene candidates have been suggested to participate in morphinan and protoberberine alkaloid biosynthesis [49], compounds belonging to these structural groups have not been detected in sacred lotus. Herein, we discuss only enzymes potentially involved in 1-benzylisoquinoline, aporphine and bisbenzylisoquinoline alkaloid pathways (Table 2). However, functional characterization of these enzymes has not been investigated. Most work has focused on the aporphine metabolism, primarily through correlational analysis of gene expression profiles and alkaloid content in different organs and developmental stages of sacred lotus [34,49,61,62,69].

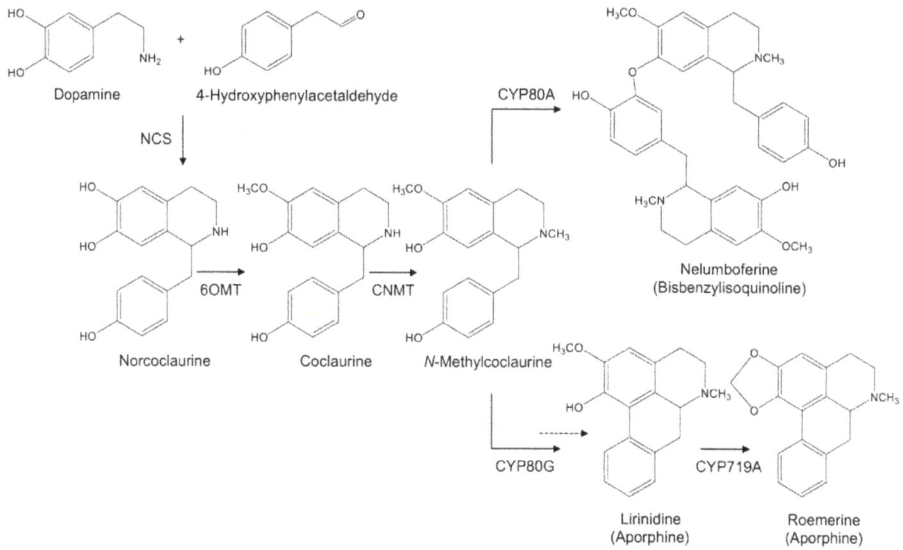

Figure 5. Suggested BIA biosynthetic pathway in sacred lotus. The scheme shows norcoclaurine as the common precursor and N-methylcoclaurine as the branch point intermediate in the formation of aporphine and bisbenzylisoquinoline alkaloids. Tailoring reactions, such as O- and N-methylations, hydroxylation, oxidation, C-C and C-O coupling (and a possible dehydration represented by the dashed arrow) yield the diverse BIAs reported in *Nelumbo nucifera*. Note that other 1-benzylisoquinolines derived from norcoclaurine could be used in the formation of aporphine and bisbenzylisoquinoline alkaloids, as this representation is merely one of many possible routes (e.g., major BIAs in sacred lotus such as nuciferine and neferine are not represented). Stereochemistry has been omitted for simplicity. Abbreviations: 6OMT, norcoclaurine 6-O-methyltransferase; CNMT, coclaurine N-methyltransferase; CYP719A, cytochrome P450 monooxygenase 719A, CYP80A, cytochrome P450 monooxygenase 80A; CYP80G: cytochrome P450 monooxygenase 80G; NCS, norcoclaurine synthase.

Table 2. BIA biosynthetic enzyme candidates potentially involved in 1-benylisoquinoline, aporphine and bisbenzylisoquinoline pathways in sacred lotus. For each enzyme a proposed substrate(s) and product are shown. Accession numbers in [a] GenBank or [b] lotus databases (lotus-db.wbgcas.cn [1]) are provided. 4-HPAA: 4-hydroxyphenylacetaldehyde, 4'OMT: 4'-O-methyltransferase, 6OMT: norcoclaurine-6-O-methyltransferase, 7OMT: 7-O-methyltransferase, CNMT: coclaurine N-methyltransferase, CYP719A: cytochrome P450 monooxygenase 719A, CYP80A: cytochrome P450 monooxygenase 80A, CYP80G: cytochrome P450 monooxygenase 80G, NCS: norcoclaurine synthase.

Class	Enzyme	Isoforms	Substrate	Product	Reference
Pictet-Spenglerase	NCS	NCS1 (KT963033) [a] NCS3 (KT963034) [a] NCS4 (KT963035) [a] NCS5 (KU234431) [a] NCS7 (KU234432) [a]	Dopamine 4-HPAA	Norcoclaurine	[34]
O-Methyltransferase	6OMT	6OMT1 (MG517493) [a] 6OMT2 (MG517492) [a] 6OMT3 (MG517491) [a] 6OMT4 (MG517490) [a]	Norcoclaurine	Coclaurine	[49,61,62]
	7OMT	7OMT1 (NNU20903) [b] 7OMT2 (NNU04966) [b] 7OMT3 (NNU09736) [b]	Coclaurine	Norarmepavine	[61]
	4'OMT	4'OMT1 (NNU15801) [b] 4'OMT2 (NNU15809) [b] 4'OMT3 (NNU24728) [b] 4'OMT4 (NNU25948) [b]	N-Methylcoclaurine	4'-O-methyl-N-methylcoclaurine	[49]
N-Methyltransferase	CNMT	CNMT1 (MG517494) [a] CNMT3 (MG517495) [a]	Coclaurine	N-Methylcoclaurine	[49,61,62]
Cytochrome P450 monooxygenase	CYP80A CYP80G CYP719A	CYP80A (NNU21373) [b] CYP80G (NNU21372) [b] CYP719A22 (XM010268782) [a]	N-Methylcoclaurine N-Methylcoclaurine Lirinidine	Nelumboferine Lirinidine Roemerine	[61] [49,61,62] [61,69]

4.1. Norcoclaurine Synthase

NCS catalyzes the condensation of dopamine and 4-hydroxyphenylacetaldehyde as the first committed step in BIA metabolism (Figure 5). In members of the Ranunculales, NCS belongs to the PR10/Bet-v1 family of proteins [54,59]. NCS activity has been detected in crude protein extracts of sacred lotus leaves, but not in petioles or roots [31]. Seven genes putatively encoding NCS have been described in the sacred lotus genome [34]. All of these genes contained two exons separated by one intron. *NnNCS1*, *NnNCS4*, and *NnNCS5* were clustered together along with two pseudogenes (*NnNCS2* and *NnNCS6*). *NnNCS3* and *NnNCS7* were not on the same genomic scaffold, but could also be part of the gene cluster. All predicted proteins contained a canonical glycine-rich loop and conserved catalytic residues (K-122 and E-110) described in the functionally and structurally characterized NCS from *T. flavum* (TfNCS) [52,56].

Correlational analysis of genes expression profiles and alkaloid content were interpreted to suggest that only NnNCS7 plays a major role in BIA biosynthesis [34]. However, even though the *NnNCS7* gene was predominantly expressed in all tested organs and developmental stages, significant variation in transcript level was detected depending on the cultivar analyzed. For example, only *NnNCS7* was (highly) expressed in mature leaves of the Xuehuou variety, although the alkaloid content was the lowest among 10 tested cultivars. In contrast, despite a low level of *NnNCS7* expression in mature leaves of the WSL40 cultivar, the alkaloid content was more than double that detected in the leaves of Xuehuou [34]. In addition, expression of *NnNCS7* has been reported to increase with leaf development, with peak levels between the folded and unfolded stages, which is prior to the detected accumulation of alkaloids [61]. However, *NnNCS7* gene expression was higher in the low-alkaloid cultivar Luming compared with the high-alkaloid cultivar WD40 [61]. Similar inconsistencies have been detected depending on the plant organ and developmental stage analyzed [34]. Inconsistencies between gene expression profiles and alkaloid content were suggested to result from the possibility that NCS in sacred lotus is a functional heterodimer composed of cultivar-dependent isoforms [34]. It is notable that TfNCS has been structurally and functionally characterized as a homodimer [52,57]. Functional characterization of putative NCS isoforms from sacred lotus is required to support their role in BIA metabolism. It is also notable that at least five putative tyrosine decarboxylase (*TYDC*) genes are expressed in lotus leaves [61]. TYDC catalyzes the decarboxylation of tyrosine and L-DOPA yielding, indirectly or directly, the NCS substrate dopamine. Putative TYDC enzymes also require functional characterization.

4.2. Methyltransferases

Norcoclaurine is modified by a series of *O*- and *N*-methylations to form the diverse 1-benzylisoquinolines reported in sacred lotus (Figure 1). Both *O*-methyltransferases (OMTs) and *N*-methyltransferases (NMTs) use S-adenosyl-L-methionine as the methyl donor [70]. Norcoclaurine contains three hydroxyl groups at C6, C7, and C4′ and a secondary nitrogen in the isoquinoline ring, all of which are susceptible to methylation.

In the Ranunculales, the 6-*O*-methylation of norcoclaurine to coclaurine is the first tailoring reaction in BIAs biosynthesis [30] and it is expected that a similar reaction occurs in sacred lotus (Figure 5). Based on sequence similarity with OMTs from members of the Ranunculales, four candidate norcoclaurine-6-*O*-methyltransferase (*Nn6OMT*) genes have been detected in the sacred lotus genome, with two of the genes (*Nn6OMT2* and *Nn6OMT3*) clustered [49,61,62]. *Nn6OMT1* showed the highest expression levels in leaves, with a peak at early stages of development, and cultivar-dependent expression aligned with cultivar-specific alkaloid content [49,61]. In addition, the *Nn6OMT1* isoform also contains conserved catalytic residues (H-256, D-257, and E-315) described in *T. flavum* 6OMT [65].

Several 1-benzylisoquinolines from sacred lotus, including norarmepavine, armepavine, and major aporphines and bisbenzylisoquinolines are *O*-methylated at C7; thus, enzymes capable of C7-*O*-methylation are also expected to occur. Five candidate genes putatively encoding 7-*O*-methyltransferases (*Nn7OMTs*) have been detected in the *N. nucifera* genome based on sequence similarity with OMTs from members of the Ranunculales. However, only *Nn7OMT1-3* genes have shown significant expression in the leaves [61]. The other two candidates *Nn7OMT4* and *Nn7OMT5* were previously proposed as *Nn4′OMT1* and *Nn4′OMT4*, respectively, along with two other genes encoding putative 4′-*O*-methyltransferases (*Nn4′OMTs*) [49]. The expression levels of the corresponding *Nn4′OMT* genes in the leaves of two cultivars were low or conflicted with the cultivar-specific alkaloid content, except for *Nn4′OMT1* [49]. Owing to the isolation of several 1-benzylisoquinoline and bisbenzylisoquinoline alkaloids containing a 4′-methoxy group, an enzyme associated with 4′OMT activity should occur in the plant. It is possible that OMTs in sacred lotus lack strict regiospecificity and enzymes that primarily function as a 6OMT or a 7OMT also catalyze 4′-*O*-methylation on certain substrates. Alternatively, the occurrence of OMT heterodimers that perform distinct *O*-methylations has recently been described in opium poppy [71]. Similarly, certain *O*-methylation activities could be associated with the possible formation of OMT heterodimers in sacred lotus.

Only a single gene candidate putatively encoding coclaurine *N*-methyltransferase (*NnCNMT1*) has been detected in the sacred lotus genome [49,61]; however, a recent report identified two additional candidates, one of which (*NnCNMT2*) is clearly a pseudogene [62]. *NnCNMT1* expression in sacred lotus leaves increased progressively with developmental stage and alkaloid content, although expression levels were 10-fold lower than *Nn6OMT1*, the preceding enzyme in the biosynthetic pathway [49]. In addition, *NnCNMTs* expression was substantially different among sacred lotus cultivars. In some cases *NnCNMTs* transcripts were undetectable in cultivars such as Bua Khem Chin1200 with a high alkaloid content [62]. CNMT catalytic activity is a critical step in sacred lotus BIA metabolism owing to the putative role of *N*-methylcoclaurine as a key branch point intermediate in the formation of aporphines and bisbenzylisoquinolines [61]. It is also possible that aporphine and bisbenzylisoquinoline, rather than 1-benzylisoquinoline intermediates, are themselves O- and/or N-methylated.

4.3. Cytochrome P450 Monooxygenases

Cytochrome P450 monooxygenases (CYPs) constitute a large group of heme proteins catalyzing diverse reactions in plant specialized metabolism. The enzymes are activated by the transfer of two electrons from NADPH via a NADPH-cytochrome P450 reductase [72]. Two main CYP families are proposed to play a key role in BIA biosynthesis in sacred lotus: CYP80 (subfamilies A and G) and CYP719A [69].

The CYP80A subfamily has been associated with bisbenzylisoquinoline alkaloids biosynthesis in the Ranunculales. For example, the enzyme CYP80A1 (berbamunine synthase) isolated from *Berberis stolonifera* catalyzes C-O phenol coupling of 1-benzylisoquinoline substrates to form (1R,1′S)-berbamunine and other dimeric BIAs [64]. In lotus genome, only one *NnCYP80A* candidate has been detected, and its expression was positively correlated with alkaloid content [61]. Curiously, the gene showed differential spatial expression, with high levels in the embryo and significantly lower levels in the leaves. In a previous study based on phylogenetic analysis, this gene was proposed as a second CYP80G isoform [49], demonstrating the need for proper functional characterization of the corresponding enzymes.

The CYP80G subfamily has been correlated with aporphine alkaloid biosynthesis. In *Coptis japonica*, CYP80G2 (corytuberine synthase) catalyzes the conversion of (S)-reticuline to (S)-corytuberine via intramolecular C-C coupling [73]. However, neither reticuline nor corytuberine have been isolated from sacred lotus; thus, other 1-benzylisoquinoline intermediates are likely involved in aporphine alkaloid biosynthesis. Transcripts of CYP80G homologs in sacred lotus leaves were detected using digital gene expression analysis and according to the observed expression pattern only one was proposed to be implicated in the aporphine biosynthesis [49]. In a recent study, the expression of this *NnCYP80G* gene was reported at high levels in leaves and transcript levels and aporphine alkaloid content were induced after mechanical wounding [62]. Likewise, the expression profile of *NnCYP80G* showed high transcript levels in the leaves but significantly lower levels in the embryos, opposite to what was observed for *NnCYP80A* [61]. Interestingly, *NnCYP80A* and *NnCYP80G* are clustered within a 20 kb region in the *N. nucifera* genome, suggesting functional divergence after duplication [61].

Members of the CYP719A subfamily typically catalyze methylenedioxy bridge formation in the Ranunculales leading to the formation of (S)-stylopine (CYP719A20), (S)-canadine (CYP719A21), and (S)-cheilanthifoline (CYP719A25) [74]. In sacred lotus, aporphines such as anonaine and roemerine (and their dehydro derivatives) contain a methylenedioxy bridge. Interestingly, only the *NnCYP719A22* gene from sacred lotus has been suggested to function in alkaloid biosynthesis [69] (Figure 5).

At least two transcript candidates encoding N-methylcoclaurine 3′-hydroxylase (NMCH; CYP80B subfamily) have been detected in sacred lotus leaves [49]. NMCH is involved in the hydroxylation of N-methylcoclaurine, which is required for reticuline biosynthesis in the Ranunculales [27]. However, as reticuline has not been detected in sacred lotus and 3′-hydroxylation is not a feature of any reported alkaloids from the plant, a functional NMCH homolog is unlikely to occur.

4.4. Other Enzymes

Expression of genes involved in the formation of morphinan (codeine 3-O-demethylase, CODM, and thebaine 6-O-demethylase, T6ODM), and protoberberine (scoulerine-9-O-methyltransferase, SOMT) alkaloids has also been considered in sacred lotus [49]. However, morphinan and protoberberine alkaloids have not been detected in *N. nucifera* [4,10]; thus, it is questionable whether these enzyme candidates are involved in BIA biosynthesis. However, it has been suggested that O- and N-demethylases could participate in tailoring reactions in aporphine biosynthesis [61].

The biosynthesis of aporphine alkaloids in sacred lotus could involve a dehydration reaction to remove the 4'-hydroxyl group from a 1-benzylisoquinoline or aporphine intermediate. Comparing the gene expression profiles of sacred lotus cultivars with markedly different aporphine profiles [33] could facilitate the detection of additional missing or unanticipated enzymes in BIA metabolism.

4.5. Functional Characterization

The elucidation of BIA biosynthetic pathways requires a thorough biochemical and physiological characterization of relevant enzymes. To date, no BIA biosynthetic enzymes from sacred lotus have been functionally analyzed. In vitro experiments using purified proteins are generally the first step in the functional characterization of enzyme candidates. Alternatively, enzyme function can be evaluated in vivo using engineered bacterial (e.g., *Escherichia coli*) and yeast (e.g., *Saccharomyces cerevisiae*) systems [51,55]. Immunoprecipitation have been used to support the physiological significance of NCS in the formation of (S)-norcoclaurine in opium poppy [54]. In planta techniques, such as candidate gene overexpression and RNA interference [75–77], and gene knockout using CRISPR/Cas9 technology [78] have also been used to demonstrate physiological relevance. Virus-induced gene silencing (VIGS) has been effective to assess the impact of candidate gene suppression on BIA biosynthesis in opium poppy [50,79,80]. Similar approaches must be developed to advance the functional characterization of biosynthetic genes and enzymes in sacred lotus.

4.6. Regulation and Localization of BIA Biosynthesis in Sacred Lotus

BIA metabolism in sacred lotus appears tightly regulated, with different organs showing specific alkaloids profiles (e.g., aporphines and bisbenzylisoquinoline accumulate in the leaves and embryos, respectively). In members of the Ranunculales, at least two transcription factors (TFs) have been implicated in the regulation of BIA metabolism: WRKY (*CjWRKY1*) and bHLH1 (*CjbHLH1*) [81,82]. MYB family TFs have been proposed to play a major role in regulating alkaloid biosynthesis in sacred lotus leaves [61]. This conclusion was based on correlations between the expression levels of putative transcription factor genes and selected genes putatively encoding biosynthetic enzymes, such as TYDC, NCS, CNMT, and CYP80G as well as TF-promoter interactions for *NnMYB6*, *NnMYB12*, and *NnMYB113* evaluated using dual luciferase assays [61]. Such deductions are compromised by the lack of functional data supporting the biochemical and physiological roles of these enzyme candidates. In addition, some variants of *NnWRKY* and *NnbHLH1* were not linked to BIA biosynthetic gene expression, although high expression levels of *NnWRKY* were detected [61].

Another aspect of BIA metabolism in sacred lotus that has received little attention is the cellular and subcellular localization of alkaloid biosynthesis. Cytosolic localization of NCS was suggested based on the absence of signal peptides on the candidate enzymes [34]. In addition, putative NCS transcripts are primarily found in leaves [34], suggesting this organ as a major site of BIA biosynthesis. If validated, this is markedly different from the abundance of NCS in the rhizome and root in *T. flavum* [59] and opium poppy [54], respectively.

In opium poppy, most BIA biosynthetic genes are expressed in companion cells, and the cognate biosynthetic enzymes are associated with sieve elements of the phloem. The final stages of BIA biosynthesis, and the ultimate storage of alkaloids occurs in specialized laticifers [83]. The rhizome, leaf, petiole, and peduncle of sacred lotus also contain laticifers associated with vascular bundles, mainly in the parenchyma between the phloem and xylem [84]. However, the roles of sacred lotus laticifers in BIA metabolism and storage are not known. Immunoblot and real-time PCR analyses using total protein and RNA extracts, respectively, from various organs of sacred lotus will provide valuable information on the localization of validated biosynthetic enzymes and corresponding gene transcripts [54]. The cell-type specific occurrence of enzymes and cognate transcripts can then be determined by immunofluorescence labeling and in situ RNA hybridization, respectively [85].

5. Conclusions

BIAs constitute a substantial part of humankind's traditional and modern medicine [27]. A vast number of BIA biosynthetic genes and enzymes have been isolated from members of the Ranunculales, especially from opium poppy [86]. The ancient aquatic plant sacred lotus has long been exploited for its medicinal properties, which are largely conferred by aporphine and bisbenzylisoquinoline alkaloids. Interestingly, most BIAs found in sacred lotus are *R*-conformers [16,17,37,39,40,46], contrary to the prevalence of *S*-conformers in the Ranunculales. Therefore, the unusual stereochemistry of alkaloids in this basal eudicot is worthy of research at the molecular and biochemical levels. The availability of a draft sacred lotus genome sequence underpins opportunities to isolate BIA biosynthetic genes and enzymes. However, a definitive elucidation of biosynthetic pathways requires thorough biochemical and physiological characterization of putative genes and enzymes.

Author Contributions: Conceptualization, I.M.M.-P. and P.J.F.; Writing-Review & Editing, I.M.M.-P. and P.J.F.; Supervision, P.J.F.

Funding: Research is funded by a Natural Sciences and Engineering Research Council of Canada Discovery Grant to P.J.F. I.M.M.-P. is the recipient of scholarships from Alberta Innovates Technology Futures and Delta Kappa Gamma Society International.

Conflicts of Interest: The authors declare no conflict of interest. The founding sponsors had no role in the design of the study; in the collection, analyses, or interpretation of data; in the writing of the manuscript, and in the decision to publish the results.

References

1. Ming, R.; VanBuren, R.; Liu, Y.; Yang, M.; Han, Y.; Li, L.T.; Zhang, Q.; Kim, M.J.; Schatz, M.C.; Campbell, M.; et al. Genome of the long-living sacred lotus (*Nelumbo nucifera* Gaertn.). *Genome Biol.* **2013**, *14*, R41. [CrossRef] [PubMed]
2. Wang, Y.; Fan, G.; Liu, Y.; Sun, F.; Shi, C.; Liu, X.; Peng, J.; Chen, W.; Huang, X.; Cheng, S.; et al. The sacred lotus genome provides insights into the evolution of flowering plants. *Plant J.* **2013**, *76*, 557–567. [CrossRef] [PubMed]
3. Xue, J.; Dong, W.; Cheng, T.; Zhou, S. Nelumbonaceae: Systematic position and species diversification revealed by the complete chloroplast genome. *J. Syst. Evol.* **2012**, *50*, 477–487. [CrossRef]
4. Sharma, B.R.; Guautam, L.N.S.; Adhikari, D.; Karki, R. A comprehensive review on chemical profiling of *Nelumbo nucifera*: Potential for drug development. *Phytother Res.* **2017**, *31*, 3–26. [CrossRef] [PubMed]
5. Ushimaru, T.; Hasegawa, T.; Amano, T.; Katayama, M.; Tanaka, S.; Tsuji, H. Chloroplasts in seeds and dark-grown seedlings of lotus. *J. Plant Physiol.* **2003**, *160*, 321–324. [CrossRef] [PubMed]
6. Grant, N.M.; Miller, R.E.; Watling, J.R.; Robinson, S.A. Synchronicity of thermogenic activity, alternative pathway respiratory flux, AOX protein content, and carbohydrates in receptacle tissues of sacred lotus during floral development. *J. Exp. Bot.* **2008**, *59*, 705–714. [CrossRef] [PubMed]
7. Koch, K.; Bhushan, B.; Jung, Y.C.; Barthlott, W. Fabrication of artificial Lotus leaves and significance of hierarchical structure for superhydrophobicity and low adhesion. *Soft Matter* **2009**, *5*, 1386–1393. [CrossRef]
8. Shen-Miller, J.; Mudgett, M.B.; Schopf, J.W.; Clarke, S.; Berger, R. Exceptional seed longevity and robust growth: Ancient sacred lotus from China. *Am. J. Bot.* **1995**, *82*, 1367–1380. [CrossRef]
9. Shen-Miller, J.; Aung, L.H.; Turek, J.; Schopf, J.W.; Tholandi, M.; Yang, M.; Czaja, A. Centuries-old viable fruit of sacred lotus *Nelumbo nucifera* Gaertn var China Antique. *Trop. Plant Biol.* **2013**, *6*, 53–68. [CrossRef]
10. Mukherjee, P.K.; Mukherjee, D.; Maji, A.K.; Rai, S.; Heinrich, M. The sacred lotus (*Nelumbo nucifera*)—Phytochemical and therapeutic profile. *J. Pharm. Pharmacol.* **2009**, *61*, 407–422. [CrossRef] [PubMed]
11. Liu, W.; Yi, D.D.; Guo, J.L.; Xiang, Z.X.; Deng, L.F.; He, L. Nuciferine, extracted from *Nelumbo nucifera* Gaertn., inhibits tumor-promoting effect of nicotine involving Wnt/beta-catenin signaling in non-small cell lung cancer. *J Ethnopharmacol.* **2015**, *165*, 83–93. [CrossRef] [PubMed]
12. Kang, E.J.; Lee, S.K.; Park, K.K.; Son, S.H.; Kim, K.R.; Chung, W.Y. Liensinine and nuciferine, bioactive components of *Nelumbo nucifera*, inhibit the growth of breast cancer cells and breast cancer-associated bone loss. *Evid. Based Complement. Altern. Med.* **2017**, *2017*, 1583185. [CrossRef] [PubMed]

13. Qi, Q.; Li, R.; Li, H.Y.; Cao, Y.B.; Bai, M.; Fan, X.J.; Wang, S.Y.; Zhang, B.; Li, S. Identification of the anti-tumor activity and mechanisms of nuciferine through a network pharmacology approach. *Acta Pharmacol. Sin.* **2016**, *37*, 963–972. [CrossRef] [PubMed]
14. Ma, C.; Li, G.; He, Y.; Xu, B.; Mi, X.; Wang, H.; Wang, Z. Pronuciferine and nuciferine inhibit lipogenesis in 3T3-L1 adipocytes by activating the AMPK signaling pathway. *Life Sci.* **2015**, *136*, 120–125. [CrossRef] [PubMed]
15. Morikawa, T.; Kitagawa, N.; Tanabe, G.; Ninomiya, K.; Okugawa, S.; Motai, C.; Kamei, I.; Yoshikawa, M.; Lee, I.-J.; Muraoka, O. Quantitative determination of alkaloids in lotus flower (flower buds of *Nelumbo nucifera*) and their melanogenesis inhibitory activity. *Molecules* **2016**, *21*, 930. [CrossRef] [PubMed]
16. Nakamura, S.; Nakashima, S.; Tanabe, G.; Oda, Y.; Yokota, N.; Fujimoto, K.; Matsumoto, T.; Sukama, R.; Ohta, T.; Ogawa, K.; et al. Alkaloid constitutens from flower buds and leaves of sacred lotus (*Nelumbo nucifera*, Nymphaeaceae) with melanogenesis inhibitory activity in B16 melanoma cells. *Bioorg. Med. Chem.* **2013**, *21*, 779–787. [CrossRef] [PubMed]
17. Liu, C.M.; Kao, C.L.; Wu, H.M.; Li, W.J.; Huang, C.T.; Li, H.T.; Chen, C.Y. Antioxidant and anticancer aporphine alkaloids from the leaves of *Nelumbo nucifera* Gaertn. cv. Rosa-plena. *Molecules* **2014**, *19*, 17829–17838. [CrossRef] [PubMed]
18. Agnihotri, V.K.; ElSohly, H.N.; Khan, S.I.; Jacob, M.R.; Joshi, V.C.; Smillie, T.; Khan, I.A.; Walker, L.A. Constituents of *Nelumbo nucifera* leaves and their antimalarial and antifungal activity. *Phytochem. Lett.* **2008**, *1*, 89–93. [CrossRef] [PubMed]
19. Qian, J.Q. Cardiovascular pharmacological effects of bisbenzylisoquinoline alkaloid derivatives. *Acta Pharmacol. Sin.* **2002**, *23*, 1086–1092. [PubMed]
20. Poornima, P.; Weng, C.F.; Padma, V.V. Neferine, an alkaloid from lotus seed embryo, inhibits human lung cancer cell growth by MAPK activation and cell cycle arrest. *Biofactors* **2014**, *40*, 121–131. [CrossRef] [PubMed]
21. Yoon, J.S.; Kim, H.M.; Yadunandam, A.K.; Kim, N.H.; Jung, H.A.; Choi, J.S.; Kim, C.Y.; Kim, G.D. Neferine isolated from *Nelumbo nucifera* enhances anti-cancer activities in Hep3B cells: Molecular mechanisms of cell cycle arrest, ER stress induced apoptosis and anti-angiogenic response. *Phytomedicine* **2013**, *20*, 1013–1022. [CrossRef] [PubMed]
22. Xu, L.; Zhang, X.; Li, Y.; Lu, S.; Li, J.; Wang, Y.; Tian, X.; Wei, J.J.; Shao, C.; Liu, Z. Neferine induces autophagy of human ovarian cancer cells via p38 MAPK/ JNK activation. *Tumour Biol.* **2016**, *37*, 8721–8729. [CrossRef] [PubMed]
23. Zhang, X.; Wang, X.; Wu, T.; Li, B.; Liu, T.; Wang, R.; Liu, Q.; Liu, Z.; Gong, Y.; Shao, C. Isoliensinine induces apoptosis in triple-negative human breast cancer cells through ROS generation and p38 MAPK/JNK activation. *Sci. Rep.* **2015**, *5*, 12579. [CrossRef] [PubMed]
24. Nishimura, K.; Horii, S.; Tanahashi, T.; Sugimoto, Y.; Yamada, J. Synthesis and pharmacological activity of alkaloids from embryo of lotus, *Nelumbo nucifera*. *Chem. Pharm. Bull.* **2013**, *61*, 59–68. [CrossRef] [PubMed]
25. Ziegler, J.; Facchini, P.J. Alkaloid biosynthesis: Metabolism and trafficking. *Annu. Rev. Plant Biol.* **2008**, *59*, 735–769. [CrossRef] [PubMed]
26. Stadler, R.; Kutchan, T.M.; Zenk, M.H. (S)-Norcoclaurine is the central intermediate in benzylisoquinoline alkaloid biosynthesis. *Phytochemistry* **1989**, *28*, 1083–1086. [CrossRef]
27. Hagel, J.M.; Facchini, P.J. Benzylisoquinoline alkaloid metabolism: A century of discovery and a brave new word. *Plant Cell Physiol.* **2013**, *54*, 647–672. [CrossRef] [PubMed]
28. Hagel, J.M.; Mandal, R.; Han, B.; Han, J.; Dinsmore, D.R.; Borchers, C.H.; Wishart, D.S.; Facchini, P.J. Metabolome analysis of 20 taxonomically related benzylisoquinoline alkaloid-producing plants. *BMC Plant Biol.* **2015**, *15*, 220. [CrossRef] [PubMed]
29. Hagel, J.M.; Morris, J.S.; Lee, E.J.; Desgagné-Penix, I.; Bross, C.D.; Chang, L.; Chen, X.; Farrow, S.C.; Zhang, Y.; Soh, J.; et al. Transcriptome analysis of 20 taxonomically related benzylisoquinoline alkaloid-producing plants. *BMC Plant Biol.* **2015**, *15*, 227. [CrossRef] [PubMed]
30. Beaudoin, G.A.W.; Facchini, P.J. Benzylisoquinoline alkaloid biosynthesis in opium poppy. *Planta* **2014**, *240*, 19–32. [CrossRef] [PubMed]
31. Liscombe, D.K.; MacLeod, B.P.; Loukanina, N.; Nandi, O.I.; Facchini, P.J. Evidence for the monophyletic evolution of benzylisoquinoline alkaloid biosynthesis in angiosperms. *Phytochemistry* **2005**, *66*, 2501–2520. [CrossRef] [PubMed]

32. Deng, X.; Zhu, L.; Fang, T.; Vimolmangkang, S.; Yang, D.; Ogutu, C.; Liu, Y.; Han, Y. Analysis of isoquinoline alkaloid composition and wound-induced variation in *Nelumbo* using HPLC-MS/MS. *J. Agric. Food Chem.* **2016**, *64*, 1130–1136. [CrossRef] [PubMed]
33. Chen, S.; Zhang, H.; Liu, Y.; Fang, J.; Li, S. Determination of lotus leaf alkaloids by solid phase extraction combined with high performance liquid chromatography with diode array and tandem mass spectrometry. *Anal. Lett.* **2013**, *46*, 2846–2859. [CrossRef]
34. Vimolmangkang, S.; Deng, X.; Owiti, A.; Meelaph, T.; Ogutu, C.; Han, Y. Evolutionary origin of the NCSI gene subfamily encoding norcoclaurine synthase is associated with the biosynthesis of benzylisoquinoline alkaloids in plants. *Sci. Rep.* **2016**, *6*, 26323. [CrossRef] [PubMed]
35. Zhou, M.; Jiang, M.; Ying, X.; Cui, Q.; Han, Y.; Hou, Y.; Gao, J.; Bai, G.; Luo, G. Identification and comparison of anti-inflammatory ingredients from different organs of *Lotus Nelumbo* by UPLC/Q-TOF and PCA coupled with a NF-κB reporter gene assay. *PLoS ONE* **2013**, *8*, e81971. [CrossRef] [PubMed]
36. Koshiyama, H.; Ohkuma, H.; Kawaguchi, H.; Hsü, H.Y.; Chen, Y.P. Isolation of 1-(*p*-hydroxybenzyl)-6,7-dihydroxy-1,2,3,4-tetrahydroisoquinoline (demethylcoclaurine), an active alkaloid from *Nelumbo nucifera*. *Chem. Pharm. Bull.* **1970**, *18*, 2564–2568. [CrossRef]
37. Kashiwada, Y.; Aoshima, A.; Ikeshiro, Y.; Chen, Y.-P.; Furukawa, H.; Itoigawa, M.; Fujioka, T.; Mishashi, K.; Cosentino, L.M.; Morris-Natschke, S.L.; et al. Anti-HIV benzylisoquinoline alkaloids and flavonoids from the leaves of *Nelumbo nucifera*, and structure-activity correlations with related alkaloids. *Bioorg. Med. Chem.* **2005**, *13*, 443–448. [CrossRef] [PubMed]
38. Lin, Z.; Yang, R.; Guan, Z.; Chen, A.; Li, W. Ultra-performance LC separation and quadrupole time-of-flight MS identification of major alkaloids in plumula nelumbinis. *Phytochem. Anal.* **2014**, *25*, 485–494. [CrossRef] [PubMed]
39. Hong, H.; Lee, Y.I.; Jin, D. Determination of *R*-(+)-higenamine enantiomer in *Nelumbo nucifera* by high-performance liquid chromatography with a fluorescent chiral tagging reagent. *Microchem. J.* **2010**, *96*, 374–379. [CrossRef]
40. Do, T.C.; Nguyen, T.D.; Tran, H.; Stuppner, H.; Ganzera, M. Analysis of alkaloids in lotus (*Nelumbo nucifera* Gaertn.) leaves by non-aqueous capillary electrophoresis using ultraviolet and mass spectrometric detection. *J. Chromatogr. A* **2013**, *1302*, 174–180. [CrossRef] [PubMed]
41. Kunitomo, J.; Yoshikawa, S.; Tanaka, Y.; Inmori, Y.; Isor, K. Alkaloids from *Nelumbo nucifera*. *Phytochemistry* **1973**, *12*, 699–701. [CrossRef]
42. Ka, S.M.; Kuo, Y.C.; Ho, P.J.; Tsai, P.Y.; Hsu, Y.J.; Tsai, W.J.; Lin, Y.L.; Shen, C.C.; Chen, A. (*S*)-armepavine from Chinese medicine improves experimental autoimmune crescentic glomerulonephritis. *Rheumatology* **2010**, *49*, 1840–1851. [CrossRef] [PubMed]
43. Guo, Y.; Chen, X.; Qi, J.; Yu, B. Simultaneous qualitative and quantitative analysis of flavonoids and alkaloids from the leaves of *Nelumbo nucifera* Gaertn. using high-performance liquid chromatography with quadrupole time-of-flight mass spectrometry. *J. Sep. Sci.* **2016**, *39*, 2499–2507. [CrossRef] [PubMed]
44. Grienke, U.; Mair, C.E.; Saxena, P.; Baburin, I.; Scheel, O.; Ganzera, M.; Schuster, D.; Hering, S.; Rollinger, J.M. Human ether-à-go-go related gene (hERG) channel blocking aporphine alkaloids from lotus leaves and their quantitative analysis in dietary weight loss supplements. *J. Agric. Food Chem.* **2015**, *63*, 5634–5639. [CrossRef] [PubMed]
45. Itoh, A.; Saitoh, T.; Tani, K.; Uchigaki, M.; Sugimoto, Y.; Yamada, J.; Nakajima, H.; Ohshiro, H.; Sun, S.; Tanahashi, T. Bisbenzylisoquinoline alkaloids from *Nelumbo nucifera*. *Chem. Pharm. Bull.* **2011**, *59*, 947–951. [CrossRef] [PubMed]
46. Yang, G.M.; Sun, J.; Pan, Y.; Zhang, J.L.; Xiao, M.; Zhu, M.S. Isolation and identification of a tribenzylisoquinoline alkaloid from *Nelumbo nucifera* Gaertn, a novel potential smooth muscle relaxant. *Fitoterapia* **2017**, *124*, 58–65. [CrossRef] [PubMed]
47. Zhang, N.; Lian, Z.; Peng, X.; Li, Z.; Zhu, H. Applications of Higenamine in pharmacology and medicine. *J. Ethnopharmacol.* **2017**, *196*, 242–252. [CrossRef] [PubMed]
48. Liu, C.P.; Tsai, W.J.; Shen, C.C.; Lin, Y.L.; Liao, J.F.; Chen, C.F.; Kuo, Y.C. Inhibition of (*S*)-armepavine from *Nelumbo nucifera* on autoimmune disease of MRL/MpJ-lpr/lpr mice. *Eur. J. Pharmacol.* **2006**, *531*, 270–279. [CrossRef] [PubMed]

49. Yang, M.; Zhu, L.; Li, L.; Li, J.; Xu, L.; Feng, J.; Liu, Y. Digital gene expression analysis provides insight into the transcript profile of the genes involved in aporphine alkaloid biosynthesis in lotus (*Nelumbo nucifera*). *Front. Plant Sci.* **2017**, *8*, 80. [CrossRef] [PubMed]
50. Morris, J.; Facchini, P.J. Isolation and characterization of reticuline N-methyltransferase involved in biosynthesis of the aporphine alkaloid magnoflorine in opium poppy. *J. Biol. Chem.* **2016**, *291*, 23416–23427. [CrossRef] [PubMed]
51. Chang, L.; Hagel, J.M.; Facchini, P.J. Isolation and characterization of O-methyltransferases involved in the biosynthesis of glaucine in *Glaucium flavum*. *Plant Physiol.* **2015**, *169*, 1127–1140. [CrossRef] [PubMed]
52. Ilari, A.; Franceschini, S.; Bonamore, A.; Arenghi, F.; Botta, B.; Macone, A.; Pasquo, A.; Bellucci, L.; Boffi, A. Structural basis of enzymatic (S)-norcoclaurine biosynthesis. *J. Biol. Chem.* **2009**, *284*, 897–904. [CrossRef] [PubMed]
53. Berkner, H.; Schweimer, K.; Matecko, I.; Rosch, P. Conformation, catalytic site, and enzymatic mechanism of the PR10 allergen-related enzyme norcoclaurine synthase. *Biochem. J.* **2008**, *413*, 281–290. [CrossRef] [PubMed]
54. Lee, E.J.; Facchini, P. Norcoclaurine synthase is a member of the pathogenesis-related 10/Bet v1 protein family. *Plant Cell.* **2010**, *22*, 3489–3503. [CrossRef] [PubMed]
55. Li, J.; Lee, E.J.; Chang, L.; Facchini, P.J. Genes encoding norcoclaurine synthase occur as tandem fusions in the Papaveraceae. *Sci. Rep.* **2016**, *6*, 39256. [CrossRef] [PubMed]
56. Lichman, B.R.; Sula, A.; Pesnot, T.; Hailes, H.C.; Ward, J.M.; Keep, N.H. Structural evidence for the dopamine-first mechanism of norcoclaurine synthase. *Biochemistry* **2017**, *56*, 5274–5277. [CrossRef] [PubMed]
57. Luk, L.Y.; Bunn, S.; Liscombe, D.K.; Facchini, P.J.; Tanner, M.E. Mechanistic studies on norcoclaurine synthase of benzylisoquinoline alkaloid biosynthesis: An enzymatic Pictet-Spengler reaction. *Biochemistry* **2007**, *46*, 10153–10161. [CrossRef] [PubMed]
58. Samanani, N.; Facchini, P.J. Purification and characterization of norcoclaurine synthase. The first committed enzyme in benzylisoquinoline alkaloid biosynthesis in plants. *J. Biol. Chem.* **2002**, *277*, 33878–33883. [CrossRef] [PubMed]
59. Samanani, N.; Liscombe, D.K.; Facchini, P.J. Molecular cloning and characterization of norcoclaurine synthase, an enzyme catalyzing the first committed step in benzylisoquinoline alkaloid biosynthesis. *Plant J.* **2004**, *40*, 302–313. [CrossRef] [PubMed]
60. Kato, E.; Iwata, R.; Kawabata, J. Synthesis and detailed examination of spectral properties of (S)- and (R)-Higenamine 4'-O-β-D-Glucoside and HPLC analytical conditions to distinguish the diastereomers. *Molecules* **2017**, *22*. [CrossRef] [PubMed]
61. Deng, X.; Zhao, L.; Fang, T.; Xiong, Y.; Ogutu, C.; Yang, D.; Vimolmangkang, S.; Liu, Y.; Han, Y. Investigation of benzylisoquinoline alkaloid biosynthetic pathway and its transcriptional regulation in lotus. *Hortic. Res.* **2018**, *5*, 29. [CrossRef] [PubMed]
62. Meelaph, T.; Kobtrakul, K.; Chansilpa, N.N.; Han, Y.; Rani, D.; De-Eknamkul, W.; Vimolmangkang, S. Coregulation of biosynthetic genes and transcription factors for aporphine-type alkaloid production in wounded lotus provides insight into the biosynthetic pathway of nuciferine. *ACS Omega* **2018**, *3*, 8794–8802. [CrossRef]
63. Park, J.E.; Kang, Y.J.; Park, M.K.; Lee, Y.S.; Kim, H.J.; Seo, H.G.; Lee, J.H.; Hye Sook, Y.C.; Shin, J.S.; Lee, H.W.; et al. Enantiomers of higenamine inhibit LPS-induced iNOS in a macrophage cell line and improve the survival of mice with experimental endotoxemia. *Int. Immunopharmacol.* **2006**, *6*, 226–233. [CrossRef] [PubMed]
64. Kraus, P.F.; Kutchan, T.M. Molecular cloning and heterologous expression of a cDNA encoding berbamunine synthase, a C-O phenol-coupling cytochrome P450 from the higher plant *Berberis stolonifera*. *Proc. Natl. Acad Sci. USA* **1995**, *92*, 2071–2075. [CrossRef] [PubMed]
65. Robin, A.Y.; Giustini, C.; Graindorge, M.; Matringe, M.; Dumas, R. Crystal structure of norcoclaurine-6-O-methyltransferase, a key rate-limiting step in the synthesis of benzylisoquinoline alkaloids. *Plant J.* **2016**, *87*, 641–653. [CrossRef] [PubMed]
66. Farrow, S.C.; Hagel, J.M.; Beaudoin, G.A.; Burns, D.C.; Facchini, P.J. Stereochemical inversion of (S)-reticuline by a cytochrome P450 fusion in opium poppy. *Nat. Chem. Biol.* **2015**, *11*, 728–732. [CrossRef] [PubMed]

67. Gui, S.; Peng, J.; Wang, X.; Wu, Z.; Cao, R.; Salse, J.; Zhang, H.; Zhu, Z.; Xia, Q.; Quan, Z.; et al. Improving *Nelumbo nucifera* genome assemblies using high-resolution genetic maps and BioNano genome mapping reveals ancient chromosome rearrangements. *Plant J.* **2018**, *94*, 721–734. [CrossRef] [PubMed]
68. Meng, Z.; Hu, X.; Zhang, Z.; Li, Z.; Lin, Q.; Yang, M.; Yang, P.; Ming, R.; Yu, Q.; Wang, K. Chromosome nomenclature and cytological characterization of sacred lotus. *Cytogenet. Genome Res.* **2017**, *153*, 223–231. [CrossRef] [PubMed]
69. Nelson, D.R.; Schuler, M.A. Cytochrome P450 genes from the sacred lotus genome. *Trop. Plant Biol.* **2013**, *6*, 138–151. [CrossRef]
70. Liscombe, D.K.; Louie, G.V.; Noel, J.P. Architectures, mechanisms and molecular evolution of natural product methyltransferases. *Nat. Prod. Rep.* **2012**, *29*, 1238–1250. [CrossRef] [PubMed]
71. Park, M.R.; Chen, X.; Lang, D.E.; Ng, K.K.S.; Facchini, P.J. Heterodimeric O-methyltransferases involved in the biosynthesis of noscapine in opium poppy. *Plant J.* **2018**, *95*, 252–267. [CrossRef] [PubMed]
72. Nelson, D.R. The cytochrome P450 homepage. *Hum. Genom.* **2009**, *4*, 59–65. [CrossRef]
73. Ikezawa, N.; Iwasa, K.; Sato, F. Molecular cloning and characterization of CYP80G2, a cytochrome P450 that catalyzes an intramolecular C-C phenol coupling of (S)-reticuline in magnoflorine biosynthesis, from cultured *Coptis japonica* cells. *J. Biol. Chem.* **2008**, *283*, 8810–8821. [CrossRef] [PubMed]
74. Dastmalchi, M.; Park, M.R.; Morris, J.S.; Facchini, P.J. Family portraits: The enzymes behind benzylisoquinoline alkaloid diversity. *Phytochem. Rev.* **2018**, *17*, 249–277. [CrossRef]
75. Gurkok, T.; Ozhuner, E.; Parmaksiz, I.; Özcan, S.; Turktas, M.; Ipek, A.; Demirtas, I.; Okay, S.; Unver, T. Functional characterization of 4′OMT and 7OMT genes in BIA biosynthesis. *Front Plant Sci.* **2016**, *7*, 98. [CrossRef] [PubMed]
76. Inui, T.; Tamura, K.I.; Fujii, N.; Morishige, T.; Sato, F. Overexpression of *Coptis japonica* norcoclaurine 6-O-methyltransferase overcomes the rate-limiting step in benzylisoquinoline alkaloid biosynthesis in cultured *Eschscholzia californica*. *Plant Cell Physiol.* **2007**, *48*, 252–262. [CrossRef] [PubMed]
77. Allen, R.S.; Miller, J.A.C.; Chitty, J.A.; Fist, A.J.; Gerlach, W.L.; Larkin, P.J. Metabolic engineering of morphian alkaloids by over-expression and RNAi suppression of salutaridinol 7-O-acetyltransferase in opium poppy. *Plant Biotechnol. J.* **2008**, *6*, 22–30. [CrossRef] [PubMed]
78. Alagoz, Y.; Gurkok, T.; Zhang, B.; Unver, T. Manipulating the biosynthesis of bioactive compound alkaloids for next-generation metabolic engineering in opium poppy using CRISP-Cas 9 genome editing technology. *Sci. Rep.* **2016**, *6*, 30910. [CrossRef] [PubMed]
79. Dang, T.T.T.; Facchini, P.J. Characterization of three O-methyltransferases involved in noscapine biosynthesis in opium poppy. *Plant Physiol.* **2012**, *159*, 618–631. [CrossRef] [PubMed]
80. Desgagné-Penix, I.; Facchini, P.J. Systematic silencing of benzylisoquinoline alkaloid biosynthetic genes reveals the major route to papaverine in opium poppy. *Plant J.* **2012**, *72*, 331–344. [CrossRef] [PubMed]
81. Kato, N.; Dubouzet, E.; Kokabu, Y.; Yoshida, S.; Taniguchi, Y.; Dubouzet, J.G.; Yazaki, K.; Sato, F. Identification of a WRKY protein as a transcriptional regulator of benzylisoquinoline alkaloid biosynthesis in *Coptis japonica*. *Plant Cell Physiol.* **2007**, *48*, 8–18. [CrossRef] [PubMed]
82. Yamada, Y.; Motomura, Y.; Sato, F. CjbHLH1 homologs regulate sanguinarine biosynthesis in *Eschscholzia californica* cells. *Plant Cell Physiol.* **2015**, *56*, 1019–1030. [CrossRef] [PubMed]
83. Lee, E.J.; Hagel, J.M.; Facchini, P.J. Role of the phloem in the biochemistry and ecophysiology of benzylisoquinoline alkaloid metabolism. *Front Plant Sci.* **2013**, *4*, 182. [CrossRef] [PubMed]
84. Esau, K.; Kosakai, H. Laticifers in *Nelumbo nucifera* Gaertn.: Distribution and structure. *Ann. Bot.* **1975**, *39*, 713–719. [CrossRef]
85. Samanani, N.; Alcantara, J.; Bourgault, R.; Zulak, K.G.; Facchini, P.J. The role of phloem sieve elements and laticifers in the biosynthesis and accumulation of alkaloids in opium poppy. *Plant J.* **2006**, *47*, 547–563. [CrossRef] [PubMed]
86. Chen, X.; Hagel, J.M.; Chang, L.; Tucker, J.E.; Shiigi, S.A.; Yelpaala, Y.; Chen, H.Y.; Estrada, R.; Colbeck, J.; Enquist-Newman, M.; et al. A pathogenesis-related 10 protein catalyzes the final step in thebaine biosynthesis. *Nat. Chem. Biol.* **2018**, *14*, 738–743. [CrossRef] [PubMed]

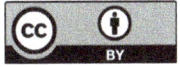

© 2018 by the authors. Licensee MDPI, Basel, Switzerland. This article is an open access article distributed under the terms and conditions of the Creative Commons Attribution (CC BY) license (http://creativecommons.org/licenses/by/4.0/).

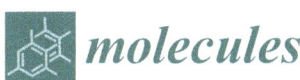

Review

Pyrrolizidine Alkaloids: Biosynthesis, Biological Activities and Occurrence in Crop Plants

Sebastian Schramm, Nikolai Köhler and Wilfried Rozhon *

Biotechnology of Horticultural Crops, TUM School of Life Sciences Weihenstephan, Technical University of Munich, Liesel-Beckmann-Straße 1, 85354 Freising, Germany; seb.schramm@tum.de (S.S.); nikolai.koehler@tum.de (N.K.)
* Correspondence: wilfried.rozhon@wzw.tum.de; Tel.: +49-8161-71-2023

Academic Editor: John C. D'Auria
Received: 20 December 2018; Accepted: 29 January 2019; Published: 30 January 2019

Abstract: Pyrrolizidine alkaloids (PAs) are heterocyclic secondary metabolites with a typical pyrrolizidine motif predominantly produced by plants as defense chemicals against herbivores. They display a wide structural diversity and occur in a vast number of species with novel structures and occurrences continuously being discovered. These alkaloids exhibit strong hepatotoxic, genotoxic, cytotoxic, tumorigenic, and neurotoxic activities, and thereby pose a serious threat to the health of humans since they are known contaminants of foods including grain, milk, honey, and eggs, as well as plant derived pharmaceuticals and food supplements. Livestock and fodder can be affected due to PA-containing plants on pastures and fields. Despite their importance as toxic contaminants of agricultural products, there is limited knowledge about their biosynthesis. While the intermediates were well defined by feeding experiments, only one enzyme involved in PA biosynthesis has been characterized so far, the homospermidine synthase catalyzing the first committed step in PA biosynthesis. This review gives an overview about structural diversity of PAs, biosynthetic pathways of necine base, and necic acid formation and how PA accumulation is regulated. Furthermore, we discuss their role in plant ecology and their modes of toxicity towards humans and animals. Finally, several examples of PA-producing crop plants are discussed.

Keywords: *Borago officinalis*; *Crassocephalum*; Copper-dependent diamine oxidase; *Gynura bicolor*; Homospermidine synthase; *Lolium perenne*; Necic acids; Necine bases; Pyrrolizidine alkaloid biosynthesis; Senecionine

---

1. Introduction

Pyrrolizidine alkaloids (PAs) are heterocyclic organic compounds synthesized by plants that are thought to act as defense compounds against herbivores [1]. Estimates indicate that approximately 6.000 plant species worldwide, representing 3% of all flowering plants, produce these secondary metabolites. In particular, members of the Asteraceae, Boraginaceae, Heliotropiaceae, Apocynaceae, and some genera of the Orchidaceae and the Fabaceae are PA producers [2]. Reported concentrations vary greatly, from trace amounts to up to 19% dry weight, and are considered to be dependent on a number of factors including the developmental stage, tissue type, environmental conditions, and extraction procedures [3].

PAs consist of a necine base esterified with a necic acid. The necine base typically includes pyrrolizidine, a bicyclic aliphatic hydrocarbon consisting of two fused five-membered rings with a nitrogen at the bridgehead [4] (Figure 1). Loline alkaloids may be formally considered as PAs since they also possess a pyrrolizidine system, although it contains an ether bridge linking carbon 2 (C-2) and carbon 7 (C-7). While *stricto sensu* PAs are exclusively formed in plants, lolines are synthesized by endophytic fungal symbionts of the genus *Epichloë* [5]. In addition, their biosynthesis is distinct from PAs [5–7]. Thus, lolines will be discussed only peripherally in this review.

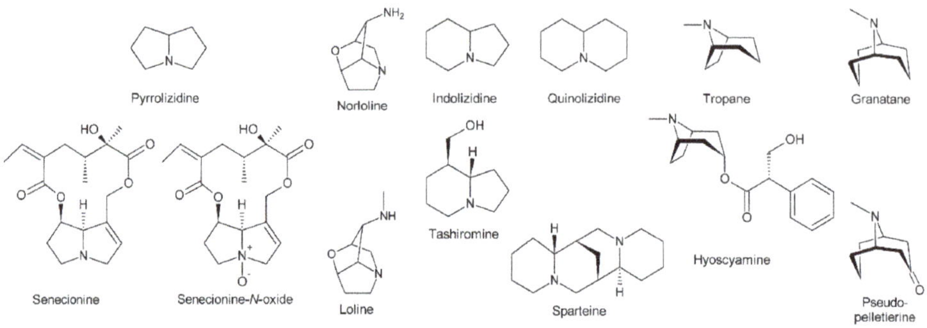

Figure 1. Core structures and examples for pyrrolizidine, loline, indolizidine, quinolizidine, tropane and granatane alkaloids. In contrast to the other alkaloids pyrrolizidine alkaloids appear mainly as N-oxides, as shown for the example of senecionine-N-oxide.

The fused bicyclic system of PAs resembles indolizidine and quinolizidine alkaloids, which contain a five and a six-membered ring or two six-membered rings, respectively [8] (Figure 1). Tropane and granatane alkaloids also show a similar structure consisting of a five and a six-membered ring or two six-membered rings, respectively [9]. However, in contrast to necine bases, the rings of tropane and granatane alkaloids are bridged rather than fused. While several tropane and quinolizidine alkaloids including atropine (the racemic mixture of (±)-hyoscyamine) and sparteine are used in medicine [9], PAs are mainly known for their hepatotoxic and potentially carcinogenic properties [10]. Nevertheless, some PAs show interesting pharmacological properties that are currently under investigation (see Section 5.3) [10,11]. While tropane and quinolizidine alkaloids are usually present in plants in their free forms, PAs are mainly present as N-oxides (Figure 1), which are highly water-soluble and considered less toxic than the free PAs.

2. Structural Diversity of Pyrrolizidine Alkaloids

Within the combination of a set of necine bases (Figures 2 and 3) and a considerable number of necic acids (Figure 4), an enormous structural diversity of PAs can be obtained. This is further amplified by modifications, including N-oxidation of the tertiary nitrogen of the necine base, hydroxylation of the necine base and/or the necic acid, and acetylation of hydroxy groups of the acid moiety. Thus, it is not surprising that several hundreds of different PAs have already been identified and each year new variants are described.

2.1. Diversity of Necine Bases

In addition to the pyrrolizidine ring system most necine bases possess a hydroxymethyl group at position 1 (Figure 2), which is a consequence of the biosynthetic pathway (see Section 3.1). Since 1-hydroxymethylpyrrolizidine contains two chiral centers, carbons C-1 and C-8, in total four compounds exist: The enantiomers (-)/(+)-trachelanthamidine and (-)/(+)-isoretronecanole (Figure 2B). Among them, (-)-trachelanthamidine and (-)-isoretronecanole are most frequently found, for instance, as the necine base of trachelanthamine (Figure 5C) and the nervosines [12] (Figure 5E), respectively. Examples for PAs containing (+)-trachelanthamidine and (+)-isoretronecanole are acetyllaburnine [13] (Figure 5G) and madhumidine A [14], respectively. The most frequent modification of saturated necine bases is hydroxylation at C-7. However, the positions C-2 and C-6 are also occasionally hydroxylated. Necine bases like (-)-platynecine, possessing hydroxy groups on C-7 and C-8, and (-)-rosmarinecine containing hydroxy groups on C-2, C7 and C-9 (Figure 2), are often esterified by dicarboxylic necic acids to form macrocyclic PAs like platyphylline and rosmarinine (Figure 5A) [15]. In general, saturated PAs are considered as non-toxic [16].

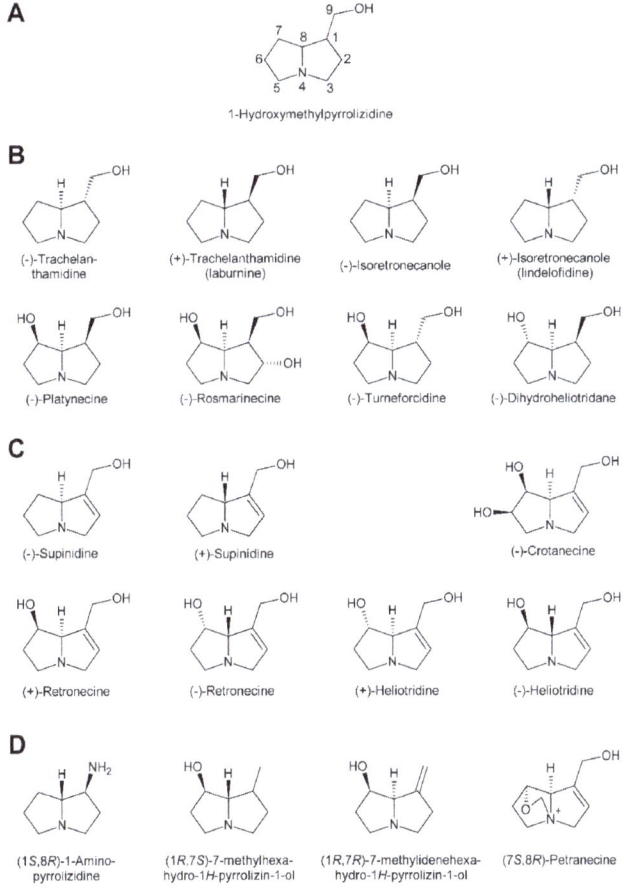

Figure 2. Structures of necine bases. (A) Basic structures and numbering of atoms in necine bases. (B) Saturated necine bases. (C) 1,2-Desaturated necine bases. (D) Unusual necine bases.

Most PAs contain a necine base possessing a double bond between C-1 and C-2 (Figure 2). Introducing that double bond eliminates the chiral centre at C-1, thus leaving only the stereocentre at C-8. Consequently, only two forms, (-)/(+)-supinidine, exist of the C-9 monohydroxalated derivatives and four, (-)/(+)-retronecine and (-)/(+)-heliotridine, of the C-7 and C-9 dihydroxylated compounds. Among them (+)-retronecine is the most frequently observed necine base in PAs.

In addition to the saturated and desaturated bases discussed above, necine bases of the otonecine type also exist. Otonecine is not a genuine bicyclus, but may act as such due to transannular interactions of the keto group and the tertiary amine (Figure 3A) [17]. These interactions are also likely for the reason that otonecine-type PAs are present in plants as free bases rather than N-oxides.

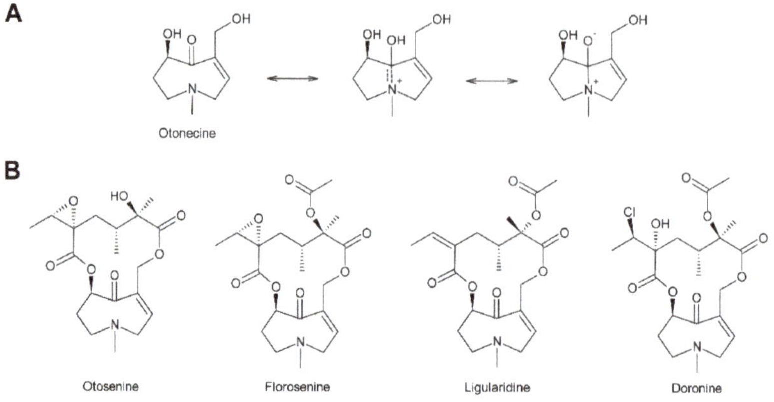

Figure 3. Otonecine and representative PAs. (**A**) Resonance structures of otonecine. (**B**) Structures of the otonecine-type PAs otosenine, florosenine, ligularidine, and doronine.

There are also several necine bases with unusual structures (Figure 2D). One of them is 1-aminopyrrolizidine, wherein the hydroxymethyl group is replaced by an amino group. This unusual necine base is found for instance in laburnamine, an alkaloid present in trace amounts in *Laburnum anagyroides* [18]. From the leaves of *Ehretia asperia*, ehretinine was isolated, which is very unusual since the 7-hydroxy group of its necine base, (1R,7S)-7-methylhexahydro-1H-pyrrolizin-1-ol, is esterified with 4-methylbenzoic acid and the typical hydroxymethyl group on C-1 is replaced by a methyl residue [19]. Similarly, *Senecio polypodioides* contains, besides sarracine N-oxide, also 7β-angeloyloxy-1-methylene-8α-pyrrolizidine, a PA with a methylene group instead of the typical hydroxymethyl residue on its necine base. The 7-hydroxy group of this PA is esterified with angelic acid [20]. In *Echium glomeratum*, PAs with a tricyclic ring were found. The 9-hydroxy group of the necine base was found to be esterified with angelic acid [21]. Another example is the necine base of tussilagine from *Tussilago farfara*, which possesses a carboxy group instead of the typical hydroxymethyl group (Figure 5H) [22].

2.2. Diversity of Necic Acids

While necine bases share a common structure, the necic acids show broad structural diversity. Some, particularly the smaller and simpler ones, are typical metabolites of plant metabolism, while others, particularly the monocarboxylic acids of the trachelanthic acid type and the dicarboxylic acids (Figure 4) are formed in specific, complex pathways.

Acetic acid (Figure 4A) is frequently observed in simple PAs, for instance 7-acetylretronecine present in *Onosma arenaria* [23] and acetyllaburnine present in *Vanda*, a genus of the Orchidaceae [13,24] (Figure 5G). Acetic acid may also esterify the second hydroxy group of the necine base in triangularine and lycopsymine-type PAs, such as 7-acetyl-9-sarracinoylretronecine present in *Alkanna tuberculata* [25] (Figure 5B) and uplandicine found in pollen of *Echium vulgare* (Figure 5C). In addition, acetic acid also frequently esterifies hydroxy groups of other necic acids in more complex PAs, for instance florosenine [26], ligularidine [27] (Figure 3B), or acetylerucifoline N-oxide [28]. In contrast to the frequently observed acetic acid, lactic acid has, so far, only been found in lactoidine, a PA of *Cynoglossum furcatum* [29].

C_5 acids of the tiglic acid type (Figure 4A) are characteristic for the triangularine group of PAs (Figure 5B). They may esterify one or two hydroxy groups of the necine base. In the former case they may appear together with acetic acid or more complex necic acids, particularly branched C_7 acids, which is seen for instance in the PAs echimidine [30] and heliosupine [31] (Figure 5F). In addition to esterifying necine bases directly, C_5 acids may also esterify hydroxy groups of other necic acids. Examples are scorpioidine, a PA of *Myosotis scorpioides* [32] (Figure 5F), and anadoline, a PA of *Symphytum orientale* [33,34]. Latifolic acid [35–37] and the closely related hackelic acid [38] are examples of cyclic C_7 acids.

Aromatic systems are rarely present in necic acids except in PAs found in the Orchidaceae. Many of them, for instance benzoic acid, salicylic acid and *p*-coumaric acid, are simple aromatic acids present as primary or secondary metabolites in most plant species. However, some aromatic necine bases, particularly those found in the genera *Phalaenopsis* and *Liparis*, show a very complex structure, for instance the phalaenopsines [39,40] and the nervosines [41] (Figures 4B and 5E).

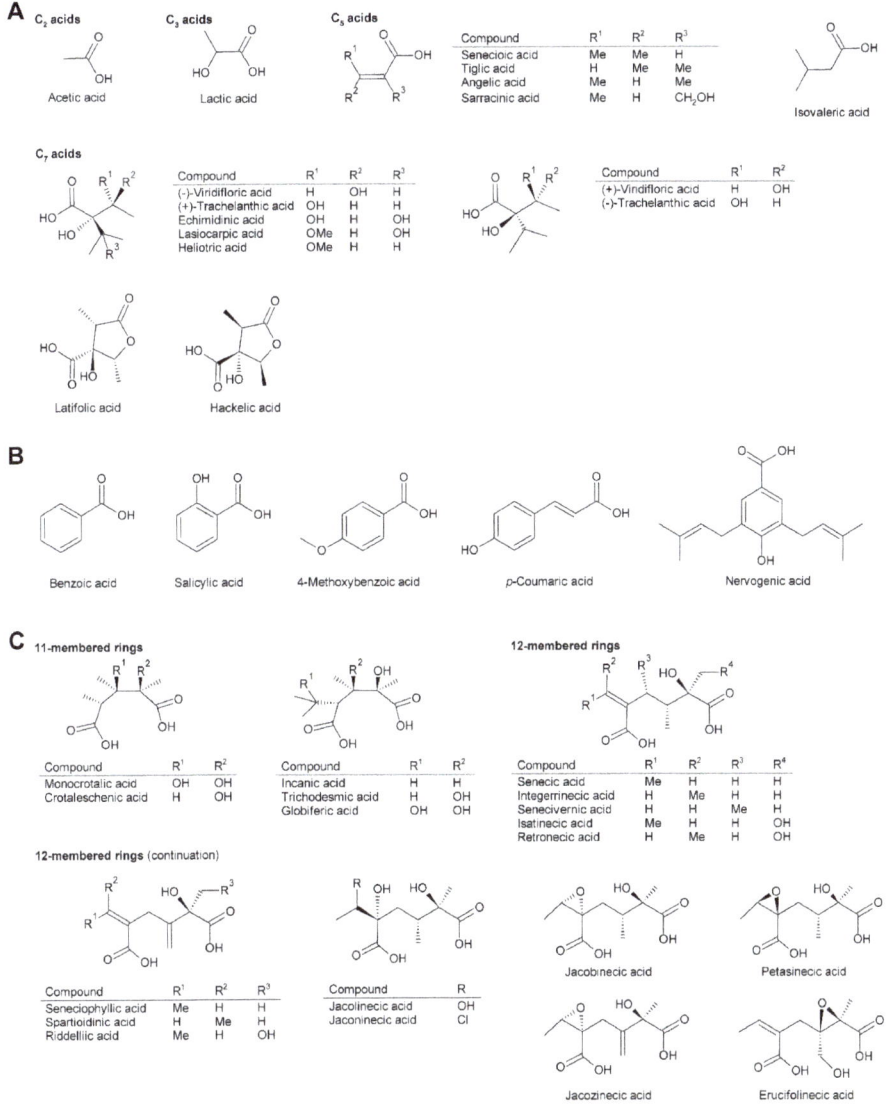

Figure 4. Examples for necic acids. (**A**) Monocarboxylic aliphatic acids. (**B**) Monocarboxylic aromatic acids. (**C**) Dicarboxylic acids forming macrocyclic PAs. Adapted from Reference [17].

The dicarboxylic necic acids (Figure 4C) are a particularly interesting group because they form macrocyclic PAs, which are considered to be the most toxic. Necic acids of the monocrotalic acid type are a relatively small group; they form 11-membered rings. In contrast, senecic acid-like necic acids typically form 12-membered rings and represent a large group. The considerable diversity is obtained by modification of the senecic acid core structure by a number of reactions (Section 3.2.4). Interestingly, a few among them contain chlorine (Figures 3B and 4C), a modification rarely observed in plant metabolites.

2.3. Linkage Patterns of Necine Bases with Necic Acids

Based on the combination of necine bases and necic acids and their linkage patterns the PAs have been classified into five groups [42]. The first and largest group are senecionine-like PAs, which consist of necine bases of the retronecine (Figure 2C), platynecine, rosmarinecine (Figure 2B), or otonecine-type (Figure 3) and typically branched C_{10} dicarboxylic necic acids (Figure 4C) derived from two molecules of L-isoleucine (see Section 3.2.4), which together form 12-membered macrocyclic rings. An exception is the small sub-group of nemorensine-like PAs [43], which form 13-membered macrocycles (Figure 5A). Typically, the necine bases are esterified at their C-7 and C-9 hydroxy groups. PAs of this type are mainly found in the tribe Senecioneae and family Fabaceae [44].

The second group is represented by triangularine-type PAs, which are open-chain mono- or diesters of necine bases with the C_5 acids tiglic, angelic, senecioic, and sarracinic acid (Figure 5B). These PAs are mainly present in Senecioneae and Boraginaceae [44].

The third type, the lycopsamine-like PAs are mainly found in Boraginaceae and Eupatorieae [44]. This type possesses branched C_7 necic acids esterifying the C-9 hydroxy group (Figure 5C). A number of PAs represent a combination of group 2 and 3 since they also possess a C_5 acid residue in addition to a C_7 necic acid. The C_5 acid residue can either be linked directly with the necine base or attached to a hydroxy group of the C_7 acid (Figure 5F).

The fourth group are the 11-membered macrocyclic PAs of the monocrotaline type. Similar to senecionine-like PAs the hydroxy groups of C-7 and C-9 are esterified with dicarboxylic necic acids (Figure 5D). This group is found predominantly in Fabaceae [44].

Phalaenopsine and ipanguline-type PAs represent the fifth group, which is characterized by the presence of an aromatic acid (Figure 4B), esterifying the usually saturated necine base (Figure 5E). The acidic compound shows a high structural diversity and includes simple aromatic acids like benzoic, salicylic and p-coumaric acid, but also very complex ones like nervogenic acid. This is the only group of PAs that are frequently glycosylated. Members of this group are found in the Orchidaceae, Convolvulaceae, and in a few representatives of other tribes including the Boraginaceae [44].

In addition to these five groups, there are also very simple PAs consisting only of the necine base and a small acid residue, particularly acetate, as illustrated by the examples shown in Figure 5G. A number of PAs show unusual linkage patterns distinct from that of the five groups discussed above. In madurensine the hydroxy group of C-9 is bridged by the dicarboxylic acid intergerrinecic acid with a hydroxy group placed at C-6 rather than the usual C-7 hydroxyl [45]. This leads to a 13-membered macrocyclic ring (Figure 5H). The structure of laburnamine [46] matches that of PAs of the triangularine type. However, since its necine base (1S,8R)-1-aminopyrrolizidine (Figure 2D) possesses an amino group instead of the hydroxy group on C-9, a reaction with isovaleric acid yields an amide rather than an ester bond (Figure 5G). Tussilagine, a PA of *Tussilago farfara* (coltsfoot), is very special since its necine base possesses, instead of the typical hydroxymethyl residue, a carboxy group on C-1, which is esterified with methanol [22]. Anhydroplatynecine is devoid of any necic acid and the C-7 and C-9 hydroxy groups of platynecine (Figure 2B) instead combine together via an ether bridge. However, anhydroplatynecine is likely not a naturally-occurring PA, but is rather formed by heating of platynecine containing PAs during isolation [47]. Finally, it is worth mentioning that several plant species also contain unmodified necine bases in their free form or as N-oxides [48].

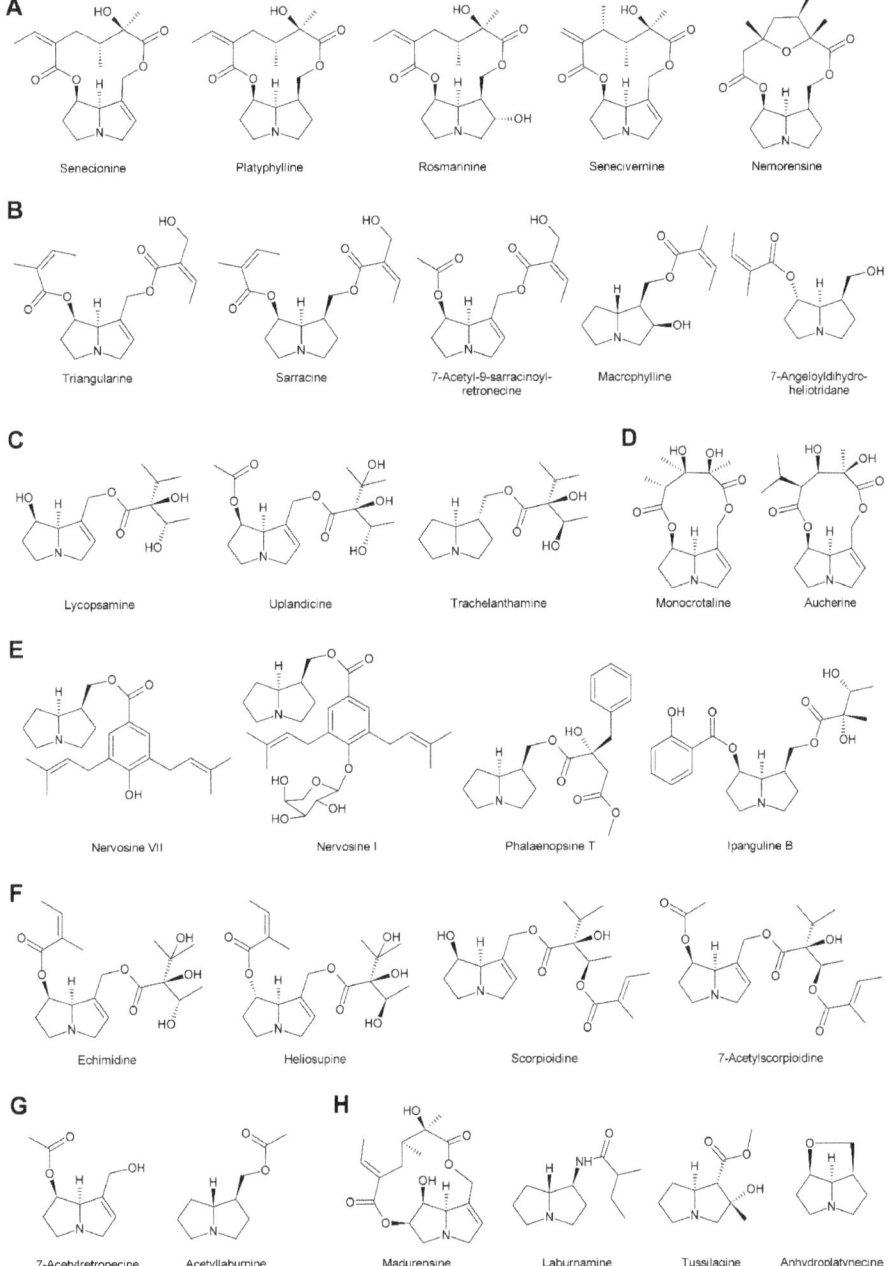

Figure 5. Linkage patterns of necic acids with necine bases. (**A**) Senecionine type. (**B**) Triangularine type. (**C**) Lycopsamine type. (**D**) Monocrotaline type. (**E**) Phalaenopsine/ipanguline type. (**F**) Compounds combining necic acids of triangularine and lycopsamine types. (**G**) Simple PAs. (**H**) PAs with unusual linkage patterns.

2.4. Modification and Conjugation of Pyrrolizidine Alkaloids

As discussed above, the astonishing diversity of PAs is achieved by hydroxylation and desaturation of necine bases and necic acids and their combination to PAs. Complete PAs might also be modified by hydroxylation, desaturation and epoxidation. The latter may be further metabolized to a diol or a chlorine-containing PA (see Section 3.2.4). In addition to these generally irreversible modifications, PAs can also be reversibly modified. By far the most frequently observed modification of this type is N-oxidation (Figure 1). In plants, the major fraction of PAs is present as N-oxides. Exceptions include seeds of several *Crotalaria* species [49] and leaves of *Crassocephalum crepidioides*, wherein the majority of the PAs are present in their basic form [50], and shoots of jacobine-chemotype plants of *Senecio jacobaea*, in which up to 50% might be present as tertiary PAs [51]. N-oxidation of the tertiary amine nitrogen changes the properties of a PA significantly. In contrast to basic tertiary amines, which are positively charged under physiological conditions, amine N-oxides are neutral and behave like very polar, highly water-soluble, salt-like compounds that are thought to be membrane impermeable. These characteristics might be important for their role in transport and storage of PAs. Accordingly, it was shown that PA transporters in membranes of plant cells have a higher affinity for PA N-oxides than for the tertiary amines [52].

In addition to N-oxidation, a number of PAs are also acetylated, particularly at hydroxy groups of the necic acid moiety. Examples are 7-acetylscorpionidine, the 7-O-acetylation product of scorpionidine (Figure 5F), and the otonecine-type PAs florosenine and ligularidine (Figure 3B), which are acetylated forms of otosenine and petasitenine, respectively.

While glycosylation is frequent among secondary metabolites, modifications of that type are rarely observed for PAs. Only among the PAs with aromatic necic acids some examples are known. They include thesinine-4'-O-α-L-glucoside present at high levels in borage seeds [53] (Section 6.1), thesinine-4'-O-α-L-rhamnoside found in *Lolium* species [54] (Section 6.4) and nervone PAs isolated from *Liparis nervosa* [41] (Figure 5E).

Other modifications are rarely seen in PAs.

3. Biosynthesis of Pyrrolizidine Alkaloids

Attempts at deciphering PA biosynthesis (Figure 6) date back to the early 1960s, when Nowacki and Byerrum performed their first feeding experiments with radiolabeled precursors [55,56]. Later, this work was continued by others, mainly the groups of Robins and Crout. Robins also introduced labeling with stable isotopes, particularly ^{13}C, ^{2}H and ^{15}N, and subsequent analysis by NMR spectroscopy for analysis of PA biosynthesis [57–59]. This technique provided detailed information about the fate of single C and H atoms during biosynthesis of the necine bases and necic acids. In the late 1990s, the first biosynthetic enzyme, homospermidine synthase, catalyzing the first committed step in PA biosynthesis, was identified [2]. Its analysis in different plant species provided interesting data about PA evolution, or more precisely, homospermidine biosynthesis.

3.1. Biosynthesis of Necine Bases

Feeding of *Crotalaria spectabilis* plants, which produce monocrotaline, with ^{14}C-labelled precursors showed that [^{14}C]-ornithine was efficiently incorporated into monocrotaline, particularly into its necine base retronecine [56]. Studies with *Senecio isatideus* [60] and *Senecio douglasii* [61] confirmed that [^{14}C]-ornithine is mainly incorporated into the necine base. Degradation studies in the latter study showed that approximately 25% of the incorporated radioactivity was present in carbon C-9 of the retronecine unit irrespective of whether [2-^{14}C]-ornithine or [5-^{14}C]-ornithine were fed, indicating that C-2 and C-5 of ornithine become equivalent during biosynthesis (at least for biosynthesis of the right-handed ring) and suggesting 1,4-diaminobutane (putrescine) as a symmetrical intermediate. Indeed, feeding of [1,4-^{14}C$_2$]-putrescine again yielded retronecine bearing approximately 25% of the radioactivity on C-9. Using *Senecio magnificus*, it was shown that arginine is also selectively incorporated into the necine base part of senecionine [62]. Subsequently, Robins and Sweeney compared the incorporation efficiency of several compounds using *Senecio isatideus* and found that putrescine, spermidine, and spermine were more efficiently incorporated than arginine and ornithine [63] and that the two latter were only effectively incorporated when present in the L configuration [64].

While these experiments established L-arginine and L-ornithine as precursors and putrescine as an intermediate, they did not allow a more comprehensive investigation since the fate of the individual C and H atoms could not be followed during biosynthesis. This problem was overcome by introduction of stable isotope labeled precursors and NMR analysis of the obtained products in combination with an improved plant feeding technique. Previously, plants were mainly fed hydroponically or as cut shoots, which resulted in incorporation rates significantly below 1%. In contrast, by absorption of aqueous solutions of the precursors directly into the xylems of freshly rooted cuttings through stem punctures, incorporation rates of up to 5% could be obtained [63]. Feeding of both [1,4-^{13}C$_2$]-putrescine and [1-^{13}C]-putrescine gave enriched ^{13}C signals for C-3, C-5, C-8 and C-9 (Figure 7A), confirming that both rings originate from putrescine [57,65].

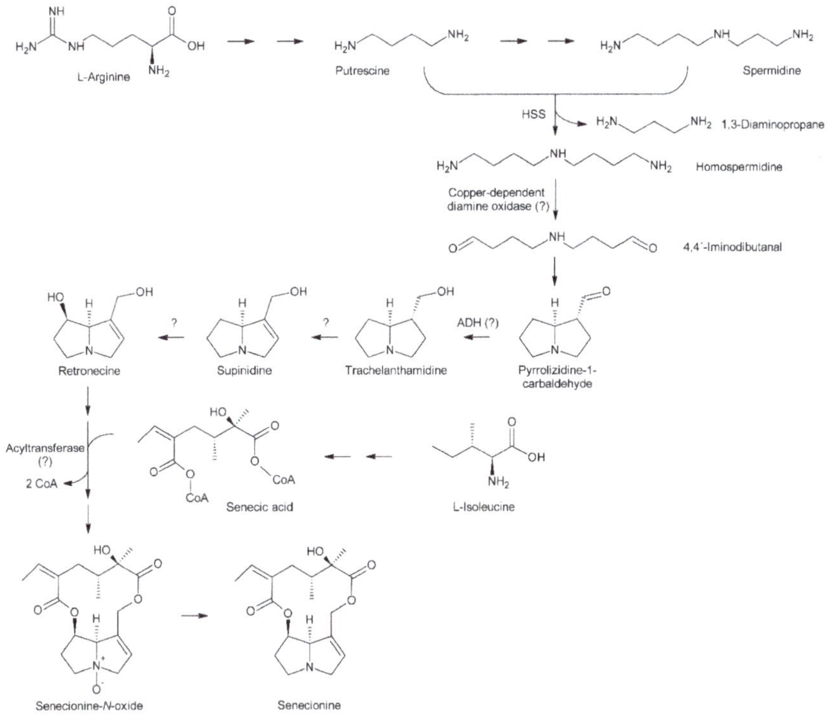

Figure 6. Biosynthesis of PAs. The polyamines putrescine and spermidine are derived from the basic amino acid arginine. Subsequently, homospermidine synthase (HSS) exchanges the 1,3-diamonopropane residue of spermidine by putrescine, which releases 1,3-diaminopropane and forms symmetric homospermidine. Oxidation of homospermidine, likely by copper-dependent diamine oxidases, to 4,4'-iminodibutanal initiates cyclization to pyrrolizidine-1-carbaldehyde, which is reduced, likely by an alcohol dehydrogenase, to 1-hydroxymethylpyrrolizidine. Desaturation and hydroxylation by unknown enzymes form retronecine, which is acylated with an activated necic acid, for instance with senecyl-CoA$_2$ as in the example shown above. Acylation might be catalyzed by an acyltransferase of the BAHD family. PA N-oxides, which are believed to be the primary products of PA biosynthesis, may be reduced to the free tertiary amine.

Because approximately 1.1% of the natural occurring carbon is the ^{13}C isotope, a ^{13}C label is easily obscured, particularly if the incorporation efficiency is moderate to low. Thus, further studies made use of double labeled precursors, where the ^{13}C-^{13}C double label can be sensitively detected by ^{13}C-NMR spectroscopy as doublet around the natural abundance signal. Feeding of [2,3-$^{13}C_2$]-putrescine gave a pair of doublets for C-1 and C-2 with a coupling constant J of 34 Hz and a second doublet pair for C-6 and C-7 with a coupling constant J of 70 Hz [65] (Figure 7B). Finally, feeding *Senecio isatideus* with [1,2-$^{13}C_2$]-putrescine gave rise to four pairs of doublets, namely C-1/C-9, C-2/C-3, C-5/C6 and C-7/C-8, with four different coupling constants (Figure 7C). To investigate which C-N bond remains intact during retronecine biosynthesis [1-^{15}N,1-^{13}C], double labeled putrescine was synthesized and fed to *Senecio vulgaris* [66,67] or *Senecio isatideus* [58,65]. Analysis of the necine base showed an equal amount of retronecine with a ^{15}N and a ^{13}C label at C-3 and retronecine with a ^{15}N and a ^{13}C label at C-5 (Figure 7D). The observation that both variants appeared at the same level confirmed the presence of a symmetric C_4-N-C_4 compound in retronecine biosynthesis. A similar series of experiments was also performed using *Senecio pleistocephalus*, which forms rosmarinine as the sole PA. Rosamarinine consists of senecic acid and the saturated necine base rosmarinecine, which has, in addition to the typical 7 and 9-hydroxy groups, an additional hydroxy group on C-2 (Figure 2B). Additionally, within this experimental system, the same result was obtained that a symmetric C_4-N-C_4 intermediate is involved in necine base biosynthesis [68].

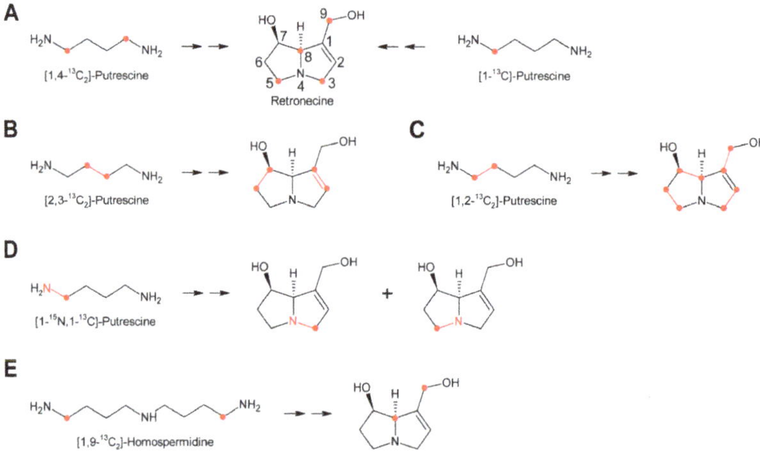

Figure 7. Investigation of necine base biosynthesis by feeding of stable isotope labeled precursors. Feeding of (**A**) [1,4-$^{13}C_2$]-putrescine and [1-^{13}C]-putrescine, (**B**) [2,3-$^{13}C_2$]-putrescine, (**C**) [1,2-$^{13}C_2$]-putrescine, (**D**) [1-^{15}N, 1-^{13}C]-putrescine and (**E**) [1,9-$^{13}C_2$]-homospermidine. Red dots symbolize ^{13}C labels, a red N symbolizes a ^{15}N label. ^{13}C-^{13}C double labels are marked with bonds in red. Please mind that the retronecine structures shown in (A), (B), and (C) are composite representations of all labeled species present.

3.1.1. Homospermidine Synthase

The most obvious candidate for the symmetric C_4-N-C_4 intermediate was homospermidine, which is known to be present in a number of plant species, particularly in such producing PAs. Initial experiments with radiolabeled homospermidine showed that this compound was incorporated into the necine base part of retrorsine in feeding experiments with *Senecio isatideus* [69]. To investigate whether the C_4-N-C_4 unit stays intact during biosynthesis ^{13}C labels were placed on the most distal carbons (Figure 7E). Feeding of [1,9-$^{13}C_2$]-homospermidine to *Senecio pleistocarpus* revealed enrichment of the label on C-8 and C-9 of the isolated retronecine [70], confirming that homospermidine is incorporated intact into necine bases.

At the same time, Bötcher et al. partially purified an enzyme with homospermidine synthase (HSS) activity from root cultures of *Eupatorium cannabinum* [71]. Enzymatic assays were performed by addition of [^{14}C]-labeled putrescine to the partially purified enzyme. The pH optimum was 9 and the enzymatic reaction was strictly dependent on the presence of NAD$^+$. The enzyme showed high selectivity for putrescine and NAD$^+$, and accepted neither NADP$^+$ as co-substrate nor any of the other tested amines including 1,3-diaminopropane, cadaverine, and pyrroline as substrate. The Michaelis-Menten constants (K_M) for putrescine and NAD$^+$ were 13.5 µM and 3 µM, respectively. In contrast to NAD$^+$, its reduced form, NADH, acted even at low concentrations (inhibition constant K_i: 2 µM) as a strong inhibitor indicating that the NADH formed in the first step of the reaction, the formation of an imine intermediate, remains bound to the enzyme and serves as electron donor for the second step, the reduction of the imine intermediate to the secondary amine. The enzymatic activity was also inhibited by 1,3-diaminopropane, spermidine, and homospermidine with K_i values of 6.3, 94 and 950 µM, respectively. While it was believed that the partially purified enzyme utilized two molecules of putrescine for formation of one molecule of homospermidine, later work with HSS purified to homogeneity showed that the enzyme instead uses putrescine and spermidine to produce homospermidine and 1,3-diaminopropane as by-products [2]. The reason for the initially wrong conclusion was that spermidine was added at all steps during enzyme purification since it was found that this compound preserves enzyme activity. Consequently, spermidine was also present in the partially purified enzyme and thus in the enzymatic reaction at sufficient concentrations allowing transfer of the radiolabeled putrescine moiety to spermidine. Thus, the first step of PA biosynthesis is transfer of the 1,4-diaminobutan part of spermidine to a specific lysine residue of HSS accompanied by release of 1,3-diaminopropane and reduction of NAD$^+$ to NADH, which remains bound to HSS (Figure 8). Subsequently, putrescine reacts with the HSS-bound 1,4-diaminobutane moiety under formation of an imine intermediate and regeneration of the lysine-NH$_2$. Finally, the imine is reduced by the HSS-bound NADH to homospermidine and released from the regenerated HSS/NAD$^+$ complex [72].

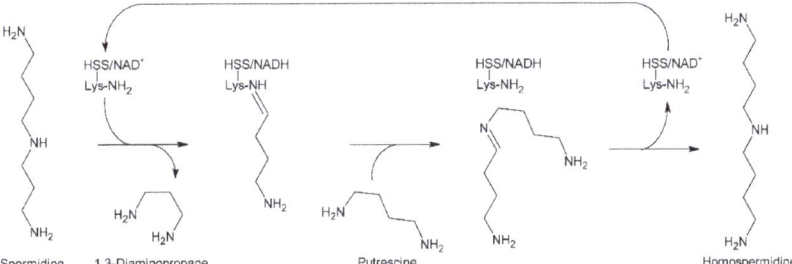

Figure 8. Mechanism of homospermidine formation by HSS. The amino group of a lysine residue of HSS reacts with spermidine, which releases 1,3-diaminopropane and reduces HSS-bound NAD$^+$ to NADH. Next, the residue is transferred to putrescine, forming an imine intermediate, which is reduced by the HSS-bound NADH to release homospermidine and recycle the HSS/NAD$^+$ complex. Adapted from [72].

Purification of HSS from *Senecio vernalis* to homogeneity allowed identification of the protein and corresponding gene. After protease treatment, four fragments were obtained that were microsequenced to give short peptide sequences. Database searches revealed close homology to deoxyhypusine synthase (DHS) [2]. DHS catalyzes the NAD$^+$-dependent transfer of an amino-butyl moiety from spermidine to a specific lysine side chain of the precursor for the eukaryotic initiation factor 5A (eIF5A), forming the amino acid deoxyhypusine. This reaction is one of the most specific post-translational modifications known [73,74] and similar to the reaction proposed for HSS except that eIF5A is replaced by spermidine (Figure 8). Subsequent PCR with redundant primers yielded the first sequences, which were completed by 3′ and 5′-RACE allowing subsequent for a cloning of the complete *Senecio vernalis* HSS coding sequence. Heterologous expression of the cloned gene as His$_{(6)}$-tagged fusion protein in *E. coli* and in vitro enzymatic assays confirmed that the enzyme for homospermidine synthesis was obtained and that putrescine and spermidine are required as substrates. With respect to that, it is worth mentioning that this may also explain the considerable incorporation of radiolabeled spermidine into homospermidine previously observed in feeding experiments using *Senecio isatideus* [63].

Since HSS catalyzes the first committed step in PA biosynthesis, thereby linking primary metabolism with PA biosynthesis, it is also interesting to study its evolution in order to deduce how PA biosynthesis was established in plants [72]. Due to 70 to 90% sequence homology—depending on the species—it was suggested that HSS evolved through gene duplication from DHS [75]. HSS has been recruited from DHS independently in different plant families at least eight times: Once in the Apocynaceae, Boraginaceae, Convolvulaceae, Fabaceae, Orchidaceae, and Poaceae, and twice in the Asteraceae [76–78]. The major difference lies in the biochemical properties of the two enzymes. DHS accepts eIF5A (lys) as well as putrescine, though with far lower efficiency, as substrate and can therefore catalyze the formation of both eIF5A(dhp) and homospermidine, the latter at a very low rate. In contrast, HSS has lost the ability to bind eIF5A, hence can only produce homospermidine [2,79,80]. This change in substrate specificity was possible because binding of putrescine occurs within the active site of DHS, while binding of eIF5A(lys) happens at the surface of the enzyme [75]. Reimann et al. [78] compared the rates of non-synonymous to synonymous mutations in HSS and DHS and found higher rates in HSS, suggesting higher selection pressure on DHS. The same study also found that it is not possible to distinguish between DHS and HSS solely by sequence data since there are no differing characteristic patterns. Despite the similar biochemical properties and sequences, the expression levels of both genes clearly differ. A study of the expression patterns of HSS and DHS in *Senecio vernalis* (Asteraceae, Senecioneae) revealed that DHS is expressed in all plant tissues in an almost constant manner throughout plant development. In contrast, HSS expression was found to be restricted to root cells, particularly to endodermis and cortex parenchyma cells [81]. In *Eupatorium cannabium* (Asteraceae, Eupatorieae) HSS expression was also found in the cortex parenchyma cells but not in the endodermis. In addition, HSS expression was shut down when the flower buds opened [82]. In contrast, in *Phalaenopsis* (Orchidaceae) HSS is expressed in the tips of aerial roots and in young flower buds [83]. In the Boraginaceae different HSS expression patterns were observed. In *Heliotropium indicum*, HSS was expressed exclusively in non-specialized cells of the lower epidermis of young leaves and shoots while in *Symphytum officinale* HSS expression was detected in the cells of the root endodermis and in leaves underneath developing inflorescences. In *Cynoglossum officinale* HSS expression was only observed in roots. In young roots, its expression was limited to cells of the endodermis, while in later developmental stages cells of the pericycle, it also showed HSS expression [84].

One theory regarding establishment of secondary metabolic pathways suggests that changes in gene function lead to subfunctionalization and a subsequent duplication event to two genes with different but complementary subfunctions, preserving the original enzyme function [75]. This complements an early suggestion by [85] that, prior to a gene duplication leading to novel protein function, the original gene was bifunctional. This theory is also supported by the bifunctionality of DHS, when considering this model for the explanation of HSS evolution. Furthermore, gene regulation and therefore gene expression patterns, might vary for the two genes, resulting from gene duplication [86]. This suggestion finds support in the varying expression patterns of DHS and HSS described above.

While extensive research on the recruitment of HSS has been conducted, there is still little knowledge about the evolution of the entire PA biosynthetic pathway, as it cannot be explained by the presence of homospermidine alone. Introduction of HSS into non-PA producing plants only results in formation of homospermidine, rather than of PAs or any precursors downstream of homospermidine [87].

3.1.2. Copper-Dependent Diamine Oxidases and Cyclization of the Dialdehyde

Early evidence for involvement of a diamine oxidase in the incorporation of homospermidine into necine bases was provided by incubating homospermidine in vitro with a diamine oxidase fraction prepared from pea. Reduction of the reaction products by sodium borohydride and subsequent analysis by GC revealed that mainly trachelanthamidine and a small amount (approximately 5%) of isoretronecanol were obtained. In another experiment, reduction of the reaction products was performed with liver alcohol dehydrogenase, which again mainly yielded trachelanthamidine and little isoretronecanol [88]. However, the stereochemical properties of the obtained products were not investigated. Subsequent studies confirmed these initial findings and suggested involvement of a copper-dependent diamine oxidase since treatment of *Senecio vulgaris* and *Heliotropium indicum* with 2-hydroxyethylhydrazine (HEH), a potent diamine oxidase inhibitor, caused homospermidine accumulation and impeded PA biosynthesis [71,89].

Oxidation of amine precursors followed by cyclisation is a common theme in alkaloid biosynthesis. In tropane biosynthesis *N*-methylputrescine is oxidized by methylputrescine oxidase to 4-methylaminobutanal, which cyclizes spontaneously to the *N*-methyl-Δ^1-pyrrolinium cation (Figure 9) [9]. This is similar to the first steps proposed for conversion of the dialdehyde 4,4'-iminodibutanal to the pyrrolium cation (Figure 10). However, biosynthesis of necine bases continues with reaction of the remaining aldehyde group for closure of the second ring via a Mannich-type reaction mechanism, which leads ultimately to pyrrolizidine-1-carbaldehyde. While cyclization in tropane alkaloid biosynthesis might be spontaneous, this is rather unlikely for necine base synthesis. Spontaneous cyclization of the dialdehyde and subsequent reduction would result in a mixture of the four saturated 1-hydroxymethylpyrrolizidines (±)-trachelanthamidine and (±)-isoretronecanol. After desaturation, a mixture of (±)-supinidine would be obtained and subsequent C-7 hydroxylation would, depending on the specificity of the hydroxylase, lead to a mixture of (+)-retronecine and (-)-heliotridine or (-)-retronecine and (+)-heliotridine. However, such mixtures are usually not observed in PA-producing plants. In contrast, plants usually contain PAs with necine bases of only a specific stereochemical configuration. For instance, *Senecio jacobaea* and *Senecio aquaticus* contain, apart from otonecine-type PAs, only senecionine-like, jacobine-like and erucifoline-like PAs, which are all (+)-retronecine-type PAs [90]. *Crassoceopahlum crepidioides* contains only jacobine, a PA of the (+)-retronecine type [50]. *Lolium perenne* contains only the (-)-isoretronecanol type PAs Z- and E-thesinine and its rhamnosides [91]. *Borago officinalis* contains only alkaloids of the (-)-isoretronecanol, (-)-supinine and (+)-retronecine-type [92], which have the same stereoconfiguration of the C-8 hydrogen. *Heliotropium europaeum* contains only (+)-heliotridine-type PAs [93]. The observed stereochemical specificity argues clearly against spontaneous cyclisation and suggests an enzymatic mechanism. Since enzyme-catalyzed cyclization must immediately follow oxidative deamination it is tempting to speculate that the copper-dependent diamine oxidase might also either support stereospecific cyclization of the dialdehyde or act in a protein complex with a second enzyme that catalyzes cyclization.

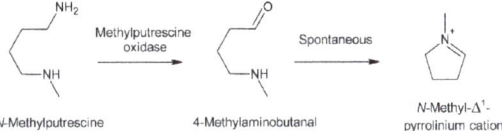

Figure 9. Cyclization in tropane alkaloid biosynthesis. The precursor *N*-methylputrescine is oxidized by methylputrescine oxidase to 4-methylaminobutanal, which cyclizes spontaneously by reaction of the amino group with the aldehyde. Adapted from Reference [9].

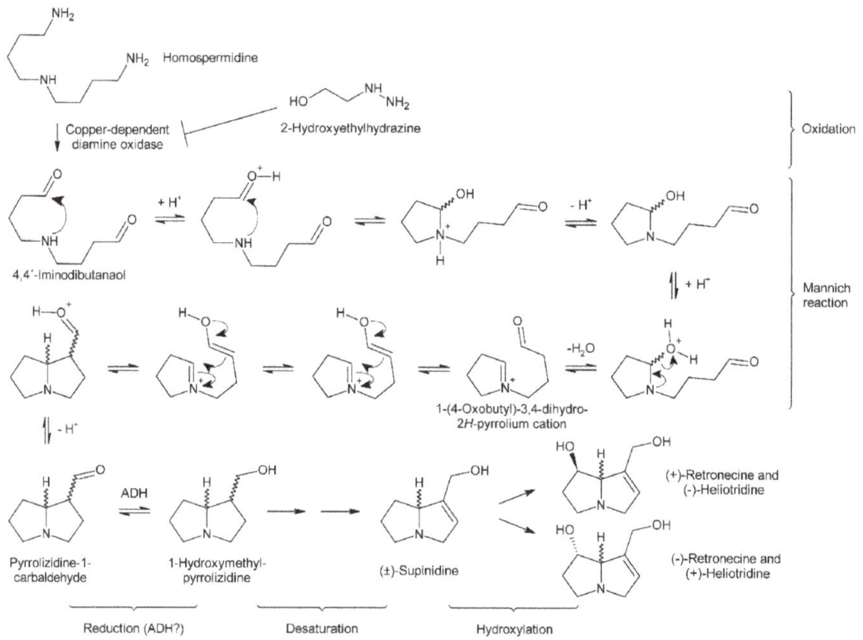

Figure 10. Cyclization in PA biosynthesis. Homospermidine is likely oxidized by a copper-dependent diamine oxidase to 4,4'-iminodibutanal, which can be inhibited by the synthetic compound 2-hydroxyethylhydrazine. The reaction product cyclizes first to the 1-(4-oxobutyl)-3,4-dihydro-2H-pyrrolium cation and further to pyrrolizidine-1-carbaldedye in a Mannich-type reaction. However, as indicated, spontaneous cyclization would lead to a mixture of the different stereomers and thus mixtures of necine bases would be obtained, arguing for enzyme-catalyzed cyclization.

3.1.3. Further Downstream Reactions

After cyclization the formed pyrrolizidine-1-carbaldehyde is reduced to the alcohol. This might be catalyzed by an alcohol dehydrogenase (ADH), since Robins showed that ADH can in principle reduce the carbaldehyde to the alcohol [88]. Additional evidence comes from a detailed stereochemical study of necine base formation. Feeding of *Senecio isatideus* with deuterium labeled [1,1,4,4-^{2}H$_4$]-putrescine and hydrolysis of the obtained PA yielded retronecine that retained three deuterium atoms on the right handed ring: Two at C-3 and one at C-9. Importantly, the latter was in the S position, which is the stereochemistry expected for an ADH-catalyzed reduction of an carbaldehyde [59].

The sequence of retronecine base interconversions was studied by Birecka and Catalfamo, using pulse-chase experiments [94]. *Heliotropium spathulatum* was used for this study since this species produces (-)-trachelanthamidine, (-)-supinidine and (-)-retronecine containing PAs. The plants were treated with [^{14}C]-carbon dioxide for 2 h prior quenching incorporation with unlabeled carbon dioxide. Samples were taken after 12 h, 24 h and 48 h and the specific activity of the necine bases analyzed. The activity of (-)-trachelanthamidine increased first, which was followed by an increase of the activity of (-)-supinidine and finally (-)-retronecine. This suggests that (-)-trachelanthamidine is first dehydrogenated at the C-1/C-2 bond to (-)-supinidine, which is subsequently hydroxylated at C-7 to (-)-retronecine. However, the involved enzymes remain elusive in addition to whether the free necine bases are modified or the, at least partially, esterified PAs.

3.2. Biosynthesis of Necic Acids

While necine bases are synthesized by a common pathway, different necic acids are formed by distinct modes. A number of acids found in PAs are normally present in plants. This includes, for instance, acetic acid, benzoic acid, and *p*-coumaric acid. These acids and their activated forms, the coenzyme A thioesters, are formed by common metabolic pathways of primary metabolism, which will not be discussed here.

3.2.1. Tiglic Acid and Related C_5 Necic Acids

C_5-acids of the tiglic acid type are frequently observed as building blocks of secondary plant metabolites. For instance, tiglic acid is the moiety of meteloidine and other tropane alkaloids formed by *Datura* species [95]. Feeding experiments in *Datura meteloides* showed that tiglic acid is derived from isoleucine [96]. Similar results were also obtained in *Cynoglossum officinale* for angelic acid, which is present as ester in the PA heliosupine [31]. Feeding of *Datura meteloides* with radiolabeled 2-methylbutanoic acid showed that the radioactivity was efficiently incorporated into the tiglic acid moiety of meteloidine, identifying 2-methylbutanoic acid as a precursor [97]. The same pathway was also established for carabid beetle [98]. Data from mammals [99] suggest that 3-hydroxy-2-methylbutyric acid acts as intermediate between 2-methylbutanoic acid and tiglic acid, and that the intermediates appear as coenzyme A thioesters. These steps are in fact part of the common L-isoleucine degradation pathway and thus it is not surprising that these metabolites including tiglyl-CoA are present in most plant tissues. McGaw and Woolley showed that angelic acid is derived by *cis-trans* isomerization from tiglic acid in *Cynoglossum officinale* [100]. These data suggest a pathway for biosynthesis of tiglic and angelic acid starting from L-isoleucine (Figure 11).

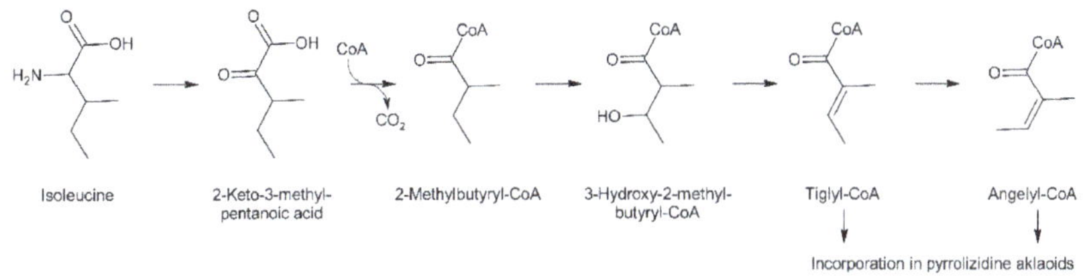

Figure 11. Biosynthesis of tiglic and angelic acid. L-Isoleucine is desaminated and the obtained ketocarboxylic acid decarboxylated to 2-methylbutyric acid, which is likely accompanied by linking with coenzyme A to yield 2-methylbutyryl-CoA. This intermediate is hydroxylated and subsequently dehydrated to form tiglyl-CoA, which can be isomerized to angelyl-CoA. The activated tiglic and angelic acid residues are finally transferred to necine bases and coenzyme A is released.

3.2.2. C_7 Necic Acids

The more complex acids are generated by specific biosynthetic pathways. The observation that many of these acids include one or two C_5 units resembles isoprenoids, although with unusual linkage and oxygenation patterns, encouraging the idea that they might be derived from mevalonate [101]. However, feeding experiments with ^{14}C-labeled acetate, acetoacetate and mevalonate did not result in specific incorporation into necic acids, excluding these compounds as direct precursors for necic acids. In contrast, feeding experiments with ^{14}C-labeled amino acids provided compelling evidence that necic acids are derived from L-isoleucine and L-valine. Additionally, [^{14}C]-L-threonine and a few further amino acids were found to be efficiently incorporated, but only since they acted as precursors for L-isoleucine or L-valine.

The PA heliosupine appearing in *Cynoglossum officinale* consists of the necine base (-)-heliotridine esterified on the 7-hydroxy group with angelic acid (which is synthesized as shown in Figure 12) and on the 9-hydroxy group with echimidinic acid, a C_7-acid (Figure 12A). Feeding experiments revealed that echimidinic acid is derived from L-valine and an additional C_2 unit of unknown origin [102].

Trachelanthic acid, which is structurally very similar to echimidinic acid, is also derived from L-valine, as revealed by feeding of ^{14}C-labeled amino acids. These results were further supported by an isotopologue study by feeding a root culture of *Eupatorium clematideum* with a mixture of ^{13}C-labeled and unlabeled glucose [103]. Subsequently, trachelanthamine and the amino acids L-arginine, L-proline, and L-valine were isolated and the ^{13}C labelling pattern analyzed by NMR spectroscopy. The ^{13}C pattern of the necine base was in agreement with that of L-arginine, while the major part of trachelanthic acid (shown in red in Figure 12B) fitted to that observed for L-valine. The remaining two carbons showed a pattern as reconstituted for hydroxyethyl-TPP. This confirmed the conclusions for echimidinic acid. However, it must be emphasized that the result that the ^{13}C pattern of the C_2 unit corresponds to that of hydroxyethyl-TPP does not mean that this compound is indeed the direct precursor. In contrast, there might be a number of metabolites in-between. Thus, the direct precursor of the C_2 unit remains to be determined.

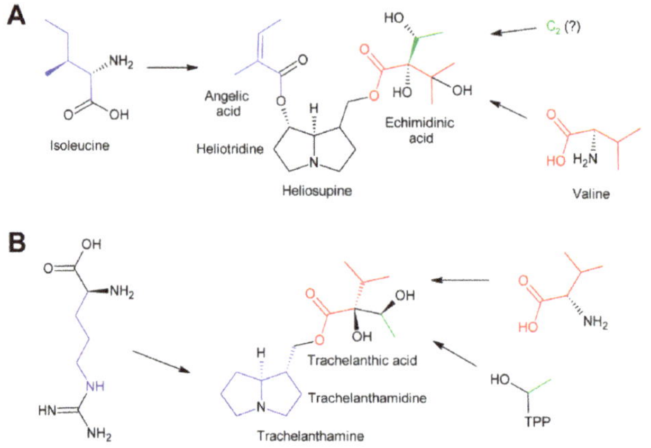

Figure 12. Biosynthesis of C_7 necic acids. (**A**) Echimidinic acid present in heliosupine is derived from L-valine (red) and a C_2 unit of unknown origin (green). Angelic acid esterifying the 7-hydroxy group of (-)-heliotridine is derived from L-isoleucine (blue) as shown in Figure 11. (**B**) Trachelanthic acid is also derived from L-valine (red) and a C_2 unit (green) that is likely derived from hydroxyethyl thiamine pyrophosphate. Adapted from References [70,103].

3.2.3. Monocrotalic Acid and Related Compounds

Biosynthesis of monocrotalic acid was analyzed in the Fabaceae *Crotalaria retusa* and *Crotalaria spectabilis* by feeding of ^{14}C-labeled acetate, DL-alanine, L-threonine, and L-isoleucine [104]. While minute incorporation was observed for acetate and DL-alanine, L-threonine and L-isoleucine were incorporated into monocrotaline to significant levels. Degradation studies showed that the necine base had incorporated little radioactivity while the necic acid monocrotalic acid contained most of the activity. More specifically, most activity was observed in fragments consisting of C-1, C-2 and C-6 and of C-3 and C-7, while the fragment consisting of C-4, C-5, and C-8 had incorporated comparatively little activity (Figure 13A). Thus, the right hand part of monocrotalic acid is derived from L-isoleucine while the origin of the left hand part remains elusive. Another study found, in addition to efficient incorporation of ^{14}C-labeled L-isoleucine and L-threonine, a significant incorporation of L-valine [105]. Since no degradation studies were performed, it remains unknown whether L-valine serves as a precursor for the left hand part.

The structure of trichodesmic acid is very similar to monocrotalic acid, except that a methyl group is replaced by an isopropyl group (Figure 13B). Thus, it was also expected that the right hand part of trichodesmic acid is derived from L-leucine (and L-threonine), which could be confirmed by feeding studies. In addition, ^{14}C-labeled L-valine and L-leucine were also efficiently incorporated, particularly into the right hand part [106]. The fact that both amino acids were incorporated to a similar level suggests that they are converted to a common precursor prior to incorporation into trichodesmic acid. However, the pathway and mechanism remain to be elucidated.

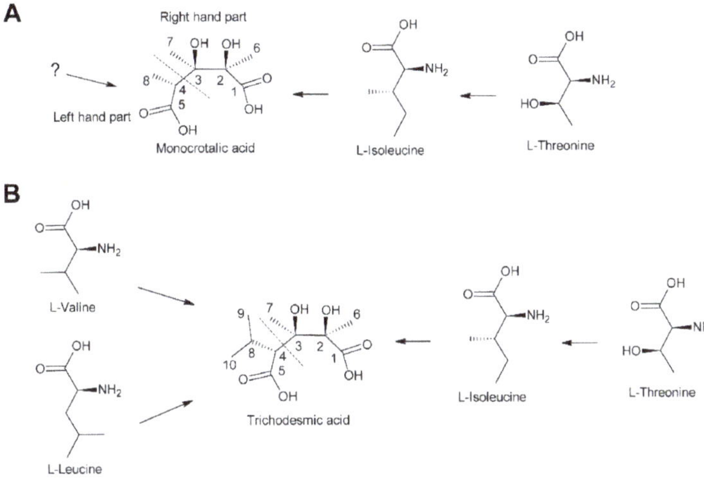

Figure 13. Biosynthesis of necic acids forming 11-membered rings. (**A**) The right hand part of monocrotalic acid is formed from L-leucine (and its precursor L-threonine). The C_3 left hand unit is of unknown origin. (**B**) The right hand side of trachelanthic acid is derived from L-leucine (and its precursor L-threonine) while the left hand side seems to be formed from L-valine or L-leucine. Dotted lines indicate the both sides. Adapted from Reference [70].

3.2.4. Senecic Acid and Senecic Acid-Derived Compounds

Among the necic acids forming 12-membered macrocyclic PAs biosynthesis of senecic acid is best characterized. Since seneciphyllic acid and isatinecic acid are derived from senecic acid, results obtained for these compounds will be discussed together with that for senecic acid. Feeding experiments of *Senecio douglasii* with ^{14}C-labeled acetate, acetoacetate and mevalonate showed that these compounds were inefficiently incorporated into senecphylline, and that the radioactivity was randomly distributed between the necine base retronecine and the necic acid seneciphyllic acid. This indicated that none of the tested compounds are direct precursors of the alkaloid. In contrast, L-threonine was efficiently incorporated and the radioactivity was found selectively in the necic acid part. Subsequent experiments showed that L-threonine was first converted to L-isoleucine prior to incorporation into seneciphyllic acid, identifying isoleucine as the direct precursor. In addition, evidence was provided that only C-2 to C-5 of L-leucine were incorporated into seneciphyllic acid, while C-1 (the carboxy group) was lost [107]. Feeding experiments using *Senecio magnificus* provided similar results for senecic acid and provided compelling evidence that the acid is derived from two molecules of L-isoleucine, both losing their C-1 during biosynthesis [108,109]. From the four possible isoleucine stereomers, L/D-isoleucine and L/D-alloisoleucine, only L-isoleucine was efficiently incorporated [110]. The loss of the carboxy groups raised the question for the five-carbon intermediate. Possible candidates were 2-methylbutanoic acid, which is an intermediate of L-isoleucine degradation and thus are present in most plant tissues, and 2-methyl-3-oxobutanoic acid and angelic acid. The latter was selected since it has the same configuration as the double bond in senecioic acid. Feeding resulted in incorporation of 0.06% (S)-[^{14}C]-2-methylbutanoate, which was a slightly lower level than for L-[^{14}C]-leucine, where incorporation rates of 0.1 to 0.4% were observed. However, analysis of the necic acid and the necine base showed random distribution of radioactivity. The two other compounds were incorporated in only trace amounts. Based on these results the idea that one of those compounds is a precursor of senecic acid was discarded. Next, ^{14}C-labeled 2-amino-3-methylenepentanoic acid (β-methylenenorvaline) was tested and efficient incorporation (0.07–0.11%) was observed with essentially only senecioic acid possessing the radio label. This observation suggested this compound as a possible intermediate (Figure 14A). Unfortunately, it could not be investigated whether the ^{14}C-label was incorporated in either or both halves of senecic acid [111].

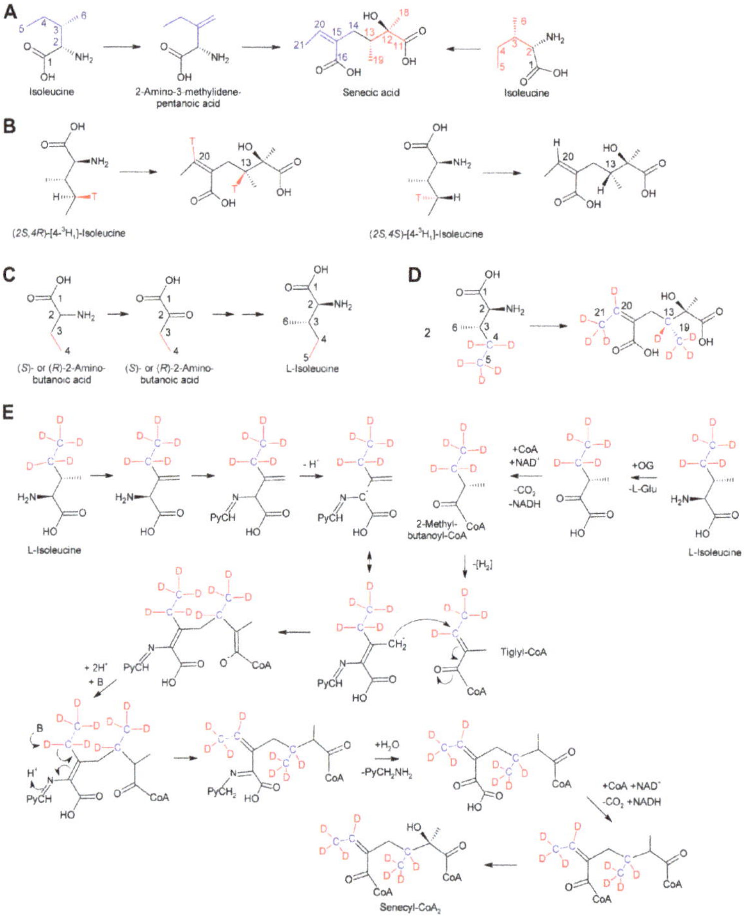

Figure 14. Biosynthesis of senecic acid. (**A**) Feeding experiments with ^{14}C-labeled compounds showed that senecic acid is formed from two L-isoleucine molecules accompanied by loss of both carboxy carbons. 2-Amino-3-methylenepentanoic acid might be an intermediate, although it is not clear whether for one or both halves of senecic acid. Carbons are numbered according to Reference [112]. (**B**) Feeding with L-isoleucine stereospecifically labeled with ^{3}H (tritium, T) at C-4 showed that only the 4R label was retained upon incorporation. (**C**) 2-Aminobutanoic acid is converted *in planta* to L-isoleucine. Due to 2-ketobutanoic acid as intermediate the initial stereochemistry of 2-aminobutyric acid is irrelevant. A label (^{13}C or ^{3}H; red) at C-3 and C-4 is retained and found on position C-5 and C-6 in L-isoleucine. (**D**) The ^{13}C-labeled C-4 and C-5 (blue) of L-leucine (obtained in planta from labeled 2-aminobutanoic acid) and most of the ^{2}H (deuterium, D; red) is retained upon incorporation into senecic acid. (**E**) Possible mechanism for formation of senecic acid. CoA, coenzyme A; L-Glu, L-glutamic acid; NAD$^+$/NAHD, oxidized/reduced nicotinamide adenine dinucleotide; OG, 2-oxoglutaric acid; and Py, pyridoxalphosphate.

The most enigmatic step in biosynthesis of senecic acid and related compounds is the mechanism for uniting C-13 and C-14 (Figure 14A). C-13 corresponds to C-4 carbons of the isoleucine precursor forming the right hand part of senecic acid. Studies with L-leucine stereospecifically labeled at C-4 with ^{3}H showed that the pro-*R* hydrogen was retained, while the pro-*S* hydrogen was lost on both L-isoleucine molecules required for synthesis of senecic acid. This demonstrates that both carbons cannot be oxidized further than the alkene or carbinol level [113]. The observation that 2-aminobutanoic acid is efficiently converted to isoleucine in feeding experiments [113] (Figure 14C) enabled feeding studies with stable isotope labelling and analysis of the produced alkaloids by NMR [112]. Feeding of *Senecio pleistocephalus* and root cultures of *Senecio vulgaris* with [3,4-^{13}C$_2$]-2-aminobutanoic acid confirmed that C-3 and C-4 of 2-aminobutyric acid carbons are the precursors of C-20 and C-21 in the left hand side of senecic acid and of C-13 and C-19 in the right hand side (Figure 14D). Analysis of alkaloids obtained by feeding of [3,4-^{2}H$_5$]-2-aminobutanoic acid revealed that three ^{2}H were retained on the methyl groups of both C-21 and C-19, and one ^{2}H was retained on each C-13 and C-20. These results show that the C-3 and C-4 positions of 2-aminobutanoic acid corresponding to C-5 and C-6 of L-isoleucine are exclusively and equally incorporated intact into the two halves of senecic acid. These results are in agreement with a mechanism proposed by Bale, where the left hand part of senecic acid is derived from L-isoleucine by conversion to β-methylenenorvaline, which reacts with pyridoxal phosphate to a Schiff's base (Figure 14E). Deprotonation would generate a mesomeric anion with a nucleophilic character at C-6 (numbering corresponding to that of L-isoleucine). This nucleophile might react with a suitable, yet unknown electrophile [111]. From the experiments with ^{3}H-labeled L-isoleucine and ^{2}H-labeled 2-aminobutanoic acid, it is clear that the electrophile cannot possess a carbonyl group at C-4 while an alkene would be in agreement with those results. An attractive candidate is tiglyl-coenzyme A since this compound is a metabolite of L-isoleucine degradation [114] and thus present in most tissues. In addition, the C-C double bond is activated due to the neighboring keto group. Attack of the nucleophile on tiglyl-CoA would create the C-13/C-14 bond. Subsequent release of the pyridoxal phosphate coenzyme would create the C-16/C-20 double bond, which is either directly or further metabolized (e.g., as epoxide, diol, etc.) almost invariably present in necic acids of the senecic acid type. It must be emphasized that feeding experiments using (*S*)-[^{14}C]-2-methylbutanoate, the precursor of tiglyl-CoA in the L-isoleucine degradation pathway, did not give conclusive results since high incorporation was observed, but the incorporation pattern was unspecific [111]. However, it might be worth reinvestigating a possible role of tiglyl-CoA in senecic acid biosynthesis by state of the art isotopologous NMR-based techniques.

First evidence for conversion of senecionine to other senecionine-type PAs came from feeding of [^{14}C]-putrescine to *Senecio vernalis* root cultures, which resulted in rapid incorporation in senecionine *N*-oxide. However, the labeled senecionine *N*-oxide was progressively converted within 10 days to senkirkine, an otonecine-type PA [28]. Pulse-chase feeding experiments of *Senecio erucifolius* root cultures with [^{14}C]-putrescine showed rapid incorporation of radioactivity in senecionine *N*-oxide and revealed absence of any significant alkaloid turnover with the exception of a slow but progressive conversion of labeled senecionine *N*-oxide to its dehydrogenation product, seneciphylline *N*-oxide [115]. Using whole *Senecio erucifolius* plants, in addition to formation of seneciphylline *N*-oxide, conversion of senecionine *N*-oxide to *O*-acetyl seneciphylline, and of erucifoline to *O*-acetyl erucifoline and to eruciflorine was also observed, indicating that the stem might be crucial for these modifications [116]. These data clearly demonstrate that the first product of PA biosynthesis in *Senecio* is senecionine *N*-oxide, which is further converted to a bouquet of senecionine-like alkaloids or their *N*-oxides (Figure 15). Such reactions mainly include simple one or two-step reactions like hydroxylations, acetylations, desaturations and epoxidations. In addition, it is tempting to speculate that the epoxide ring of jacobine and similar compounds might undergo further metabolization by hydrolysis or addition of hydrochloric acid to yield jacoline *N*-oxide or jaconine *N*-oxide, respectively. Thus, senecionine-like alkaloids are derived by modification of senecionine *N*-oxide rather than combination of necine bases with different necic acids.

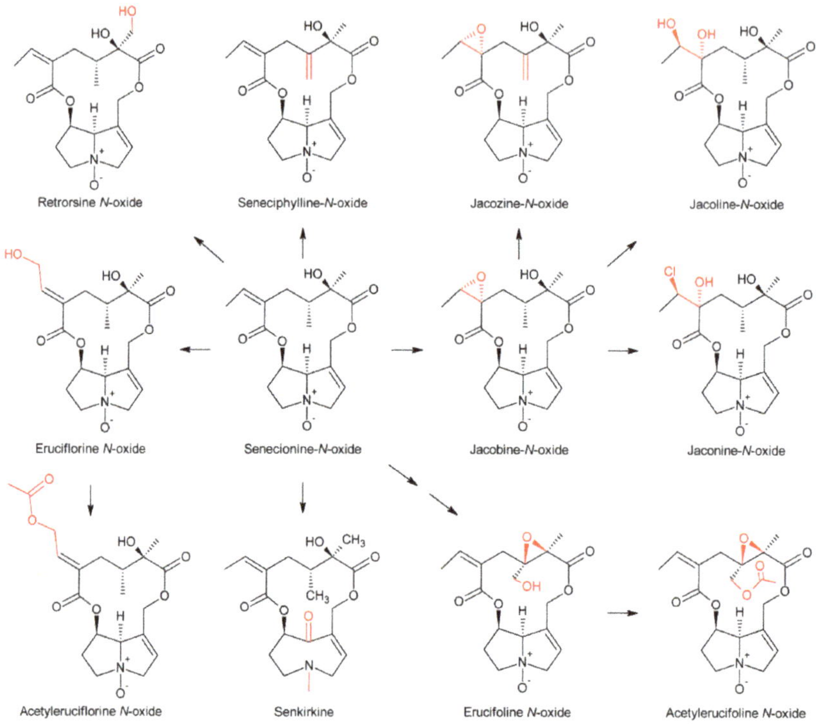

Figure 15. Diversification of senecionine-like PAs. Modifications of the senecionine N-oxide structure are shown in red. Adapted from Reference [116].

4. Regulation of Pyrrolizidine Alkaloid Levels and Biosynthesis

PA biosynthesis is known to be regulated differently during plant development. For example, in *Eupatorium cannabium* HSS expression is restricted to young roots with close correlation to plant growth [82]. HSS is only detectable in newly grown, white roots until the produced biomass peaks and flowers open. When these plant parts die off at the end of the vegetation period, de novo alkaloid biosynthesis is required at the beginning of the next growth period. In contrast, plants of the species *Symphytum officinale* can activate a second site of HSS expression once inflorescence development begins in leaves subtending emerging flowers [117]. The same study could also demonstrate that not only HSS but the whole PA biosynthetic pathway are active in these young leaves. This second site of PA biosynthesis allows for drastically increased PA levels within the inflorescences ensuring optimal protection of the reproductive structures against herbivores.

Furthermore, PA expression is influenced by nutrient and water supply as well as herbivore infestation [118–120]. On the effects of nutrient availability, a general proposal is that a higher NPK supply reduces the PA content in *Senecio jacobaea*, *Senecio vulgaris*, and *Senecio aquaticus*, presumably due to dilution effects in shoots and roots, whereas PA levels in flowers are not affected [118]. These findings are further supported by results of PA analysis in *Senecio jacobaea* and *Senecio aquaticus* on marginal, sandy soils showing that low nutrient supply increases relative PA amounts [119]. Nevertheless, the same study found a significant change in PA composition on fertilized soils, as they reported a high rise in jacobine contents, while the total PA amount remained constant under nutrient rich conditions. One reason for increased jacobine levels could be the role of jacobine in insect herbivore resistance. Research on root herbivore damage in *Senecio jacobaea* has revealed no change in total PA content in the whole plant, but a translocation of PAs from shoot to the root, mostly of N-oxides, also causing the ratio of N-oxide to free PAs to drop from 2:1 to 1:1 in the shoot [120]. Moreover, plants stabilize free PA levels in aerial plant parts by converting PA N-oxide into free bases [120].

There is substantial evidence for the genetic control and heritability of PA biosynthesis. A study by Vrieling et al. [121] using a diallel cross of *Senecio jacobaea* revealed that 48% of the variation in total PA content was caused by genotypic variation. Half-sib analysis from natural progenies combined with drought and nutrient deficiency treatments indicated that 85–90% of the differences in total PA concentration were caused by additive genetic variation. Heritability for individual PAs was significant as well. van Dam et al. [122] estimated that 33–43% of the variation in PA levels between selfed families of *Cynoglossum officinale* is due to broad-sense heritability and found that the inducibility of PA production by wounding of leaves differs significantly between families. Macel et al. [123] evaluated the variations in PA profiles within clonal families of *Senecio jacobaea* and found significant differences in the relative percentages and absolute concentrations of individual PAs between clonal families. The variation in PA composition within clonal families was smaller than the variation among families, indicating a strong genetic influence. Furthermore, Joosten et al. [51] found that the presence of pyrrolizidine alkaloids in the tertiary amine form in *Senecio jacobaea* is genotype-dependent as well. Pelser et al. [124] reconstructed the evolutionary history of qualitative PA variation in the *Jacobaea* section of *Senecio*. They concluded that the variations in PA profiles are not caused by simple gain and loss of PA-specific genes, but rather by changes in transient expression of PA biosynthesis genes, since the large intra and interspecific variation in PA distribution seems to be largely incidental and nearly all of the PAs identified in the *Jacobaea* section are also present in species of other sections of the genus.

Hybridization can result in the occurrence of novel PA structures through inter-specific epistatic interactions between enzymes and substrates, as demonstrated by Kirk et al. [119]. They observed that F1 hybrids between *Senecio jacobaea* and *Senecio aquaticus* produce florosenine, which is not present in parent populations. Since florosenine is formed by O-acetylation of otosenine, the capacity of *Senecio aquaticus* to synthesise otosenine and the ability of *Senecio jacobaea* for PA acetylation could be combined in the hybrids. A study by Cheng et al. [125] using F1 and F2 hybrids of *Senecio jacobaea* and *Senecio aquaticus* showed that hybrid roots contained acetylated otosenine-like PAs, while roots of the parental lines did not. Additionally, shoots of F2 hybrids exhibited an over-expression of otosenine-like PAs with contents reaching >20% of total PAs. In contrast, otosenine-like PAs have not been previously reported as a major fraction of the PA bouquet in *Senecio jacobaea* or *Senecio aquaticus*. Furthermore, some F2 hybrids contained higher relative proportions of erucifoline-like PAs in shoots compared to the parental genotypes where jacobine or senecionine-type PAs dominated. These findings indicate that hybridization contributes to the increase of the structural diversity of PAs.

There is little knowledge about the regulation of PA biosynthesis by plant hormones. Methyl-jasmonate is thought to play a part because of its role as an elicitor of induced responses and anti-herbivory resistance. Wei et al. [126] conducted a study with *Senecio jacobaea* and *Senecio aquaticus* grown aseptically on medium containing methyl jasmonate. In treated *Senecio jacobaea* plants, the total concentration of PAs increased in shoots but decreased in roots. A similar non-significant trend was observed for *Senecio aquaticus*. The application of methyl jasmonate leads to a strong shift from senecionine to erucifoline-like PAs, while the jacobine and otosenine-like PAs were not affected. This indicates that methyl jasmonate does not necessarily induce *de novo* synthesis, but rather leads to reallocation of certain PAs from roots to shoots and a conversion of PA structures. Sievert et al. [127] tested the influence of methyl jasmonate on PA levels and on the transcript levels of homospermidine synthase in *Heliotropium indicum*, *Symphytum officinale*, and *Cynoglossum officinale*, but could not detect any significant effects. The only case where a clear influence of methyl jasmonate on PAs was observed was in hairy root cultures of *Echium rauwolfii* [128]. Root culture medium, supplemented with 100 µM of methyl jasmonate, lead to a 19-fold increase of total PAs, while the flavonoid quercetin boosted the PA accumulation 6-fold at 50 µM. When the root cultures were pre-incubated with salicylic acid, the inducing effect of both compounds could be suppressed.

Regarding PA transport within the plant it has been shown for *Senecio vernalis* that translocation from roots to shoots occurs through phloem cells, located opposite to specialized HSS-expressing cells of the endodermis and the adjoining cortex parenchyma [81,129]. These cells are likely to execute the entire biosynthesis of PAs which can then be transported as *N*-oxides through the pericycle into the phloem, from there into the shoot and finally to the sites of storage, thereby uncoupling sites of PA synthesis from sites of activity. PA *N*-oxides are more soluble than free PA bases and are thus very phloem mobile, enabling transport between different storage tissues when necessary [130]. Also, the shoot is suggested to harbor the ability to diversify the chemical composition of PAs by simple hydroxylation, epoxidation, dehydrogenation, or *O*-acetylation reactions [89,116].

In a study by van Dam et al. [131], the inducibility of PA production after leaf damage was tested in two different plants species, namely *Senecio jacobaea* and *Cynoglossum officinale*, by cutting off 50% of their leaf area. PA concentrations were measured at different time points after damage and the cut-off leaf tips were used as controls for diurnal fluctuations. In *Senecio jacobaea* leaf damage significantly decreased PA concentrations. PA levels reached a minimum 12 h after the treatment and went back to initial values 24 h after. PA levels in *Cynoglossum officinale* steadily increased with time after damage. The authors hypothesize that the different responses might be due to adaptations related to the type and severity of herbivory occurring under natural conditions as *Senecio jacobaea* is adapted to initiate regrowth after severe defoliation by specialist herbivores. Therefore, a decrease of PAs in the leaves after damage could be caused by a reallocation of defense resources for future regrowth. *Cynoglossum officinale* on the other hand is not adapted to severe herbivory and does not recover as quickly following damage. Thus, it might be advantageous for this species to boost its chemical defense in order to reduce herbivore-inflicted damage.

5. Biological Activity

5.1. Role in Plant Ecology

The parallel evolvement of PA synthesis in phylogenetically unrelated plant families suggests an evolutionary advantage from PA presence. One important aspect in this context is, as for the evolution of many other secondary metabolites, a defense against insect herbivores [132,133]. Support for this hypothesis is found by studying insects specialized on PA-containing plants, which are found in a number of families, such as Lepidoptera, Coleoptera, Orthoptera, and Homoptera [134]. Additionally, grazing animals are known to only consume PA plants in times of low feed supply and generalist insect herbivores are suggested to be deterred by different PAs whereas adapted insects are thought to be attracted [131,134–136]. The general PA metabolism in insects is similar to human PA metabolism, including the negative physiological effects. Various studies regarding the effects of single PAs and general PA content on both specialist and generalist herbivore feeding have been conducted. Wei et al. [137] and Macel et al. [138] showed that the influence on different generalist species depends on PA-type and concentration. While Macel et al. [138] only observed effects under certain dietary conditions, Wei et al. [137] performed bioassays with *Senecio jacobaea* x *Senecio aquaticus* F2 hybrids with varying PA contents to draw conclusions about the correlation between the presence and abundance of different PAs and feeding damage. The results indicate that, for instance, thrips prefer leaves with lower jacobine-like PA contents, while for slugs, low senecionine-like PA levels are important. Furthermore, single PAs of both types were correlated to feeding behavior. These results are particularly interesting because presence of a C-13/C-19 double bond seems to play an important role in generalist herbivore resistance [137]. However, also jacobine *N*-oxide, although not carrying the C-13/C-19 double bond, has been shown to deter western flower thrips (*Frankliniella occidentalis*) and higher amounts were shown to be a characteristic trait of thrips resistant PA plants [90,139].

There are several reports stating that PA *N*-oxides are less bioactive against insect herbivores than the corresponding free bases [131,140–142]. Contrarily, PAs are mostly present in plants as *N*-oxides [129] with some jacobine-like PAs occurring up to 50% as free base in *Senecio jacobaea* [51] and

Crassocephalum crepidioides [50]. An advantage of N-oxides is their higher solubility resulting in more efficient storage and transport [130,143,144]. Another possible explanation suggested by Liu et al. [145] are synergistic effects of PA N-oxides with other plant metabolites. They showed that PA free bases and chlorogenic acid act antagonistically on western flower thrips (*Frankliniella occidentalis*) mortality, while in contrast, PA N-oxides showed synergistic interactions with chlorogenic acid on thrips mortality. In the absence of chlorogenic acid, PA free bases decreased thrips survival more severely than PA N-oxides, but when chlorogenic acid was added, this effect was reversed. Thus, the bioactivity of individual PAs seems to be influenced by the natural chemical background in which they occur. This aspect is further supported by a study of Liu et al. [146], which demonstrated that fractions of a methanol extract from *Senecio jacobaea* all showed a higher survival rate of western flower thrips than the whole extract. Additionally, the expected combined effect of the single fractions on survival, assuming no interaction, was lower than that of the methanol extract. Furthermore, retrorsine and retrorsine N-oxide were added alone and in combination to the five fractions; the effects on thrips survival depended on the fraction to which the PAs were added. These studies highlight the relevance of synergistic effects of PAs and other plant metabolites on herbivores. In contrast, different PAs (free amines and N-oxides) do not show synergistic effects on one another [141].

While the correlation of PA content and feeding is generally negative for generalists, the exact opposite is reported for specialists, indicating an attraction by PA in plants. In fact, several cases of adaption and utilization of PAs by insects have been reported [1,147,148]. The oviposition of *Tyria jacobaea*, a well-studied member of the Lepidoptera, also called the cinnabar moth, was shown to be positively influenced by the concentration of jacobine-like PAs [136]. This finding suggests an advantage for *Tyria jacobaea* larvae from PA ingestion. Frequently, PAs are sequestered and stored as N-oxides in specialist beetles, moths, butterflies and grasshoppers [1,147–149]. With the storage of PA N-oxides insects have developed a strategy of using plant defense chemicals for their own defense against predators. An astonishing example for this adaption are neotropic Ithomiinae butterflies which, unlike moths, neither feed on PA plants nor sequester them from larvae stage on, but rather take up PAs solely through nectar or withered twigs [135,138]. This habit protects them from the spider *Nephila clavipes*, which cuts out butterflies that had previously ingested PAs, of her own net [150,151]. In *Utetheisa ornatrix* the male butterflies are able to transfer their PA storage during mating onto females, who then utilize them to protect their eggs [152]. Sequestered PAs play an important role in the mating process of some tribes of the Lepidoptera family, because they serve as a precursor for male pheromones [135,153]. Another impressive adaption was found in *Tyria jacobaea* and *Creatonotos transiens*. These two arctiids are able to synthesize their own PAs by esterifying a necine base of plant origin with a necic acid derived from isoleucine by their own metabolism [42,154,155]. Kubitza et al. [156] provided a high-resolution crystal structure of the flavin-dependent monooxygenase from the African locust (*Zonocerus variegatus*). This locust expresses three flavin-dependent monooxygenase isoforms contributing to a counterstrategy against PAs. By N-oxidation of PAs and accumulation of PA N-oxides within its hemolymph the locust circumvents the chemical plant defense and uses PA N-oxides to protect itself against predators. By such mechanisms specialized insects may gain advantages from PA-containing plants. Macel and Klinkhamer [157] reported positive correlations between the jacobine N-oxide and free base content of *Senecio jacobaea* with damage from specialist insect herbivores. Moreover, a study by Joshi and Vrieling [158] reported higher jacobine concentrations in *Senecio jacobaea* growing in invasive areas, indicating fitness advantage of lower PA amounts in areas with specialist herbivores compared to areas with exclusively generalist insects, wherein higher contents are advantageous.

Livshultz et al. [77] studied the evolution of PAs in species of the Apocynaceae family, which are larval host plants for PA-adapted butterflies of the Danainae family. The phylogenetic analysis showed a monophyletic origin of the HSS sequences early in the evolution of one Apocynaceae lineage. They found HSS orthologues, pseudogenes and multiple losses of HSS amino acid motifs in several non-PA producing species consistent with multiple independent losses of PAs. This indicates a selection for the loss of PA biosynthesis by PA-adapted specialist herbivores in the Apocynaceae family.

Despite their contribution in defense against insects, PAs have also been reported to influence interactions with symbiotic and pathogenic fungi. An inhibitory effect of PAs was measurable on *Fusarium* and *Trichoderma*, with PA mixtures exhibiting the highest inhibition [159]. Interestingly, in the same study an enhancement of growth by PAs was quantifiable for strains isolated from *Senecio jacobaea* indicating specialization. PA chemotypes of *Senecio jacobaea* also influence the diversity of fungal communities in soil, as shown by Kowalchuk et al. [119]. It was possible to distinguish fungal communities associated with high-PA jacobine chemotypes from low PA samples as well as senecionine/seneciphylline chemotypes. Additionally, a trend towards lower diversity in the rhizosphere of high-PA plants was observed compared to low-PA plants. This shows that PA chemotypes of *Senecio jacobaea* influence fungal communities in the rhizosphere, with jacobine types selecting more intensely than senecionine/seneciphylline types. In another study, artificial root colonization of *Senecio jacobaea* by *Rhizophagus irregularis* increased concentrations of senecionine, jacoline N-oxide, jaconine N-oxide, and usaramine N-oxide in roots but not in shoots. Only the amount of senecionine was significantly correlated with root length colonized [160]. On the other hand, Reidinger et al. [161] observed a negative correlation between natural colonization levels of roots of *Senecio jacobaea* by vesicles and the concentrations of both jacoline and total PAs. The authors suggest that the natural variations in PA concentrations between individual plants might have affected arbuscular mycorrhizal fungi colonization.

In the Fabaceae member *Crotalaria* PA production can also be influenced by root nodulation as demonstrated by Irmer et al. [162]. Only nodulating *Crotalaria spectabilis* plants infected with their rhizobial partner produce the PA monocrotaline, which is not regarded as being functionally involved in the symbiosis. The absolute amounts of PA per plant were highest in leaves, followed by nodules, roots, and stems, while the concentration was highest in the nodules (1.97 mg/g dry weight), exhibiting a 10-fold higher concentration than in leaves (0.21 mg/g dry weight). A plant derived HSS sequence was identified suggesting that the plant and not the microbiont is the PA producer. HSS transcripts were only detectable in nodules, indicating that they are the only location of alkaloid biosynthesis and the source from which the PAs are transported to above ground parts of the plant.

Plants which are not producing PAs can still accumulate them if they grow on soil containing decomposing PA-containing plants according to a study by Nowak et al. [163]. Various plant species commonly used as herbal teas or spices, i.e., melissa (*Melissa officinalis*), peppermint (*Mentha x piperita*), chamomile (*Matricaria chamomilla*), and parsley (*Petroselinum crispum*), were grown on soil mulched with 1 g of dried *Senecio jacobaea* plant material to investigate the uptake of PAs. Seven days after application, all mulched plants exhibited marked concentrations of PA in their leaves while the untreated controls were PA-free. The maximum PA levels in peppermint, melissa and chamomile were 0.1–0.15 mg/kg dry weight, whereas PA levels in parsley were up to five times higher (>0.5 mg/kg). Fourteen days after mulching, PA concentrations severely decreased, especially the N-oxide forms. The composition of the imported PAs in parsley, chamomile and melissa, showed a similar pattern to that of *Senecio jacobaea* with erucifoline being the most abundant alkaloid, followed by seneciphylline and jacobine, whereas in peppermint erucifoline occurred only in traces. This observation is probably due to species dependent differences in PA degradation or modification in the acceptor plants. While PA free bases can pass the membranes of the roots by simple diffusion, the uptake of PA N-oxides might be catalyzed by transporters normally responsible for the uptake of other compounds. Since the flowers of treated chamomile plants did not contain any PAs it was assumed that the transport to the leaves of acceptor plants happens via the xylem. These findings are significant for the production of herbal teas, spices, and plant derived pharmaceuticals as PA-contaminations can occur due to decomposing PA-containing plants in the fields.

5.2. Toxicity of Pyrrolizidine Alkaloids and Mechanisms for their Detoxification

Toxicity and pharmacology of PAs has recently been discussed in a detailed review by Moreira et al. [10]. Thus, we summarize toxicity here only very briefly and focus more on detoxification mechanisms.

PAs are one of the most important classes of naturally occurring toxins due to their wide distribution and high risk of unwitting consumption of contaminated natural products like grains, honey, milk, herbal teas, and medicines [3,164–171]. Numerous studies have demonstrated the hepatotoxic [172], genotoxic [173], cytotoxic [173,174], tumorigenic [175], and neurotoxic [176] potential of naturally occurring PAs. Possible symptoms of PA toxicity are hepatic veno-occlusive disease, liver cirrhosis, megalocystosis and cancer. Furthermore, they can cause chronic pulmonary arterial hypertension and congenital anomalies [3,177]. Several cases of poisonings and poisoning outbreaks caused by PA contaminated food have been documented [3,178]. The two main sources of intoxication for humans are the consumption of cereal grain contaminated with seeds from PA-containing weeds and the use of alkaloid-forming herbs or herbal remedies for medicinal and dietary purposes [17,177].

The degree of harm caused by a specific PA relies on its necine base structure, since toxic PAs, like the retronecine, otonecine and heliotridine-types, generally carry a 1,2-unsaturated necine base. The first step of metabolic activation of PAs after ingestion and absorption is dehydrogenation catalyzed by cytochrome P450 monooxygenases (CYP3A4 and CYP2C19) of the liver (Figure 16) [179]. In retronecine and heliotridine-type PAs hydroxylation of the necine base occurs at the C-3 and C-8 position to form 3- or 8-hydroxynecine derivatives followed by spontaneous dehydration [180–182]. For otonecine-type PAs, oxidative N-demethylation of the necine base occurs, followed by ring closure and dehydration [183,184]. Those reactions lead to the formation of reactive dehydropyrrolizidine intermediates, also known as pyrroles or pyrrolic esters, followed by the formation of pyrrolizinium ions. The electrophilic metabolites are capable of binding nucleophilic -OH, -SH, or -NH functional groups on physiologically important macromolecules like glutathione (GSH), DNA and proteins [173,185–189]. Nucleophilic substitution of one or two glutathione molecules produces the GSH conjugates 7-, 7,9-di- and 9-glutathionyl-6,7-dihydro-1-hydroxymethyl-5*H*-pyrrolizine for excretion [173,183,190,191]. These GSH conjugates are considered to be detoxification metabolites but it has been reported that they also act as reactive metabolites, causing DNA adduct formation [172]. Additionally, glutathione S-transferases (GSTs) can mediate these reactions leading to species-dependent toxicity effects, as it has been observed that guinea pig hepatic GSTs catalyze GSH conjugation of the pyrrolic metabolites of jacobine whereas rat hepatic GST did not affect the reaction [192]. GSH conjugation is one of the most important detoxification reactions of PAs. If the levels of reactive intermediates are high enough, the cellular GSH pool can be depleted causing severe oxidative damage of liver tissues [193–195]. Dehydro-PAs, including 6,7-dihydro-7-hydroxy-1-hydroxymethyl-5*H*-pyrrolizine (DHP) [196,197], their C-7 and C-9 hydrolysis product, and the dehydration product (3*H*-pyrrolizin-7-yl)methanol [198] are all reactive alkylating species. They can bind to liver cellular proteins and DNA resulting in the formation of DNA and/or protein adducts as well as DNA-protein cross links, which are all associated with genotoxicity and carcinogenicity ultimately leading to veno-occlusive disease and/or tumors [175,199,200].

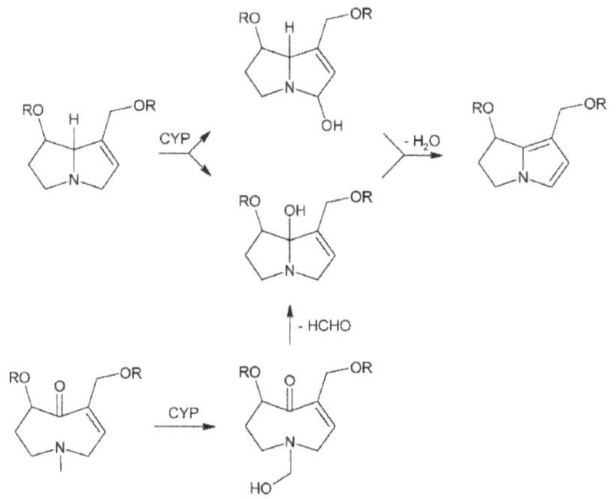

Figure 16. Metabolic activation of pyrrolizidine alkaloids. PAs are oxidized by cytochrome P450 enzymes (CYP), which converts them to the reactive and toxic pyrrole derivatives. Adapted from Reference [11].

A study on the in vitro metabolism of lasiocarpine in liver microsomes of humans, pigs, rats, mice, rabbits, and sheep was compared and a tendency towards species-dependent toxicity was observed [201]. The highest levels of reactive metabolites like (3H-pyrrolizin-7-yl)methanol and GSH conjugates were detected in human microsomes, followed by pig, rat and mouse, all known to be susceptible to PA intoxication. The microsomes of rabbit and sheep, known to be more PA-resistant, exhibited lower metabolite levels. Interestingly, the scale of PA toxicity also depends on age and gender, since male rats are more prone to clavinorine and isoline intoxication than female rats [194,202,203] and young mice are more susceptible to retrorsine in comparison to adult mice [204].

One mode of detoxification catalyzed by flavin-containing monooxygenase (FMOs) is the N-oxidation of the necine bases of retronecine and heliotridine-type PAs to form PA N-oxides [205,206]. Otonecine-type PAs on the other hand cannot form PA N-oxides due to methylation of the necine base nitrogen. PA N-oxides can be conjugated for excretion and are therefore generally regarded as detoxification products, although they may also be converted back to their toxic parent PAs [181,207–209]. As it was demonstrated for senecionine, the susceptibility of an animal species to PA exposure depends on the rate of FMO-catalyzed conversion of the PA into its N-oxide leading to detoxification as well as the P450-catalyzed formation of DHP leading to toxicity [210]. In susceptible species such as rats, cattle, horses, and chickens, a high glutathione–DHP conjugation is observed. However, in sheep, a resistant species, low rates of glutathione conjugation combined with high rates of FMO-catalyzed conversion of senecionine into its N-oxide occur.

Another mode of detoxification in mammal metabolism is the cleavage of the necine base-necine acid bond, mediated by unspecific esterases followed by phase II-conjugation and excretion. This process was shown to contribute to guinea pig resistance to PA toxicity and rat susceptibility, as guinea pigs have higher liver esterase activity in contrast to rats [211–214].

Recently, N-glucuronidation has been identified as a potential new metabolic pathway in humans and several animal species for the activation and detoxication of PAs [215].

PAs with a saturated necine base like platynecine-type PAs are known to be nontoxic. It has been demonstrated that in hepatocytes treated with platyphylline the metabolites being formed are mainly dehydroplatyphylline carboxylic acid and in lower amounts, platyphylline epoxide as well as platyphylline N-oxide [216]. Disparate in comparison to unsaturated PAs, which are activated to reactive pyrrolic esters causing the formation of hepatotoxic protein and/or DNA adducts, the saturated structure of the platynecine-type PAs causes the P450-mediated oxidative metabolism to generate nonreactive polar compounds that are water-soluble and easily excreted.

5.3. Beneficial Properties of Certain PAs

Despite the toxic properties of 1,2-unsaturated PAs and their negative implications on human and animal health, some PAs have the potential to be used for the treatment of diseases and infections. One of the most consequential and positive characteristics of these PAs is their glycosidase inhibitory activity [217,218], potentially leading to antidiabetic, anticancer, fungicidal, and antiviral effects [219]. Glycosidases are a class of enzymes involved in selective hydrolysis of sugar bonds in glycoconjugates as well as the covalent attachment of carbohydrates to lipids, proteins, and peptides on the cell surfaces [220–223]. Disfunctional glycosidases can reduce the proliferation of malignant cells and tumor growth [219,224]. Furthermore, inhibited glycosidases can cause the formation of disorganized oligosaccharides, thereby interrupting cell–cell and cell–virus recognition [219,225]. Thus, certain PAs may be used for the treatment of cancer, diabetes, and infections [226,227]. Some of the most potent glycosidase inhibitors are polyhydroxylated PAs since they mimic the pyranosyl and furanosyl core of the natural glycosidase substrates [226,228]. It has been demonstrated that the polyhydroxylated PAs alexine from *Alexa leiopetala* and australine from *Castanospermum australe* exhibit a strong glycosidase inhibition [229–231] and show promising potential to be used as chemotherapeutic [219], antiviral [228], and immunomodulatory drugs.

A pair of PAs with antitumor as well as antibiotic properties are (-)-clazamycin A and (+)-clazamycin B, which were isolated from *Streptomyces puniceus* [232,233]. These compounds show activity against *Herpes simplex* virus in vitro [233], as well as a strong inhibition of *Pseudomonas* species [232]. Moreover, in some fungus species, PAs with potent activity against Gram-positive and Gram-negative bacteria, as well as tumor cells have been isolated [234,235].

6. Occurrence of Pyrrolizidine Alkaloids in Crop Plants

While many plant species are PA producers, few of them are used by humans, which is likely related to PA toxicity. Among them, most are used in traditional medicine for treatment of diverse diseases, which is discussed in detail in a number of review articles [16,17,177,236–239]. However, there are also several PA-producing plants used as food or as forage crops. While intake of medicinal plants is usually minute, vegetables and herbs may be consumed at substantial amounts, making presence of PAs very critical. Thus, we will focus here on plant species that are consumed as food or used as livestock feed in different regions of the world.

6.1. Borago officinalis

Borage (*Borago officinalis*), which originated from the Mediterranean area, is a common annual garden herb used in salads and teas and is widely cultivated for seed oil production. The oil contains high amounts of the essential fatty acid γ-linolenic acid (18–25%), and is therefore used for nutritional, medical, and cosmetic purposes. Larson et al. [240] first identified the pyrrolizidine alkaloids lycopsamine and amabiline (Figure 17) in fresh and dried leaves and stems of *B. officinalis* with a total alkaloid amount of less than 0.001% dry weight. They also showed that in roots the alkaloids are mainly present as the free base, while fresh leaves contain mainly N-oxides. Lüthy et al. [241] did not only detect lycopsamine and amabiline but also intermedine, supinine and the isomer pair acetyllycopsamine/acetylintermedine in the range of 2-10 mg/kg in vegetative tissues. Dodson et al. [92] determined thesinine as the only alkaloid in the flowers and the major alkaloid in seeds. Mature seeds were found to contain thesinine and minute amounts of lycopsamine. Immature seeds contained only thesinine. The first glycosylated pyrrolizidine alkaloid reported in plants, namely thesinine-4′-O-β-D-glucoside, was discovered in dried and defatted borage seeds [53]. Seeds contain approximately 0.1% to 0.5% thesinine-4′-O-β-D-glucoside.

Wretensjö and Karlberg [242] analyzed crude borage oil as well as borage oil from different processing stages and found no pyrrolizidine alkaloids present above a detection limit of 20 µg/kg. Additionally, they could demonstrate by spiking experiments with crotaline that the pyrrolizidine content in crude borage oil was reduced overall by a factor of approximately 30,000 in the refining process. Additionally, Vacillotto et al. [243] could not detect any pyrrolizidine alkaloids above a detection limit of 0.2 µg/kg in seed oil.

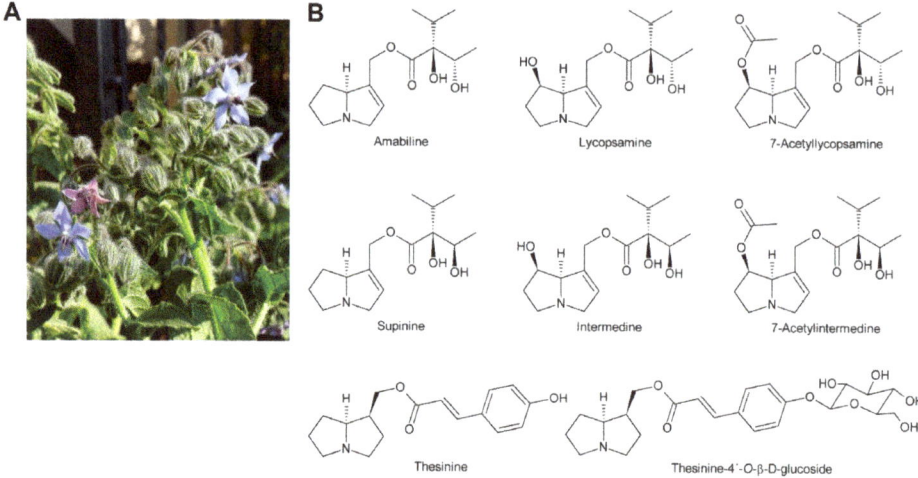

Figure 17. Pyrrolizidine alkaloids found in *Borago officinalis* (borage): (**A**) Flower of *B. officinalis*. Young flowers show a bright blue color while older flowers exhibit, because of a lower pH, a slightly reddish coloration. (**B**) Leaves of *B. officinalis* contain the supinidine-type PAs amabiline and supinine and the retronecine-type lycopsamine and intermedine as well as their 7-acetylated derivatives. Seeds contain mainly the (-)-isoretronecanol-type PA thesinine and its glucoside thesinine-4'-O-β-D-glucoside.

6.2. Crassocephalum crepidioides

The genus *Crassocephalum* belongs to the Asteraceae family (subfamily Asteroideae, tribe Senecioneae) [244] and includes approximately 100 plant species growing in Africa, tropical and subtropical regions of Asia and Australia and locally in America [245,246]. Both *Crassocephalum crepidioides* (Figure 18A) and *Crassocephalum rubens* are erect annual herbs used as leafy vegetables [245,247–249].

C. crepidioides and *C. rubens* are used fresh or dried for preparation of sauces, soups and stews [250]. *C. crepidioides* is also eaten raw, for example in Australia in salad dishes [245]. A factor making particularly *C. crepidioides* interesting for food production is its high yield of up to 25-27 t/ha per year even on soils with low nutrient supply [245]. Moreover, it has desirable nutritional properties since dried leaves contain about 27% protein, 8% fiber, 42% carbohydrates, and 3% lipids [248,251]. These values suggest that *C. crepidioides* is a good source of fiber while the relatively high amount of carbohydrates makes it a good source of energy. *C. crepidioides* and *C. rubens* contain also high levels of minerals including potassium, magnesium, calcium, phosphorous, iron, copper and manganese [251]. Both plant species are also used in traditional medicine due to supposed medicinal properties, such as antibiotic, antioxidant, anti-fungal, anti-inflammatory, anti-diabetic and blood regulative effects. They are included in traditional treatment of hepatic insufficiency, intestinal worms, stomach disorders and open wounds [245,252,253]. Furthermore, in Africa *C. crepidioides* is traditionally part of diets of pregnant and breast-feeding women as it is believed to prevent anemia and stimulate milk production [252]. In addition to human consumption and application in traditional medicine, *C. crepidioides* is also used as livestock feed, for instance for poultry [245].

Based on brine shrimp lethality tests and application of Mayer's reagent Adjatin et al. considered both *C. crepidioides* and *C. rubens* as safe for human consumption [254]. In sharp contrast, Asada et al. reported isolation of significant amounts of jacobine and jacoline (Figure 18C) from *C. crepidioides* [255]. The reason for these divergent results might be the low sensitivity of Mayer's reagent for PAs, which are in fact usually detected with Dragendorff's reagent, or with higher sensitivity and specificity, by chromatographic techniques. Indeed, presence of high amounts of jacobine in *C. crepidioides* was recently confirmed by cation exchange chromatography [50]. Interestingly, the content of jacobine depended highly on the tissue. In young leaves jacobine was present at levels exceeding 200 mg/kg fresh weight while it was below 1 mg/kg fresh weight in old leaves. In addition, the jacobine content was under developmental control since six-week-old plants showed contents of approximately 27 mg/kg fresh weight while 10-week-old plants had contents of 260 mg/kg. Also, the growth conditions had a significant impact since incubator-grown plants had high levels while jacobine was below the detection limit (1 mg/kg) in greenhouse grown plants [50]. Production of alkaloids has also been reported for *C. rubens* [256]. These results clearly show that *C. crepidioides* and *C. rubens* cannot be considered safe for human consumption and that PA-free varieties have to be identified prior to utilization of these species as food or forage crops.

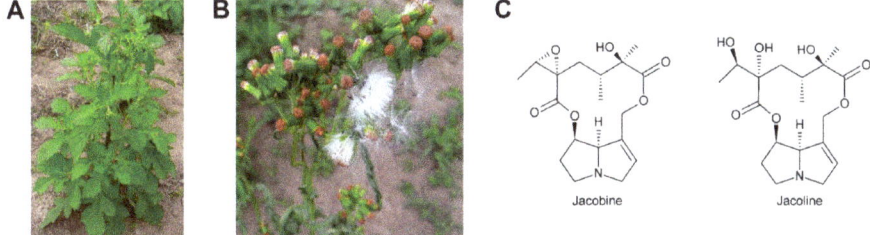

Figure 18. *Crassocephalum crepidioides*. *C. crepidioides* plant (**A**) and flowers (**B**). (**C**) The retronecine-type PAs jacobine and jacoline were reported in *C. crepidioides*. Pictures shown in (**A**) and (**B**): Courtesy of N. Adebimpe Adedej.

6.3. Gynura

Gynura, a genus of the Asteraceae family, contains several edible species native to Asia like *G. bicolor*, *G. divaricata* and *G. procumbens* which are used in Asian cuisine and traditional medicine. The species *G. bicolor* for example, has great nutraceutical potential, containing high levels of phenolic acids, flavonoids, carotenoids and anthocyanins and exhibits anti-oxidative as well as anti-inflammatory properties [257]. Furthermore, it can be used for the treatment of diabetes mellitus [258] and cancer [259,260]. Even though the use of *Gynura* may have numerous beneficial effects on health, its consumption is not without risk because of the presence of PAs. Intergerrimine and usaramine were first identified in *G. divaricata* by Roeder et al. [261]. Chen et al. [262] compared the PA profiles of *G. bicolor* and *G. divaricata* collected from five different provinces of China. They found 27 PAs consisting of five different types in the two species. Known PAs that were identified are retrorsine, spartioidine, seneciphylline, integerrimine, senecionine, senkirkine, retrorsine N-oxide, senecionine N-oxide, and seneciphylline N-oxide (Figure 19). Additionally, 18 other unidentified PAs were detected in both species. *G. divaricata* collected in the Jiangsu province showed the highest concentration (39.7 µg/g) of retronecine type PAs while *G. bicolor* from Fujian contained the lowest concentration (1.4 µg/g). *G. divaricata* always contained higher amounts of retronecine type PAs in comparison to *G. bicolor* from the same locality and harvest time. Both species collected from Jiangsu contained the most diverse PA profile, while *G. divaricata* from Fujian showed the lowest variety of

PAs. A weak cytotoxic activity was detected in alkaloid extracts of both species collected from Jiangsu. These results show that the amount and variety of PAs in *Gynura* depends on the species as well as the growing region, indicating that environmental factors likely play a role in PA accumulation in *Gynura*. Another *Gynura* species traditionally used in Chinese medicine is *Gynura segetum*, also known as Jusanqi. It has been shown to have anti-angiogenic [263] as well as antioxidative and anti-inflammatory properties [264]. Its medicinal use is risky though as there have been several reports of hepatic veno-occlusive disease linked to the consumption of *G. segetum* [265–268]. Liang and Roeder were the first to characterize senecionine from *G. segetum* [269]. The presence of senecionine was confirmed by Yuan et al. [270], who could additionally detect seneciphylline as well as seneciphyllinine and E-seneciphylline. Qi et al. [271] analyzed whole plants of *G. segetum* collected from Zhejiang province of China and could unequivocally identify seneciphylline, senecionine, seneciphyllinine, and seneciphyllinine N-oxide using HPLC / ITMS. 16 further PA or PANO structures were tentatively assigned, among them E-seneciphylline, E-seneciphylline N-oxide, senecannabine, senecannabine N-oxide, a yamataimine isomer, jacoline, and tetrahydrosenecionine, which has been reported for the first time from a natural source. Considering the present research about PAs in *Gynura* indicates that caution is required concerning its use for dietary and medicinal purposes.

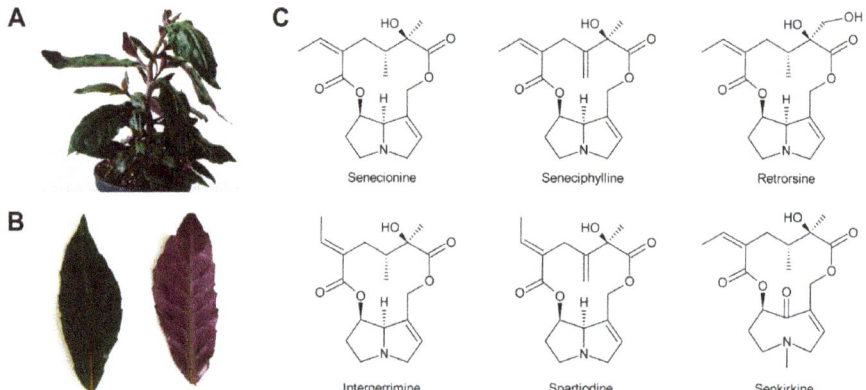

Figure 19. Pyrrolizidine alkaloids observed in *Gynura bicolor*. (**A**) *G. bicolor* plant. (**B**) *G. bicolor* leaves from the upper (green) and lower (ruby-colored) side. (**B**) Senecionine, seneciphylline and retrorsine were reported in *G. bicolor* in both, their free forms (shown above) and as N-oxides, while intergerrimine, spartiodine, and senkirkine were only found as free alkaloids.

6.4. Lolium

Lolium species, commonly known as ryegrass, are important pasture grass species serving as main feed for grazing livestock in numerous countries and regions, for example Australia, New Zealand, North America and Europe. These species can have toxic effects on mammals that graze them and are related to a syndrome known as ryegrass staggers. Therefore, their chemical composition has been analyzed intensively.

Interestingly, the originally identified toxins, lolitrem B [272], ergovaline [273], and loline alkaloids are produced by endophytic fungi [5]. The loline alkaloids represent a special class of PAs, which are characterized by the presence of an ether bridge (Figure 1). In contrast to classical PAs, which are produced by plants, lolines are metabolic products of fungi, particularly of the genus *Epichloë* [5,274,275].

In addition, several *Lolium* species can also produce PAs of the thesinine type themself. Koulman et al. [54] were the first to isolate and elucidate the stereoisomers E-thesinine-O-4′-α-rhamnoside and Z-thesinine-O-4′-α-rhamnoside from *Lolium perenne* (Figure 20), thereby providing the first report of PAs in the Poaceae family which are synthesized by the plant itself. Furthermore, they could detect those two compounds together with the aglycone and a hexoside in *Festuca arundinacea*, a species of grasses closely related to *L. perenne*. In *L. perenne* the highest concentrations of E/Z-thesinine-O-4'-α-rhamnoside were found in sheath tissue, followed by blade tissue while immature tissue contained the lowest amounts. Infection with the endophytic fungus *Neotyphodium lolii* increased the concentrations only slightly. The authors analyzed plants grown in a greenhouse and found variations in the ratios of E-thesinine-O-4'-α-rhamnoside to Z-thesinine-O-4'-α-rhamnoside between 0.2 and 1. When clonal material was grown in a climate room under controlled conditions the variation was severely reduced, indicating a strong environmental influence on the accumulation of E/Z-thesinine-rhamnoside. Since the identified alkaloid conjugates do not possess a C-1/C-2 unsaturation and a hydroxy group at C-7, they likely exhibit a limited toxicity to mammals. The common occurrence of these PAs in several widely used commercial *L. perenne* and *F. arundinacea* cultivars further demonstrates their non-toxicity or low toxicity to grazing livestock, but detoxification by rumen bacteria might play a role as well [276]. It is currently unknown if the thesinine-rhamnoside PAs play any role in insect deterrence or if they enhance plant fitness by any other means. Wesseling et al. [91] analyzed various Pooideae species grown under controlled conditions and found that PA biosynthesis is restricted to a small group of species producing only a narrow range of thesinine conjugates. The three closely related outbreeding *Lolium* species *L. perenne*, *L. multiflorum*, and *L. rigidum* were shown to accumulate PAs while the inbreeding *L. temulentum* and *L. remotum* do not. Furthermore, *F. arundinacea* contained PAs while in the closely related *F. pratensis* they were absent. Potential explanations for this pattern might be the independent evolution of PA biosynthesis in *F. arundinacea* or a secondary loss in the inbreeding *Lolium* species. Hybridization of PA producing *Lolium* species with *Festuca* could be another possibility of how PA production was acquired in *Festuca*. Additionally, the inter and intra-specific PA patterns are highly variable. *L. rigidum* contained the highest average amounts of PAs, followed by *L. perenne* and *F. arundinacea*, while *L. multiflorum* showed the lowest concentrations. *F. arundinacea* was the only species which contained the aglycone thesinine in significant amounts. In *L. perenne* and *L. multiflorum* PAs were restricted to only a few of the tested individuals, while all samples of *L. rigidum* and *F. arundinacea* were tested positive. It seems like PA biosynthesis is a constitutive trait in some species, while in others it occurs only infrequently and might possibly be induced by external stimuli or occur in later developmental stages. Gill et al. [76] identified two putative HSS genes in perennial ryegrass, one of them (*LpHSS1*) occurring only sporadically. A significant association of absence of the *LpHSS1* gene with lower levels of thesinine-rhamnoside PAs was found. This provides the possibility of developing genetic markers for future breeding efforts in regard to PA presence and enables investigations about the role of PAs in deterring herbivore pests. Further HSS-like gene sequences were identified in other Poaceae species, including tall fescue, wheat, maize, and sorghum. Therefore, PA biosynthesis might be even more widespread in the grass family than it is known to date with unknown PA structures still to be discovered.

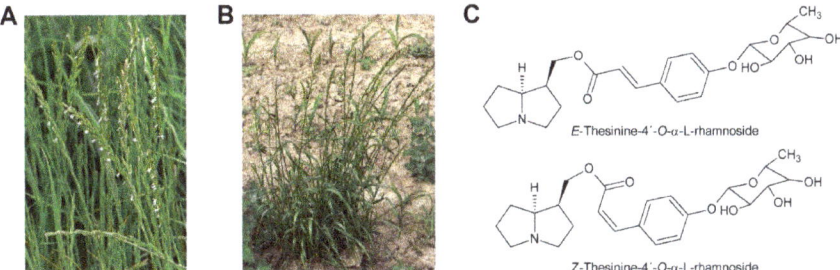

Figure 20. Pyrrolizidine alkaloids reported for *Lolium* species. (**A**) *Lolium perenne* (ray grass). (**B**) *Lolium multiflorum* (Italian rye-grass). (**C**) Structures of *E*- and *Z*-thesinine-4'-*O*-α-L-rhamnoside. Pictures shown in (A) and (B): Courtesy of Leo Michels.

Author Contributions: Conceptualization, W.R., S.S.; writing and original draft preparation W.R., S.S. and N.K.; figure preparation, W.R. and S.S.

Funding: The publication costs were covered by the German Research Foundation (DFG) and the Technical University of Munich (TUM) in the framework of the Open Access Publishing Program.

Acknowledgments: Thanks to N. Adebimpe Adedej for providing pictures used in Figure 18 and for help with editing. Thanks to Leo Michels for providing pictures used in Figure 20. Thanks to Brigitte Poppenberger and Veronica Ramirez for critical reading of the manuscript.

Conflicts of Interest: The authors declare no conflict of interest.

References

1. Macel, M. Attract and deter: A dual role for pyrrolizidine alkaloids in plant-insect interactions. *Phytochem. Rev.* **2011**, *10*, 75–82. [CrossRef] [PubMed]
2. Ober, D.; Hartmann, T. Homospermidine synthase, the first pathway-specific enzyme of pyrrolizidine alkaloid biosynthesis, evolved from deoxyhypusine synthase. *Proc. Natl. Acad. Sci. USA* **1999**, *96*, 14777–14782. [CrossRef] [PubMed]
3. EFSA. Scientific opinion on pyrrolizidine alkaloids in food and feed. *EFSA J.* **2011**, *9*, 2406. [CrossRef]
4. Molyneux, R.J.; Gardner, D.L.; Colegate, S.M.; Edgar, J.A. Pyrrolizidine alkaloid toxicity in livestock: A paradigm for human poisoning? *Food Addit. Contam. Part A Chem. Anal. Control Expo. Risk Assess.* **2011**, *28*, 293–307. [CrossRef] [PubMed]
5. Schardl, C.L.; Grossman, R.B.; Nagabhyru, P.; Faulkner, J.R.; Mallik, U.P. Loline alkaloids: Currencies of mutualism. *Phytochemistry* **2007**, *68*, 980–996. [CrossRef] [PubMed]
6. Pan, J.; Bhardwaj, M.; Faulkner, J.R.; Nagabhyru, P.; Charlton, N.D.; Higashi, R.M.; Miller, A.F.; Young, C.A.; Grossman, R.B.; Schardl, C.L. Ether bridge formation in loline alkaloid biosynthesis. *Phytochemistry* **2014**, *98*, 60–68. [CrossRef]
7. Pan, J.; Bhardwaj, M.; Nagabhyru, P.; Grossman, R.B.; Schardl, C.L. Enzymes from fungal and plant origin required for chemical diversification of insecticidal loline alkaloids in grass-*Epichloe* symbiota. *PLoS ONE* **2014**, *9*, e115590. [CrossRef]
8. Bunsupa, S.; Yamazaki, M.; Saito, K. Quinolizidine alkaloid biosynthesis: Recent advances and future prospects. *Front. Plant Sci.* **2012**, *3*, 239. [CrossRef]
9. Kim, N.; Estrada, O.; Chavez, B.; Stewart, C.; D'Auria, J.C. Tropane and Granatane Alkaloid Biosynthesis: A Systematic Analysis. *Molecules* **2016**, *21*, 1510. [CrossRef]
10. Moreira, R.; Pereira, D.M.; Valentao, P.; Andrade, P.B. Pyrrolizidine Alkaloids: Chemistry, Pharmacology, Toxicology and Food Safety. *Int. J. Mol. Sci.* **2018**, *19*, 1668. [CrossRef]
11. Robertson, J.; Stevens, K. Pyrrolizidine alkaloids: Occurrence, biology, and chemical synthesis. *Nat. Prod. Rep.* **2017**, *34*, 62–89. [CrossRef] [PubMed]
12. Ikeda, Y.; Nonaka, H.; Furumai, T.; Igarashi, Y. Cremastrine, a pyrrolizidine alkaloid from *Cremastra appendiculata*. *J. Nat. Prod.* **2005**, *68*, 572–573. [CrossRef] [PubMed]
13. Lindström, B.; Lüning, B. Studies on Orchidaceae alkaloids XIII. A new alkaloid, laburnine acetate, from *Vanda cristata* Lindl. *Acta Chem. Scand.* **1969**, *23*, 3352–3354. [CrossRef]
14. Hoang le, S.; Tran, M.H.; Lee, J.S.; To, D.C.; Nguyen, V.T.; Kim, J.A.; Lee, J.H.; Woo, M.H.; Min, B.S. Anti-inflammatory Activity of Pyrrolizidine Alkaloids from the Leaves of *Madhuca pasquieri* (Dubard). *Chem. Pharm. Bull.* **2015**, *63*, 481–484. [CrossRef] [PubMed]
15. Freer, A.A.; Kelly, H.A.; Robins, D.J. Rosmarinine: A pyrrolizidine alkaloid. *Acta Cryst. C* **1986**, *42*, 1348–1350. [CrossRef]
16. Roeder, E.; Wiedenfeld, H. Pyrrolizidine alkaloids in medicinal plants of Mongolia, Nepal and Tibet. *Pharmazie* **2009**, *64*, 699–716. [CrossRef]
17. Roeder, E. Medicinal plants in Europe containing pyrrolizidine alkaloids. *Pharmazie* **1995**, *50*, 83–98. [PubMed]
18. Tasso, B.; Novelli, F.; Sparatore, F.; Fasoli, F.; Gotti, C. (+)-Laburnamine, a natural selective ligand and partial agonist for the alpha4beta2 nicotinic receptor subtype. *J. Nat. Prod.* **2013**, *76*, 727–731. [CrossRef]
19. Suri, O.P.; Jamwal, R.S.; Suri, K.A.; Atal, C.K. Ehretinine, a novel pyrrolizidine alkaloid from *Ehretia aspera*. *Phytochemistry* **1980**, *19*, 1273–1274. [CrossRef]

20. Villanueva-Canongo, C.; Perez-Hernandez, N.; Hernandez-Carlos, B.; Cedillo-Portugal, E.; Joseph-Nathan, P.; Burgueno-Tapia, E. Complete ^{1}H NMR assignments of pyrrolizidine alkaloids and a new eudesmanoid from *Senecio polypodioides*. *Magn. Reson. Chem.* **2014**, *52*, 251–257. [CrossRef]
21. Alali, F.Q.; Tahboub, Y.R.; Ibrahim, E.S.; Qandil, A.M.; Tawaha, K.; Burgess, J.P.; Sy, A.; Nakanishi, Y.; Kroll, D.J.; Oberlies, N.H. Pyrrolizidine alkaloids from *Echium glomeratum* (Boraginaceae). *Phytochemistry* **2008**, *69*, 2341–2346. [CrossRef] [PubMed]
22. Roeder, E.; Wiedenfeld, H.; Jost, E.J. Tussilagine—A new pyrrolizidine alkaloid from *Tussilago farfara*. *Planta Med.* **1981**, *43*, 99–102. [CrossRef] [PubMed]
23. El-Shazly, A.; Abdel-Ghani, A.; Wink, M. Pyrrolizidine alkaloids from *Onosma arenaria* (Boraginaceae). *Biochem. Syst. Ecol.* **2003**, *31*, 477–485. [CrossRef]
24. Brandänge, S.; Granelli, I.; Johanson, R.; Hytta, R.; van der Hoeven, M.G.; Swahn, C.G. Studies on Orchidaceae Alkaloids. XXXVI. Alkaloids from some *Vanda* and *Vandopsis* Species. *Acta Chem. Scand.* **1973**, *27*, 1096–1097. [CrossRef]
25. El-Shazly, A.; El-Domiaty, M.; Witte, L.; Wink, M. Pyrrolizidine alkaloids in members of the Boraginaceae from Sinai (Egypt). *Biochem. Syst. Ecol.* **1998**, *26*, 619–636. [CrossRef]
26. Roeder, E.; Wiedenfeld, H.; Hoenig, A. Pyrrolizidinalkaloide aus *Senecio aureus*. *Planta Med.* **1983**, *49*, 57–59. [CrossRef]
27. Hikichi, M.; Asada, Y.; Furuya, T. Ligularidine, a new pyrrolizidine alkaloid from *Ligularia dentata*. *Tetrahedron Lett.* **1979**, *20*, 1233–1236. [CrossRef]
28. Toppel, G.; Witte, L.; Riebesehl, B.; Borstel, K.V.; Hartmann, T. Alkaloid patterns and biosynthetic capacity of root cultures from some pyrrolizidine alkaloid producing *Senecio* species. *Plant Cell Rep.* **1987**, *6*, 466–469. [CrossRef]
29. Ravi, S.; Ravikumar, R.; Lakshmanan, A.J. Pyrrolizidine alkaloids from *Cynoglossum furcatum*. *J. Asian Nat. Prod. Res.* **2008**, *10*, 349–354. [CrossRef]
30. Culvenor, C.C.; Edgar, J.A.; Smith, L.W. Pyrrolizidine alkaloids in honey from *Echium plantagineum* L. *J. Agric. Food Chem.* **1981**, *29*, 958–960. [CrossRef]
31. Crout, D.H. Pyrrolizidine alkaloids. Biosynthesis of the angelate component of heliosupine. *J. Chem. Soc. Perkin Trans. 1* **1967**, *13*, 1233–1234. [CrossRef] [PubMed]
32. Resch, J.F.; Rosberger, D.F.; Meinwald, J.; Appling, J.W. Biologically active pyrrolizidine alkaloids from the true forget-me-not, *Myosotis scorpioides*. *J. Nat. Prod.* **1982**, *45*, 358–362. [CrossRef] [PubMed]
33. Culvenor, C.C.J.; Edgar, J.A.; Frahn, J.L.; Smith, L.W.; Ulubelen, A.; Doganca, S. The structure of anadoline. *Aust. J. Chem.* **1975**, *28*, 173–178. [CrossRef]
34. Ulubelen, A.; Doganca, S. Anadoline, a new senecio alkaloid from *Symphytum orientale*. *Tetrahedron Lett.* **1970**, *11*, 2583–2585. [CrossRef]
35. Crowley, H.C.; Culvenor, C.C.J. Alkaloids of *Cynoglossum latifolium* R.Br. Latifoline and 7-Angelylretronecine. *Aust. J. Chem.* **1962**, *15*, 139–144. [CrossRef]
36. Hagglund, K.M.; L'Empereur, K.M.; Roby, M.R.; Stermitz, F.R. Latifoline and Latifoline-*N*-Oxide from *Hackelia floribunda*, the Western False Forget-Me-Not. *J. Nat. Prod.* **1985**, *48*, 638–639. [CrossRef]
37. Roitman, J.N.; Wong, R.Y. Revised Absolute Configurations of Latifolic Acid and the Pyrrolizidine Alkaloid Latifoline. *Aust. J. Chem.* **1988**, *41*, 1781–1787. [CrossRef]
38. L'Empereur, K.M.; Li, Y.; Stermitz, F.R.; Crabtree, L. Pyrrolizidine Alkaloids from *Hackelia californica* and *Gnophaela latipennis*, an *H. californica*-Hosted Arctiid Moth. *J. Nat. Prod.* **1989**, *52*, 360–366. [CrossRef]
39. Frolich, C.; Hartmann, T.; Ober, D. Tissue distribution and biosynthesis of 1,2-saturated pyrrolizidine alkaloids in *Phalaenopsis* hybrids (Orchidaceae). *Phytochemistry* **2006**, *67*, 1493–1502. [CrossRef]
40. Luning, B.; Trankner, H.; Brandange, S. Studies on orchidaceae alkaloids V. A new alkaloid from *Phalaenopsis amabilis* Bl. *Acta Chem. Scand.* **1966**, *20*, 2011. [CrossRef]
41. Huang, S.; Zhou, X.L.; Wang, C.J.; Wang, Y.S.; Xiao, F.; Shan, L.H.; Guo, Z.Y.; Weng, J. Pyrrolizidine alkaloids from *Liparis nervosa* with inhibitory activities against LPS-induced NO production in RAW264.7 macrophages. *Phytochemistry* **2013**, *93*, 154–161. [CrossRef] [PubMed]
42. Hartmann, T.; Witte, L. Pyrrolizidine alkaloids: Chemical, biological and chemoecological aspects. In *Alkaloids: Chemical and Biological Perspectives*; Pergamon Press: Oxford, UK, 1995; Volume 9, pp. 155–233.
43. Klásek, A.; Sedmera, P.; Boeva, A.; Šantavý, F. Pyrrolizidine alkaloids. XX. Nemorensine, an alkaloid from *Senecio nemorensis* L. *Collect. Czech. Chem. Commun.* **1973**, *38*, 2504–2512. [CrossRef]

44. Langel, D.; Ober, D.; Pelser, P. The evolution of pyrrolizidine alkaloid biosynthesis and diversity in the Senecioneae. *Phytochem. Rev.* **2011**, *10*, 3–74. [CrossRef]
45. Culvenor, C.C.J.; Smith, L.W.; Willing, R.I. Madurensine, a macrocyclic pyrrolizidine diester with the secondary ester attachment at C-6. *J. Chem. Soc. D* **1970**, 65–66. [CrossRef]
46. Neuner-Jehle, N.; Nesvadba, H.; Spiteller, G. Application of mass spectrometry to structure elucidation of alkaloids, 6th center: Pyrrolizidine alkaloids from laburnum. *Chem. Mon.* **1965**, *96*, 321–338. [CrossRef]
47. Stelljes, M.E.; Kelley, R.B.; Molyneux, R.J.; Seiber, J.N. GC-MS Determination of Pyrrolizidine Alkaloids in Four *Senecio* Species. *J. Nat. Prod.* **1991**, *54*, 759–773. [CrossRef]
48. El-Shazly, A.; Wink, M. Diversity of Pyrrolizidine Alkaloids in the Boraginaceae Structures, Distribution, and Biological Properties. *Diversity* **2014**, *6*, 188–282. [CrossRef]
49. Mattocks, A.R.; Jukes, R. Improved field tests for toxic pyrrolizidine alkaloids. *J. Nat. Prod.* **1987**, *50*, 161–166. [CrossRef]
50. Rozhon, W.; Kammermeier, L.; Schramm, S.; Towfique, N.; Adebimpe Adedeji, N.; Adesola Ajayi, S.; Poppenberger, B. Quantification of the Pyrrolizidine Alkaloid Jacobine in *Crassocephalum crepidioides* by Cation Exchange High-Performance Liquid Chromatography. *Phytochem. Anal.* **2017**, *29*, 48–58. [CrossRef]
51. Joosten, L.; Cheng, D.; Mulder, P.P.; Vrieling, K.; van Veen, J.A.; Klinkhamer, P.G. The genotype dependent presence of pyrrolizidine alkaloids as tertiary amine in *Jacobaea vulgaris*. *Phytochemistry* **2011**, *72*, 214–222. [CrossRef]
52. Ehmke, A.; von Borstel, K.; Hartmann, T. Alkaloid N-oxides as transport and vacuolar storage compounds of pyrrolizidine alkaloids in *Senecio vulgaris* L. *Planta* **1988**, *176*, 83–90. [CrossRef] [PubMed]
53. Herrmann, M.; Joppe, H.; Schmaus, G. Thesinine-4'-O-beta-D-glucoside the first glycosylated plant pyrrolizidine alkaloid from *Borago officinalis*. *Phytochemistry* **2002**, *60*, 399–402. [CrossRef]
54. Koulman, A.; Seeliger, C.; Edwards, P.J.; Fraser, K.; Simpson, W.; Johnson, L.; Cao, M.; Rasmussen, S.; Lane, G.A. E/Z-Thesinine-O-4'-alpha-rhamnoside, pyrrolizidine conjugates produced by grasses (Poaceae). *Phytochemistry* **2008**, *69*, 1927–1932. [CrossRef] [PubMed]
55. Nowacki, E.; Byerrum, R.U. Biosynthesis of lupanine from lysine and other labeled compounds. *Biochem. Biophys. Res. Commun.* **1962**, *7*, 58–61. [CrossRef]
56. Nowacki, E.; Byerrum, R.U. A study on the biosynthesis of the *Crotalaria* alkaloids. *Life Sci.* **1962**, *1*, 157–161. [CrossRef]
57. Khan, H.A.; Robins, D.J. Pyrrolizidine alkaloid biosynthesis; incorporation of ^{13}C-labelled putrescines into retronecine. *J. Chem. Soc. Chem. Commun.* **1981**, 146–147. [CrossRef]
58. Khan, H.A.; Robins, D.J. Pyrrolizidine alkaloids: Evidence for N-(4-aminobutyl)-1,4-diaminobutane (homospermidine) as an intermediate in retronecine biosynthesis. *J. Chem. Soc. Chem. Commun.* **1981**, 554–556. [CrossRef]
59. Rana, J.; Robins, D.J. Application of ^{2}H n.m.r. Spectroscopy to study the incorporation of ^{2}H-labelled putrescines into the pyrrolizidine alkaloid retrorsine. *J. Chem. Soc. Perkin Trans. 1* **1986**, 983–988. [CrossRef]
60. Hughes, C.A.; Letcher, R.; Warren, F.L. 956. The Senecio alkaloids. Part XVI. The biosynthesis of the "necine" bases from carbon-14 precursors. *J. Chem. Soc.* **1964**, 4974–4978. [CrossRef]
61. Bottomley, W.; Gheissman, T.A. Pyrrolizidine alkaloids. The biosynthesis of retronecine. *Phytochemistry* **1964**, *3*, 357–360. [CrossRef]
62. Bale, N.M.; Crout, D.H.G. Determination of the relative rates of incorporation of arginine and ornithine into retronecine during pyrrolizidine alkaloid biosynthesis. *Phytochemistry* **1975**, *14*, 2617–2622. [CrossRef]
63. Robins, D.J.; Sweeney, J.R. Pyrrolizidine alkaloid biosynthesis. Incorporation of ^{14}C-labelled precursors into retronecine. *J. Chem. Soc. Perkin Trans. 1* **1981**, 3083–3086. [CrossRef]
64. Robins, D.J.; Sweeney, J.R. Pyrrolizidine alkaloid biosynthesis: Derivation of retronecine from L-arginine and L-ornithine. *Phytochemistry* **1983**, *22*, 457–459. [CrossRef]
65. Khan, H.A.; Robins, D.J. Pyrrolizidine alkaloid biosynthesis. Synthesis of ^{13}C-labelled putrescines and their incorporation into retronecine. *J. Chem. Soc. Perkin Trans. 1* **1985**, 101–105. [CrossRef]
66. Grue-Soerensen, G.; Spenser, I.D. Biosynthesis of retronecine. *J. Am. Chem. Soc.* **1981**, *103*, 3208–3210. [CrossRef]
67. Grue-Sørensen, G.; Spenser, I.D. The biosynthesis of retronecine. *Can. J. Chem.* **1982**, *60*, 643–662. [CrossRef]
68. Kelly, H.A.; Robins, D.J. Pyrrolizidine alkaloid biosynthesis. Incorporation of ^{13}C-labelled precursors into rosmarinine. *J. Chem. Soc. Perkin Trans. 1* **1987**, 177–180. [CrossRef]

69. Khan, H.A.; Robins, D.J. Pyrrolizidine alkaloid biosynthesis. Synthesis of ^{14}C-labelled homospermidines and their incorporation into retronecine. *J. Chem. Soc. Perkin Trans. 1* **1985**, 819–824. [CrossRef]
70. Robins, D.J. Chapter 1 Biosynthesis of Pyrrolizidine and Quinolizidine Alkaloids. In *The Alkaloids: Chemistry and Pharmacology*; Cordell, G.A., Ed.; Academic Press: Cambridge, MA, USA, 1995; Volume 46, pp. 1–61.
71. Böttcher, F.; Adolph, R.D.; Hartmann, T. Homospermidine synthase, the first pathway-specific enzyme in pyrrolizidine alkaloid biosynthesis. *Phytochemistry* **1993**, *32*, 679–689. [CrossRef]
72. Ober, D.; Hartmann, T. Phylogenetic origin of a secondary pathway: The case of pyrrolizidine alkaloids. *Plant Mol. Biol.* **2000**, *44*, 445–450. [CrossRef]
73. Krishna, R.G.; Wold, F. Post-translational modification of proteins. *Adv. Enzymol. Relat. Areas Mol. Biol.* **1993**, *67*, 265–298. [CrossRef] [PubMed]
74. Park, M.H.; Lee, Y.B.; Joe, Y.A. Hypusine is essential for eukaryotic cell proliferation. *Neurosignals* **1997**, *6*, 115–123. [CrossRef]
75. Ober, D.; Kaltenegger, E. Pyrrolizidine alkaloid biosynthesis, evolution of a pathway in plant secondary metabolism. *Phytochemistry* **2009**, *70*, 1687–1695. [CrossRef] [PubMed]
76. Gill, G.P.; Bryant, C.J.; Fokin, M.; Huege, J.; Fraser, K.; Jones, C.; Cao, M.; Faville, M.J. Low pyrrolizidine alkaloid levels in perennial ryegrass is associated with the absence of a homospermidine synthase gene. *BMC Plant Biol.* **2018**, *18*, 56. [CrossRef] [PubMed]
77. Livshultz, T.; Kaltenegger, E.; Straub, S.C.K.; Weitemier, K.; Hirsch, E.; Koval, K.; Mema, L.; Liston, A. Evolution of pyrrolizidine alkaloid biosynthesis in Apocynaceae: Revisiting the defence de-escalation hypothesis. *New Phytol.* **2018**, *218*, 762–773. [CrossRef] [PubMed]
78. Reimann, A.; Nurhayati, N.; Backenkohler, A.; Ober, D. Repeated evolution of the pyrrolizidine alkaloid-mediated defense system in separate angiosperm lineages. *Plant Cell* **2004**, *16*, 2772–2784. [CrossRef] [PubMed]
79. Ober, D.; Harms, R.; Witte, L.; Hartmann, T. Molecular evolution by change of function. Alkaloid-specific homospermidine synthase retained all properties of deoxyhypusine synthase except binding the eIF5A precursor protein. *J. Biol. Chem.* **2003**, *278*, 12805–12812. [CrossRef] [PubMed]
80. Ober, D.; Hartmann, T. Deoxyhypusine synthase from tobacco. cDNA isolation, characterization, and bacterial expression of an enzyme with extended substrate specificity. *J. Biol. Chem.* **1999**, *274*, 32040–32047. [CrossRef]
81. Moll, S.; Anke, S.; Kahmann, U.; Hansch, R.; Hartmann, T.; Ober, D. Cell-specific expression of homospermidine synthase, the entry enzyme of the pyrrolizidine alkaloid pathway in *Senecio vernalis*, in comparison with its ancestor, deoxyhypusine synthase. *Plant Physiol.* **2002**, *130*, 47–57. [CrossRef]
82. Anke, S.; Niemuller, D.; Moll, S.; Hansch, R.; Ober, D. Polyphyletic origin of pyrrolizidine alkaloids within the Asteraceae. Evidence from differential tissue expression of homospermidine synthase. *Plant Physiol.* **2004**, *136*, 4037–4047. [CrossRef]
83. Anke, S.; Gonde, D.; Kaltenegger, E.; Hansch, R.; Theuring, C.; Ober, D. Pyrrolizidine alkaloid biosynthesis in Phalaenopsis orchids: Developmental expression of alkaloid-specific homospermidine synthase in root tips and young flower buds. *Plant Physiol.* **2008**, *148*, 751–760. [CrossRef] [PubMed]
84. Niemuller, D.; Reimann, A.; Ober, D. Distinct cell-specific expression of homospermidine synthase involved in pyrrolizidine alkaloid biosynthesis in three species of the boraginales. *Plant Physiol.* **2012**, *159*, 920–929. [CrossRef] [PubMed]
85. Hughes, A.L. The evolution of functionally novel proteins after gene duplication. *Proc. Biol. Sci.* **1994**, *256*, 119–124. [CrossRef] [PubMed]
86. Zhang, J. Evolution by gene duplication: An update. *Trends Ecol. Evol.* **2003**, *18*, 292–298. [CrossRef]
87. Abdelhady, M.I.; Beuerle, T.; Ober, D. Homospermidine in transgenic tobacco results in considerably reduced spermidine levels but is not converted to pyrrolizidine alkaloid precursors. *Plant Mol. Biol.* **2009**, *71*, 145–155. [CrossRef]
88. Robins, D.J. The pyrrolizidine alkaloids. *Fortschr. Chem. Org. Naturst.* **1982**, *41*, 115–203.
89. Frolich, C.; Ober, D.; Hartmann, T. Tissue distribution, core biosynthesis and diversification of pyrrolizidine alkaloids of the lycopsamine type in three *Boraginaceae* species. *Phytochemistry* **2007**, *68*, 1026–1037. [CrossRef]
90. Cheng, D.; Kirk, H.; Vrieling, K.; Mulder, P.P.; Klinkhamer, P.G. The relationship between structurally different pyrrolizidine alkaloids and western flower thrips resistance in F(2) hybrids of *Jacobaea vulgaris* and *Jacobaea aquatica*. *J. Chem. Ecol.* **2011**, *37*, 1071–1080. [CrossRef]

91. Wesseling, A.M.; Demetrowitsch, T.J.; Schwarz, K.; Ober, D. Variability of Pyrrolizidine Alkaloid Occurrence in Species of the Grass Subfamily Pooideae (Poaceae). *Front. Plant Sci.* **2017**, *8*, 2046. [CrossRef]
92. Dodson, C.D.; Stermitz, F.R. Pyrrolizidine Alkaloids from Borage (*Borago officinalis*) Seeds and Flowers. *J. Nat. Prod.* **1986**, *49*, 727–728. [CrossRef]
93. O'Dowd, D.J.; Edgar, J.A. Seasonal dynamics in the pyrrolizidine alkaloids of *Heliotropium europaeum*. *Aust. J. Ecol.* **1989**, *14*, 95–105. [CrossRef]
94. Birecka, H.; Catalfamo, J.L. Incorporation of assimilated carbon into aminoalcohols of *Heliotropium spathulatum*. *Phytochemistry* **1982**, *21*, 2645–2651. [CrossRef]
95. Leete, E. Biosynthesis and metabolism of the tropane alkaloids. *Planta Med.* **1979**, *36*, 97–112. [CrossRef]
96. Leete, E.; Murrill, J.B. Biosynthesis of the tiglic acid moiety of meteloidine in *Datura meteloides*. *Tetrahedron Lett.* **1967**, *18*, 1727–1730. [CrossRef]
97. Leete, E. Biosynthetic conversion of α-methylbutyric acid to tiglic acid in *Datura meteloides*. *Phytochemistry* **1973**, *12*, 2203–2205. [CrossRef]
98. Attygalle, A.B.; Wu, X.; Will, K.W. Biosynthesis of tiglic, ethacrylic, and 2-methylbutyric acids in a carabid beetle, *Pterostichus* (Hypherpes) *californicus*. *J. Chem. Ecol.* **2007**, *33*, 963–970. [CrossRef] [PubMed]
99. Robinson, W.G.; Bachhawat, B.K.; Coon, M.J. Tiglyl coenzyme A and alpha-methylacetoacetyl coenzyme A, intermediates in the enzymatic degradation of isoleucine. *J. Biol. Chem.* **1956**, *218*, 391–400.
100. Mcgaw, B.A.; Woolley, J.G. The biosynthesis of angelic acid in *Cynoglossum officinale*. *Phytochemistry* **1979**, *18*, 1647–1649. [CrossRef]
101. Hughes, C.; Warren, F.L. The Senecio alkaloids. Part XIV. The biological synthesis of the "necic" acids using carbon-14. *J. Chem. Soc.* **1962**, 34–37. [CrossRef]
102. Crout, D.H. Pyrrolizidine alkaloids. The biosynthesis of echimidinic acid. *J. Chem. Soc. Perkin Trans. 1* **1966**, *21*, 1968–1972. [CrossRef]
103. Weber, S.; Eisenreich, W.; Bacher, A.; Hartmann, T. Pyrrolizidine alkaloids of the lycopsamine type: Biosynthesis of trachelanthic acid. *Phytochemistry* **1999**, *50*, 1005–1014. [CrossRef]
104. Robins, D.J.; Bale, N.M.; Crout, D.H. Pyrrolizidine alkaloids. Biosynthesis of monocrotalic acid, the necic acid component of monocrotaline. *J. Chem. Soc. Perkin Trans. 1* **1974**, 2082–2086. [CrossRef]
105. Rao, P.G.; Zutshi, U.; Soni, A.; Atal, C.K. Studies on Incorporation of ^{14}C–Labelled Precursors in Monocrotaline. *Planta Med.* **1979**, *35*, 279–282. [CrossRef]
106. Devlin, J.A.; Robins, D.J. Pyrrolizidine alkaloids. Biosynthesis of trichodesmic acid. *J. Chem. Soc. Perkin Trans. 1* **1984**, 1329–1332. [CrossRef]
107. Crout, D.H.G.; Benn, M.H.; Imaseki, H.; Geissman, T.A. Pyrrolizidine alkaloids: The biosynthesis of seneciphyllic acid. *Phytochemistry* **1966**, *5*, 1–21. [CrossRef]
108. Crout, D.H.; Smith, E.H.; Davies, N.M.; Whitehouse, D. Pyrrolizidine alkaloids. The biosynthesis of senecic acid. *J. Chem. Soc. Perkin Trans. 1* **1972**, *5*, 671–680. [CrossRef]
109. Crout, D.H.G.; Davies, N.M.; Smith, E.H.; Whitehouse, D. Biosynthesis of the C10 necic acids of the pyrrolizidine alkaloids. *J. Chem. Soc. D* **1970**, 635–636. [CrossRef]
110. Davies, N.M.; Crout, D.H. Pyrrolizidine alkaloid biosynthesis. Relative rates of incorporation of the isomers of isoleucine into the necic acid component of senecionine. *J. Chem. Soc. Perkin Trans. 1* **1974**, 2079–2082. [CrossRef]
111. Bale, N.M.; Cahill, R.; Davies, N.M.; Mitchell, M.B.; Smith, E.H.; Crout, D.H.G. Biosynthesis of the necic acids of the pyrrolizidine alkaloids. Further investigations of the formation of senecic and isatinecic acids in *Senecio* species. *J. Chem. Soc. Perkin Trans. 1* **1978**, 101–110. [CrossRef]
112. Stirling, I.R.; Freer, I.K.A.; Robins, D.J. Pyrrolizidine Alkaloid Biosynthesis. Incorporation of 2-Aminobutanoic Acid Labeled with ^{13}C or ^{2}H into the Senecic Acid Portion of Rosmarinine and Senecionine. *J. Chem. Soc. Perkin Trans. 1* **1997**, *1*, 677–680. [CrossRef]
113. Cahill, R.; Crout, D.H.G.; Gregorio, M.V.M.; Mitchell, M.B.; Muller, U.S. Pyrrolizidine alkaloid biosynthesis: Stereochemistry of the formation of isoleucine in *Senecio* species and of its conversion into necic acids. *J. Chem. Soc. Perkin Trans. 1* **1983**, 173–180. [CrossRef]
114. Binder, S. Branched-Chain Amino Acid Metabolism in *Arabidopsis thaliana*. *Arabidopsis Book* **2010**, *8*, e0137. [CrossRef]
115. Sander, H.; Hartmann, T. Site of synthesis, metabolism and translocation of senecionine N-oxide in cultured roots of *Senecio erucifolius*. *Plant Cell Tissue Organ Cult.* **1989**, *18*, 19–31. [CrossRef]

116. Hartmann, T.; Dierich, B. Chemical diversity and variation of pyrrolizidine alkaloids of the senecionine type: Biological need or coincidence? *Planta* **1998**, *206*, 443–451. [CrossRef]
117. Kruse, L.H.; Stegemann, T.; Sievert, C.; Ober, D. Identification of a Second Site of Pyrrolizidine Alkaloid Biosynthesis in Comfrey to Boost Plant Defense in Floral Stage. *Plant Physiol.* **2017**, *174*, 47–55. [CrossRef]
118. Hol, W.H. The effect of nutrients on pyrrolizidine alkaloids in *Senecio* plants and their interactions with herbivores and pathogens. *Phytochem. Rev.* **2011**, *10*, 119–126. [CrossRef]
119. Kirk, H.; Vrieling, K.; Van Der Meijden, E.; Klinkhamer, P.G. Species by environment interactions affect pyrrolizidine alkaloid expression in *Senecio jacobaea, Senecio aquaticus*, and their hybrids. *J. Chem. Ecol.* **2010**, *36*, 378–387. [CrossRef]
120. Kostenko, O.; Mulder, P.P.; Bezemer, T.M. Effects of root herbivory on pyrrolizidine alkaloid content and aboveground plant-herbivore-parasitoid interactions in *Jacobaea vulgaris*. *J. Chem. Ecol.* **2013**, *39*, 109–119. [CrossRef]
121. Vrieling, K.; de Vos, H.; van Wijk, C.A. Genetic analysis of the concentrations of pyrrolizidine alkaloids in *Senecio jacobaea*. *Phytochemistry* **1993**, *32*, 1141–1144. [CrossRef]
122. Van Dam, N.M.; Vrieling, K. Genetic variation in constitutive and inducible pyrrolizidine alkaloid levels in *Cynoglossum officinale* L. *Oecologia* **1994**, *99*, 374–378. [CrossRef]
123. Macel, M.; Vrieling, K.; Klinkhamer, P.G. Variation in pyrrolizidine alkaloid patterns of *Senecio jacobaea*. *Phytochemistry* **2004**, *65*, 865–873. [CrossRef] [PubMed]
124. Pelser, P.B.; de Vos, H.; Theuring, C.; Beuerle, T.; Vrieling, K.; Hartmann, T. Frequent gain and loss of pyrrolizidine alkaloids in the evolution of *Senecio* section *Jacobaea* (Asteraceae). *Phytochemistry* **2005**, *66*, 1285–1295. [CrossRef] [PubMed]
125. Cheng, D.; Kirk, H.; Mulder, P.P.; Vrieling, K.; Klinkhamer, P.G. Pyrrolizidine alkaloid variation in shoots and roots of segregating hybrids between *Jacobaea vulgaris* and *Jacobaea aquatica*. *New Phytol.* **2011**, *192*, 1010–1023. [CrossRef]
126. Wei, X.; Vrieling, K.; Mulder, P.P.J.; Klinkhamer, P.G.L. Methyl Jasmonate Changes the Composition and Distribution Rather than the Concentration of Defence Compounds: A Study on Pyrrolizidine Alkaloids. *J. Chem. Ecol.* **2018**. [CrossRef] [PubMed]
127. Sievert, C.; Beuerle, T.; Hollmann, J.; Ober, D. Single cell subtractive transcriptomics for identification of cell-specifically expressed candidate genes of pyrrolizidine alkaloid biosynthesis. *Phytochemistry* **2015**, *117*, 17–24. [CrossRef] [PubMed]
128. Abd El-Mawla, A.M. Effect of certain elicitors on production of pyrrolizidine alkaloids in hairy root cultures of *Echium rauwolfii*. *Pharmazie* **2010**, *65*, 224–226. [CrossRef] [PubMed]
129. Hartmann, T.; Ehmke, A.; Eilert, U.; von Borstel, K.; Theuring, C. Sites of synthesis, translocation and accumulation of pyrrolizidine alkaloid N-oxides in *Senecio vulgaris* L. *Planta* **1989**, *177*, 98–107. [CrossRef] [PubMed]
130. Hartmann, T.; Toppel, G. Senecionine N-oxide, the primary product of pyrrolizidine alkaloid biosynthesis in root cultures of *Senecio vulgaris*. *Phytochemistry* **1987**, *26*, 1639–1643. [CrossRef]
131. Van Dam, N.M.; Vuister, L.W.; Bergshoeff, C.; de Vos, H.; van Der Meijden, E. The "Raison D'etre" of pyrrolizidine alkaloids in *Cynoglossum officinale*: Deterrent effects against generalist herbivores. *J. Chem. Ecol.* **1995**, *21*, 507–523. [CrossRef]
132. Bennett, R.N.; Wallsgrove, R.M. Secondary Metabolites in Plant Defense-Mechanisms. *New Phytol.* **1994**, *127*, 617–633. [CrossRef]
133. Van der Meijden, E. Plant defence, an evolutionary dilemma: Contrasting effects of (specialist and generalist) herbivores and natural enemies. In Proceedings of the 9th International Symposium on Insect-Plant Relationships; Städler, E., Rowell-Rahier, M., Bauer, R., Eds.; Springer Netherlands: Dordrecht, The Netherlands, 1996; pp. 307–310.
134. Hartmann, T. Chemical ecology of pyrrolizidine alkaloids. *Planta* **1999**, *207*, 483–495. [CrossRef]
135. Boppré, M. Insects pharmacophagously utilizing defensive plant chemicals (*Pyrrolizidine alkaloids*). *Naturwissenschaften* **1986**, *73*, 17–26. [CrossRef]
136. Cheng, D.; van der Meijden, E.; Mulder, P.P.; Vrieling, K.; Klinkhamer, P.G. Pyrrolizidine alkaloid composition influences cinnabar moth oviposition preferences in *Jacobaea* hybrids. *J. Chem. Ecol.* **2013**, *39*, 430–437. [CrossRef] [PubMed]

137. Wei, X.; Vrieling, K.; Mulder, P.P.; Klinkhamer, P.G. Testing the generalist-specialist dilemma: The role of pyrrolizidine alkaloids in resistance to invertebrate herbivores in *Jacobaea* species. *J. Chem. Ecol.* **2015**, *41*, 159–167. [CrossRef] [PubMed]
138. Macel, M.; Bruinsma, M.; Dijkstra, S.M.; Ooijendijk, T.; Niemeyer, H.M.; Klinkhamer, P.G. Differences in effects of pyrrolizidine alkaloids on five generalist insect herbivore species. *J. Chem. Ecol.* **2005**, *31*, 1493–1508. [CrossRef]
139. Leiss, K.A.; Choi, Y.H.; Abdel-Farid, I.B.; Verpoorte, R.; Klinkhamer, P.G. NMR metabolomics of thrips (*Frankliniella occidentalis*) resistance in *Senecio* hybrids. *J. Chem. Ecol.* **2009**, *35*, 219–229. [CrossRef]
140. Dreyer, D.L.; Jones, K.C.; Molyneux, R.J. Feeding deterrency of some pyrrolizidine, indolizidine, and quinolizidine alkaloids towards pea aphid (*Acyrthosiphon pisum*) and evidence for phloem transport of indolizidine alkaloid swainsonine. *J. Chem. Ecol.* **1985**, *11*, 1045–1051. [CrossRef]
141. Liu, X.; Klinkhamer, P.G.L.; Vrieling, K. The effect of structurally related metabolites on insect herbivores: A case study on pyrrolizidine alkaloids and western flower thrips. *Phytochemistry* **2017**, *138*, 93–103. [CrossRef]
142. Nuringtyas, T.R.; Verpoorte, R.; Klinkhamer, P.G.L.; van Oers, M.M.; Leiss, K.A. Toxicity of Pyrrolizidine Alkaloids to *Spodoptera exigua* Using Insect Cell Lines and Injection Bioassays. *J. Chem. Ecol.* **2014**, *40*, 609–616. [CrossRef]
143. Lindigkeit, R.; Biller, A.; Buch, M.; Schiebel, H.M.; Boppre, M.; Hartmann, T. The two facies of pyrrolizidine alkaloids: The role of the tertiary amine and its N-oxide in chemical defense of insects with acquired plant alkaloids. *Eur. J. Biochem.* **1997**, *245*, 626–636. [CrossRef]
144. Von Borstel, K.; Hartmann, T. Selective uptake of pyrrolizidine N-oxides by cell suspension cultures from pyrrolizidine alkaloid producing plants. *Plant Cell Rep.* **1986**, *5*, 39–42. [CrossRef] [PubMed]
145. Liu, X.; Vrieling, K.; Klinkhamer, P.G.L. Interactions between Plant Metabolites Affect Herbivores: A Study with Pyrrolizidine Alkaloids and Chlorogenic Acid. *Front. Plant Sci.* **2017**, *8*, 903. [CrossRef] [PubMed]
146. Liu, X.; Vrieling, K.; Klinkhamer, P.G.L. Phytochemical Background Mediates Effects of Pyrrolizidine Alkaloids on Western Flower Thrips. *J. Chem. Ecol.* **2018**. [CrossRef] [PubMed]
147. Eisner, T.; Meinwald, J. The chemistry of sexual selection. *Proc. Natl. Acad. Sci. USA* **1995**, *92*, 50–55. [CrossRef] [PubMed]
148. Trigo, J. Effects of pyrrolizidine alkaloids through different trophic levels. *Phytochem. Rev.* **2011**, *10*, 83–98. [CrossRef]
149. Martins, C.H.; Cunha, B.P.; Solferini, V.N.; Trigo, J.R. Feeding on Host Plants with Different Concentrations and Structures of Pyrrolizidine Alkaloids Impacts the Chemical-Defense Effectiveness of a Specialist Herbivore. *PLoS ONE* **2015**, *10*, e0141480. [CrossRef]
150. Masters, A.R. Pyrrolizidine Alkaloids in Artificial Nectar Protect Adult Ithomiine Butterflies from a Spider Predator. *Biotropica* **1990**, *22*, 298–304. [CrossRef]
151. Silva, K.L.; Trigo, J.R. Structure-activity relationships of pyrrolizidine alkaloids in insect chemical defense against the orb-weaving spider *Nephila clavipes*. *J. Chem. Ecol.* **2002**, *28*, 657–668. [CrossRef]
152. Brown, K.S. Chemistry at the Solanaceae/Ithomiinae Interface. *Ann. Mo. Bot. Garden* **1987**, *74*, 359–397. [CrossRef]
153. Boppré, M. Lepidoptera and pyrrolizidine alkaloids Exemplification of complexity in chemical ecology. *J. Chem. Ecol.* **1990**, *16*, 165–185. [CrossRef]
154. Ehmke, A.; Witte, L.; Biller, A.; Hartmann, T. Sequestration, N-Oxidation and Transformation of Plant Pyrrolizidine Alkaloids by the Arctiid Moth *Tyria jacobaeae* L. *Z. Naturforsch. C* **1990**, *45*, 1185. [CrossRef]
155. Hartmann, T.; Biller, A.; Witte, L.; Ernst, L.; Boppré, M. Transformation of plant pyrrolizidine alkaloids into novel insect alkaloids by Arctiid moths (Lepidoptera). *Biochem. Syst. Ecol.* **1990**, *18*, 549–554. [CrossRef]
156. Kubitza, C.; Faust, A.; Gutt, M.; Gath, L.; Ober, D.; Scheidig, A.J. Crystal structure of pyrrolizidine alkaloid N-oxygenase from the grasshopper *Zonocerus variegatus*. *Acta Crystallogr. D Struct. Biol.* **2018**, *74*, 422–432. [CrossRef] [PubMed]
157. Macel, M.; Klinkhamer, P.G.L. Chemotype of *Senecio jacobaea* affects damage by pathogens and insect herbivores in the field. *Evol. Ecol.* **2010**, *24*, 237–250. [CrossRef]
158. Joshi, J.; Vrieling, K. The Enemy Release and EICA hypothesis revisited: Incorporating the fundamental difference between specialist and generalist herbivores. *Ecol. Lett.* **2005**, *8*, 704–714. [CrossRef]

159. Hol, W.H.; Van Veen, A. Pyrrolizidine alkaloids from *Senecio jacobaea* affect fungal growth. *J. Chem. Ecol.* **2002**, *28*, 1763–1772. [CrossRef] [PubMed]
160. Hill, E.M.; Robinson, L.A.; Abdul-Sada, A.; Vanbergen, A.J.; Hodge, A.; Hartley, S.E. Arbuscular Mycorrhizal Fungi and Plant Chemical Defence: Effects of Colonisation on Aboveground and Belowground Metabolomes. *J. Chem. Ecol.* **2018**, *44*, 198–208. [CrossRef] [PubMed]
161. Reidinger, S.; Eschen, R.; Gange, A.C.; Finch, P.; Bezemer, T.M. Arbuscular mycorrhizal colonization, plant chemistry, and aboveground herbivory on *Senecio jacobaea*. *Acta Oecol.* **2012**, *38*, 8–16. [CrossRef]
162. Irmer, S.; Podzun, N.; Langel, D.; Heidemann, F.; Kaltenegger, E.; Schemmerling, B.; Geilfus, C.M.; Zorb, C.; Ober, D. New aspect of plant-rhizobia interaction: Alkaloid biosynthesis in *Crotalaria* depends on nodulation. *Proc. Natl. Acad. Sci. USA* **2015**, *112*, 4164–4169. [CrossRef] [PubMed]
163. Nowak, M.; Wittke, C.; Lederer, I.; Klier, B.; Kleinwachter, M.; Selmar, D. Interspecific transfer of pyrrolizidine alkaloids: An unconsidered source of contaminations of phytopharmaceuticals and plant derived commodities. *Food Chem.* **2016**, *213*, 163–168. [CrossRef] [PubMed]
164. Mathon, C.; Edder, P.; Bieri, S.; Christen, P. Survey of pyrrolizidine alkaloids in teas and herbal teas on the Swiss market using HPLC-MS/MS. *Anal. Bioanal. Chem.* **2014**, *406*, 7345–7354. [CrossRef] [PubMed]
165. Kokalj, M.; Prikerznik, M.; Kreft, S. FTIR spectroscopy as a tool to detect contamination of rocket (*Eruca sativa* and *Diplotaxis tenuifolia*) salad with common groundsel (*Senecio vulgaris*) leaves. *J. Sci. Food Agric.* **2017**, *97*, 2238–2244. [CrossRef] [PubMed]
166. Dubecke, A.; Beckh, G.; Lullmann, C. Pyrrolizidine alkaloids in honey and bee pollen. *Food Addit. Contam. Part A Chem. Anal. Control Expo. Risk Assess.* **2011**, *28*, 348–358. [CrossRef] [PubMed]
167. Kempf, M.; Beuerle, T.; Buhringer, M.; Denner, M.; Trost, D.; von der Ohe, K.; Bhavanam, V.B.; Schreier, P. Pyrrolizidine alkaloids in honey: Risk analysis by gas chromatography-mass spectrometry. *Mol. Nutr. Food Res.* **2008**, *52*, 1193–1200. [CrossRef] [PubMed]
168. Kempf, M.; Wittig, M.; Reinhard, A.; von der Ohe, K.; Blacquiere, T.; Raezke, K.P.; Michel, R.; Schreier, P.; Beuerle, T. Pyrrolizidine alkaloids in honey: Comparison of analytical methods. *Food Addit. Contam. Part A Chem. Anal. Control Expo. Risk Assess.* **2011**, *28*, 332–347. [CrossRef] [PubMed]
169. Betz, J.M.; Eppley, R.M.; Taylor, W.C.; Andrzejewski, D. Determination of pyrrolizidine alkaloids in commercial comfrey products (*Symphytum* sp.). *J. Pharm. Sci.* **1994**, *83*, 649–653. [CrossRef] [PubMed]
170. Edgar, J.A.; Colegate, S.M.; Boppre, M.; Molyneux, R.J. Pyrrolizidine alkaloids in food: A spectrum of potential health consequences. *Food Addit. Contam. Part A Chem. Anal. Control Expo. Risk Assess.* **2011**, *28*, 308–324. [CrossRef] [PubMed]
171. Prakash, A.S.; Pereira, T.N.; Reilly, P.E.; Seawright, A.A. Pyrrolizidine alkaloids in human diet. *Mutat. Res.* **1999**, *443*, 53–67. [CrossRef]
172. Xia, Q.; Ma, L.; He, X.; Cai, L.; Fu, P.P. 7-Glutathione pyrrole adduct: A potential DNA reactive metabolite of pyrrolizidine alkaloids. *Chem. Res. Toxicol.* **2015**, *28*, 615–620. [CrossRef] [PubMed]
173. Fu, P.P.; Xia, Q.; Lin, G.; Chou, M.W. Pyrrolizidine alkaloids—Genotoxicity, metabolism enzymes, metabolic activation, and mechanisms. *Drug Metab. Rev.* **2004**, *36*, 1–55. [CrossRef]
174. Kim, H.Y.; Stermitz, F.R.; Coulombe, R.A., Jr. Pyrrolizidine alkaloid-induced DNA-protein cross-links. *Carcinogenesis* **1995**, *16*, 2691–2697. [CrossRef] [PubMed]
175. Xia, Q.; Zhao, Y.; Von Tungeln, L.S.; Doerge, D.R.; Lin, G.; Cai, L.; Fu, P.P. Pyrrolizidine alkaloid-derived DNA adducts as a common biological biomarker of pyrrolizidine alkaloid-induced tumorigenicity. *Chem. Res. Toxicol.* **2013**, *26*, 1384–1396. [CrossRef] [PubMed]
176. Huxtable, R.J.; Yan, C.C.; Wild, S.; Maxwell, S.; Cooper, R. Physicochemical and metabolic basis for the differing neurotoxicity of the pyrrolizidine alkaloids, trichodesmine and monocrotaline. *Neurochem. Res.* **1996**, *21*, 141–146. [CrossRef] [PubMed]
177. Fu, P.P.; Yang, Y.C.; Xia, Q.; Chou, M.W.; Cui, Y.Y.; Lin, G. Pyrrolizidine Alkaloids -Tumorigenic Components in Chinese Herbal Medicines and Dietary Supplements. *J. Food Drug Anal.* **2002**, *10*, 198–211.
178. FAO/WHO. Discussion paper on pyrrolizidine alkaloids, Joint FAO/WHO food standards programme. In *CODEX Committee on Contaminants in Foods*, 5th ed.; FAO: The Hague, The Netherlands, 2011.
179. Xia, Q.; Chou, M.W.; Kadlubar, F.F.; Chan, P.C.; Fu, P.P. Human liver microsomal metabolism and DNA adduct formation of the tumorigenic pyrrolizidine alkaloid, riddelliine. *Chem. Res. Toxicol.* **2003**, *16*, 66–73. [CrossRef] [PubMed]
180. Mattocks, A.R. Toxicity of pyrrolizidine alkaloids. *Nature* **1968**, *217*, 723–728. [CrossRef] [PubMed]

181. Mattocks, A.R. Hepatotoxic effects due to pyrrolizidine alkaloid N-oxides. *Xenobiotica* **1971**, *1*, 563–565. [CrossRef]
182. White, I.N.; Mattocks, A.R. Some factors affecting the conversion of pyrrolizidine alkaloids to N-oxides and to pyrrolic derivatives *in vitro*. *Xenobiotica* **1971**, *1*, 503–505. [CrossRef]
183. Lin, G.; Cui, Y.Y.; Hawes, E.M. Microsomal formation of a pyrrolic alcohol glutathione conjugate of clivorine. Firm evidence for the formation of a pyrrolic metabolite of an otonecine-type pyrrolizidine alkaloid. *Drug Metab. Dispos.* **1998**, *26*, 181–184.
184. Mattocks, A.R.; White, I.N. The conversion of pyrrolizidine alkaloids to N-oxides and to dihydropyrrolizine derivatives by rat-liver microsomes *in vitro*. *Chem. Biol. Interact.* **1971**, *3*, 383–396. [CrossRef]
185. Edgar, J.A.; Molyneux, R.J.; Colegate, S.M. Pyrrolizidine Alkaloids: Potential Role in the Etiology of Cancers, Pulmonary Hypertension, Congenital Anomalies, and Liver Disease. *Chem. Res. Toxicol.* **2015**, *28*, 4–20. [CrossRef] [PubMed]
186. Fu, P.P. Pyrrolizidine Alkaloids: Metabolic Activation Pathways Leading to Liver Tumor Initiation. *Chem. Res. Toxicol.* **2017**, *30*, 81–93. [CrossRef] [PubMed]
187. Li, N.; Xia, Q.; Ruan, J.; Fu, P.P.; Lin, G. Hepatotoxicity and tumorigenicity induced by metabolic activation of pyrrolizidine alkaloids in herbs. *Curr. Drug Metab.* **2011**, *12*, 823–834. [CrossRef] [PubMed]
188. Nigra, L.; Huxtable, R.J. Hepatic glutathione concentrations and the release of pyrrolic metabolites of the pyrrolizidine alkaloid, monocrotaline, from the isolated perfused liver. *Toxicon* **1992**, *30*, 1195–1202. [CrossRef]
189. Pereira, T.N.; Webb, R.I.; Reilly, P.E.; Seawright, A.A.; Prakash, A.S. Dehydromonocrotaline generates sequence-selective N-7 guanine alkylation and heat and alkali stable multiple fragment DNA crosslinks. *Nucleic Acids Res.* **1998**, *26*, 5441–5447. [CrossRef] [PubMed]
190. Chen, M.; Li, L.; Zhong, D.; Shen, S.; Zheng, J.; Chen, X. 9-Glutathionyl-6,7-dihydro-1-hydroxymethyl-5H-pyrrolizine Is the Major Pyrrolic Glutathione Conjugate of Retronecine-Type Pyrrolizidine Alkaloids in Liver Microsomes and in Rats. *Chem. Res. Toxicol.* **2016**, *29*, 180–189. [CrossRef] [PubMed]
191. Robertson, K.A.; Seymour, J.L.; Hsia, M.T.; Allen, J.R. Covalent interaction of dehydroretronecine, a carcinogenic metabolite of the pyrrolizidine alkaloid monocrotaline, with cysteine and glutathione. *Cancer Res.* **1977**, *37*, 3141–3144. [PubMed]
192. Dueker, S.R.; Lame, M.W.; Jones, A.D.; Morin, D.; Segall, H.J. Glutathione conjugation with the pyrrolizidine alkaloid, jacobine. *Biochem. Biophys. Res. Commun.* **1994**, *198*, 516–522. [CrossRef] [PubMed]
193. Ji, L.; Liu, T.; Wang, Z. Pyrrolizidine alkaloid clivorine induced oxidative injury on primary cultured rat hepatocytes. *Hum. Exp. Toxicol.* **2010**, *29*, 303–309. [CrossRef] [PubMed]
194. Liang, Q.; Sheng, Y.; Jiang, P.; Ji, L.; Xia, Y.; Min, Y.; Wang, Z. The gender-dependent difference of liver GSH antioxidant system in mice and its influence on isoline-induced liver injury. *Toxicology* **2011**, *280*, 61–69. [CrossRef] [PubMed]
195. Liu, T.Y.; Chen, Y.; Wang, Z.Y.; Ji, L.L.; Wang, Z.T. Pyrrolizidine alkaloid isoline-induced oxidative injury in various mouse tissues. *Exp. Toxicol. Pathol.* **2010**, *62*, 251–257. [CrossRef] [PubMed]
196. Hsu, I.C.; Allen, J.R.; Chesney, C.F. Identification and toxicological effects of dehydroretronecine, a metabolite of monocrotaline. *Proc. Soc. Exp. Biol. Med.* **1973**, *144*, 834–838. [CrossRef] [PubMed]
197. Jago, M.V.; Edgar, J.A.; Smith, L.W.; Culvenor, C.C. Metabolic conversion of heliotridine-based pyrrolizidine alkaloids to dehydroheliotridine. *Mol. Pharmacol.* **1970**, *6*, 402–406. [PubMed]
198. Fashe, M.M.; Juvonen, R.O.; Petsalo, A.; Rahnasto-Rilla, M.; Auriola, S.; Soininen, P.; Vepsalainen, J.; Pasanen, M. Identification of a new reactive metabolite of pyrrolizidine alkaloid retrorsine: (3H-pyrrolizin-7-yl)methanol. *Chem. Res. Toxicol.* **2014**, *27*, 1950–1957. [CrossRef] [PubMed]
199. Chen, T.; Mei, N.; Fu, P.P. Genotoxicity of pyrrolizidine alkaloids. *J. Appl. Toxicol.* **2010**, *30*, 183–196. [CrossRef]
200. Yang, Y.C.; Yan, J.; Doerge, D.R.; Chan, P.C.; Fu, P.P.; Chou, M.W. Metabolic activation of the tumorigenic pyrrolizidine alkaloid, riddelliine, leading to DNA adduct formation *in vivo*. *Chem. Res. Toxicol.* **2001**, *14*, 101–109. [CrossRef]
201. Fashe, M.M.; Juvonen, R.O.; Petsalo, A.; Rasanen, J.; Pasanen, M. Species-Specific Differences in the in Vitro Metabolism of Lasiocarpine. *Chem. Res. Toxicol.* **2015**, *28*, 2034–2044. [CrossRef]
202. Lin, G.; Cui, Y.Y.; Liu, X.Q. Gender differences in microsomal metabolic activation of hepatotoxic clivorine in rat. *Chem. Res. Toxicol.* **2003**, *16*, 768–774. [CrossRef]

203. Lin, G.; Tang, J.; Liu, X.Q.; Jiang, Y.; Zheng, J. Deacetylclivorine: A gender-selective metabolite of clivorine formed in female Sprague-Dawley rat liver microsomes. *Drug Metab. Dispos.* **2007**, *35*, 607–613. [CrossRef]
204. Yang, X.; Li, W.; Li, H.; Wang, X.; Chen, Y.; Guo, X.; Peng, Y.; Zheng, J. A Difference in Internal Exposure Makes Newly Weaned Mice More Susceptible to the Hepatotoxicity of Retrorsine Than Adult Mice. *Chem. Res. Toxicol.* **2018**. [CrossRef]
205. Williams, D.E.; Reed, R.L.; Kedzierski, B.; Dannan, G.A.; Guengerich, F.P.; Buhler, D.R. Bioactivation and detoxication of the pyrrolizidine alkaloid senecionine by cytochrome P-450 enzymes in rat liver. *Drug Metab. Dispos.* **1989**, *17*, 387–392. [PubMed]
206. Williams, D.E.; Reed, R.L.; Kedzierski, B.; Ziegler, D.M.; Buhler, D.R. The role of flavin-containing monooxygenase in the N-oxidation of the pyrrolizidine alkaloid senecionine. *Drug Metab. Dispos.* **1989**, *17*, 380–386. [PubMed]
207. Chou, M.W.; Wang, Y.P.; Yan, J.; Yang, Y.C.; Beger, R.D.; Williams, L.D.; Doerge, D.R.; Fu, P.P. Riddelliine N-oxide is a phytochemical and mammalian metabolite with genotoxic activity that is comparable to the parent pyrrolizidine alkaloid riddelliine. *Toxicol. Lett.* **2003**, *145*, 239–247. [CrossRef]
208. Wang, Y.P.; Yan, J.; Fu, P.P.; Chou, M.W. Human liver microsomal reduction of pyrrolizidine alkaloid N-oxides to form the corresponding carcinogenic parent alkaloid. *Toxicol. Lett.* **2005**, *155*, 411–420. [CrossRef] [PubMed]
209. Yan, J.; Xia, Q.; Chou, M.W.; Fu, P.P. Metabolic activation of retronecine and retronecine N-oxide - formation of DHP-derived DNA adducts. *Toxicol. Ind. Health* **2008**, *24*, 181–188. [CrossRef] [PubMed]
210. Huan, J.Y.; Miranda, C.L.; Buhler, D.R.; Cheeke, P.R. Species differences in the hepatic microsomal enzyme metabolism of the pyrrolizidine alkaloids. *Toxicol. Lett.* **1998**, *99*, 127–137. [CrossRef]
211. Chung, W.G.; Buhler, D.R. Major factors for the susceptibility of guinea pig to the pyrrolizidine alkaloid jacobine. *Drug Metab. Dispos.* **1995**, *23*, 1263–1267. [PubMed]
212. Dueker, S.R.; Lame, M.W.; Morin, D.; Wilson, D.W.; Segall, H.J. Guinea pig and rat hepatic microsomal metabolism of monocrotaline. *Drug Metab. Dispos.* **1992**, *20*, 275–280.
213. Dueker, S.R.; Lame, M.W.; Segall, H.J. Hydrolysis of pyrrolizidine alkaloids by guinea pig hepatic carboxylesterases. *Toxicol. Appl. Pharmacol.* **1992**, *117*, 116–121. [CrossRef]
214. Tang, J.; Akao, T.; Nakamura, N.; Wang, Z.T.; Takagawa, K.; Sasahara, M.; Hattori, M. In vitro metabolism of isoline, a pyrrolizidine alkaloid from Ligularia duciformis, by rodent liver microsomal esterase and enhanced hepatotoxicity by esterase inhibitors. *Drug Metab. Dispos.* **2007**, *35*, 1832–1839. [CrossRef]
215. He, Y.Q.; Yang, L.; Liu, H.X.; Zhang, J.W.; Liu, Y.; Fong, A.; Xiong, A.Z.; Lu, Y.L.; Yang, L.; Wang, C.H.; et al. Glucuronidation, a new metabolic pathway for pyrrolizidine alkaloids. *Chem. Res. Toxicol.* **2010**, *23*, 591–599. [CrossRef] [PubMed]
216. Ruan, J.; Liao, C.; Ye, Y.; Lin, G. Lack of metabolic activation and predominant formation of an excreted metabolite of nontoxic platynecine-type pyrrolizidine alkaloids. *Chem. Res. Toxicol.* **2014**, *27*, 7–16. [CrossRef] [PubMed]
217. Lahiri, R.; Ansari, A.A.; Vankar, Y.D. Recent developments in design and synthesis of bicyclic azasugars, carbasugars and related molecules as glycosidase inhibitors. *Chem. Soc. Rev.* **2013**, *42*, 5102–5118. [CrossRef] [PubMed]
218. Winchester, B.; Fleet, G.W.J. Amino-sugar glycosidase inhibitors: Versatile tools for glycobiologists. *Glycobiology* **1992**, *2*, 199–210. [CrossRef] [PubMed]
219. Asano, N.; Nash, R.J.; Molyneux, R.J.; Fleet, G.W.J. Sugar-mimic glycosidase inhibitors: Natural occurrence, biological activity and prospects for therapeutic application. *Tetrahedron* **2000**, *11*, 1645–1680. [CrossRef]
220. Wong, C.-H.; Halcomb, R.L.; Ichikawa, Y.; Kajimoto, T. Enzymes in Organic Synthesis: Application to the Problems of Carbohydrate Recognition (Part 2). *Angew. Chem. Int. Ed.* **1995**, *34*, 521–546. [CrossRef]
221. Davies, G.J.; Gloster, T.M.; Henrissat, B. Recent structural insights into the expanding world of carbohydrate-active enzymes. *Curr. Opin. Struct. Biol.* **2005**, *15*, 637–645. [CrossRef] [PubMed]
222. Compain, P.; Bodlenner, A. The multivalent effect in glycosidase inhibition: A new, rapidly emerging topic in glycoscience. *ChemBioChem* **2014**, *15*, 1239–1251. [CrossRef] [PubMed]
223. Asano, N. Sugar-mimicking glycosidase inhibitors: Bioactivity and application. *Cell. Mol. Life Sci.* **2009**, *66*, 1479–1492. [CrossRef] [PubMed]
224. Wrodnigg, T.M.; Steiner, A.J.; Ueberbacher, B.J. Natural and synthetic iminosugars as carbohydrate processing enzyme inhibitors for cancer therapy. *Anticancer Agents Med. Chem.* **2008**, *8*, 77–85. [CrossRef] [PubMed]

225. Rempel, B.P.; Withers, S.G. Covalent inhibitors of glycosidases and their applications in biochemistry and biology. *Glycobiology* **2008**, *18*, 570–586. [CrossRef] [PubMed]
226. Watson, A.A.; Fleet, G.W.; Asano, N.; Molyneux, R.J.; Nash, R.J. Polyhydroxylated alkaloids - natural occurrence and therapeutic applications. *Phytochemistry* **2001**, *56*, 265–295. [CrossRef]
227. Vlietinck, A.J.; De Bruyne, T.; Apers, S.; Pieters, L.A. Plant-derived leading compounds for chemotherapy of human immunodeficiency virus (HIV) infection. *Planta Med.* **1998**, *64*, 97–109. [CrossRef] [PubMed]
228. Tropea, J.E.; Molyneux, R.J.; Kaushal, G.P.; Pan, Y.T.; Mitchell, M.; Elbein, A.D. Australine, a pyrrolizidine alkaloid that inhibits amyloglucosidase and glycoprotein processing. *Biochemistry* **1989**, *28*, 2027–2034. [CrossRef] [PubMed]
229. Kato, A.; Kano, E.; Adachi, I.; Molyneux, R.J.; Watson, A.A.; Nash, R.J.; Fleet, G.W.J.; Wormald, M.R.; Kizu, H.; Ikeda, K.; et al. Australine and related alkaloids: Easy structural confirmation by ^{13}C NMR spectral data and biological activities. *Tetrahedron* **2003**, *14*, 325–331. [CrossRef]
230. Nash, R.J.; Fellows, L.E.; Dring, J.V.; Fleet, G.W.J.; Derome, A.E.; Hamor, T.A.; Scofield, A.M.; Watkin, D.J. Isolation from alexaleiopetala and X-ray crystal structure of alexine, (1r,2r,3r,7s,8s)-3-hydroxymethyl-1,2,7-trihydroxypyrrolizidine [(2r,3r,4r,5s,6s)-2-hydroxymethyl-1-azabicyclo 3.3.0 octan-3,4,6-triol], a unique pyrrolizidine alkaloid. *Tetrahedron Lett.* **1988**, *29*, 2487–2490. [CrossRef]
231. Nash, R.J.; Fellows, L.E.; Dring, J.V.; Fleet, G.W.J.; Girdhar, A.; Ramsden, N.G.; Peach, J.M.; Hegarty, M.P.; Scofield, A.M. Two alexines 3-hydroxymethyl-1,2,7-trihydroxypyrrolizidines from *Castanospermum australe*. *Phytochemistry* **1990**, *29*, 111–114. [CrossRef]
232. Horiuchi, Y.; Kondo, S.; Ikeda, T.; Ikeda, D.; Miura, K.; Hamada, M.; Takeuchi, T.; Umezawa, H. New antibiotics clazamycins A and B. *J. Antibiot.* **1979**, *32*, 762–764. [CrossRef]
233. Dolak, L.A.; DeBoer, C. Clazamycin B is antibiotic 354. *J. Antibiot.* **1980**, *33*, 83–84. [CrossRef]
234. Sugie, Y.; Hirai, H.; Kachi-Tonai, H.; Kim, Y.J.; Kojima, Y.; Shiomi, Y.; Sugiura, A.; Sugiura, A.; Suzuki, Y.; Yoshikawa, N.; et al. New pyrrolizidinone antibiotics CJ-16,264 and CJ-16,367. *J. Antibiot.* **2001**, *54*, 917–925. [CrossRef]
235. Nakai, R.; Ogawa, H.; Asai, A.; Ando, K.; Agatsuma, T.; Matsumiya, S.; Akinaga, S.; Yamashita, Y.; Mizukami, T. UCS1025A, a novel antibiotic produced by *Acremonium* sp. *J. Antibiot.* **2000**, *53*, 294–296. [CrossRef] [PubMed]
236. Roeder, E. Medicinal plants in China containing pyrrolizidine alkaloids. *Pharmazie* **2000**, *55*, 711–726. [PubMed]
237. Roeder, E.; Wiedenfeld, H. Plants containing pyrrolizidine alkaloids used in the Traditional Indian medicine—Including Ayurveda. *Pharmazie* **2013**, *68*, 83–92. [CrossRef] [PubMed]
238. Roeder, E.; Wiedenfeld, H. Pyrrolizidine alkaloids in plants used in the traditional medicine of Madagascar and the Mascarene islands. *Pharmazie* **2011**, *66*, 637–647. [CrossRef] [PubMed]
239. Roeder, E.; Wiedenfeld, H.; Edgar, J.A. Pyrrolizidine alkaloids in medicinal plants from North America. *Pharmazie* **2015**, *70*, 357–367. [CrossRef] [PubMed]
240. Larson, K.M.; Roby, M.R.; Stermitz, F.R. Unsaturated Pyrrolizidines from Borage (*Borago officinalis*), a Common Garden Herb. *J. Nat. Prod.* **1984**, *47*, 747–748. [CrossRef]
241. Luthy, J.; Brauchli, J.; Zweifel, U.; Schmid, P.; Schlatter, C. Pyrrolizidine alkaloids in medicinal plants of Boraginaceal: *Borago officinalis* L. and *Pulmonaria officinalis* L. *Pharm. Acta Helv.* **1984**, *59*, 242–246. [PubMed]
242. Wretensjö, I.; Karlberg, B. Pyrrolizidine alkaloid content in crude and processed borage oil from different processing stages. *J. Am. Oil Chem. Soc.* **2003**, *80*, 963–970. [CrossRef]
243. Vacillotto, G.; Favretto, D.; Seraglia, R.; Pagiotti, R.; Traldi, P.; Mattoli, L. A rapid and highly specific method to evaluate the presence of pyrrolizidine alkaloids in *Borago officinalis* seed oil. *J. Mass Spectrom.* **2013**, *48*, 1078–1082. [CrossRef] [PubMed]
244. Pelser, P.B.; Nordenstam, B.; Kadereit, J.W.; Watson, L.E. An ITS Phylogeny of Tribe Senecioneae (Asteraceae) and a New Delimitation of *Senecio* L. *Taxon* **2007**, *56*, 1077–1104. [CrossRef]
245. Denton, O.A. *Crassocephalum crepidioides* (Benth.) S. Moore. In *Plant Resources of Tropical Africa 2. Vegetables*; Grubben, G.J.H., Denton, O.A., Eds.; PROTA Foundation: Wageningen, The Netherlands, 2004; pp. 226–228.
246. Joshi, R.K. Study on essential oil composition of the roots of *Crassocephalum crepidioides* (benth.) S. Moore. *J. Chin. Chem. Soc.* **2014**, *59*, 2363–2365. [CrossRef]
247. Bosch, C.H. *Crassocephalum rubens* (Juss. ex Jacq.) S.Moore. In *Plant Resources of Tropical Africa 2. Vegetables*; Grubben, G.J.H., Denton, O.A., Eds.; PROTA Foundation: Wageningen, The Netherlands, 2004; pp. 228–229.

248. Dairo, F.; Adanlawo, I. Nutritional Quality of *Crassocephalum crepidioides* and *Senecio biafrae*. *Pak. J. Nutr.* **2007**, *6*, 35–39. [CrossRef]
249. Nakamura, I.; Hossain, M.A. Factors affecting seed gemination and seedling emergence of redflower ragleaf (*Crassocephalum crepidioides*). *Weed Biol. Manag.* **2009**, *9*, 315–322. [CrossRef]
250. Adedayo, B.C.; Oboh, G.; Oyeleye, S.I.; Ejakpovi, I.I.; Boligon, A.A.; Athayde, M.L. Blanching alters the phenolic constituents and in vitro antioxidant and anticholinesterases properties of fireweed (*Crassocephalum crepidioides*). *J. Taibah Univ. Med. Sci.* **2015**, *10*, 419–426. [CrossRef]
251. Adjatin, A.; Dansi, A.; Badoussi, M.E.; Sanoussi, F.; Dansi, M.; Azokpota, P.; Ahissou, H.; Akouegninou, A.; Koffi, A.; Sanni, A. Proximate, mineral and vitamin C composition of vegetable Gbolo [*Crassocephalum rubens* (Juss. ex Jacq.) S. Moore and *C. crepidioides* (Benth.) S. Moore] in Benin. *Int. J. Biol. Chem. Sci.* **2013**, *7*, 319–331. [CrossRef]
252. Adjatin, A.; Dansi, A.; Eze, S.; Assogba, P.; Dossou-Aminon, I.; Koffi, A.; Akoègninou, A.; Sanni, A. Ethnobotanical investigation and diversity of Gbolo (*Crassocephalum rubens* (Juss. ex Jacq.) S. Moore and *Crassocephalum crepidioides* (Benth.) S. Moore), a traditional leafy vegetable under domestication in Benin. *Genet. Resour. Crop. Evol.* **2012**, *59*, 1867–1881. [CrossRef]
253. Dansi, A.; Adjatin, A.; Adoukonou-Sagbadja, H.; Faladé, V.; Yedomonhan, H.; Odou, D.; Dossou, B. Traditional leafy vegetables and their use in the Benin Republic. *Genet. Resour. Crop. Evol.* **2008**, *55*, 1239–1256. [CrossRef]
254. Adjatin, A.; Dansi, A.; Badoussi, M.E.; Loko, L.; Dansi, M.; Azokpota, P.; Gbaguidi, F.; Ahissou, H.; Akoègninou, A.; Koffi, A.; et al. Phytochemical screening and toxicity studies of *Crassocephalum rubens* (Juss. ex Jacq.) S. Moore and *Crassocephalum crepidioides* (Benth.) S. Moore consumed as vegetable in Benin. *J. Chem. Pharm. Res.* **2013**, *2*, 1–13.
255. Asada, Y.; Shiraishi, M.; Takeuchi, T.; Osawa, Y.; Furuya, T. Pyrrolizidine Alkaloids from *Crassocephalum crepidioides*. *Planta Med.* **1985**, *51*, 539–540. [CrossRef]
256. Adegoke, E.A.; Akinsaya, A.; Naqvi, H.Z. Studies of Nigerian medicinal plants: A preliminary survey of plant alkaloid. *J. West Afr. Sci. Assoc.* **1968**, *13*, 13–33.
257. Chao, C.Y.; Liu, W.H.; Wu, J.J.; Yin, M.C. Phytochemical profile, antioxidative and anti-inflammatory potentials of *Gynura bicolor* DC. *J. Sci. Food Agric.* **2015**, *95*, 1088–1093. [CrossRef] [PubMed]
258. Li, W.L.; Ren, B.R.; Min, Z.; Hu, Y.; Lu, C.G.; Wu, J.L.; Chen, J.; Sun, S. The anti-hyperglycemic effect of plants in genus Gynura Cass. *Am. J. Chin. Med.* **2009**, *37*, 961–966. [CrossRef] [PubMed]
259. Teoh, W.Y.; Sim, K.S.; Moses Richardson, J.S.; Abdul Wahab, N.; Hoe, S.Z. Antioxidant Capacity, Cytotoxicity, and Acute Oral Toxicity of *Gynura bicolor*. *Evid. Based Complement. Altern. Med.* **2013**, *2013*, 958407. [CrossRef] [PubMed]
260. Teoh, W.Y.; Tan, H.P.; Ling, S.K.; Abdul Wahab, N.; Sim, K.S. Phytochemical investigation of *Gynura bicolor* leaves and cytotoxicity evaluation of the chemical constituents against HCT 116 cells. *Nat. Prod. Res.* **2016**, *30*, 448–451. [CrossRef] [PubMed]
261. Roeder, E.; Eckert, A.; Wiedenfeld, H. Pyrrolizidine alkaloids from *Gynura divaricata*. *Planta Med.* **1996**, *62*, 386. [CrossRef] [PubMed]
262. Chen, J.; Lu, H.; Fang, L.X.; Li, W.L.; Verschaeve, L.; Wang, Z.T.; De Kimpe, N.; Mangelinckx, S. Detection and Toxicity Evaluation of Pyrrolizidine Alkaloids in Medicinal Plants *Gynura bicolor* and *Gynura divaricata* Collected from Different Chinese Locations. *Chem. Biodivers.* **2017**, *14*. [CrossRef] [PubMed]
263. Seow, L.J.; Beh, H.K.; Majid, A.M.; Murugaiyah, V.; Ismail, N.; Asmawi, M.Z. Anti-angiogenic activity of *Gynura segetum* leaf extracts and its fractions. *J. Ethnopharmacol.* **2011**, *134*, 221–227. [CrossRef] [PubMed]
264. Seow, L.J.; Beh, H.K.; Umar, M.I.; Sadikun, A.; Asmawi, M.Z. Anti-inflammatory and antioxidant activities of the methanol extract of *Gynura segetum* leaf. *Int. Immunopharmacol.* **2014**, *23*, 186–191. [CrossRef] [PubMed]
265. Dai, N.; Yu, Y.C.; Ren, T.H.; Wu, J.G.; Jiang, Y.; Shen, L.G.; Zhang, J. Gynura root induces hepatic veno-occlusive disease: A case report and review of the literature. *World J. Gastroenterol.* **2007**, *13*, 1628–1631. [CrossRef] [PubMed]
266. Fang, J.; Zhang, G.; Teng, X.; Zhang, Z.; Pan, J.; Shou, Q.; Chen, M. Hematologic toxicity of *Gynura segetum* and effects on vascular endothelium in a rat model of hepatic veno-occlusive disease. *Zhonghua Gan Zang Bing Za Zhi* **2015**, *23*, 59–63. [CrossRef]

267. Lin, G.; Wang, J.Y.; Li, N.; Li, M.; Gao, H.; Ji, Y.; Zhang, F.; Wang, H.; Zhou, Y.; Ye, Y.; et al. Hepatic sinusoidal obstruction syndrome associated with consumption of *Gynura segetum*. *J. Hepatol.* **2011**, *54*, 666–673. [CrossRef] [PubMed]
268. Yu, X.Z.; Ji, T.; Bai, X.L.; Liang, L.; Wang, L.Y.; Chen, W.; Liang, T.B. Expression of MMP-9 in hepatic sinusoidal obstruction syndrome induced by *Gynura segetum*. *J. Zhejiang Univ. Sci. B* **2013**, *14*, 68–75. [CrossRef] [PubMed]
269. Liang, X.T.; Roeder, E. Senecionine from *Gynura segetum*. *Planta Med.* **1984**, *50*, 362. [CrossRef] [PubMed]
270. Yuan, S.Q.; Gu, G.M.; Wei, T.T. Studies on the alkaloids of *Gynura segetum* (Lour.) Merr. *Yao Xue Xue Bao* **1990**, *25*, 191–197. [PubMed]
271. Qi, X.; Wu, B.; Cheng, Y.; Qu, H. Simultaneous characterization of pyrrolizidine alkaloids and *N*-oxides in *Gynura segetum* by liquid chromatography/ion trap mass spectrometry. *Rapid Commun. Mass Spectrom.* **2009**, *23*, 291–302. [CrossRef] [PubMed]
272. Gallagher, R.T.; White, E.P.; Mortimer, P.H. Ryegrass staggers: Isolation of potent neurotoxins lolitrem A and lolitrem B from staggers-producing pastures. *N. Z. Vet. J.* **1981**, *29*, 189–190. [CrossRef]
273. Lyons, P.C.; Plattner, R.D.; Bacon, C.W. Occurrence of peptide and clavine ergot alkaloids in tall fescue grass. *Science* **1986**, *232*, 487–489. [CrossRef]
274. Luo, H.; Xie, L.; Zeng, J.; Xie, J. Biosynthesis and Regulation of Bioprotective Alkaloids in the Gramineae Endophytic Fungi with Implications for Herbivores Deterrents. *Curr. Microbiol.* **2015**, *71*, 719–724. [CrossRef]
275. Guerre, P. Ergot alkaloids produced by endophytic fungi of the genus Epichloe. *Toxins* **2015**, *7*, 773–790. [CrossRef]
276. Wachenheim, D.E.; Blythe, L.L.; Craig, A.M. Characterization of rumen bacterial pyrrolizidine alkaloid biotransformation in ruminants of various species. *Vet. Hum. Toxicol.* **1992**, *34*, 513–517.

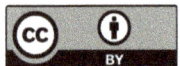

© 2019 by the authors. Licensee MDPI, Basel, Switzerland. This article is an open access article distributed under the terms and conditions of the Creative Commons Attribution (CC BY) license (http://creativecommons.org/licenses/by/4.0/).

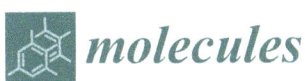

Review

Tropane Alkaloids: Chemistry, Pharmacology, Biosynthesis and Production

Kathrin Laura Kohnen-Johannsen and Oliver Kayser *

Technical Biochemistry, Department of Biochemical and Chemical Engineering, Technical University Dortmund, D-44227 Dortmund, Germany; Laura.Kohnen@tu-dortmund.de
* Correspondence: Oliver.Kayser@tu-dortmund.de; Tel.: +49-231-755-7487

Received: 15 January 2019; Accepted: 18 February 2019; Published: 22 February 2019

Abstract: Tropane alkaloids (TA) are valuable secondary plant metabolites which are mostly found in high concentrations in the Solanaceae and Erythroxylaceae families. The TAs, which are characterized by their unique bicyclic tropane ring system, can be divided into three major groups: hyoscyamine and scopolamine, cocaine and calystegines. Although all TAs have the same basic structure, they differ immensely in their biological, chemical and pharmacological properties. Scopolamine, also known as hyoscine, has the largest legitimate market as a pharmacological agent due to its treatment of nausea, vomiting, motion sickness, as well as smooth muscle spasms while cocaine is the 2nd most frequently consumed illicit drug globally. This review provides a comprehensive overview of TAs, highlighting their structural diversity, use in pharmaceutical therapy from both historical and modern perspectives, natural biosynthesis *in planta* and emerging production possibilities using tissue culture and microbial biosynthesis of these compounds.

Keywords: tropane alkaloids; scopolamine; cocaine; calystegine; chemistry; pharmacology; biosynthesis; biotechnological production

1. Introduction

Alkaloids are naturally occurring compounds containing one or more nitrogen atoms. The name is derived from the basic nature of many members of this group, alkaloids from "alkaline-like". The definition of alkaloids is complex as many nitrogen-containing molecules do not necessarily belong to this group. Biogenic amines or amino sugars, for example, are natural plant products and N-containing but not defined as alkaloids. Tropane alkaloids (TAs) are a specific class of alkaloid and can be more specifically defined as all molecules that possess a tropane ring system (Figure 1 Structure of the tropane skeleton (green box) and the three major groups of TAs derived from, green box) [1].

TAs are either esters of 3α-tropanole (tropine) or, to a lesser extent, 3β-tropanole (pseudotropine) and can be distinguished into three groups: TAs from Solanaceae plants like hyoscyamine and scopolamine, coca alkaloids like cocaine from *Erythoxylum coca* and the recently discovered calystegines group, which are polyhydroxylated nortropane alkaloids (NTAs) mainly occurring in Convolvulaceae, Solanaceae, Moraceae, Erythrocylaceae and Brassicaceae (Figure 1 Structure of the tropane skeleton (green box) and the three major groups of TAs derived from) [2]. In total, ~200 different TAs have been described [3].

Biosynthesis of the tropane ring system is homologous in organisms which produce these three TA classes. TA biosynthesis begins with the amino acids ornithine or arginine and their intermediate putrescine, continuing to the common N-methyl-Δ^1-pyrrolinium cation precursor of all TAs. This is the branch point of cocaine, hyoscyamine/scopolamine and calystegine as well as nicotine biosynthesis [4].

Although all TAs have a high degree of structural similarity due to their tropane ring, the pharmacological effects of these compounds differ significantly. Cocaine and hyoscyamine/scopolamine are able to pass the blood-brain barrier and commit dose-dependent hallucination and psychoactive effects. Calystegines do not cause these effects due to their polarity as well as hydrophilicity and consequent inability to pass this barrier.

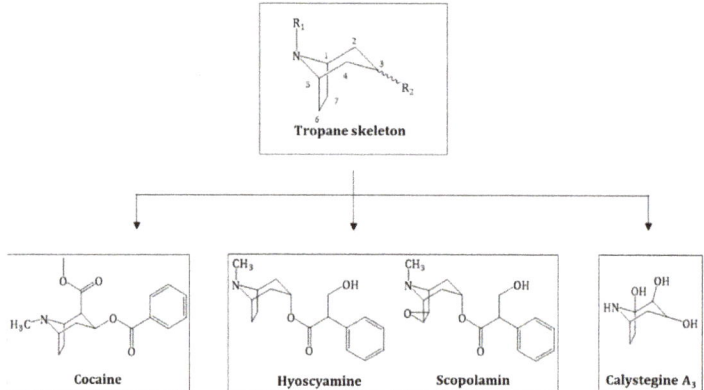

Figure 1. Structure of the tropane skeleton (green box) and the three major groups of TAs derived from this skeleton.

The cultivation of coca plants, the extraction of cocaine and production of other cocaine-containing drugs as well as their trade, with a few exceptions, is illegal and cocaine is the 2nd most frequently consumed illicit drug globally [5]. Due its legal designation, research has only been conducted on pathway elucidation in order to understand cocaine biosynthesis, however, research of large-scale commercial production has not been conducted (legally). As the calystegines are a newly discovered group of TAs without any pharmaceutical, medicinal or economic interest, little research has thus far been performed on this group of TAs. In contrast, the cultivation and production of scopolamine is of major economic interest due to its miscellaneous pharmaceutical applications. Indeed, global demand for this compound is increasing. Moreover, scopolamine is one of the Essential Medicines of the World Health Organization (WHO) [6]. Hyoscyamine and scopolamine are extracted from the *Duboisia* plants being cultivated on large plantations in Queensland, Australia [1]. Climate change and resulting new biotic and abiotic factors challenge the pharmaceutical industry to produce consistently high volumes of scopolamine. To overcome this issue, alternative production methods have been also tested.

This review seeks to provide a comprehensive overview of current knowledge on medicinal and pharmaceutical applications of TAs, a comparative analysis of TA biosynthesis and future strategies for elucidation of biosynthetic pathways, with special focus placed on the production of scopolamine as well as derivatives and enhancement of their production.

2. History and Chemical Elucidation of Tropane Alkaloids

The TAs cocaine, scopolamine and calystegines share a common tropane moiety. Nevertheless, these compounds cause very different physiological effects in humans. Cocaine manifests its effects in the synaptic cleft by inhibiting the dopamine, noradrenaline and serotonin reuptake while scopolamine acts as a competitive muscarinic receptor antagonist. The ingestion of both substances may lead to hallucinations and psychoactive effects or death [7,8]. Calystegines, on the other hand, are not absorbed into the central nervous system (CNS) due to their hydrophilicity and consequently, exhibit no psychoactive effects in humans [9].

2.1. Hyoscyamine and Scopolamine

TA producing Solanaceae plants are distributed globally. *Duboisia* plants are found in Australia and New Caledonia, while *Datura* plants, which had their origin in Asia and America, grow worldwide except in polar und subpolar climate zones. Members of the genus *Atropa* and *Hyoscyamus* have origins in Europe, Asia, as well as North Africa and were introduced to the USA, Canada and Australia [10]. All plants are simple to cultivate and readily found in nature, highly potent, and, consequently, have a long history in traditional medicines from different cultures. Until single compounds were isolated, whole plant or herbal preparations of these plants including extracts, ointments or teas were used for medicinal applications. Earliest reports of hyoscyamine or scopolamine-induced states of perception reach back into antiquity. Over 3000 years ago, *Mandragora* extracts were added to beer in Egypt to lower amounts of alcohol in these beverages. In Russia and China, *Datura* extracts and in Europe *Hyoscyamus* was added to enhance the thrilling effect of beer. A physician in Babylonia documented the analgesic property of the nightshades to reduce toothache [11]. In addition to hallucinogenic and analgesic effects, nightshades have a history of being used as poisons, for example, a wave of unexplainable mortality in the French high-society during was attributed to these plants [12]. In Australia, indigenous people exploited the TA-containing *Duboisia* plants for centuries for their cholinergic activity [13]. *Hopwoodii*, also called pituri, produces the alkaloid nicotine, which is arguably more widely popular for common use than the *Duboisia* plants *leichhardtii* and *myoporoides* [14].

Solanaceae plants have been given several names due to their historical and widespread use. These names often reflect the type of application and respective pharmacological action. *Datura stramonium*, which was introduced to European medicine by Romany immigrants, is called asthma herb due to its application in mitigating the symptoms of asthma. If *Datura* herb is smoked, a bronchorelaxation effect has been documented. Further names are "thornapple" after the hooked capsule or "horse poison" due to the toxic effects after ingestion on equines that are particularly sensitive to TAs [15]. The common *Datura* name jimsonweed is derived from Jamestown, a town in Virginia (USA) and it was reported that in 1676, settlers ingested this weed with fatal results. The intoxications were described and documented vividly leading to this additional name [10,16]. *Atropa* is named after the Greek goddess of fate and the goddess of the kingdom of the dead, Atropos. The species name belladonna is derived from its pharmacological effect, the mydriasis. Applying the extract into the eye, enflames beautiful eyes - with the disadvantage that the eye is unable to accommodate and one cannot see properly [11]. *Mandragora* and *Hyoscyamus* plants have historically played essential roles as the major active substances in the ointments of "witches" [17]. As TAs can easily be absorbed through the skin, it has been documented that the witches' flying ointment was rubbed onto broomsticks, so the toxins were absorbed through the rectum and vagina. The intoxicating effects of these ointments have been reported as a feeling of lightness of being, followed by strong and vivid delirium and hallucinations. These effects were so pronounced that many users thought themselves to fly and the skill to fly was associated with witchcraft [18]. Solanaceae TAs were also used for love potion, exploiting the aphrodisiac qualities which could evoke sexual feelings [19].

The isolation and structural elucidation of TAs from Solanaceae plants began with the discovery of atropine. In 1832, this alkaloid was isolated by the German pharmacist H. F. G. Mein, however, he did not publish his results [20]. One year later, P. L. Geiger and O. Hesse (1833) published the isolation of atropine, a nitrogen containing, alkaline substance, from *Atropa belladonna* and *Hyoscyamus niger*. They described early investigations regarding the medicinal use, different isolation methods and chemical properties [21]. The stereochemical relation between atropine and hyoscyamine was elucidated by K. Kraut and W. Lossen almost fifty years later [22,23]. They were able to elucidate the reaction mechanism of the alkaline hydrolyzation of hyoscyamine and detected that the cleavage products of both, hyoscyamine and atropine, are tropic acid and tropine. From this it was concluded that atropine is the racemate of hyoscyamine [23]. A. Ladenburg (1879) discovered that the reverse reaction of the hydrolysis is possible by boiling the educts in hydrochloric acid and established a frequently used method of esterifying tropine with numerous organic acids [24].

2.2. Cocaine

The first reports of the use of cocaine date back to 3000 B.C. in Ecuador. The cultivation and chewing of coca plant leaves is assumed to have originated on the Eastern slope of the Ecuadorian or Peruvian Andes by the Inca peoples. Tribesmen traditionally chewed the leaves of the coca plant together with lime to release the alkaloids, both for spiritual purposes such as burial ceremonies or to give strength and energy and also to tolerate thin air high at high altitudes in the mountains. The coca plant and its invigorating effect was believed to be a mysterious gift of the gods. Before the Spanish soldiers entered South America, chewing coca leaves was reserved only for the tribal leaders. After the Spanish conquest of South America, its use was spread of over the continent and no longer socially limited. Cocaine was isolated for the first time in 1855 by F. Gaedecke. He published his results in the journal Archiv der Pharmacie and called the substance, isolated from coca leaves, Erythroxyline [25]. Working on cocaine was an interesting field but due to the limited access to plant samples available in Europe, little research could be conducted. Albert Niemann, who received enough supply of coca leaves for research, was able to proceed his study and improved the isolation process as well as the general knowledge of cocaine and its mode of action [26]. The chemical formula of cocaine was determined in 1862 by W. Lossen, who also dealt with the analysis of atropine. Subsequently, the first chemical synthesis and the elucidation of its chemical structure was achieved by R. Willstätter in 1898. About fifty years later, the stereochemistry was elucidated by the Swiss chemists E. Hardegger and H. Ott [27]. However, not all published reports on cocaine and its chemistry were scientifically or ethically correct. In 1885, S. Freud published his work "Über Coca" and recommended cocaine as an almost miracle medicine, with local anaesthetic properties, which is best for the treatment for postnatal depression and morphine addiction—a dangerous application for a substance with such high addictive potential [28].

2.3. Calystegines

Polyhydroxylated NTAs like calystegine do not show any psychoactive effects due to their inability to pass the blood-brain barrier based on their hydrophilicity. In addition, they exhibit minimal pharmacological activity. As a result, this class of NTAs have not found use in ancient medicines. Recently, researchers proposed that these compounds inhibit mammalian and plant glucosidases, although until now they do not have any pharmacological application and have received little research attention [29]. The first structures of polyhydroxylated NTAs were published in 1990 [2].

3. Pharmacology of TAs and Their Role as Drug Lead Substances

3.1. Scopolamine, Hyoscyamine and Anisodamine and Their Derived Drugs

Hyoscyamine and scopolamine are widely used as anticholinergic drugs. They affect the central and peripheral nervous system as competitive, non-selective muscarinic acetylcholine receptor (mAChR) antagonists, that prevent binding of the physiological neurotransmitter acetylcholine. In humans, two acetylcholine receptor types are known: Muscarinic and nicotinic receptors, which are named after their agonists, muscarine (Figure 2) and nicotine. Muscarine is a poison of the toadstool mushroom *Amanita muscaria* and acts on the mAChR of the synapses like acetylcholine, with the difference that the acetylcholinesterase does not metabolize it.

The mAChRs are a subclass of the G-protein-coupled receptors (GPCRs) family, containing five subtypes (M1–M5). M1, M3 and M5 that are coupled with the stimulating Gq receptors and generate cytosolic calcium transients via the phospholipase C signalling pathway. M2 and M4, on the other hand, couple with the Gi protein and inhibit the adenylyl cyclase [7]. In particular, M1 receptors occur in the central nervous system and ganglia where they are involved in memory and learning processes. M2 receptors are found in the heart and are lower in abundance than M1 receptors. M3 receptors are involved in the contraction of the smooth muscles. M4 receptors were detected in the forebrain, hippocampus and striatum, they are likely involved in pain processes [30]. The physiological action of M5 receptors is not yet elucidated, however, it is assumed that these receptors are involved in brain microcirculation and mediate vasoconstriction, vasodilatation and activation of nitric oxide synthase [31].

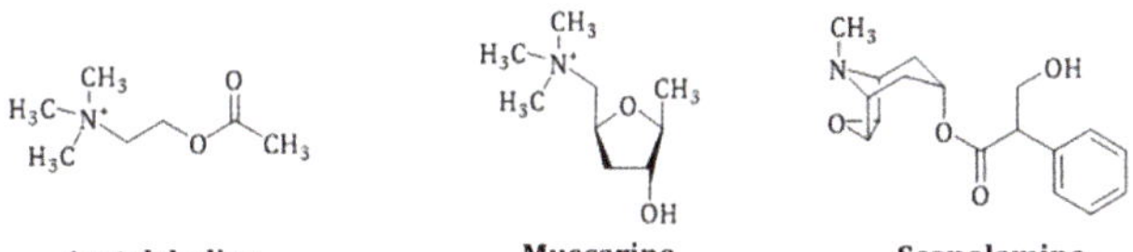

Figure 2. Comparison of the chemical structures of acetylcholine, muscarine and scopolamine. Scopolamine is protonated in the body due to the physiological pH and is present as a quaternary ammonium salt.

TAs are absorbed from the gastrointestinal tract, rapidly distributed into the tissues and excreted predominantly through the renal system [32]. The short half-life in plasma and dose-dependent adverse effects limit the administration of scopolamine to transdermal application [33]. After absorption, scopolamine experiences a significant first-pass effect, because only a minor amount (2.6%) is excreted in the urine in the pharmacologically active form [34]. Cytochrome P450 enzymes seem to be especially involved in the metabolism of scopolamine by oxidative demethylation. Inhibition of CYP3A by ingestion of grapefruit juice prolonged the t_{max} and increased the AUC_{0-24h} value of scopolamine metabolization [33]. Additionally, it has been observed that scopolamine and its apo- and nor-metabolites are conjugated to glucuronide (glucuronidation) or sulphate during phase II metabolism for excretion into urine. Scopolamine and hyoscyamine do not accumulate in the human body, nor exhibit genotoxic or chronic toxicity, an adverse effect due to long-term exposure have not been reported (EFSA, 2013).

Occurring side effects of anticholinergic drug substances occur from inhibition of the parasympathetic nervous system. Symptoms include decelerated heart rate, dry mouth and reduced perspiration. At higher therapeutic oral doses, increased heart rate, inhibition of the respiratory tract secretory activity as well as bronchodilation and mydriasis have been observed. Sweating is also inhibited which is accompanied by a consequent rise in body temperature.

A dysfunction of muscarinic cholinergic system has been drawn in various diseases like depression, epilepsy, Parkinson's and Alzheimer's disease. Therefore, antagonists of the muscarinic system such as the TAs remain of great interest as potential lead CNS drug substances. In addition to the properties described above, hyoscyamine serves as an antidote against toxins such as organothiophosphates, for example the pesticide parathion (E605) [35]. The organic phosphorous derivates are used as insecticides and as nerve gases applied in military weapons. The antidote against scopolamine and hyoscyamine intoxications is physostigmine, a pyrolo-indole alkaloid. Physostigmine naturally occurs in the Calabar bean (*Physostigma venenosum*, Fabaceae) and acts as parasympathomimetic drug by reversible inhibition of the cholinesterase [36].

3.1.1. Scopolamine

Scopolamine causes mydriatic, spasmolytic and local anaesthetics effects yet exhibits side effects which can be hallucinogenic and even lethal. The most important mode of application for scopolamine is transdermal, a technology which was developed as transdermal therapeutic systems (TTS) in 1981. Scopoderm TTS® is the trade name for a scopolamine delivery system used in the treatment of motion sickness. During the Second World War, scopolamine was used to treat shell shock, psychoactive side effects and also motion sickness [13]. The drawbacks of scopolamine lay in the manifold peripheral and central nervous system side effects. To overcome these issues, scopolamine derivates have been developed, leading to its classification as a drug lead substance.

3.1.2. Hyoscyamine and Atropine

Hyoscyamine and atropine have similar modes of action and effects as scopolamine. The pharmacological action of TAs is stereoselective, due to the difference of the stereoisomers concerning affinity and binding to muscarinic receptors. This results in different potency between S-(−)- and R-(+)- isomers of hyoscyamine: The S-(−)- isomer is estimated to be 30–300 fold more potent than the R-(+)- isomer [37]. The S-(−)-isomer of hyoscyamine is not stable and is racemized rapidly to atropine, which is a 1:1 mixture of the two forms. Atropine is very stable over time and hence, it used for medicinal applications instead of hyoscyamine. Both, atropine and scopolamine have a characteristic, dose dependent action on the cardiovascular system, which is clinically useful for resuscitation.

3.1.3. Anisodamine

Anisodamine, which is isolated from *Anisodus tanguticus*, a Tibetan regional plant, is less toxic than atropine and scopolamine. It has a long tradition in folkloric Asian medicine especially in the treatment of septic shock by improvement of blood flow in microcirculation and also in various circulatory as well as gastric disorders with similar effects to atropine and scopolamine.

3.1.4. Homatropine, Cyclopentolate and Tropicamide

Homatropine, the mandelic acid ester of tropine, is used in ophthalmology to evoke a more rapid and less paralytically effect than atropine. This is a major advantage over atropine and, consequently, homatropine was launched as a new mydriatic by Merck Darmstadt in 1883 as one of the first synthetic drugs [38]. Other modified mydriatic agents are cyclopentolate, which is used especially for paediatric eye examinations and tropicamide, which has been approved in ophthalmology since 2005.

3.1.5. Trospium Chloride

Trospium chloride is a quaternary ammonium 3α-nortropane derivate esterified with benzylic acid. This synthetic anticholinergic is not able to cross blood-brain barrier and relaxes the smooth muscle in the bladder. Its main application is to treat urgency and reflex incontinence [39].

3.1.6. Tropisetron

Tropisetron possesses a tropane skeleton but due to its mechanism of action it belongs to the serotonin receptor antagonist. It is applied to antiemetic therapy in cases of nausea and vomiting during chemotherapy and additionally as analgesic in fibromyalgia [40].

3.1.7. N-butylscopolamine

To minimize adverse effects on the central nervous system, scopolamine has been modified by N-butylation and, in this form, it cannot longer pass the blood-brain barrier. N-butylscopolamine is used to treat abdominal pain from cramping, renal colic and bladder spasms [41]. Available dosage forms are as tablets or film-coated tablets (also available in combination with paracetamol), rectal suppositories (also available in combination with paracetamol) or solutions for injection and the according drug products are Buscopan® or Buscofem®.

3.1.8. Tiotropium Bromide, Ipratropium Bromide and Oxitropium Bromide

In traditional medicine, smoking of *Datura* leaves have been frequently used to treat asthmatic symptoms. Bronchodilation is caused by blocking of M3 receptors located on smooth muscle cells in the bronchi. Scopolamine and hyoscyamine are the TAs responsible for this effect. To reduce the adverse and intoxicating effects of this treatment, tiotropium bromide and ipratropium bromide were developed and are also administered by inhalation. Tiotropium bromide (Spiriva®; released on the market in 2005) is dominantly used in the treatment of chronic obstructive pulmonary disease

(COPD) while ipratropium bromide (Atrovent®; released 1975) is used in the treatment of COPD (in combination with salbutamol, a β2-adrenergic receptor agonist) and asthma [42]. Oxitropium bromide is less known and less used than the previous ones but also acts as an anticholinergic bronchodilator for the treatment of asthma and COPD.

3.1.9. Benzatropine

Benzatropine is a selective M1 muscarinic acetylcholine receptor antagonist with central nervous effects. Chemically, it is a combination of the tropine skeleton of atropine and the benzohydryl skeleton of diphenhydramine. It partially blocks cholinergic activity in the basal ganglia and increases the availability of dopamine by blocking its reuptake. This increases dopaminergic activity, therefore, it has found use in the treatment of early stages of Parkinson's disease [43].

3.1.10. Scopolamine and Its Use as an Antidepressant

Scopolamine may also be suitable for the application in central nervous system (CNS) diseases. It is known that scopolamine and other muscarinic receptor antagonists have an effect on the cognition processes, sensory functions (for example pain perception) and stress responses. As there is considerable evidence supporting the cholinergic-adrenergic hypothesis of mania and depression, the clinical effects of scopolamine as a central acting inhibitor of the muscarinic receptor has been tested. Several randomized double-blind studies have been performed and demonstrated contrasting outcomes. Some studies found scopolamine to have a rapid and prominent effect [44] while others found no benefit from scopolamine over placebo [45] for the treatment of these conditions. The contrasting findings indicate that more extensive studies are needed to verify the use of scopolamine for treatment of CNS diseases.

3.2. Cocaine Derived Drugs

Although cocaine has been used for a long time and by many people, little is known about it is use in treatment of neurobiology and pharmacology. The application of cocaine is legally restricted and consequently, the research is limited. It is known that cocaine exhibits different pharmaceutical modes of action like local anaesthetic properties, CNS stimulating actions and cardiovascular effects. However, these modes of action may alter according to the way of application—oral, nasal, by chewing, inhalation or by injection [46].

The central nervous effects such as euphoria, relief of fatigue and boredom as well as psychic stimulation are mainly explained by the resulting excess of dopamine after cocaine consumption. Cocaine inhibits the reuptake of dopamine, noradrenaline and serotonin, thus increasing their concentration in the synaptic cleft of the limbic system [8]. The intake of cocaine has an influence on the brain which is detectable in an electroencephalogram (EEG). However, the effects are inconsistent and may appear as increased or lowered signals in EEGs [47]. The local anaesthetic properties of cocaine by topical application are achieved by blocking the ion channels in neural membranes. Cocaine is absorbed by the mucosa after application and paralysis rapidly occurs in the peripheral ends of sensory nerves. It was widely applied in dentistry as a local anaesthetic but has been substituted by safer drugs. Nevertheless, it served as a lead substance for different local anaesthetics and painkillers. Procaine was the first major analogue of cocaine which was mainly used in dentistry. Nowadays, more potent local anaesthetics are available and so, its use has declined. A huge disadvantage of procaine is instability of the ester to hydrolysis. Tetracaine, a further development of procaine, is used for minor face surgeries and in ophthalmology. It is almost 10-times more potent than procaine, however, its toxicity increased proportionately to its potency [48]. Lidocaine is an amino amide analogue to the ester type of cocaine and was synthesized in 1943 by the Swedish chemists Nils Löfgren and Bengt Lundqvist [49]. Its advantages are the better stability towards hydrolysis in aqueous solution or esterase catalysis [48]. Beside its local anaesthetic properties, it is used as an Ib type antiarrhythmic medication due to its positive cardiovascular effects.

3.3. Calystegine Derived Drugs

Until now, no drug products derived from calystegines are available, although the inhibition of mammalian glucosides by these compounds may be a promising lead in the development of new active pharmaceutical ingredients.

4. TA Biosynthesis *In Planta*

4.1. Early Steps in TA Biosynthesis—A United Way

The different classes of TAs: cocaine, scopolamine/hyoscyamine and the calystegines share a common precursor biosynthetic route (Figure 3) beginning with the amino acids L-ornithine (Orn) and L-arginine (Arg). In planta, Orn and Arg are formed from glutamate (Glu), an amino acid which is directly connected to the nitrogen assimilation. Ammonia (absorbed from the soil or synthesized from nitrate) is incorporated into Glu via the glutamine synthetase-glutamate synthase (GS-GOGAT) pathway. Glu is the precursor in several polyamine (PA) pathways. The regulation of PAs is very complex and not fully elucidated due to their pleiotropic functions [50] and PA concentration in plants can be used as indicators of various forms of abiotic stress.

In order to form putrescine (1,4-diaminobutane) from the amino acids Orn or Arg, Orn is decarboxylated by the ODC (ornithine decarboxylase; EC 4.1.1.17) and Arg undergoes a three-step reaction, including decarboxylation, hydrolysis of the imine functionality of guanidine and hydrolysis of urea which is catalysed by the enzymes ADC (arginine decarboxylase; EC 4.1.1.19), AIH (agmatine deiminase; EC 3.5.3.12) and CPA (N-carbamoylputrescine amidase; EC 3.5.1.53), respectively. The activities of ADC and ODC were suppressed in *Datura* plants by using the specific irreversible inhibitors DL-α-difluoromethylarginine and DL-α-difluoromethylornithine, respectively in order to probe the nature of these two routes to putrescine biosynthesis. These experiments indicated that the two routes do not act independently from each other and that the ADC exhibited a higher activity than the ODC [51]. Putrescine (tetramethylenediamine) is an intermediate in several metabolic pathways. It can be formed to spermidine by a spermidine synthase (SPDS; EC. 2.5.1.16) catalysed reaction using S-adenosyl methioninamine (decarboxylated S-adenosyl methionine) and putrescine as substrates.

Putrescine can also be methylated to N-methylputrescine by the enzyme PMT (putrescine N-methyltransferase; EC 2.1.1.53) [52] using SAM (S-adenosyl methionine). The next step in TA biosynthesis is the oxidative deamination of N-methylputrescine to 4-methylaminobutanal which is catalysed by a N-methylputrescine oxidase (MPO; EC 1.4.3.6) [53]. This diamine oxidase requires copper as a cofactor. N-methyl-Δ^1-pyrrolinium, a central intermediate, is formed by spontaneous cyclization of N-methylputrescine. Chemically, this reaction is an intramolecular Schiff base formation. N-methyl-Δ^1-pyrrolinium cation is a branchpoint in TA and nicotine biosynthesis [54]. In Figure 3. Joint steps of the early TA biosynthesis; ACD = arginine decarboxylase; AIH = agmatine deiminase; OCD = ornithine decarboxylase; CPA = N-carbamoylputrescine amidase; PMT = putrescine N-methyltransferase; SPDS = spermidine synthase; SMS = spermine synthase; MPO = N-methylputrescine oxidase; * = spontaneous cyclization, the joint biosynthesis is depicted. The condensation of nicotinic acid or more precisely its reactive derivate 2,5-Dihydropyrindine with N-methyl-Δ^1-pyrrolinium cation yields nicotine.

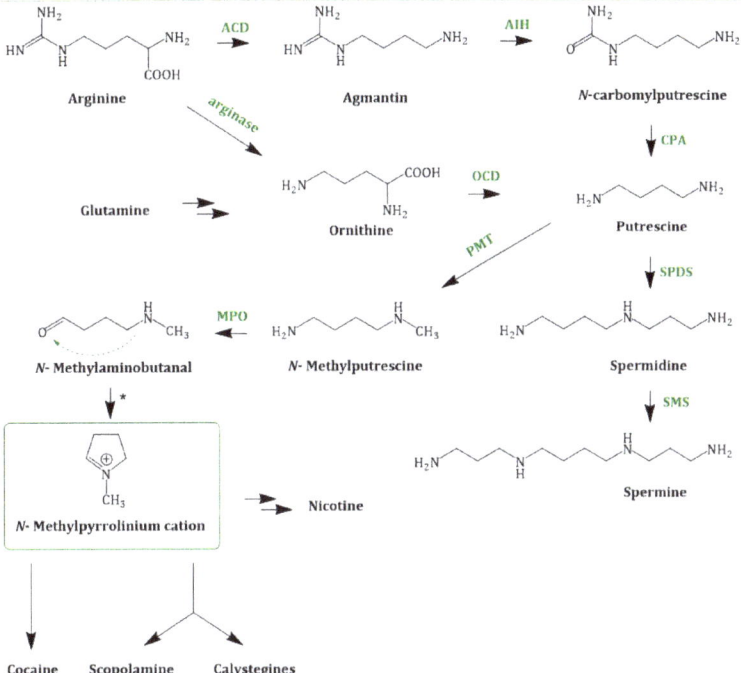

Figure 3. Joint steps of the early TA biosynthesis; ACD = arginine decarboxylase; AIH = agmatine deiminase; OCD = ornithine decarboxylase; CPA = N-carbamoylputrescine amidase; PMT = putrescine N-methyltransferase; SPDS = spermidine synthase; SMS = spermine synthase; MPO = N-methylputrescine oxidase; * = spontaneous cyclization.

4.2. Hyoscyamine and Scopolamine Biosynthesis

Originating from N-methyl-Δ^1-pyrrolinium, the next steps in the scopolamine biosynthesis (Figure 4) were not elucidated for a long time. Recently in 2018, Bedewitz et al. (2018) identified an atypical polyketide synthase from *A. belladonna* which catalyses the formation of the intermediate 4-(1-methyl-2-pyrrolidinyl)-3-oxobutanoic acid [55]. This intermediate is subsequently formed to tropinone by a malonyl-Coenzyme A mediated decarboxylative condensation catalysed by a cytochrome P450 enzyme, named AbCYP82M3. Tropinone serves as substrate for two stereospecific reductases: the tropinone reductase I (TR-I; EC 1.1.1.206) and the tropinone reductase II (TR-II; EC 1.1.1.236) [56]. TR-I catalyses its reduction to tropine (3α-tropanol), whereas TR-II catalyses tropinone reduction to pseudotropine (3β-tropanol), respectively. Pseudotropine is the precursor of calystegine biosynthesis while tropine is used to produce scopolamine.

Tropine is assumed to undergo condensation with activated (R)-phenyllactate (phenyllactyl-CoA), which delivers the third ring intermediate to littorine. Phenyllactate is derived from phenylalanine, an intermediate of the shikimate pathway, which is transaminated to phenylpyruvate. Bedewitz et al. (2014) discovered the coding sequence of a distinct aromatic amino acid aminotransferase (ArAT) that is co-expressed with known tropane alkaloid biosynthesis genes [57]. Silencing of ArAT4 in *A. belladonna* disrupted scopolamine biosynthesis by reduction of phenyllactate levels. The next step, the reduction of ketone function, is catalysed by a recently discovered phenylpyruvic acid reductase (AbPPAR). This reductase exhibited cell-specific expression also and was detected in root pericycle as well as the endodermis [58].

Although no enzymatic activity had been described, it is likely that an enzyme related to the cocaine synthase may be involved [59,60] in the formation of littorine. Littorine is rearranged via the littorine mutase/monooxygenase (CYP80F1; EC 1.6.2.4) to hyoscyamine aldehyde, which is subsequently reduced to the corresponding alcohol hyoscyamine [61]. Hyoscyamine is converted via the enzyme H6H (hyoscyamine 6β-hydroxylase; EC 1.14.11.11). The H6H is a 2-oxoglutarate dependent dioxygenase [62] which catalyses two reactions: first, the hydroxylation of hyoscyamine to 6β-hydroxy hyoscyamine and second, the epoxidation of 6β-hydroxy hyoscyamine to scopolamine. The bifunctional dioxygenase exhibits a strong hydroxylase activity in comparison to the rate limiting epoxidase activity [63].

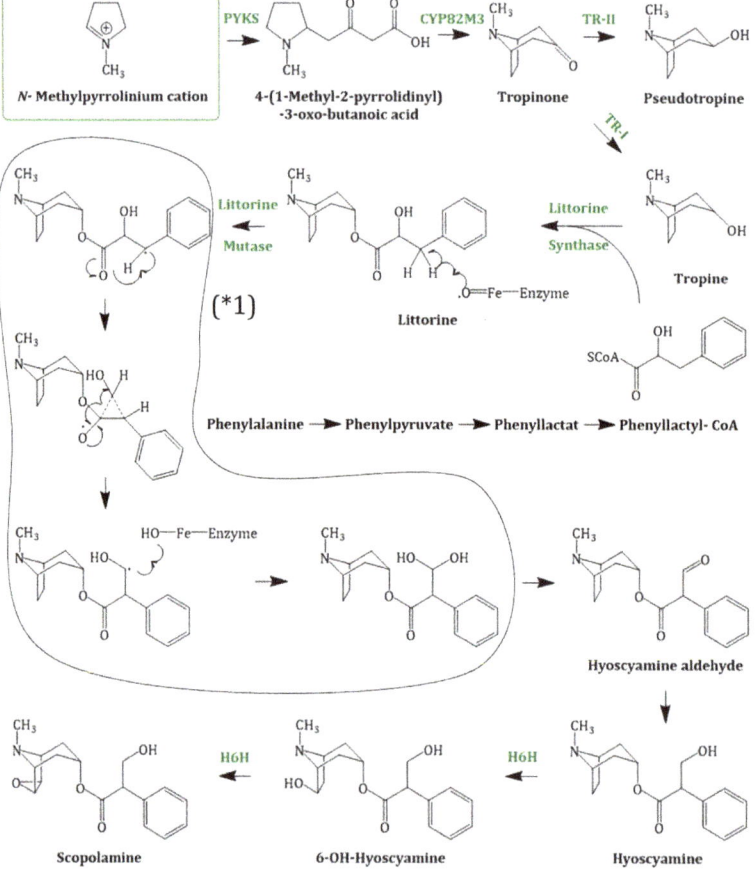

Figure 4. Scopolamine biosynthesis, starting with the N-methylpyrrolinium cation; PYKS = polyketide synthase; CYP82M3 = cytochrome P450 enzyme; TR-I/II = tropinone reductase I/II; littorine synthase (sequence not known); littorine mutase/monooxygenase (CYP80F1); (*1) = proposed mechanism of littorine rearrangement; H6H = hyoscyamine 6β-hydroxylase.

4.2.1. Enzymes Involved in Scopolamine Formation and Their Regulation

Putrescine Methyltransferase

The amino acid sequence of putrescine methyltransferase (PMT) is evolutionary related to those of plant spermidine and spermine synthases (SPMS, EC 2.5.1.22; converts spermidine into spermine; cofactor: decarboxylated S-adenosyl methionine). These enzymes are grouped in the spermidine synthase family by the Prosite database and contain a polyamine biosynthesis (PABS) domain. The PABS domain consists of two subdomains: I) *N*-terminal subdomain composed of six β-strands and II) Rossmann-like *C*-terminal subdomain [64]. It is assumed that PMT evolved from SPDS [65,66]. Teuber et al. (2007) performed a kinetic study of heterologous PMTs from different plants and measured K_{cat} values between 0.16 and 0.39 s^{-1}.

Tropinone Reductase I and Tropinone Reductase II

Tropinone reductase I and II (TR-I (EC 1.1.1.206) and TR-II (EC 1.1.1.236)) are small proteins belonging to the short chain dehydrogenase/reductase (SDR) family and catalyze NADPH + H$^+$-dependent conversion of tropinone into tropine or pseudotropine, respectively. They share the characteristic motifs of the SDR family, such as TGXXXGXG, a motif involved in NADPH binding, a NNAG motif and the catalytic sequence motif SYK [67]. Kushwaha et al. (2013) expressed the cDNA of *tr-I* from *Withania coagulans* in *Escherichia coli* and purified the protein to investigate its functional and catalytic properties [68]. They investigated the pH optimum, the thermostability, substrate saturations kinetics and specificity, as well as the effect of salts. A K_{cat} value of 16.74 s^{-1} for tropinone was determined. Additional work was performed by Qiang et al. (2016) on TR-I from *Brugmansia arborea* and *D. stramonium* [69]. The K_{cat} of BaTR-I for tropinone was 2.93 s^{-1} at pH 6.4 and the K_{cat} of DsTR-I was determined to be 2.40 s^{-1} at pH 6.4.

Putative Littorine Synthase

In 2015, Schmidt et al. published that the final step in the cocaine biosynthesis in *Erythoxylum coca*, the esterification of methylecgonine (2-carbomethoxy-3b-tropine) with benzoic acid, is catalyzed by a member of the benzylalcohol *O*-acetyl-, anthocyanin-*O*-hydroxycinnamoyl-, anthranilate-*N*-hydroxycinnamoyl/benzoyl- and deacetylvindoline 4-*O*-acetyltransferase (BAHD) family. This cocaine synthase is a plant acyltransferase, capable of producing both cocaine and cinnamoylcocaine via the activated benzoyl- or cinnamoyl-CoA thioesters. This esterification seems to be similar to the esterification of tropine with phenyllactic acid from scopolamine biosynthesis and hence, it can be assumed that the littorine synthase may also belong to the BAHD family. Enzymes of the BAHD family utilize CoA thioesters and catalyse the formation of numerous plant metabolites All identified members so far are monomeric, cytosolic enzymes with a molecular mass ranging from 48 to 55 kDa. The enzymes of this family share two conserved domains: The first is the HXXXDG domain, which is located near the center portion of each enzyme and is responsible for the utilization of CoA thioesters. The second highly conserved region is a DFGWG motif that is localized near the carboxyl terminus. These two motifs were identified in almost every functional enzyme of the BAHD family [70].

Littorine Mutase/Monooxygenase//CYP80F1

After the esterification of tropine with phenyllactic acid, the (R)-littorine formed is rearranged to (S)-hyoscyamine. Although the substrates for this isomerization were already identified in 1995 [71], the enzyme involved and its mechanism remained unknown until recently. Due to the similarity of this step to rearrangement reactions of comparable substances, it was speculated that this reaction is a coenzyme-B12 mediated isomerization. As no traces of vitamin B12 have ever been found in plants, this idea has been rejected [72]. Moreover, it was discovered that SAM is involved in the rearrangement of littorine to hyoscyamine. In 2006, Li et al. demonstrated in vitro that CYP80F1 (EC 1.6.2.4) converts littorine mainly to hyoscyamine aldehyde. Moreover, they showed that the suppression of the CYP80F1 gene by virus-induced gene silencing and RNAi results in the accumulation of littorine and reduction of hyoscyamine levels in planta.

Hyoscyamine 6β-hydroxylase

Hyoscyamine 6β-hydroxylase (H6H) is assumed to be the determining factor in many plants that accumulate hyoscyamine instead of scopolamine. H6H (EC 1.14.11.11) is a monomeric α-ketoglutarate dependent dioxygenase and the final enzyme of the TA pathway. This enzyme catalyses a two-step reaction, the hydroxylation of L-hyoscyamine to 6-hydroxy hyoscyamine and the epoxidation of 6-hydroxy hyoscyamine to scopolamine, exhibiting low epoxidase activity compared to hydroxylase activity [73]. The enzyme has an average molecular mass of 41 kDa and exhibits maximum activity at pH 7.8. L-hyoscyamine, oxygen and α-ketoglutarate are required for the enzyme activity, with respective K_m values of 35 µM and 43 µM. Iron ions (Fe^{2+}), catalase and ascorbate (as a reductant) increase reaction catalysis. H6H is inhibited by EDTA and completely by other divalent cations, including Ca^{2+}, Cd^{2+}, Co^{2+}, Cu^{2+}, Hg^{2+}, Mn^{2+}, Ni^{2+}, Zn^{2+}, as well as by Fe^{3+}. Several alkaloids which are structurally related to L-hyoscyamine have also been shown to be hydroxylated at the C-6 position of the tropane moiety by H6H. This enzyme also epoxidizes 6,7-dehydrohyoscyamine to scopolamine (K_m 10 µM) [74].

4.2.2. Localization and Organization of Scopolamine Biosynthesis in Plants

The spatial localization of TA biosynthesis and their organization is diverse and complex. In Solanaceae plants, TA biosynthesis takes place in the roots and the alkaloids are then transported to the aerial parts where they are stored. Not much information regarding the transport and the transport form is available but it is assumed that the TAs are transported through the xylem. Cell-specific compartmentalization of scopolamine biosynthesis was previously observed in the root tissue pericycle, where expression of the genes *pmt* in *A. belladonna* [75] and *h6h* in *Hyoscyamus niger* [76] were detected. The enzyme TR-I, however, resides in the endodermis and nearby cortical cells in *H. niger* [56,77]. In potatoes, the TR-II, which provides pseudotropine for calystegine biosynthesis, was detected in the cortex and phloem parenchyma of roots and stolons; in tuber spouts, the protein was detected in companion cells. TR-I, whose function in potatoes is not yet elucidated, was also detected in protein extracts of tuber tissue, however, in quantities too low to permit localization to single cells [78]. The enzyme PMT also catalyses the first step in nicotine biosynthesis (discussed above). In *Nicotiana sylvestris*, a nicotine producing plant, *pmt* is expressed in the endodermis, outer cortex and found in root xylem [79]. This compartmentalization in biosynthesis in planta may complicate future attempts at heterologous production in single-celled microbial systems (discussed below). It may be that eukaryotic host cells such as yeasts or microalgae may be suitable host organisms for their biosynthesis as these cells exhibit compartmentalization of organelles and have been used for effective metabolic engineering of complex metabolites [80].

4.3. Cocaine Biosynthesis

Cocaine biosynthesis (Figure 5), past its branch point with common intermediates shared with other TAs, is still under investigation and not fully elucidated. In literature, two different possibilities of the pathway towards cocaine biosynthesis have been reported. According to the classical hypothesis, the bridgehead carbon atom C-1 of methylecgonine is derived from an N-methyl-Δ^1-pyrrolinium cation and that of C-2 originates from acetoacetate. However, feeding experiments with labelled N-methyl-Δ^1-pyrrolinium cation were inconclusive in planta and could not confirm this theory. It was, therefore, suggested that the observed regiochemistry of incorporation of the labelled N-methyl-Δ^1-pyrrolinium cation into cocaine was compatible with the stepwise introduction of C2 units into the ecgonine skeleton, derived from acetate [81]. Consequently, this hypothesis proposes a new intermediate in cocaine biosynthesis, N-methyl-2-pyrrolidineacetic acid. Although this compound was detected in several plants, all attempts at incorporation of it into the ester or thioester forms have been so far unsuccessful [82]. Chemically, nucleophilic addition of the first acetyl-CoA moiety reaction is assumed to be a Mannich-like reaction using the enolate anion; the side-chain extension occurs via Claisen condensation [48]. The (S)-enantiomer cyclizes and forms the bicyclic structure of the cocaine tropane ring skeleton by an intramolecular Mannich reaction [83]. Hydrolysis of the CoA-ester, followed by SAM-dependent methylation and reduction yield methylecgonine (2-carbomethoxy-3β-tropine). Methylecgonine in its turn condenses with benzoyl-CoA, which is derived from L-phenylalanine [84], to cocaine. Schmidt et al. (2015) described an enzyme catalysing this reaction and termed it the cocaine synthase. This synthase belongs to the BAHD family, which catalyses the transfer of CoA-activated acyl thioesters to oxygen- or nitrogen-containing acceptor molecules [70].

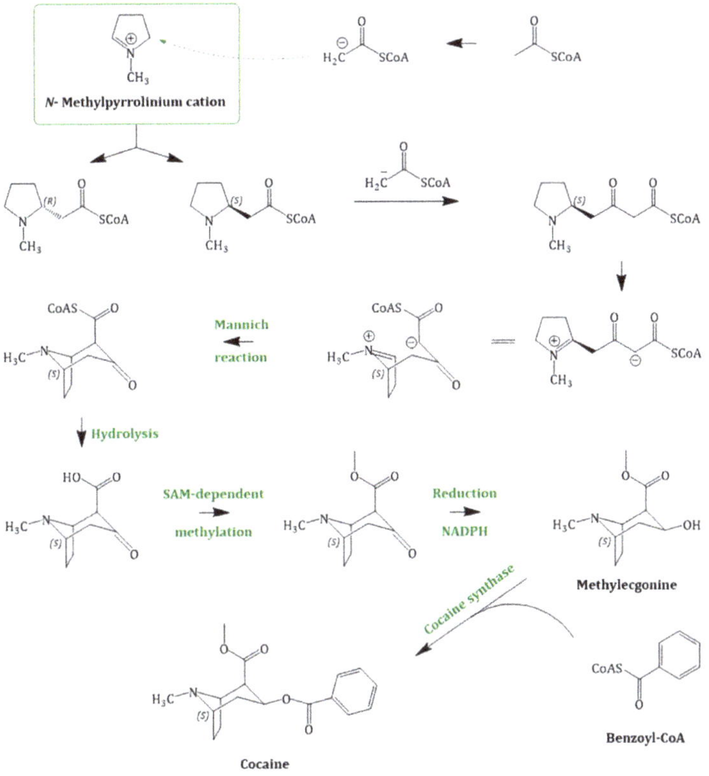

Figure 5. Cocaine biosynthesis, starting with the intermediate N-methyl-Δ^1-pyrrolinium cation; only less information regarding the enzymatically involvement is proven. The iminium cation reacts with two acetyl-CoA moieties to an intermediate that cyclizes in an intramolecular Mannich reaction. After hydrolysis, methylation and reduction methylecgonine is formed. The cocaine synthase catalyses the last step in the pathway: the condensation of methylecgonine with benzoyl-CoA.

Cocaine and scopolamine differ mainly in two structures: First, the retention of the C-1 carboxyl group of acetoacetate, which is subsequently methylated and second, the different stereochemistry of the C-3 hydroxy group.

4.4. Calystegine Biosynthesis

Comparable to the hyoscyamine/scopolamine and cocaine pathways, the detailed processes of calystegine biosynthesis are not known. Tropinone is assumed to be involved and which should be reduced to pseudotropine, a reaction catalysed by TR-II. No further information regarding the biosynthesis is available so far [85]. To date, no attempts at elucidation of the hydroxylation or the demethylation of these compounds has been reported. This may be due to the relatively recent discovery of calystegines in 1990 [2] and reduced interest in medical applications compared to scopolamine or cocaine. In contrast to cocaine and scopolamine, the calystegine skeleton (8-azabicyclo [3.2.1] octane) is not N-methylated, rather, it is polyhydroxylated. These compounds are classified into different groups, depending on the number of hydroxy groups: subgroup A consists three, subgroup B four and subgroup C have five [86].

5. Biotechnological Approaches of Scopolamine Production and Alternative Methods of Raw Material Supply

5.1. Scopolamine Production in Cell Suspension and Hairy Root Cultures

The quality of *Duboisia* spp. plant material and the quantity of scopolamine in agricultural production depends on different abiotic factors such as climate, sunlight, soil fertilization and biotic factors [87,88]. In times of climate change, abiotic influences may become less predictable and more extreme. This in turn influences the biomass and results in variability alkaloid content and production potentials [89]. To establish a more independent production system, different plant cell cultures have been developed—especially callus cultures, cell suspension cultures and hairy root cultures. The advantage of these cell cultures is the possibility to control TA biosynthesis via process design in order to achieve increased or altered tropane alkaloid yields. However, to date, the produced amounts of TAs by tissue culture are not competitive to the production of scopolamine by agricultural farming of *Duboisia* hybrids. This difference in production arises due to complicated scale-up of tissue culture production and associated costs. Additionally, the cell-specific compartmentalization of TA biosynthesis as discussed in previous sections likely reduces tissue-culture specific production as callus and cell suspension cultures are totipotent, undifferentiated cells [90].

Hairy roots are disease manifestations developed by plants that are wounded and infected by *Agrobacterium rhizogenes* [91]. In contrast to undifferentiated cell cultures, hairy root cultures can usually synthesize the same metabolites as unmodified roots and may also produce desired secondary metabolites [92]. In nightshades, TA biosynthesis is localized in the root and this plant organ has been exploited for TA production. Early experiments were performed in the late 1980s and reports are continuing to be published on this process. The hairy root system itself is stable for several years with steady growth and alkaloid production rates [93], however, scale-up of this system remains technically challenging. Table 1 presents a brief overview of TA concentrations in engineered and untreated hairy root cultures from different plants:

Table 1. Overview of TA concentrations in engineered and untreated hairy cultures from different plants. TAs content in leaves of regenerated plants; n.d. = not determined, DW = dry weight.

Plant	Overexpression of	Amount		Citation
		Hyoscyamine	Scopolamine	
Atropa belladonna	-	0.371 ± 0.013% DW	0.024 ± 0.010% DW	Kamada et al., 1986 [94]
	H. niger h6h	0.02% *)	0.45% *)	Hashimoto et al., 1993b [95]
Hyoscyamus niger	-	2.1 + 0.2 mg g^{-1} DW	n.d.	Falk and Doran, 1996 [96]
	**)	0.31 mg g^{-1} DW	0.27 mg g^{-1} DW	Vakili et al., 2012 [97]
	-	1.6 mg g^{-1} DW	5.3 mg g^{-1} DW	Jaremicz et al., 2014 [98]
	pmt, h6h	n.d.	411 mg L^{-1}	Zhang et al., 2004 [99]
Anisodus acutangulus	h6h	0.789 ± 0.078 mg g^{-1} DW	0.070 ± 0.003 mg g^{-1} DW	Kai et al., 2012 [100]
	tr-I	2.479 ± 0.432 mg g^{-1} DW	0.023 ± 0.004 mg g^{-1} DW	
	tr-I, h6h	2.286 ± 0.46 mg g^{-1} DW	0.072 ± 0.018 mg g^{-1} DW	
Brugmansia candida ***)	-	0.35 ± 0.07 mg g^{-1} DW	1.05 mg g^{-1} DW	Cardillo et al., 2010 [101]
Hyoscyamus muticus	h6h	287.7 mg L^{-1}	14.41 mg L^{-1}	Jouhikainen et al., 1999 [102]
Duboisia myoporoides	pmt	no increase observed		Moyano et al., 2002 [103]
	h6h	n.d.	24.93 mg g^{-1} DW	Palazón et al., 2003 [104]

*) TAs content in leaves of regenerated plants **) chromium treatment ***) *B. candida* hairy roots grown in a special bioreactor.

A further development of the hairy roots cultures is the exploitation of TAs by "milking the plant." After stimulation of aeroponically cultivated plants, roots were "extracted" by putting the roots into physiological extraction medium without harming or destroying them and desired secondary metabolites were isolated. After "milking," plants are returned to their cultivation apparatus to regenerate and produce more secondary metabolites which can be subsequently extracted in further cycles. This promising approach still needs to be optimized to be economically competitive [105].

Transgenic plants have also been generated and cultivated for TA production. Recently, Xia et al. (2016) overexpressed *pmt* from *Nicotiana tabacum* (NtPMT) and *h6h* from *H. niger* (HnH6H) in *A. belladonna* and reached high scopolamine levels (2.94–5.13 mg g^{-1} DW) in field conditions [106]. Almost thirty years previously, Wang et al. (1985) also overexpressed *pmt* and *h6h* in *A. belladonna*, although a scopolamine concentration of only 1.2 mg g^{-1} DW was achieved [107].

To date, cell suspension cultures, callus cultures or hairy root cultures have been demonstrated to be competitive for TA production in comparison to agricultural means. In comparison to these alternative production options, the conventional field cropping of *Duboisia* species in Australia provides up to 15 tons fresh leaves per hectare, with three harvests annually. The total TA concentration of these plants is about 2–4% (equivalent to 20–40 mg g^{-1} DW) with ca. 60% scopolamine [1]. Obtaining these yields in terms of concentration and total amount is not yet competitive with biotechnological approaches.

5.2. Microbial Production of Scopolamine and Enzyme Engineering Approaches

Plants and plant cell suspension cultures are often slow growing and difficult to handle. In comparison, microbial cultures such as bacteria, for example, *E. coli* or yeast, for example, *Saccharomyces cerevisiae*, are straightforward to cultivate and are well characterized model organisms with fully developed molecular toolkits. Cultivation of these organisms can be readily scaled in existing fermentation infrastructure, which makes their cultivation more economically favourable than plant tissue culture. Therefore, heterologous production of TAs such as scopolamine in these hosts may represent an attractive alternative given transfer of the molecular pathways is possible.

Most research in this area has been performed on understanding and optimizing H6H by metabolic engineering. Cardillo et al. (2017) expressed recombinant *Brugmansia candida h6h* in *S. cerevisiae* and performed bioassays using isolated enzymes [108]. Untagged H6H was able to produce 83.3% 6β-hydroxy hyoscyamine and 7.6% scopolamine from hyoscyamine after 15 h of incubation. Additionally, specific hydroxylase and epoxidase activity: 2.60 ± 0.19 nKat mg^{-1} and 0.24 ± 0.02 nKat mg^{-1} for these two compounds were observed, respectively. The H6H from *Anisodus acutangulus* was cloned and expressed in *E. coli* fused with either a His- or GST-tag at the N-terminus [109]. A bifunctional assay revealed that both recombinant enzymes converted up to 80% of fed hyoscyamine to scopolamine, however, reaction kinetics were not analysed. Li et al., (2012) expressed *h6h* from *A. belladonna* (AbH6H) in *E. coli* and determined that the K_m value for hyoscyamine under optimal conditions was 52.1 ± 11.5 µM [110]. Compared with former experiments it revealed that the K_m of AbH6H is higher than that of HnH6H from *H. niger* (35 µM; [74]) and from *A. tanguticus* AtH6H (15.1 ± 0.3 µM; [111]), which implies that AbH6H has lower affinity for the substrate than HnH6H. Furthermore, it has been shown that epoxidation is slower than hydroxylation by this enzyme [63]. Pramod et al. (2010) characterized the H6H from *D. metel* and obtained K_m values for hyoscyamine and 2-oxoglutarate to be 50 µM each. In 2018, Fischer et. al., published results of SUMO-tagged H6H from *Brugmansia sanguinea* to have a K_m value of ~60µM [112].

First promising results concerning protein engineering of H6H were published in 2015. Cao et al. (2015) used random mutagenesis and site-directed saturation mutagenesis to increase the hydroxylation activity of H6H from *A. acutangulus* [113]. They developed a double mutant, AaH6HM1 (S14P/K97A), which has a 3.4-fold increased hydroxylation and 2.3 times higher epoxidase activity than the native enzyme, a conversion rate of 97% was achieved in vitro.

The main challenge of the heterologous TA production is that the native biosynthesis of most target compounds in planta are not fully elucidated to date. It is not known if the condensation of tropine with phenyllactic acid-CoA reacts spontaneously or is enzymatically catalysed. Therefore, it is currently not yet possible to engineer the complete biosynthesis heterologously. The goal of microbial production of scopolamine is still in its early stages and will require complete pathway elucidation before it can be seriously considered as an alternative to conventional farming practices. Future efforts will require intense bioinformatic analysis of genomes and transcriptomic data to aid in identification of the complete biochemical pathways towards TA biosynthesis. Once identified, the pathways can be engineered into heterologous hosts and optimized for the generation of these desired products. More details on the application of bioinformatics in this field are discussed in Section 6.

5.3. Additional Methods of Scopolamine Production

To increase the scopolamine level in planta, polyploid plants have been developed TA yields determined. An impressive example was published by Dehghan et al. (2017) [114]. The authors produced stable tetraploid hairy root lines of *H. muticus* that exhibited lower biomass production than diploids, however, higher scopolamine (13.87 mg L^{-1}) and hyoscyamine levels (107.7 mg L^{-1}), up to 200% more scopolamine than in diploid plants. However, the total yield of scopolamine from these plants was rather low due to the slow growth rates and results were only reported for growth conditions in optimized Murashige and Skoog (MS) or Gamborg's B5 media which are not competitive to conventional field cultivation. And moreover, other *Hyoscyamus* species like *H. senecionis* exhibit higher scopolamine then hyoscyamine levels in the leaves [115] which may be favourable for breeding and optimization approaches. Nonetheless, these initial trials are promising and polyploid plants of other species such as *D. myoporoides* may be interesting alternatives. In order for this strategy to realize economic potential, a polyploid clone must be able to be cultivated under the same conditions as the current plants, produce the same (or higher) biomass and be genetically is stable over a period of at least 10 years.

In 2017, Naik et al. published the first report regarding TA producing endophytes, namely *Colletotrichum boninense*, *Phomopsis* sp., *Fusarium solani*, *Colletotrichum incarnatum*, *Colletotrichum siamense* and *Colletotrichum gloeosporioides*, that are found in *D. metel* and possess the enzymes PMT, TR-I and H6H [116]. It was reported that these fungi produce a remarkable amount of scopolamine (4.1 mg L^{-1}) and hyoscyamine (3.9 g L^{-1}). Perhaps independent cultivation of these fungal species may represent a natural alternative to heterologous hosts or agricultural cultivation. It may also be possible to identify the biosynthetic pathways of TAs in these hosts, which could either be optimized in the fungi themselves and enhanced or transferred into heterologous microbial hosts.

6. Big Data—The Use of "Omics" in Plant Science and Pathway Elucidation

The biosynthesis of different TAs have not yet been fully elucidated. The further biosynthetic steps starting from the shared precursor N-methyl-Δ^1-pyrrolinium cation are still uncertain. The latter stages of scopolamine biosynthesis are quite well elucidated, however, the formation of littorine is still unknown. Considerable progress was achieved in the elucidation of the cocaine biosynthesis by identification of the cocaine synthase, however many other steps in its biosynthesis have not yet been described. Calystegine biosynthesis is poorly investigated and consequently, very little information is known about its biosynthesis. Remaining metabolic steps may be elucidated through the concerted efforts of genomic, transcriptomic, metabolomic and proteomic data analysis, together "omics" coupled to biochemical and heterologous enzyme characterization.

The field of computational research is increasing and so are the potential applications and the ability to support laboratory investigations. With the help of powerful computing power, it is possible to process large amounts of data and filter relevant information. The four major disciplines—genomics, transcriptomics, metabolomics and proteomics—investigate the genetics, transcripts (messenger RNA/mRNA), complete proteins and metabolites in a biological sample, respectively. The four fields are connected indispensably: during protein biosynthesis or gene expression, which is a multi-layered process, two major steps are performed. In the first step, the information in DNA, the genes, is transferred to mRNA by transcription. The mRNA is then translated into proteins or peptides. Parts of these proteins are involved in different biosynthetic pathways, which produce then again different metabolites. The comprehensive data from these four disciplines are collected in a variety of ways but they come together in the sense that an evaluation can only be done with the help of computer science.

The genome of an organism usually remains constant throughout its lifetime; hence it is difficult to receive new information regarding biotic and abiotic regulation. The transcriptome, however, changes directly with the environmental conditions of the organism and so does the proteome and metabolome. This opens the possibility to use controlled lines of the appropriate organism and evaluation of its behaviour with respect to different parameters. Changing different parameters can for example provide information about gene regulation, help to elucidate biosynthesis, identify candidate genes or even possibilities for genetic engineering to enhance the production of desired metabolites. In literature, several examples for successful pathway elucidation using new techniques are described. Comparative transcript analyses identify candidate genes for secondary metabolism. In 2014, De Luca et al. reviewed how candidate genes for the monoterpenoid indole alkaloids (MIA) biosynthesis were identified by comparative transcript analyses [117]. Their roles in secondary metabolism were demonstrated by virus induced gene silencing and corresponding changes in metabolic profiles. Subsequently, these gene candidates could be heterologously expressed, purified and their biochemical roles characterized. Another example is the identification of candidate genes involved in betalain (tyrosine-derived pigments) biosynthesis. In this study, the authors combined transcriptomic analysis and metabolic profiling in *Mirabilis jalapa* and other betalain-producing species [118]. As these research fields are increasing, much more data also regarding other plants and the valuable secondary metabolites is available. As mentioned, the TA biosynthesis is not elucidated completely and important steps like the reaction of hygrine to tropinone as well as the synthase of littorine formation are not illuminated up to now. The application of "omics" with regard to the candidate gene isolation and the understanding of the process in detail will be enlightening.

7. Conclusions

TAs are a large and diverse group of plant secondary metabolites that can be divided into three major groups: hyoscyamine and scopolamine, cocaine and calystegines. The cultivation of coca, the source plant of cocaine, is illegal and no relevant pharmacological activity has been found for calystegine, therefore, only the cultivation of scopolamine containing plants is currently of legitimate economic interest. The demand for scopolamine is currently growing due to its various therapeutic applications and increasing market demand. Unfortunately, climate change and consequent variable abiotic and biotic stressors are resulting in challenges for agricultural production of this compound at high quantities in adequate quality. Investigations have been conducted in alternative production systems such as engineered plants, climate-independent production systems such as plant cell cultures or heterologous microbial production. To date, none of these alternative approaches has been economically competitive to the conventional scopolamine production from agricultural cultivation of *D. myoporoides* plants. The main issue preventing these new approaches from being successful is insufficient elucidation of the biosynthetic pathways towards different classes of TA biosynthesis. Not all enzymes have been described yet, the corresponding genes are unknown, rate-limiting steps have not been identified and the interaction of metabolic flux is not known. Newly available "omics" techniques will assist in the elucidation of these pathways, a strategy which has already been applied with other chemical classes from a variety of plant species.

Transfer of TA biosynthesis to heterologous hosts may present other challenges. For example, for some TAs, the production site in planta is not the storage site and compartmentalized production systems such as yeast or algal cells may be required to duplicate biosynthetic environments in microbial hosts. In addition, TA producing plant cells are specialized and only certain cells express their biosynthetic pathways, limiting the applications of undifferentiated plant-cell culture for TA production. Promising findings have recently been published which detail the potential for endophyte fungi to produce TAs and may be an interesting new source of these compounds separate from their plant hosts. Indeed, the production of scopolamine, in native plants or endophytes, in plant cell cultures or heterologously in microbial hosts is an exciting and dynamic field in which many new insights can be expected in the upcoming years, especially due to the application of modern "omics" technologies for pathway elucidation.

Author Contributions: Writing-Original Draft Preparation, K.L.K.-J. and O.K.; Writing-Review & Editing, K.L.K.-J. and O.K.

Funding: This project has received funding from the European Union's Seventh Framework Programme for research, technological development and demonstration [grant No. 613513].

Acknowledgments: We acknowledge financial support by Deutsche Forschungsgemeinschaft and Technische Universität Dortmund/TU Dortmund University within the funding programme Open Access Publishing.

Conflicts of Interest: This work was supported by Boehringer Ingelheim Pharma GmbH & Co. KG.

References

1. Grynkiewicz, G.; Gadzikowska, M. Tropane alkaloids as medicinally useful natural products and their synthetic derivatives as new drugs. *Pharmacol. Rep.* **2008**, *60*, 439–463. [PubMed]
2. Dräger, B. Chemistry and Biology of calystegines. *Nat. Prod. Rep.* **2003**, 211–223. [CrossRef] [PubMed]
3. Gadzikowska, M.; Grynkiewicz, G. Tropane alkaloids in pharmaceutical and phytochemical analysis. *Acta Pol. Pharm.* **2001**, *58*, 481–492.
4. Ziegler, J.; Facchini, P.J. Alkaloid biosynthesis: Metabolism and trafficking. *Annu. Rev. Plant Biol.* **2008**, *59*, 735–769. [CrossRef] [PubMed]
5. Schultze-Kraft, M. *Evolution of Estimated Coca Cultivation and Cocaine Production in South America (Bolivia, Colombia and Peru) and of the Actors, Modalities and Routes of Cocaine Trafficking to Europe*; Background Paper Commissioned by the EMCDDA for the 2016 EU Drug Marke; European Monitoring Centre for Drugs and Drug Addiction: Lisbon, Portugal, 2016; pp. 1–15.
6. WHO. *Annex 1 19th WHO Model List of Essential Medicines*; WHO: Geneva, Switzerland, 2015.
7. Langmead, C.J.; Watson, J.; Reavill, C. Muscarinic acetylcholine receptors as CNS drug targets. *Pharmacol. Ther.* **2008**, *117*, 232–243. [CrossRef] [PubMed]
8. Rothman, R.B.; Baumann, M.H.; Dersch, C.M.; Romero, D.V.; Rice, K.C.; Carroll, F.I.V.Y.; Partilla, J.S. Amphetamine-Type Central Nervous Norepinephrine More Potently Than They Release Dopamine and Serotonin. *Synapse* **2001**, *39*, 32–41. [CrossRef]
9. Dräger, B. Identification and Quantification of Calystegines, Polyhydroxyl Nortropane Alkaloids. *Phytochem. Anal.* **1994**, *6*, 31–37. [CrossRef]
10. Griffin, W.J.; Lin, G.D. Chemotaxonomy and geographical distribution of tropane alkaloids. *Phytochemistry* **2000**, *53*, 623–637. [CrossRef]
11. Müller, J. Hexensalben und Liebestränke: Ein Beitrag zur Kulturgeschichte der Nachtschattengewächse Hexensalben und Liebestränke. *Gesnerus Swiss J. Hist. Med. Sci.* **1998**, *55*, 205–220.
12. Ulbricht, C.; Basch, E.; Hammerness, P.; Vora, M.; Wylie, J.; Woods, J. An Evidence-Based Systematic Review of Belladonna by the Natural Standard Research Collaboration. *J. Herb. Pharmacother.* **2005**, *4*, 61–90. [CrossRef]
13. Heinrich, M.; Jäger, A.K. *Ethnopharmacology*; Wiley: West Sussex, UK, 2015; ISBN 9781118930748.
14. Endo, T.; Yamada, Y. Alkaloid production in cultured roots of three species of *Duboisia*. *Phytochemistry* **1985**, *24*, 1233–1236. [CrossRef]
15. Naudé, T.W. *Datura spp. and Other Related Plants*; Elsevier Inc.: Atlanta, GA, USA, 2007; ISBN 9780123704672.
16. Bobick, J.E.; Balaban, N.E. *The Handy Science Answer Book*; Science and Technology Department of the Carnegie Library of Pittsburgh: Pittsburgh, PA, USA, 2011; ISBN 1578593212.
17. Wiart, C. *Ethnopharmacology of Medicinal Plants*; Humana Press: Totowa, NJ, USA, 2006; ISBN 1588297489.
18. Pearn, J.; Thearle, J. The history of hyoscine. *Hist. Sci. Med.* **1982**, *17*, 257–261.

19. Kim, N.; Estrada, O.; Chavez, B.; Stewart, C.; D'Auria, J. Tropane and Granatane Alkaloid Biosynthesis: A Systematic Analysis. *Molecules* **2016**, *21*, 1510. [CrossRef] [PubMed]
20. Döbereiner, J.W. *Deutsches Apothekerbuch; zum Gebrauche bei Vorlesungen und zum Selbstunterrichte für Apotheker, Droguisten, Aerzte und Medicin-Studirende*; Walz: Stuttgart, Germany, 1847.
21. Geiger, P.L.; Hesse, O. Über das Atropin. *Pharm. Cent.* **1833**, *49*, 768.
22. Lossen, W. Ueber das Atropin. *Ann. der Chemie und Pharm.* **1864**. [CrossRef]
23. Wolffenstein, R. *Die Pflanzenalkaloide*; Julius Springer Verlag: Heidelberg, Germany, 1922.
24. Ladenburg, A. Künstliches Atropin. *Berichte der Dtsch. Chem. Gesellschaft* **1879**, *12*, 941–944. [CrossRef]
25. Gaedcke, F. Ueber das Erythroxylin. *Arch. der Pharm.* **1855**, *132*, 141–150. [CrossRef]
26. Niemann, A. Ueber eine neue organische Base in den Cocablättern. *Arch. Der Pharm.* **1860**, *153*, 129–155. [CrossRef]
27. Hardegger, E.; Ott, H. Konfiguration des Cocains und Derivate der Ecgoninsäure. *Helv. Chim. Acta* **1954**, *331*, 312–320. [CrossRef]
28. Freud, S. *Über Coca*; Moritz Perles Verlag: Wien, Austria, 1885; ISBN 978-3226009682.
29. Jocković, N.; Fischer, W.; Brandsch, M.; Brandt, W.; Dräger, B. Inhibition of human intestinal b-glucosidases by calystegines. *J. Agric. Food Chem.* **2013**, *61*, 5550–5557. [CrossRef] [PubMed]
30. Wess, J.; Duttaroy, A.; Zhang, W.; Gomeza, J.; Cui, Y.; Miyakawa, T.; Bymaster, F.P.; Mckinzie, L.; Felder, C.C.; Lamping, K.G.; et al. M 1 -M 5 Muscarinic Receptor Knockout Mice as Novel Tools to Study the Physiological Roles of the Muscarinic Cholinergic System. *Recept. Channels* **2003**, *9*, 279–290. [CrossRef]
31. Watts, S.W.; Kanagy, N.L.; Lombard, J.H. Receptor-Mediated Events in the Microcirculation. *Microcirculation* **2008**, 285–348. [CrossRef]
32. EFSA Scientific Opinion on Tropane alkaloids in food and feed. *EFSA J.* **2013**, *9*, 1–134. [CrossRef]
33. Renner, U.D.; Oertel, R.; Kirch, W. Pharmacokinetics and pharmacodynamics in clinical use of scopolamine. *Ther. Drug Monit.* **2005**, *27*, 655–665. [CrossRef]
34. Kanto, J.; Kentala, E.; Kaila, T.; Pihlajamäki, K. Pharmacokinetics of scopolamine during caesarean section: Relationship between serum concentration and effect. *Acta Anaesthesiol. Scand.* **1989**, *33*, 482–486. [CrossRef] [PubMed]
35. Boffa, J.-M.; Yarnéogo, G.; Nikiéma, P.; Knudson, D.M. *Domestication and Commercialization of Non-Timber Forest Products in Agroforestry Systems*; Food and Agriculture Organization of the United Nations: Rome, Italy, 1996; ISBN 9251039356.
36. Robenshtok, E.; Luria, S.; Tashma, Z.; Hourvitz, A. Adverse reaction to atropine and the treatment of organophosphate intoxication. *Isr. Med. Assoc. J.* **2002**, *4*, 535–539. [PubMed]
37. Gyermek, L. Structure-activity relationships among derivatives of dicarboxylic acid esters of tropine. *Pharmacol. Ther.* **2002**, *96*, 1–21. [CrossRef]
38. Sneader, W. *Drug Discovery: A History*; Wiley: West Sussex, UK, 2005; ISBN 0471899798.
39. Rudy, D.; Cline, K.; Harris, R.; Goldberg, K.; Dmochowski, R. Multicenter phase III trial studying trospium chloride in patients with overactive bladder. *Urology* **2006**, *67*, 275–280. [CrossRef]
40. Sorbe, B.; Andersson, H.; Schmidt, M.; Söderberg, M.; Högberg, T.; Wernstedt, L.; Janson, E.T.; Ehrnström, B.; Kjaer, M.; Havsteen, H.; et al. Tropisetron (Navoban) in the prevention of chemotherapy-induced nausea and vomiting—the Nordic experience. *Support. Care Cancer* **1994**, *2*, 393–399. [CrossRef]
41. Mutschler, E.; Geisslinger, G.; Kroemer, H.; Ruth, P.; Schäfer-Korting, M. *Mutschler Arzneimittelwirkungen*, 9th ed.; WVG: Stuttgart, Germany, 2008; ISBN 978-3-8047-1952-1.
42. Barnes, P.J. The Pharmacological Properties of Tiotropium. *Chest* **2000**, *117*, 63S–66S. [CrossRef]
43. Schlagmann, C.; Remien, J. Klinische Schrift Zur Behandlung der Parkinson-Krankheit. *Klin. Wochenschr.* **1986**, *64*, 939–942. [CrossRef] [PubMed]
44. Yu, H.; Lv, D.; Shen, M.; Zhang, Y.; Zhou, D.; Chen, Z.; Wang, C. BDNF mediates the protective effects of scopolamine in reserpine-induced depression-like behaviors via up-regulation of 5-HTT and TPH1. *Psychiatry Res.* **2019**, *271*, 328–334. [CrossRef] [PubMed]
45. Park, L.; Furey, M.; Nugent, A.; Farmer, C.; Ellis, J.; Szczepanik, J.; Lener, M.; Zarate, C. F173. Negative Trial of Scopolamine in Major Depressive Disorder Does Not Demonstrate Neurophysiological Changes Seen With the Antidepressant Response of Ketamine. *Biol. Psychiatry* **2018**, *83*, S305–S306. [CrossRef]
46. Williams, N. Cocaine and Metabolites: Relationship between pharmacological activity and inhibitory action on dopamine uptake into struatal synaptosomes. *Prog. Neuropsychopharmacol.* **1977**, *1*, 265–269. [CrossRef]

47. Berger, H. Archiv Für Psychiatrie Und Nervenkrankheiten. *Clin. Neurophysiol.* **1931**, *28*, 95–132.
48. Dewick, P.M. Medicinal Natural Products. *Pharm. Sci.* **2002**, *0471496405*, 514.
49. Sinatra, R.S.; Jahr, J.S.; Watkins-Pitchford, M. *The Essence of Analgesia and Analgesics*; Cambridge University Press: Cambridge, UK, 2010; ISBN 9780511841378.
50. Agostinelli, E. Polyamines and transglutaminases: Biological, clinical and biotechnological perspectives. *Amino Acids* **2014**, *46*, 475–485. [CrossRef] [PubMed]
51. Robins, R.J.; Parr, A.J.; Walton, N.J. Studies on the biosynthesis of tropane alkaloids in *Datura stramonium* L. transformed root cultures. *Planta* **1991**, *183*, 196–201. [CrossRef]
52. Biastoff, S.; Brandt, W.; Dräger, B. Putrescine N-methyltransferase—The start for alkaloids. *Phytochemistry* **2009**, *70*, 1708–1718. [CrossRef]
53. Mizusaki, S.; Tanabe, Y.; Noguchi, M.; Tamaki, E. N-methylputrescine oxidase from tobacco roots. *Phytochemistry* **1972**, *11*, 2757–2762. [CrossRef]
54. Courdavault, V. Biosynthesis and Regulation of Alkaloids. In *Plant Developmental Biology*; Humana Press: Totowa, NJ, USA, 2010; Volume 655, pp. 139–160. ISBN 978-1-60761-764-8.
55. Bedewitz, M.A.; Jones, A.D.; D'Auria, J.C.; Barry, C.S. Tropinone synthesis via an atypical polyketide synthase and P450-mediated cyclization. *Nat. Commun.* **2018**, *9*, 5281. [CrossRef] [PubMed]
56. Hashimoto, T.; Nakajima, K.; Ongena, G.; Yasuyuki, Y. Two Tropinone Reductases with Distinct Stereospecificities from Cultured Roots of *Hyoscyamus niger*. *Plant Physiol.* **1992**, *100*, 836–845. [CrossRef] [PubMed]
57. Bedewitz, M.A.; Gongora-Castillo, E.; Uebler, J.B.; Gonzales-Vigil, E.; Wiegert-Rininger, K.E.; Childs, K.L.; Hamilton, J.P.; Vaillancourt, B.; Yeo, Y.-S.; Chappell, J.; et al. A Root-Expressed L-Phenylalanine:4-Hydroxyphenylpyruvate Aminotransferase Is Required for Tropane Alkaloid Biosynthesis in *Atropa belladonna*. *Plant Cell* **2014**, *26*, 3745–3762. [CrossRef] [PubMed]
58. Qiu, F.; Yang, C.; Yuan, L.; Xiang, D.; Lan, X.; Chen, M.; Liao, Z. A Phenylpyruvic Acid Reductase Is Required for Biosynthesis of Tropane Alkaloids. *Org. Lett.* **2018**, *20*, 7807–7810. [CrossRef] [PubMed]
59. Schmidt, G.W.; Jirschitzka, J.; Porta, T.; Reichelt, M.; Luck, K.; Torre, J.C.P.; Dolke, F.; Varesio, E.; Hopfgartner, G.; Gershenzon, J.; et al. The Last Step in Cocaine Biosynthesis Is Catalyzed by a BAHD Acyltransferase. *Plant Physiol.* **2015**, *167*, 89–101. [CrossRef] [PubMed]
60. Robins, R.J.; Bachmann, P.; Robinson, T.; Rhodes, M.J.; Yamada, Y. The formation of 3 alpha- and 3 beta-acetoxytropanes by *Datura stramonium* transformed root cultures involves two acetyl-CoA-dependent acyltransferases. *FEBS Lett.* **1991**, *292*, 293–297. [PubMed]
61. Li, R.; Reed, D.W.; Liu, E.; Nowak, J.; Pelcher, L.E.; Page, J.E.; Covello, P.S. Functional genomic analysis of alkaloid biosynthesis in *Hyoscyamus niger* reveals a cytochrome P450 involved in littorine rearrangement. *Chem. Biol.* **2006**, *13*, 513–520. [CrossRef] [PubMed]
62. Hashimoto, T.; Yamada, Y. Hyoscyamine 6b-Hydroxylase, a 2-Oxoglutarate-Dependent Dioxygenase, in Alkaloid Producing Root Cultures. *Plant Physiol.* **1985**, *81*, 619–625. [CrossRef]
63. Hashimoto, T.; Matsuda, J.; Yamada, Y. Two-step epoxidation of hyoscyamine to scopolamine is catalyzed by bifunctional hyoscyamine-6β-hydroxylase. *FEBS Lett.* **1993**, *329*, 35–39. [CrossRef]
64. Korolev, S.; Ikeguchi, Y.; Skarina, T.; Beasley, S.; Arrowsmith, C.; Edwards, A.; Joachimiak, A.; Pegg, A.E.; Savchenko, A. The crystal structure of spermidine synthase with a multisubstrate adduct inhibitor. *Nat. Struct. Biol.* **2002**, *9*, 27–31. [CrossRef]
65. Biastoff, S.; Reinhardt, N.; Reva, V.; Brandt, W.; Draeger, B. Evolution of putrescine N-methyltransferase from spermidine synthase demanded alterations in substrate binding. *FEBS Lett.* **2009**, *583*, 3367–3374. [CrossRef] [PubMed]
66. Teuber, M.; Azemi, M.E.; Namjoyan, F.; Meier, A.C.; Wodak, A.; Brandt, W.; Draeger, B. Putrescine N-methyltransferases—A structure-function analysis. *Plant Mol. Biol.* **2007**, *63*, 787–801. [CrossRef]
67. Oppermann, U.; Filling, C.; Hult, M.; Shafqat, N.; Wu, X.; Lindh, M.; Shafqat, J.; Nordling, E.; Kallberg, Y.; Persson, B.; et al. Short-chain dehydrogenases/reductases (SDR): The 2002 update. *Chem. Biol. Interact.* **2003**, *143–144*, 247–253. [CrossRef]
68. Kushwaha, A.K.; Sangwan, N.S.; Tripathi, S.; Sangwan, R.S. Molecular cloning and catalytic characterization of a recombinant tropine biosynthetic tropinone reductase from *Withania coagulans* leaf. *Gene* **2013**, *516*, 238–247. [CrossRef]

69. Qiang, W.; Xia, K.; Zhang, Q.; Zeng, J.; Huang, Y.; Yang, C.; Chen, M.; Liu, X.; Lan, X.; Liao, Z. Functional characterisation of a tropine-forming reductase gene from *Brugmansia arborea*, a woody plant species producing tropane alkaloids. *Phytochemistry* **2016**, *127*, 12–22. [CrossRef]
70. D'Auria, J.C. Acyltransferases in plants: A good time to be BAHD. *Curr. Opin. Plant Biol.* **2006**, *9*, 331–340. [CrossRef] [PubMed]
71. Chesters, N.C.J.E.; O'Hagan, D.; Robins, R.J. The biosynthesis of tropic acid: The (R)-D-phenyllactyl moiety is processed by the mutase involved in hyoscyamine biosynthesis in *Datura stramonium*. *J. Chem. Soc. Chem. Commun.* **1995**, *0*, 127–128. [CrossRef]
72. Ollagnier, S.; Kervio, E.; Rétey, J. The role and source of 5′-deoxyadenosyl radical in a carbon skeleton rearrangement catalyzed by a plant enzyme. *FEBS Lett.* **1998**, *437*, 309–312. [CrossRef]
73. Pramod, K.K.; Singh, S.; Jayabaskaran, C. Biochemical and structural characterization of recombinant hyoscyamine 6β-hydroxylase from *Datura metel*. *Plant Physiol. Biochem.* **2010**, *48*, 966–970. [CrossRef]
74. Hashimoto, T.; Yamada, Y. Purification and characterization of hyoscyamine 6 beta-hydroxylase from root cultures of *Hyoscyamus niger* L. Hydroxylase and epoxidase activities in the enzyme preparation. *Eur. J. Biochem.* **1987**, *164*, 277–285. [CrossRef]
75. Suzuki, K.; Yamada, Y.; Hashimoto, T. Expression of *Atropa belladonna* putrescine N-methyltransferase gene in root pericycle. *Plant Cell Physiol.* **1999**, *40*, 289–297. [CrossRef] [PubMed]
76. Kanegae, T.; Kajiya, H.; Amano, Y.; Hashimoto, T.; Yamada, Y. Species-dependent expression of the hyoscyamine 6 beta-hydroxylase gene in the pericycle. *Plant Physiol.* **1994**, *105*, 483–490. [CrossRef] [PubMed]
77. Nakajima, K.; Hashimoto, T. Two tropinone reductases, that catalyze opposite stereospecific reductions in tropane alkaloid biosynthesis, are localized in plant root with different cell-specific patterns. *Plant Cell Physiol.* **1999**, *40*, 1099–1107. [CrossRef] [PubMed]
78. Kaiser, H.; Richter, U.; Keiner, R.; Brabant, A.; Hause, B.; Draeger, B. Immunolocalisation of two tropinone reductases in potato (*Solanum tuberosum* L.) root, stolon and tuber sprouts. *Planta* **2006**, *225*, 127–137. [CrossRef] [PubMed]
79. Shoji, T.; Yamada, Y.; Hashimoto, T. Jasmonate induction of putrescine N-methyltransferase genes in the root of *Nicotiana sylvestris*. *Plant Cell Physiol.* **2000**, *41*, 831–839. [CrossRef] [PubMed]
80. Lauersen, K.J. Eukaryotic microalgae as hosts for light-driven heterologous isoprenoid production. *Planta* **2018**, *249*, 155–180. [CrossRef] [PubMed]
81. Leete, E.; Endo, T.; Yamada, Y. Biosynthesis of nicotine and scopolamine in a root culture of *Duboisia leichhardtii*. *Phytochemistry* **1990**, *29*, 1847–1851. [CrossRef]
82. Hemscheidt, T.; Spenser, I.D. Biosynthesis of 6β.-hydroxytropine in *Datura stramonium*: Nonregiospecific incorporation of [1,2-13C2]acetate. *J. Am. Chem. Soc.* **1992**, *114*, 5472–5473. [CrossRef]
83. Hoye, T.R.; Bjorklund, J.A.; Koltun, D.O.; Renner, M.K. N-methylputrescine oxidation during cocaine biosynthesis: Study of prochiral methylene hydrogen discrimination using the remote isotope method. *Org. Lett.* **2000**, *2*, 3–5. [CrossRef]
84. Leete, E.; Bjorklund, J.A.; Sung, H.K. The biosynthesis of the benzoyl moiety of cocaine. *Phytochemistry* **1988**, *27*, 2553–2556. [CrossRef]
85. Scholl, Y.; Höke, D.; Dräger, B. Calystegines in *Calystegia sepium* derive from the tropane alkaloid pathway. *Phytochemistry* **2001**, *58*, 883–889. [CrossRef]
86. Goldmann, A.; Message, B.; Tepfer, D.; Molyneux, R.J.; Duclos, O. Biological Activities of the Nortropane Alkaloid, Calystegine B 2 and Analogs: Structure—Function Relationships. *J. Nat. Prod.* **1996**, *59*, 1137–1142. [CrossRef]
87. Luanratana, O.; Griffin, W.J. Cultivation of a *Duboisia* Hybrid—Part A. *J. Nat. Prod.* **1980**, *43*, 477–491. [CrossRef]
88. Ullrich, S.F.; Hagels, H.; Kayser, O. Scopolamine: a journey from the field to clinics. *Phytochem. Rev.* **2017**, *16*, 333–353. [CrossRef]
89. Ullrich, S.F.; Rothauer, A.; Hagels, H.; Kayser, O. Influence of Light, Temperature and Macronutrients on Growth and Scopolamine Biosynthesis in *Duboisia* species. *Planta Med.* **2017**, *83*, 937–945. [CrossRef] [PubMed]
90. Oksman-Caldentey, K.-M.; Strauss, A. Somaclonal Variation of Scopolamine Content in Protoplast-Derived Cell Culture Clones of *Hyoscyamus muticus*. *Planta Med.* **1986**, *52*, 6–12. [CrossRef]

91. Wang, K. *Agrobacterium Protocols*; Humana Press: Totowa, NJ, USA, 2007; ISBN 1588298434.
92. Georgiev, M.I.; Agostini, E.; Ludwig-Müller, J.; Xu, J. Genetically transformed roots: From plant disease to biotechnological resource. *Trends Biotechnol.* **2012**, *30*, 528–537. [CrossRef]
93. Maldonado-Mendoza, I.E.; Ayora-Talavera, T.; Loyola-Vargas, V.M. Establishment of hairy root cultures of *Datura stramonium*. Characterization and stability of tropane alkaloid production during long periods of subculturing. *Plant Cell. Tissue Organ Cult.* **1993**, *33*, 321–329. [CrossRef]
94. Kamada, H.; Okamura, N.; Satake, M.; Harada, H.; Shimomura, K. Alkaloid production by hairy root cultures in *Atropa belladonna*. *Plant Cell Rep.* **1986**, *5*, 239–242. [CrossRef]
95. Hashimoto, T.; Yun, D.J.; Yamada, Y. Production of tropane alkaloids in genetically engineered root cultures. *Phytochemistry* **1993**, *32*, 713–718. [CrossRef]
96. Falk, L.R.; Doran, P.M. Influence of inoculum morphology on growth of *Atropa belladonna* hairy roots and production of tropane alkaloids. *Biotechnol. Lett.* **1996**, *18*, 1099–1104. [CrossRef]
97. Vakili, B.; Karimi, F.; Sharifi, M.; Behmanesh, M. Chromium-induced tropane alkaloid production and H6H gene expression in *Atropa belladonna* L. (Solanaceae) invitro-propagated plantlets. *Plant Physiol. Biochem.* **2012**, *52*, 98–103. [CrossRef] [PubMed]
98. Jaremicz, Z.; Luczkiewicz, M.; Kokotkiewicz, A.; Krolicka, A.; Sowinski, P. Production of tropane alkaloids in *Hyoscyamus niger* (black henbane) hairy roots grown in bubble-column and spray bioreactors. *Biotechnol. Lett.* **2014**, *36*, 843–853. [CrossRef] [PubMed]
99. Zhang, L.; Ding, R.; Chai, Y.; Bonfill, M.; Moyano, E.; Oksman-Caldentey, K.-M.; Xu, T.; Pi, Y.; Wang, Z.; Zhang, H.; et al. Engineering tropane biosynthetic pathway in *Hyoscyamus niger* hairy root cultures. *Proc. Natl. Acad. Sci. USA* **2004**, *101*, 6786–6791. [CrossRef] [PubMed]
100. Kai, G.; Zhang, A.; Guo, Y.; Li, L.; Cui, L.; Luo, X.; Lin, C.; Xiao, J. Enhancing the production of tropane alkaloids in transgenic *Anisodus acutangulus* hairy root cultures by over-expressing tropinone reductase I and hyoscyamine-6β-hydroxylase. *Mol. Biosyst.* **2012**, *8*, 2883–2890. [CrossRef] [PubMed]
101. Cardillo, A.B.; Otálvaro, A.Á.M.; Busto, V.D.; Talou, J.R.; Velásquez, L.M.E.; Giulietti, A.M. Scopolamine, anisodamine and hyoscyamine production by *Brugmansia candida* hairy root cultures in bioreactors. *Process Biochem.* **2010**, *45*, 1577–1581. [CrossRef]
102. Jouhikainen, K.; Lindgren, L.; Jokelainen, T.; Hiltunen, R.; Teeri, T.H.; Oksman-Caldentey, K.-M. Enhancement of scopolamine production in *Hyoscyamus muticus* L. hairy root cultures by genetic engineering. *Planta* **1999**, *208*, 545–551. [CrossRef]
103. Moyano, E.; Fornalé, S.; Palazón, J.; Cusidó, R.M.; Bagni, N.; Piñol, M.T. Alkaloid production in *Duboisia* hybrid hairy root cultures overexpressing the pmt gene. *Phytochemistry* **2002**, *59*, 697–702. [CrossRef]
104. Palazón, J.; Moyano, E.; Cusidó, R.M.; Bonfill, M.; Oksman-Caldentey, K.M.; Piñol, M.T. Alkaloid production in *Duboisia* hybrid hairy roots and plants overexpressing the h6h gene. *Plant Sci.* **2003**, *165*, 1289–1295. [CrossRef]
105. Bourgaud, F.; Benoit, M.; De Picardie, U.; Verne, J. Développement D' un Nouveau Procédé de Production D'actifs Pharmaceutiques à Partir de Plantes Médicinales: La Technologie des Plantes à Traire. Conference Paper: Les Rencontres du Végétal. Angers, France, 2013. Available online: http://agris.fao.org/agris-search/search.do?recordID=FR2016219199 (accessed on 28 December 2018).
106. Xia, K.; Liu, X.; Zhang, Q.; Qiang, W.; Guo, J.; Lan, X.; Chen, M.; Liao, Z. Promoting scopolamine biosynthesis in transgenic *Atropa belladonna* plants with pmt and h6h overexpression under field conditions. *Plant Physiol. Biochem.* **2016**, *106*, 46–53. [CrossRef] [PubMed]
107. Wang, X.; Chen, M.; Yang, C.; Liu, X.; Zhang, L.; Lan, X.; Tang, K.; Liao, Z. Enhancing the scopolamine production in transgenic plants of *Atropa belladonna* by overexpressing *pmt* and *h6h* genes. *Physiol. Plant.* **2011**, *143*, 309–315. [CrossRef] [PubMed]
108. Cardillo, A.B.; Talou, J.R.; Giulietti, A.M. Expression of *Brugmansia candida* Hyoscyamine 6beta-Hydroxylase gene in *Saccharomyces cerevisiae* and its potential use as biocatalyst. *Microb. Cell Fact.* **2008**, *7*, 17. [CrossRef] [PubMed]
109. Kai, G.; Liu, Y.; Wang, X.; Yang, S.; Fu, X.; Luo, X.; Liao, P. Functional identification of hyoscyamine 6β-hydroxylase from *Anisodus acutangulus* and overproduction of scopolamine in genetically-engineered *Escherichia coli*. *Biotechnol. Lett.* **2011**, *33*, 1361–1365. [CrossRef] [PubMed]
110. Li, J.; Van Belkum, M.J.; Vederas, J.C. Functional characterization of recombinant hyoscyamine 6β-hydroxylase from *Atropa belladonna*. *Bioorganic Med. Chem.* **2012**, *20*, 4356–4363. [CrossRef] [PubMed]

111. Liu, T.; Zhu, P.; Meng, C.; Cheng, K.D.; He, H.X. Molecular cloning, expression and characterization of hyoscyamine 6beta-hydroxylase from hairy roots of *Anisodus tanguticus*. *Planta* **2005**, *71*, 249–253. [CrossRef]
112. Fischer, C.; Kwon, M.; Ro, D.; Van Belkum, M.J.; Vederas, J.C. Isolation, expression and biochemical characterization of recombinant hyoscyamine-6β- hydroxylase from *Brugmansia sanguinea*—Tuning the scopolamine production. *Med. Chem. Commun.* **2018**, *9*, 888–892. [CrossRef]
113. Cao, Y.; He, Y.; Li, H.; Kai, G.; Xu, J.; Yu, H. Efficient biosynthesis of rare natural product scopolamine using *E. coli* cells expressing a S14P/K97A mutant of hyoscyamine 6b -hydroxylase. *J. Biotechnol.* **2015**, *211*, 123–129. [CrossRef]
114. Dehghan, E.; Reed, D.W.; Covello, P.S.; Hasanpour, Z.; Palazon, J.; Oksman-Caldentey, K.M.; Ahmadi, F.S. Genetically engineered hairy root cultures of *Hyoscyamus senecionis* and *H. muticus*: Ploidy as a promising parameter in the metabolic engineering of tropane alkaloids. *Plant Cell Rep.* **2017**, *36*, 1615–1626. [CrossRef]
115. Dehghan, E.; Shahriari Ahmadi, F.; Ghotbi Ravandi, E.; Reed, D.W.; Covello, P.S.; Bahrami, A.R. An atypical pattern of accumulation of scopolamine and other tropane alkaloids and expression of alkaloid pathway genes in *Hyoscyamus senecionis*. *Plant Physiol. Biochem.* **2013**, *70*, 188–194. [CrossRef]
116. Naik, T.; Vanitha, S.C.; Rajvanshi, P.K.; Chandrika, M.; Kamalraj, S.; Jayabaskaran, C. Novel Microbial Sources of Tropane Alkaloids: First Report of Production by Endophytic Fungi Isolated from *Datura metel* L. *Curr. Microbiol.* **2017**, *75*, 1–7. [CrossRef]
117. De Luca, V.; Salim, V.; Thamm, A.; Masada, S.A.; Yu, F. Making iridoids/secoiridoids and monoterpenoid indole alkaloids: Progress on pathway elucidation. *Curr. Opin. Plant Biol.* **2014**, *19*, 35–42. [CrossRef] [PubMed]
118. Polturak, G.; Heinig, U.; Grossman, N.; Battat, M.; Leshkowitz, D.; Malitsky, S.; Rogachev, I.; Aharoni, A. Transcriptome and Metabolic Profiling Provides Insights into Betalain Biosynthesis and Evolution in *Mirabilis jalapa*. *Mol. Plant* **2018**, *11*, 189–204. [CrossRef] [PubMed]

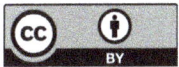

© 2019 by the authors. Licensee MDPI, Basel, Switzerland. This article is an open access article distributed under the terms and conditions of the Creative Commons Attribution (CC BY) license (http://creativecommons.org/licenses/by/4.0/).

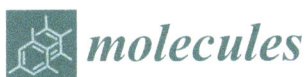

Review

Erythroxylum in Focus: An Interdisciplinary Review of an Overlooked Genus

David A. Restrepo [1,†], Ernesto Saenz [2,†], Orlando Adolfo Jara-Muñoz [3], Iván F. Calixto-Botía [4], Sioly Rodríguez-Suárez [1], Pablo Zuleta [1], Benjamin G. Chavez [5], Juan A. Sanchez [1,2] and John C. D'Auria [5,*]

[1] Centro de Estudios sobre Seguridad y Drogas, Facultad de Economía, Universidad de los Andes, Bogota 111711, Colombia; d.restrepod@uniandes.edu.co (D.A.R.); sirodriguezsu@unal.edu.co (S.R.-S.); p.zuleta@uniandes.edu.co (P.Z.); juansanc@uniandes.edu.co (J.A.S.)
[2] Departamento Ciencias Biológicas, Facultad de Ciencias, Universidad de los Andes, Bogota 111711, Colombia; je.saenz1181@uniandes.edu.co
[3] Jardín Botánico de Bogotá José Celestino Mutis, Bogota 111071, Colombia; ojara@jbb.gov.co
[4] CEMarin student, Escuela de Biología, Universidad Pedagógica y Tecnológica de Colombia, Tunja 150003, Colombia; ivan.calixto@uptc.edu.co
[5] Department of Molecular Genetics, Leibniz Institute of Plant Genetics and Crop Plant Research (IPK), 06466 Gatersleben, Germany; chavez@ipk-gatersleben.de
* Correspondence: dauria@ipk-gatersleben.de; Tel.: +49-394-825-176
† These authors contributed equally to this work.

Academic Editor: John C. D'Auria.
Received: 2 September 2019; Accepted: 18 October 2019; Published: 21 October 2019

Abstract: The genus *Erythroxylum* contains species used by indigenous people of South America long before the domestication of plants. Two species, *E. coca* and *E. novogranatense*, have been utilized for thousands of years specifically for their tropane alkaloid content. While abuse of the narcotic cocaine has impacted society on many levels, these species and their wild relatives contain untapped resources for the benefit of mankind in the form of foods, pharmaceuticals, phytotherapeutic products, and other high-value plant-derived metabolites. In this review, we describe the current state of knowledge of members within the genus and the recent advances in the realm of molecular biology and biochemistry.

Keywords: Erythroxylaceae; *Erythroxylum coca*; next generation sequencing; traditional medicine; bioprospecting; tropane

---

1. Introduction

Humanity has an enduring and intimate relationship with medicinal plants. From prehistoric times through to the modern era, the use of plant specialized metabolites has helped treat diseases, steer religious ceremonies, and cosmetically augment the body. While modern synthetic chemical methods often provide quicker, safer and more cost-effective production of economically important compounds, many plants remain the sole source of such molecules [1,2]. In addition, several plants containing mind altering hallucinogenic or narcotic chemicals have become infamous for the detrimental societal impacts of illicit drugs derived from them [3]. Nonetheless, it is imperative to obtain a deeper understanding of how these plants synthesize their compounds for the future prospects of synthetic biology, metabolic engineering, and potential applications in as far-ranging fields as green medicine and space exploration.

Few plant genera are as rich as *Erythroxylum* L. in their contribution to both highly lucrative legal industries (soft drinks) and one of the largest illicit markets on the planet (cocaine trafficking). The integration of *Erythroxylum* species into the fabric of South American societies makes any discussion of eliminating these plants exceedingly controversial and difficult, with many counterproductive consequences [4]. Indeed, after decades of seemingly fruitless eradication policies, it appears productive and prudent to explore the development of the beneficial uses of these plants, which is an approach that is already being implemented by communities, companies, and governments in South America, within the growing scope of legality provided by the current laws in the Andean region [5]. This approach appears to carry significant potential, given the promising applications indicated by both traditional cultures and the scientific research available. Additionally, recent advances in our knowledge about the biosynthesis of tropane alkaloids, and a growing body of molecular phylogeny studies are revealing a dynamic system of interactions and compounds that justifies further research. Indeed, the use of beneficial products from these plants for medicinal, nutritional, agricultural, and cosmetic purposes is becoming the focus of several countries and scientific groups. In addition, with the ever-increasing capabilities of chemical and genetic analyses, wild species of Erythroxylum are being described and subjected to new studies identifying their potential for future development of medicines. In this review, we consolidate the most recent advances and knowledge in species found within the genus *Erythroxylum*.

2. History and Evolution of the *Erythroxylum* Genus

The genus *Erythroxylum* includes approximately 230 species, distributed across the tropics [6]. Two species in this genus, *Erythroxylum coca* Lam. and *Erythroxylum novogranatense* (D. Morris) Hieron., are particularly salient. They have been cultivated for thousands of years by traditional South American societies and, more recently, have become sources for the production of the tropane alkaloid cocaine (commonly diverted into the global illicit trade).

Each one of these two species commonly referred to as "coca" can be subdivided into two regionally and phenotypically defined varieties, *E. coca* var. *ipadu* Plowman and *E. novogranatense* var. *truxillense* (Rusby) Plowman. The typical variety of *E. coca* is also known as Huánuco or Bolivian Coca (*E. coca* var. *coca*). According to Plowman (1986) [7] this variety probably originated from the eastern Andes of Perú and Bolivia, particularly in the Huállaga Valley, where wild coca plants can be found. The typical altitude of coca crops in this region is between 500 and 1500 m above sea level, but reaching 2000 m in some areas [7]. *E. coca* var. *coca* is the most common cultivar used in cocaine production for the drug trade in Perú and Colombia. Amazonian coca, or Ipadú coca (*E. coca* var. *ipadu*) is grown in the Amazonian region, which includes Colombia, Brazil, and Perú. Colombian coca (*E. novogranatense* var. *novogranatense*) is cultivated in the inter-Andean valleys of Colombia, and in the Sierra Nevada de Santa Marta region. It can also be found as a domestic garden plant in urban settings. Finally, Trujillo coca (*E. novogranatense* var. *truxillense*), which grows mainly in northern Perú, and is the variety best adapted to the dry, arid climates of Perú's coastal deserts.

Coca is among the oldest cultivated medicinal plant species, with evidence of its use dating back at least 8000 years in South America [8,9]. Traditional coca consumption remains prevalent across scores of Andean and Amazonian communities. In 2012, Bolivia's traditional coca-using population was estimated at around three million people [10], while in 2013, Perú's coca-using population numbered around 3.5 million [11]. In addition, significant traditional coca-using populations are also found in Argentina, Brazil, Chile, and Colombia, although their numbers are unknown [12].

Coca leaves contain the highest amounts of cocaine and other tropanes in the plant [13]. The total alkaloid content of coca leaves varies by variety and climate. For example, Bolivian coca contains on average 0.63% dry weight cocaine in the leaves [14], whereas, *E. coca* var. ipadu (Amazonian coca) contains between 0.11% and 0.41% cocaine content. No significant differences were witnessed between laboratory and field grown Amazonian coca plants, suggesting that the biosynthesis of tropane alkaloids is regulated at the molecular genetic level. The highest cocaine levels identified in common cultivars of coca are obtained from the *E. novogranatense* varieties. In this species, cocaine levels vary from an average of 0.77% in Colombian coca to 0.72% in Trujillo coca. A study by Acock et al. (1996) [15] revealed that while light intensity (photosynthetic photon flux density) did not seem to have much of an effect on alkaloid production, temperature did have an effect. Lower temperatures seemed to adversely affect alkaloid content in all studied cultivars.

Coca leaves are traditionally consumed by forming a quid in the cheek (i.e., in English this is called "coca chewing", although little chewing is involved). Frequently, the coca leaf quid is complemented with a basified material or alkaline adjuvants. These are generally processed (usually burnt) from diverse sources such as plant ashes (i.e., quinoa, tree leaves, and cinnamon), animal bones, seashells, mineral deposits, and sodium bicarbonate. These alkaline adjuvants bear a multitude of names across South America (i.e., cal, llipta, ilucta, mambe, tocra, lejía, etc.) [16]. The mode of traditional coca consumption varies according to the coca variety and the alkaline substance used. For example, Huánuco coca leaves are chewed directly following the addition of the alkaline powder (cal), which is alternated with additional leaves and cal. The alkaline powder is often substituted with sodium bicarbonate or other adjuvants, especially for non-native consumers. Colombian coca and Trujillo coca are both chewed with ashes made from incinerated seashells, bones, or mineral deposits found in limestone rock formations. Amazonian coca is processed more extensively, presumably with the aim of strengthening the release of its lower alkaloid content, via a complex process that includes the mild roasting and powdering of the leaves, followed by filtering with a fine mesh or fabric and mixing with dried leaf ashes of the species *Cecropia sciadophylla* Mart. Other species of the Cecropiaceae, such as *Cecropia peltata* L. and *Pouruma cecropiifolia* Mart. are occasionally used when C. sciadophylla is unavailable [7,17]. Schultes (1981) [17] makes reference to the addition of other plants to the coca powder to increase its effects or improve flavor. For example, several species within the genus *Costus* L., one species of *Styrax* L., and the palms *Cocratea exorrhiza* (Mart.) H.Wendl. and *Astrocaryum gynacanthum* Mart. (=*Astrocaryum munbaca* Mart.) have all been documented for this purpose. The subjective effect on human consumers is described as energizing and mood enhancing, as well as providing a sense of well-being, while suppressing feelings of appetite and thirst [18].

Coca has a rich social, cultural and medicinal significance in the traditional South American cultures where it is cultivated and used [12]. It is employed, disproportionately by adult men, to promote individual work performance and self-discipline as well as to strengthen community ties via work-related social gatherings, "town hall" style meetings, religious ceremonies, and important life events (such as weddings and funerals), where sharing and using coca are central activities [19–21]. Coca also bears metaphysical significance, as it is used as an offering to nature, in divinatory practices, and as part of rituals believed to help sustain the balance between the human and natural worlds [19].

In traditional medicine, coca is utilized as a remedy for a wide variety of conditions, ranging from alleviating oral pains, digestive maladies, hunger, altitude sickness, muscular and skeletal aches, as well as sadness and sexual impotence [22]. The uses and potential of coca in traditional and contemporary medicine, nutrition, and agriculture are further explored in Section 4.

2.1. The Phylogeny of Erythroxylum and Related Genera

The families Erythroxylaceae and Rhizophoraceae make up a well-supported clade in the order Malpighiales [23]. Both families share numerous morphological characteristics [24], as well as specific types of alkaloids that are rare in other groups of angiosperms, such as hygroline, tropane alkaloids, and pyrrolizidines [25]. In the Erythroxylaceae, *Erythroxylum* is placed adjacent to the clade formed by the African genera *Nectaropetalum* Engl., *Pinacopodium* Exell and Mendonça, and *Aneulophus* Benth. The clade formed by these three genera is sister to the genus *Aneulophus* Benth., also endemic to Africa [26]. A phylogenetic framework of *Erythroxylum* has been recently reported by Islam (2011) [27] and White et al. (2019) [28]. This work provides a greater understanding of the subgeneric relationships within the genus and complements the original monograph written over 100 years ago [29]. Recent phylogenetic studies agree with earlier work, suggesting that most of the sections proposed by Schulz (1907) [29] are not monophyletic [14,30–32].

The phylogeny presented by Islam (2011) [27] is based on two loci, the intergenic spacer of the chloroplast rpL32-trnL, and the intergenic spacer of the Ribosome (ITS), whereas the tree presented by

White et al. (2019) [28] is based on 547 nuclear genes. These studies are consistent with each other when considering the position of the cultivated species. In both phylogenies, *E. novogranatense* and *E. coca* are not sister species, contradicting the results from Bohm et al. (1982) [33]. According to White et al. (2019) [28], cultivated species stay in a clade with approximately 24 species (see Figure 1), distributed mainly in the northwestern region of the Neotropics, which in turn includes a mainly Caribbean clade, with species such as, *Erythroxylum brevipes* DC., *Erythroxylum carthagenense* Jacq., *Erythroxylum cumanense* Jacq., and *Erythroxylum havanense* Jacq., and a mainly Amazonian and Andean clade which includes the two cultivated species, as well as *Erythroxylum cataractarum* Spruce ex Peyr., and *Erythroxylum gracilipes* Peyr.

Erythroxylum species, with current or potential biomedical applications, belong to a variety of clades within the genus's phylogeny. The American species are grouped in sections of *Erythroxylum*, *Archerythroxylum*, and *Macrocalyx*. *Archerythroxylum* is a paraphyletic grouping, containing at least seven American sections [28]. *Macrocalyx* is polyphyletic and nested within the *Archerythroxylum* species [30]. Species belonging to *Archerythroxylum* include *Erythroxylum vacciniifolium* Mart. which is located in clade I (sensu [28]), *Erythroxylum caatingae* Plowman which is a sister species in clade V (also containing the cultivated species), and *Erythroxylum ovaliifolium* Peyr. whose phylogenetic location is unknown. *Erythroxylum subsessile* (Mart.) O.E. Schulz belongs to *Erythroxylum* and is located also in clade I. *Erythroxylum suberosum* A.St.-Hill., A.Juss. and Cambess has not been included in molecular phylogenies, but there is morphological and anatomical evidence to place it near *Erythroxylum macrophyllum* var. *savannarum* Plowman in clade III [30].

Few African species have been included in phylogenetic analyses, however, it can be inferred from White et al. (2019) [28] that these species do not constitute a monophyletic grouping. At least one of these groups, which includes *Erythroxylum nitidulum* Baker, is sister to the rest of the genus. The African species with biomedical applications belongs in two sections as follows: *Erythroxylum macrocarpum* O.E. Schulz and *Erythroxylum laurifolium* Lam. can be found in the *Pachylobus* section and *Erythroxylum pervillei* Baill. belongs to the *Eurysepalum* section. Finally, the Asian *Erythroxylum cuneatum* (Miq.) belongs to the *Coelocarpus* section, which is morphologically diverse and possibly not monophyletic, with species present in Australia, Southeast Asia, and West Africa.

Most *Erythroxylum* species are distyle, featuring individuals whose flowers have short styles and long stamens (brevistyles) and long styles and short stamens (longistyles). This characteristic was first described by Darwin [34]. Such floral dimorphism is associated with self-incompatibility in the genus, which has been shown experimentally to be stronger in *E. coca* than in *E. novogranatense* [33,35]. Crossing has been successful between *E. novogranatense* varieties, whereas crossing is only successful between species when one of the individuals is a staminated *E. coca*. Crosses are much more frequent when they involve *E. novogranatense* var. *truxillense* [33].

In studies of wild and distyle species in the genus, it has been shown that *Erythroxylum havanense* Jacq. is self-incompatible [36], while *Erythroxylum amazonicum* Peyr. is self-compatible [37]. More detailed *E. havanense* analyses have proven the existence of sharp pollen fertility differences across flower types, suggesting an active evolutionary transition toward dioicity [38–40]. A similar loss of the distyle condition, expressed as seed production without pollination (agamospermy), was detected for *Erythroxylum undulatum* Plowman at the embryological level [41].

2.2. Domestication of the Coca Plant

The first explicit hypothesis about coca domestication was based mainly on the results of hybridization experiments and flavonoid profiles of the cultivated varieties [33]. Under this hypothesis, Bohm et al. (1982) [33] proposed a linear process of domestication of the cultivated varieties. This postulated series of domestication events started with *E. coca*, which is thought to have originated from a wild relative, presumably in the Amazonian foothills of Perú and Bolivia. In this domestication model, the Amazonian variety Ipadú originated from the Andean-adapted species. Trujillo Coca was then developed independently as an adaptation to the dryer conditions of the northern regions of Perú.

Finally, Colombian coca was selected from Trujillo coca, with an adaptation to the wetter environments of the inter-Andean valleys of Colombia.

Phylogenies based on amplified fragment length polymorphism (AFLP) fingerprinting [42,43], support the monophyly of each cultivated species, *E. coca* and *E. novogranatense*. Johnson et al. (2005) [43] reported that both cultivated species are genetically well separated and have similar intraspecific variability, which is a pattern that contradicts the linear hypothesis of domestication. This genetic structure pattern, combined with the allopatric distribution of both species, suggests an independent origin, which makes both species sister groups. At the intraspecific level, AFLP data showed little variation in *E. coca* var. *ipadu*, which is consistent with the clonal mode of propagation in this variety [9,44,45], and with the domestication hypothesis of Bohm et al. (1982) [33]. Genetic distance between varieties of *E. novogranatense* was negligible, however, because differences in ecological preferences and leaf flavonoid chemotypes are clearly distinguished, taxonomic status of these varieties was not rejected [46–49].

The most robust taxonomically-sampled phylogenies produced by Islam et al. (2011) [27] and White et al. (2019) [28] indicate that the cultivated species of coca are not sister groups, contradicting the results of the studies mentioned above. According to White et al. (2019) [28] *E. coca* is located in a clade that includes *E. gracilipes* (paraphyletic) and *E. cataractarum* (Figure 1), while *E. novogranatense* is the sister species of the clade formed by these three species. Under this scenario, White et al. (2019) [28], proposed a new hypothesis, with independent domestication events, one of these from *E. cataractarum* to produce *E. novogranatense*, and the second one from *E. gracilipes* to produce *E. coca*. This view is supported by the phylogenetic position of the taxa, and by the geographical distribution of the potential ancestor species, with *E. cataractarum* closer to *E. novogranatense*, and *E. gracilipes* closer to *E. coca*. More genetic evidence at the population level could help produce a more conclusive hypothesis of coca domestication. In addition, improving the taxonomic sampling in section *Archerythroxylum* would also help resolve the question of the proper placement of species in this clade.

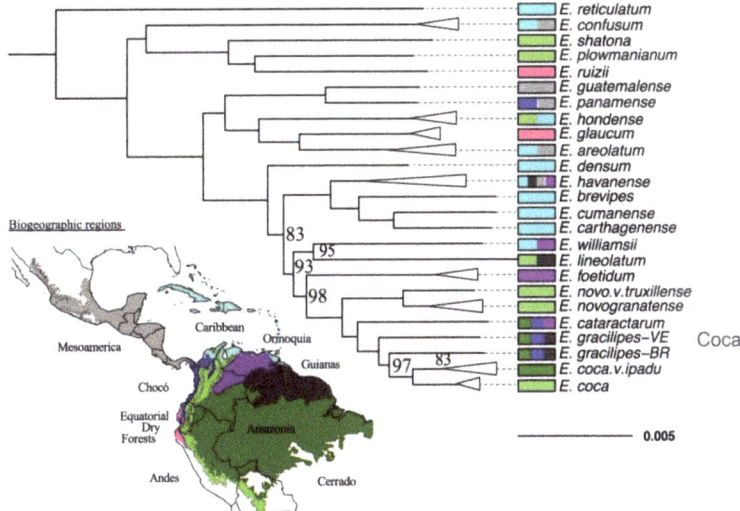

Figure 1. Phylogeny of the *Erythroxylum* genus. Colors on the map and the bars next to the names indicate the biogeographic regions where the species are naturally distributed. Numbers on the nodes indicate bootstrap support, which is 100% where not indicated. Modification of the phylogeny, inferred by White et al. (2019) [28] in the American Journal of Botany, 106(1), p. 158, is republished with permission from the Botanical Society of America.

2.3. Omic Studies on Erythroxylum to Shed Light on Evolution and Functional Background

Next-generation sequencing (NGS) technologies have revolutionized the acquisition of genetic information and the understanding of molecular processes. Recovering high-throughput genetic data in *Erythroxylum* can provide an integral perspective regarding key components of its genome. For instance, this data can uncover the basis of current diversification patterns by shedding light on the functional meaning (i.e., the function of DNA sequences), structural organization (including the genetic mapping and sequencing of entire chromosomes or genomes), and the scale of genomic differences (such as constructing multiple genome alignments to assess major evolutionary events such as chromosomal rearrangements). Population and phylogenetic studies are migrating from traditional molecular markers such as microsatellites and AFLP [42,43], to screening methodologies coupled to NGS platforms. To date, few efforts have been reported regarding the use of omic data for *Erythroxylum* species. Noteworthy exceptions are the Sanger library of sequenced cDNA and the 454 transcriptome data both made from biosynthetically active young leaf tissue [50,51], which characterize the biosynthesis of alkaloids. In addition, there is a reported chloroplast genome for *E. novogranatense* (NCBI accession number NC_030601.1), produced from whole genome sequencing using a short-read high-throughput strategy via an Illumina platform. Finally, there is the previously mentioned study of White et al. (2019) [28] across *Acherythroxylum* members, which utilized a gene-target sequencing strategy (exome sequencing) and a draft genome assembly for *E. coca* as a reference for phylogenetic purposes.

A cost-effective strategy to obtain genomic information is reduced representation sequencing (RRS), where thousands of single nucleotide polymorphisms (SNP) are homogeneously screened with genotype neutral loci and adaptive loci detected as outliers from the genomic background (for extended literature see [52–54]). Neutral loci can provide a measure of genetic differentiation to address several questions in demography, phylogeography, or population genetics based on how the genetic diversity is partitioned across individuals, populations, and species in *Erythroxylum*. In addition to supporting our knowledge of evolutionary processes, these types of studies can provide new approaches for tracing gene flow dynamics, allowing the development of marker-based tools. These can help the identification of new cultigens, as well as the loci involved in the biosynthesis of compounds of interest (such as alkaloids).

Omics data also have the potential to produce useful information for several bioprospecting targets in *Erythroxylum*, such as the ones referenced in the next two chapters. This information can serve as a platform for gene discovery, the development of breeding programs (where phenotypic traits are linked to specific sites or genes, using strategies such as marker assisted selection, MAS), and even the development of pharmaceutical products using gene editing tools. Nevertheless, limited published data on these efforts is available, particularly in comparison to other species that produce specialized metabolites and are also used as illicit substances. The most conspicuous example is the research on *Cannabis*, which is at least a decade ahead in available omic information (genomes, transcriptomes, genetic maps, metabolic pathways, etc.) and is already succeeding in using this data to generate desirable plant characteristics for industrial purposes. This includes the development of plant lines where the biosynthesis of tetrahydrocannabinol (THC, the molecule producing psychoactive effects) is minimized, and cannabidiol (CBD, with broad medical applications) biosynthesis is enhanced [55,56], boosting a growing pharmaceutical and phytotherapeutic market.

Cannabis research demonstrates the importance of modern omics technologies in deciphering and making productive use of genetic resources. Within the bioprospection studies in *Erythroxylum*, such endeavors involve reconstructing the overall metabolic network of tropane biosynthesis, where association studies between particular phenotypes of *E. coca* and *E. novogranatense* are coupled with whole genomes (both assembled and annotated), transcriptional profiles, SNP screens (for putative genes of interest), and whole metabolomic data. This type of biological information could serve as a knowledge platform with multiple productive applications. These range from detailing the history and evolution of *Erythroxylum* species to identifying the metabolic pathways (as well as promoters and inhibitors) of key compounds (such as alkaloids and flavonoids) to enabling more effective crop management strategies.

3. An Overview of Bioprospection and Pharmacological Research in the *Erythroxylum* Genus

The widespread distribution of the *Erythroxylum* genus has led its member species to face diverse climates, herbivore pressures, and soil nutrient conditions, resulting in a wide array of adaptations. These include the evolution of multiple general and specialized metabolites with nutritional and biomedical potential. Such a large reservoir of molecules offers an opportunity for the use of up-to-date "screening" tools that can help identify the productive applications of this genus across many biochemical pathways. Table 1 summarizes the applications of *Erythroxylum* metabolites found across the health literature.

Table 1. Bioactive properties within some members of the genus *Erythroxylum*.

Species	Distribution	Type of Study	Bioactive Properties	Extract Source	Active Compounds	References
Erythroxylum vacciniifolium Mart.	Brazilian northeast, Atlantic Forest	Pre-clinical testing: Lymphotropic virus type I (HTLV-1) positive MT-4 cells and mice	- Aphrodisiac - Tonic - Antimicrobial - Anticancer	Stem bark	C-3 α ester; C-3 3,4,5 trimethoxybenzoic acid; pyrrole-2-carboxylic acid; cinchonains 1a and 1b	Zanolari et al. (2003) Graf et al. (1978) Manabe et al. (1992) Satoh et al. (2000)
Erythroxylum ovalifolium Peyr.	Restinga (sandbanks) in the state of Rio de Janeiro (Brazil)	Pre-clinical testing: Swiss mice	- Neutralize toxicity of snake venom - Treat edemas and hemorrhages - Anti-fungal	Stem bark	Friedelin and Lupeol	Coriolano de Olivero et al. (2016)
Erythroxylum pervillei Baill.	Endemic to Madagascar	Testing: Human ovarian adenocarcinoma (SKVLB) cells and multidrug-resistance oral epidermoid carcinoma (KB-V1) cells	- Anticancer - Treat abdominal pain	Stem bark and roots	- Previlleine A, G and H - Aromtic sters	Chin et al. (2006) Silva et al. (2001)
Erythroxylum macrocarpum O.E. Schulz	Endemic to Mauritius	Pre-clinical testing: Swis albino rats	- Antibacterial - Diuretic	Leaves and twigs	- Tannins - Flavonoids - Tropan-3α-ol - tropan-3β-ol - 6β-diol	Mahomoodally et al. (2005) Al-said et al. (1986)
Erythroxylum caatingae Plowman	Dry forest in northeastern Brazil known as Caatinga	Pre-clinical testing: Swiss mice and human cancer cells from leukemia (K562), lung (NCI-H292) and larynx (Hep-2)	- Anticancer - Antimicrobial	Stem	- 6β-Benzoyloxy-3α-(3,4,5-trimethoxybenzoyloxy)	Aguiar et al. (2012)
Erythroxylum suberosum A.St.-Hill., A.Juss & Cambess.	Savannahs in Brazil, Bolivia, Paraguay, Venezuela and the Guyanas.	Testing: Human cancer cells of oral squamous carcinoma (SCC-9), hypopharynx squamous carcinoma (FaDu) and human keratinocyte (HaCaT)	- Antidiarrhea - Astringent - Antirheumatoid - Anesthetic - Antioxidant	Leaves	- Coumarins - Flavonoids - Isoquercitrin - Catechin	Riberio et al. (2015) Barros et al. (2017) Macedo et al. (2016)
Erythroxylum laurifolium Lam.	Endemic to Mauritius	Testing: Kidney epithelial cells (VERO)	- Anti-diabetic - Anti-hypertension - Effects against Herpes I virus	Leaves	- Afzelin - Quercitrin - Tannins - Flavonoids	Picot et al. (2014) Hansen et al. (1996) Lohezic et al. (1999) Jelager et al. (1998)

3.1. *Erythroxylum vacciniifolium* Mart.

E. vacciniifolium is a popular medicinal plant in Brazil. An infusion made with this plant is called "catuaba" (a name also applied to infusions of plants belonging to other genera). *E. vacciniifolium* stands out for having tonic and aphrodisiac properties. According to Zanolari et al. (2003) [57], these effects are linked to the plant's tropane content, including catuabines **A**, **B**, and **C**. Extensive research has been conducted on *E. vacciniifolium* and other species in this genus to identify bioactive compounds with medicinal properties. These bioactive properties are linked to the compounds' chemical structure, such as the presence of C-3 α ester, a moiety not often found in tropanes of the

Erythroxylaceae. For catuabines **A** and **B**, this is C-3 3,4,5 trimethoxybenzoic acid and for catuabine C it is pyrrole-2-carboxylic acid [58]. Novel tropane alkaloids are shown in Figure 2.

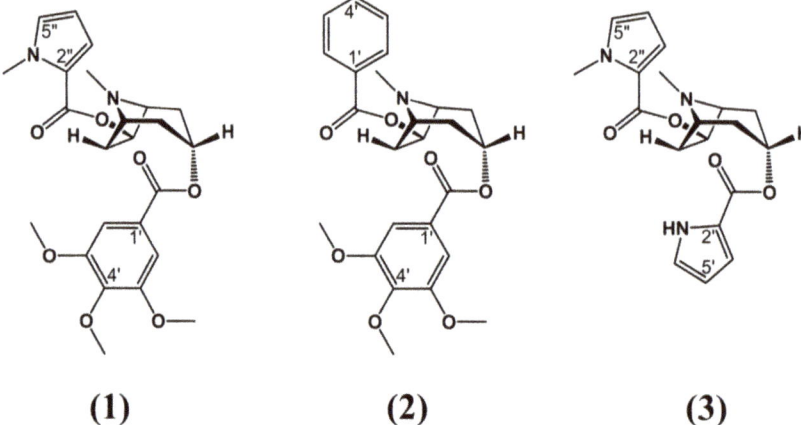

Figure 2. Example of novel tropane alkaloids found in extracts of *E. vacciniifolium*. Structural data was determined using high-resolution electrospray ion cyclotron resonance mass spectroscopic analysis [57].

Indigenous people utilize the leaves of the plant as a stimulant. In addition, its bark is used as a remedy for erectile dysfunction. Alkaline extracts and teas made with *E. vacciniifolium* appear to act on the human immunodeficiency virus (HIV) and against opportunistic infections [57]. This may stem from the antimicrobial activity of the *E. vacciniiifolium* extract against *Escherichia coli* and *Staphylococcus aureus*, which can cause lethal infections especially in patients with compromised immune systems [59]. Catuaba's cytotoxic activity has also been studied, as it yields two cytotoxic flavonoids, cinchonains [DR1] 1a (**4**) and 1b (**5**). Applying these flavonoids to L1210 mouse leukemia cell cultures results in a significant reduction in the number of cancerous cells. [60] (Figure 3).

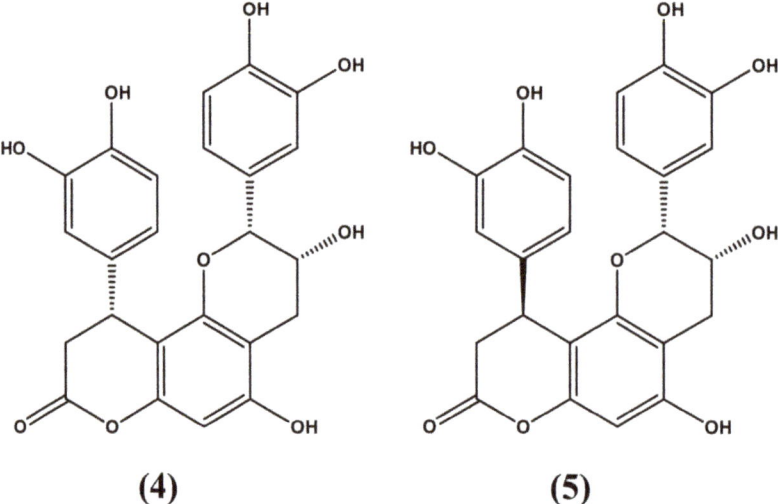

Figure 3. Cinchonains 1a (**4**) and 1b (**5**) as reported in Satoh et al. (2000) [60].

3.2. Erythroxylum ovalifolium Peyr.

E. ovalifolium is a woody shrub extensively distributed along Brazil's coastal plains. As with other species in the genus, this shrub has attracted research interest due to its medicinal bioactive properties. E. ovalifolium extracts can significantly neutralize the toxic effects of snake venom, such as the one produced by the Southern American bushmaster Lachesis muta. Additionally, these extracts also minimize edemas and hemorrhages, symptoms associated with snake venom exposure. Pure E. ovalifolium extracts have been noted for their antifungal properties against fibrous fungi such as Fusarium guttiforme and Chalara paradoxa. Along with other species in the genus, E. ovalifolium can produce tropane alkaloids. Medicinal triterpenoids, such as friedelin (**6**) and lupeol (**7**) Figure 4, and a host of flavonoids have also been detected in E. ovalifolium extracts [61].

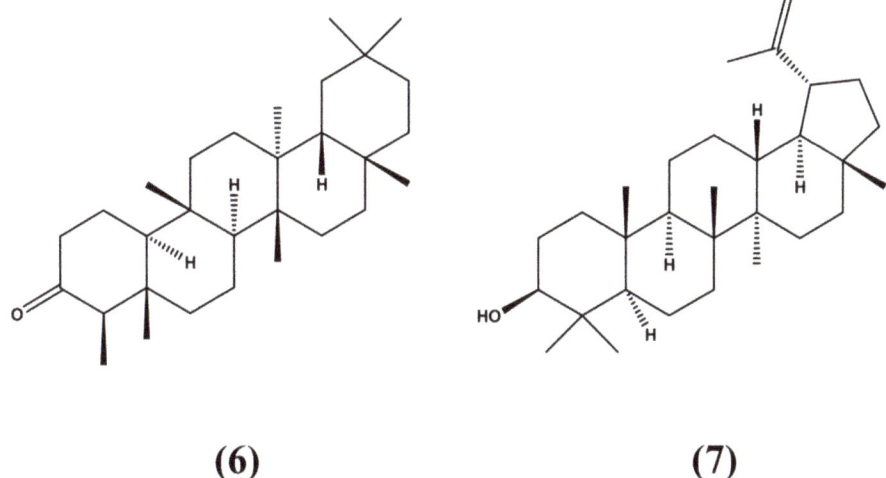

Figure 4. The triterpenoids friedelin (**6**) and lupeol (**7**) isolated and described in E. ovalifolium extracts [61].

3.3. Erythroxylum pervillei Baill.

E. pervillei stands out in its genus for having the most applications across both biotechnology and medicine. Several isolated compounds from E. pervillei are used to counteract drug resistance in tumor-based diseases [62].

For instance, pervilleines such as pervilleine A (**8**) with N-oxide are used to revert pharmacological resistance in small tumor panels. These compounds are known for their trimethoxycinnamate group at C-6, which confers the cytotoxic and antitumor properties commonly found in these plants. Additionally, these compounds restore vinblastine and colchicine sensitivity in several cell lines. Furthermore, methanolic extracts and tropane alkaloids from E. pervillei preparations are used in traditional medicine for their cytotoxic properties and as antineoplastic agents, inhibiting malignant tumor growth [52]. In traditional medicine, E. pervillei preparations are used for their cytotoxic properties and as antineoplastic agents, inhibiting malignant tumor growth. Traditional communities also use E. pervillei roots for treating abdominal pain. Among certain cultures, this plant is known as "Tsivano" and is employed as a fish poison [63,64]. This research resulted in the identification of novel aromatic esters shown in Figure 5.

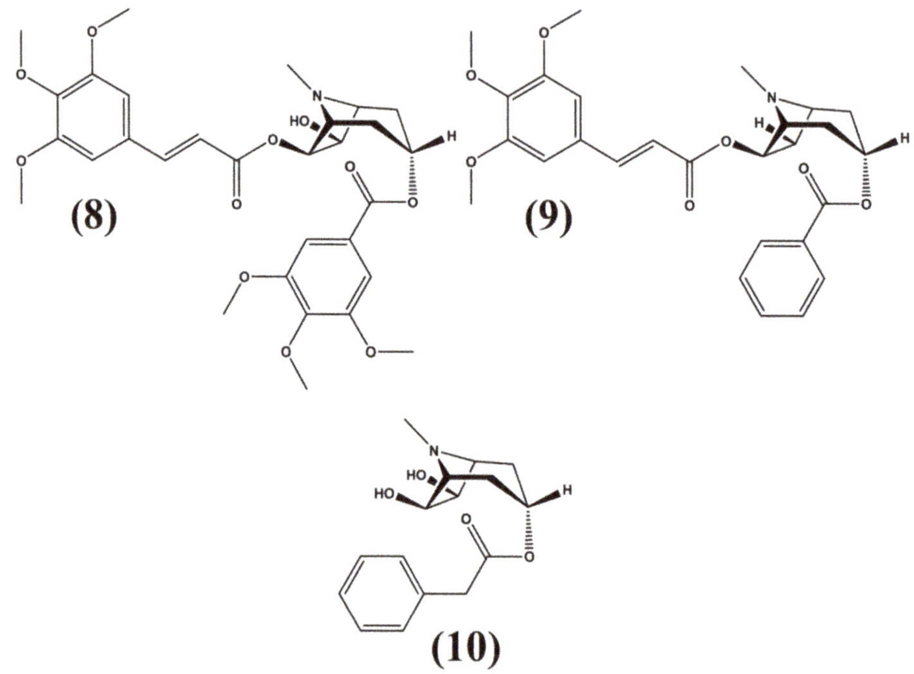

Figure 5. Pervilleine A (**8**) and other aromatic esters isolated from extracts of *E. pervillei* [64].

3.4. Erythroxylum macrocarpum O.E. Schulz

Several studies have produced descriptions of *E. macrocarpum*'s components and medicinal properties. The plant is rich in tannins, phenols, flavonoids, and alkaloids, with the latter displaying antimicrobial activity. Aqueous extracts of *E. macrocarpum* feature a wide spectrum antibiotic activity against test organisms like *Staphylococcus aureus*, however, there are no reports of antifungal properties associated with these extracts. It is noteworthy that most of the antibacterial compounds are found in the plant's leaves, and less frequently in branches or roots [65].

Several studies suggest that *E. macrocarpum* displays a notable diuretic effect (i.e., it augments the flow of urine), which may have clinical value in several kidney disorders. This activity is achieved by means of compounds that limit the Na+ permeability of enterocytes, reducing the electrochemical gradient and minimizing the force that propels fluid through the small intestine. In this manner, the liquid reabsorption is inhibited across the nephron's proximate, distal and collector ducts, which leads to the production of high urine quantities [66]. The plant's main alkaloids are benzoyl esters of tropan-3α-ol, tropan-3β-ol and tropan-3α, 6β-diol, as well as their Nor-derivatives, which contribute to this plant's medicinal characteristics [67]. Examples of these structures can be found in Figure 6.

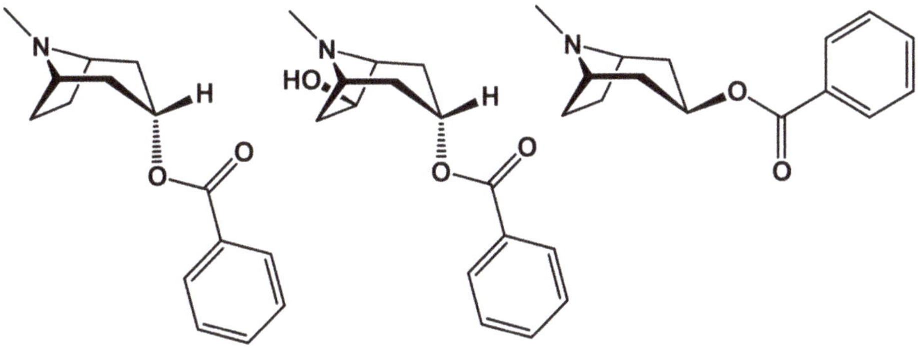

(11)   **(12)**   **(13)**

Figure 6. Examples of tropanes found in *Erythroxylum macrocarpum* [67].

3.5. *Erythroxylum caatingae* Plowman

E. caatingae, another species found in Brazil was reported to have antifungal and antimicrobial activity with little cytotoxic activity in mice [63]. In particular, the tropane catuabine B, 6β-benzoyloxy-3α-(3,4,5-trimethoxybenzoyloxy), elucidated by De Oliveira et al. (2011) [68], induced a rise in early apoptosis in cells from 53.0% to 74.8% [63].

3.6. *Erythroxylum Suberosum* A.St.-Hill., A.Juss and Cambess

E. suberosum is a small and woody shrub popular in Brazil as a medicinal plant. It is claimed to have anti-diarrhea, astringent, anti-rheumatoid, and anesthetic properties among others. There has been little research to ascertain the chemistry behind these effects. Nonetheless, Ribeiro et al. 2015 [69] highlights some of the properties of *E. suberosum* extracts and suggests the presence of alkaloids, coumarins, flavonoids, anthocyanins, tannins, and tri-terpenes as causal agents. He also mentions that the *E. suberosum* extract displays high antioxidant effects through DPPH reduction, mediated by the phenolic compounds from this plant [69]. This last claim is confirmed in Barros et al. 2017 [70], wherein he isolates isoquercitrin, quercetin, catechin, and epicatechin isomers displaying antioxidant activities. Additionally, extracts from this plant show cytotoxic activity from these compounds in head and neck cancers, particularly tongue and hypopharynx carcinomas [71].

3.7. *Erythroxylum laurifolium* Lam.

Found in the Mauricio region in Brazil, this plant is thought to have antidiabetic medicinal properties. One mechanistic study reported the plant's inhibitory effect on important carbohydrate hydrolysis enzymes, including amylase and α-glucosidase. Additionally, the plant's extracts appear to trap glucose via its kinetic effect on amylosis. These extracts show stronger medicinal effects if prepared with methanol rather than water [72]. Ethanol extracts from *E. laurifolium* inhibit angiotensin enzymes, an effect used in treating arterial hypertension from heart and kidney failure. The effect is linked to *E. laurifolium*'s proanthocyanidins or condensed tannins and flavonoids quercitrin and afzelin [73]. Additionally, its oligomeric and polymeric proanthocyanidins act against the Herpes simplex type I virus, by disrupting its replication via enzyme inhibition [74]. Similarly, the plant extracts' antimicrobial activity has been evaluated against *Staphylococcus aureus*, *Escherichia coli*, *Pseudomonas aeruginosa*, and *Salmonella typhi*. These effects are attributed to the isolated tannins found in *E. laurifolium* extracts [75].

4. *Erythroxylum coca* and *E. novogranatense*: Coca's Productive Uses

4.1. Context of Coca's Uses

Coca's traditional use as a natural stimulant among native South Americans prompted a boom in scientific interest during the 19th and early 20th century. This history is extensively researched by Gootemberg (2008) [76]. This initial scientific interest led to the isolation of cocaine and its derivatives, the first anesthetics identified by science, contributing to the rise of modern anesthetic-assisted surgery and pharmaceuticals, as well as the emergence of the soft-beverage industry (including Coca Cola, which still contains decocainized coca leaf extracts).

Nevertheless, the early 20th century backlash against cocaine, due to its toxicity and potential for addiction, drove the stigmatization of whole coca [76] and has held back research and development activity regarding its potential applications. Indeed, legal hurdles, stigma, and conflation with cocaine, compounded by the lack of awareness regarding coca's unique characteristics, have impeded research on whole coca and its non-cocaine components [77,78]. To this day, the science regarding whole coca's risk profile and productive applications remains limited, both due to the paucity of research on this topic and the need to replicate and enhance existing studies [79]. For instance, the available articles on coca's physiological and health effects (referenced throughout this section) consist of case studies rather than clinical trials. This is unsurprising given the obstacles to performing coca research thus far. That said, traditional medicine, the incipient research available on coca, and the findings from related *Erythroxylum* species indicate that there is potential for addressing the coca research gap and developing coca's productive applications.

4.2. Whole Coca versus Isolated Cocaine

Coca's safety profile, due to its cocaine content, is a key consideration when pondering the development of coca's productive applications. The Biondich and Joslin (2016) [79] review explores coca's safety profile and finds several factors that may contribute to the safety of whole coca leaf products as compared to the health risks associated with cocaine isolates. First, whole coca leaf products expose humans to significantly lower cocaine content. Whole leaves average 0.1% to 0.9% cocaine weight and, typically, traditional coca chewers consume 60 g of leaf over the span of a day, resulting in gradual, partial absorption of coca's alkaloids. Secondly, because the cocaine present in whole leaf is not as readily absorbed as cocaine isolates (particularly, the soluble cocaine hydrochloride salt), peak cocaine concentrations in the blood are approximately 50 times lower than when cocaine isolates are consumed. Third, whole coca is believed to contain three endogenous alkaloids, as well as yield some 17 other alkaloids [80,81], belonging to the tropanes, pyrrolidines, and pyridines. According to Novák et al. (1984) [82], coca's other alkaloids are significantly less toxic and active than cocaine and, based on Rubio et al. (2015) [83], at least some of these are also significantly absorbed. Potentially, these alkaloids interact with similar receptors as cocaine and may contribute to different, and possibly milder, pharmacological outcomes.

A topic that has not received significant scientific attention is the pharmacokinetic activity of whole coca alkaloids. As whole coca's endogenous cocaine and related alkaloids are not stabilized as a cocaine salt (i.e., cocaine hydrochloride), whole coca's endogenous cocaine may react in the presence of saliva and alkali solutions in the oral mucus. This could result in the partial breakdown of cocaine into other alkaloids that also contribute to different pharmacological outcomes vis-à-vis cocaine isolates. Similarly, the presence of other phytochemicals (such as flavonoids) with significant metabolic activity is poorly documented and their effects and interactions with coca's other components remains unexamined in the literature.

Nersesyan et al. (2013) [84] produced a case study of whole coca's oral cancer risk and found indications that it was potentially lower than other psychoactive plants used orally. Nersesyan et al. (2013) [84] detected no nuclear DNA damage resulting from coca use, however, they noted some acute cytotoxicity when coca is accompanied with alkaline adjuvants [84]. The extent to which these effects may or may not increase cancer risk is unknown.

The multiple factors that reduce coca's risks vis-à-vis isolated cocaine may explain the absence of reports regarding whole coca harms. The WHO/UNICRI Cocaine Project 1995 [85], which allegedly reviewed coca and cocaine, could not identify evidence of negative health consequences for coca leaf chewing or whole coca product formats [85], however, this review went unpublished due to political pressures and was only recovered for general dissemination after lobbying efforts by civil society organizations [86]. It should be noted that this WHO project did not conduct extensive epidemiological research on coca leaf consumption, which remains a gap in the scientific evidence.

4.3. Potential Uses in Contemporary Medicine

The potential value of coca leaf in contemporary medicine is hypothesized based on both traditional medicine reports and the small number of studies that have managed to overcome the legal constraints, logistic barriers, and stigma surrounding this plant. As mentioned earlier, the literature is limited in volume and constitutes a low level of evidence across all of coca's applications but may indicate a significant opportunity to use updated techniques exploring hypotheses about coca. Additionally, more work is needed to explore the molecules and interactions behind the physiological effects observed (Figure 7). Though coca's alkaloids may well drive many of the observations, other chemical families (such as flavonoids) could play an important part as well, however, a full characterization of coca's alkaloid and nutrient content with contemporary techniques remains absent and thus hinders further research studies in this area.

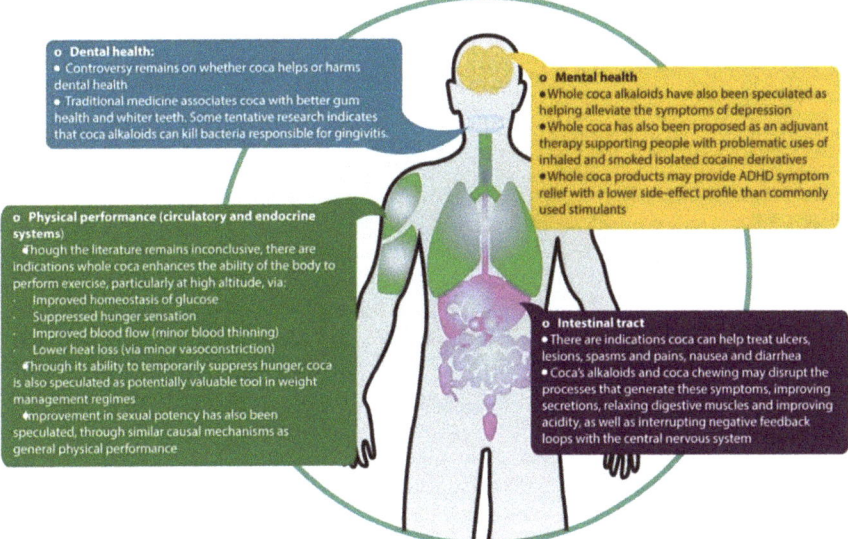

Figure 7. Potential biomedical uses of the coca plant across mental health, dental health, physical performance, and intestinal tract.

It is worth noting that some of the available research on whole coca does not appear to account for the challenge that novice coca chewers may encounter in mastering the techniques of traditional coca consumption. This may limit research participants' ability to fully realize coca's effects. Anthropological reports point out that learning these techniques takes time, even among members of traditional cultures [16,19]. Future research may require methods or product formats that facilitate product adoption to assess the full effects of coca and the variation of these effects among novice and experienced users.

4.3.1. Coca and Physical Performance: Metabolic and Cardiovascular Effects

Among the areas of interest for contemporary medicine, a key topic explored in the literature has been coca's value as a stimulant and its effect on physical performance, which is the application most akin to coca's traditional use.

The available literature explores several whole coca effects on the endocrine and vascular systems, associated with physical performance enhancement. First, there is the presumed increase in glucose availability, especially during physical exertion [87–92], which may be achieved via coca's effects on promoting fatty acid metabolism [93]. Secondly, Weil's (1981) [22] review identified a subjectively reported temporary appetite suppression, which may be linked to coca's promotion of higher glucose availability. Third, there are hypotheses that coca use is associated with improved blood flow and reduced heat loss [94,95], possibly connected with mild vasoconstriction, higher hemoglobin levels, and blood thinning effects [96]. These may stem from coca's alkaloids atropine-like behavior, that temporarily reduces the rate of red blood cell production, resulting in lower blood viscosity [97].

Overall, coca's physical performance effects are relatively mild, but potentially clinically significant. Biondich and Joslin (2015) [98] and Biondich and Joslin (2016) [79] indicated that coca's impact on glucose availability appears to be coca's most scientifically-validated metabolic effect [93]. They reported the value of using coca in reducing the symptoms of altitude sickness. The effects on glucose metabolism may provide a basis for the appetite suppression that Weil (1981) [22] hypothesizes could support coca's use in weight management regimes, as well as, potentially, diabetes management. Coca's blood thinning effects, speculated in Fuchs (1978) [97], may also contribute to the low incidence of thrombosis in native Bolivian populations, as noted by Rodriguez (1997) [96]. This would indicate the potential of coca products for stroke prevention, as long as coca's vasoconstrictive effects are properly accounted for and managed.

4.3.2. Coca and Digestive and Oral Health

Weil (1981) [22] reported coca's digestive health application in traditional Andean medicine, where it was used for alleviating gastric tract ulcers, lesions, spasms and pains, nausea, and diarrhea. It can be hypothesized that coca's tropane alkaloids may employ similar metabolic pathways as hyoscine, with proven clinical value in managing digestive symptoms. Montesinos (1965) [99] and Weil (1981) [22] speculated that coca's anesthetic alkaloids may disrupt the negative feedback loops between the central nervous system and the digestive tract that generate these symptoms, thereby improving secretions, relaxing digestive muscles and regulating acidity.

Traditional Andean cultures ascribe positive dental effects to coca, claiming it whitens teeth, improves gum health, and treats tooth aches, oral infections, and sores [22], however, the potentially corrosive effect on tooth enamel of the lime often used as an adjuvant in coca chewing may undermine this effect. Indeed, archeological analysis in Odin (1996) [100] indicates that ancient coca chewing populations displayed worse dental health than their non-coca chewing counterparts, although other factors, such as differences in diet, may have played an important role. Initial case studies indicated that coca extracts kill the main bacteria responsible for gingivitis [101] and has general antiseptic effects [102]. Less corrosive alkaline adjuvants, such as sodium bicarbonate and calcium carbonate from ash, are also common in many coca cultures [16] and may prevent dental harm. To settle this controversy, additional research is required on coca's composition (especially tooth-staining tannin content), its antimicrobial effects, and the role of alkaline adjuvants.

4.3.3. Sexual Impotence

Though there is no confirmatory research on coca's impact on sexual performance, there are ample anecdotal and documented reports claiming coca's value for this application [103,104].

The improvement in sexual performance may be linked to coca's effect on glucose metabolism, mood, and blood flow linked to its alkaloid, flavonoid, and nutrient content. In any case, aphrodisiac properties, such as improved erectile function, have also been claimed for congener species like *E. vacciniifolium* [57].

4.3.4. Mental Health and Problematic Drug Use

There are initial proposals for coca's role in providing tools for several important mental health conditions. Weil (1981) [22] indicated that coca may act as a fast-acting antidepressant, owing to the mood-enhancing effects of its main alkaloids. This would imply the potential value of integrating whole coca products into depression treatment pathways. In terms of attention deficit and hyperactivity disorder (ADHD), it can be hypothesized that coca may provide analogous clinical benefits to current treatments available. As whole coca contains several stimulants in the tropane family, whole coca products and isolated alkaloids could well provide similar outcomes to those achieved by methylphenidate and amphetamines, which are currently used in ADHD management [105], however, it may be necessary to determine whether coca and coca alkaloids act on both dopamine and noradrenaline neuron receptors, which are key targets in the pharmacological treatment of ADHD [106].

Finally, Hurtado Gumucio (1995) [107] reported the potential value in using coca leaf products to treat addictions to stimulants. This study featured a case study with 50 subjects displaying problematic use of insufflated cocaine hydrochloride and smoked cocaine sulphates (coca paste). Subjects were given psychotherapeutic support and whole coca products as part of a harm reduction strategy aimed at improving participants' social functionality. The case study indicated significantly higher scores on social functionality measures after interventions using whole coca products.

4.4. Potential Uses in Nutrition

Several studies have provided insight into coca's comparatively high nutritional contents [108–110]. Particularly, coca leaf contains significant quantities of protein, carbohydrates, fiber, minerals (especially calcium, phosphorus, and iron), and vitamins, such as thiamine, riboflavin, and carotene [108,109,111]. When consumed as tea, coca provides minerals such as calcium, magnesium, potassium, iron, manganese, zinc, phosphorus, copper, sulfur, sodium, and aluminum. Potentially harmful minerals are found in such low quantities that they do not appear to pose a health risk [110].

Despite coca's high nutritional density, Penny et al. (2009) [111] questioned coca nutrient bioavailability, due to the presence of absorption inhibitors common across green vegetables and leaves like coca. Although research on bioavailability of coca minerals and protein is limited, Collazos, Uriquieta, and Alvistur (1965) [108], one of the few reported clinical studies, provides an initial basis for assessing the bioavailability of coca's vitamins. It found that coca chewing extracted 100% of thiamine, 37% of riboflavin, and 62% of carotene available in the leaf. Additionally, absorption capacity can be improved via certain additives. Extrapolating from Hallberg and Huthén (2000) [112], ascorbic acid can be used as an additive to promote the absorption of plant minerals, such as iron, and this strategy may be applicable to whole coca-based products.

Although coca's nutritional contents are insufficient for a whole diet, they may be valuable in dietary supplementation [109,110]. These may be particularly relevant in traditional and indigenous communities in South America, where malnutrition remains a concern. To fully establish the potential of whole coca products as a dietary supplement, it would also be necessary to confirm the low risk of coca's alkaloid contents and their effect on nutritional outcomes [111].

4.5. Potential Uses in Agriculture

There are reports of coca's potential for organic fertilizers, animal feed, and pesticides. The case for using coca for plant and animal nutrition is based on its high macro- and micronutrient contents, particularly its significant amounts of vegetable protein. Several rural initiatives for turning coca leaf into organic fertilizers are mentioned in the media across the Andean region. Coca-based fertilizers are proposed as a strategy for rural communities to improve local food production and reduce fertilization costs [113]. In terms of animal feed, a rodent case study found coca protein to be less nutritious than cow's milk protein, but of sufficient quality to provide adequate rodent nutrition [114]. This contrasts with research cited in Penny et al. (2009) [111], which observed that rodents did not gain sufficient weight and showed liver abnormalities when offered whole coca-based diets. Further work on coca animal feed is required to settle the controversy. Finally, Nathanson et al. (1993) [115] claimed coca alkaloids act as a pesticide with insecticidal effects at naturally-occurring concentrations. This indicates that coca-based insecticidal sprays may provide crop protection against pests.

4.6. Legality and Development of the Coca Industry in the Andean Region and Beyond

The coca plant and ecgonine-bearing *Erythroxylum* species are prohibited globally for cultivation, transformation, and consumption under the UN's international drug control regime [77], despite their potential for productive applications. The only exemptions are medical and scientific uses of coca, as well as decocainized coca leaf extracts (utilized by Coca Cola) [76]. However, the main coca growing countries, Bolivia, Colombia, and Perú, have invoked international laws guaranteeing indigenous people their right to defend and promote their cultural practices and have thereby created a space of legality for coca products [116]. Indeed, fully legal markets for whole coca products have operated in Bolivia and Perú for decades [117], while in Colombia these markets operate in a more tenuous grey area [77]. In all three countries, the space of legality coexists alongside eradication and crop substitution policies targeting coca farmers and aimed at curtailing coca cultivation for the trade in illicit cocaine. The legitimacy of these policies is questioned, as they are associated with exacerbating violence and causing social, public health, and environmental harms. These policies are also considered ineffective, as they focus a disproportionate amount of resources on the least lucrative and most readily replaceable section of the illicit cocaine supply chain [118].

Despite the legal barriers, numerous formal and informal companies have emerged across the Andean region selling whole coca products, across food and personal care categories. These are registered by or operate through government agencies in Perú and Bolivia [12,117,119] or are licensed via indigenous authorities in Colombia [77]. In terms of food products, coca is sold as whole dried leaf, pulverized leaf, or as an infusion. It is also used as an ingredient in soft drinks, alcoholic beverages, breads, pastries, and confectionery (including coca chocolates and sweets). There are also a variety of personal care products, such toothpastes, gels and ointments in which coca is used as an ingredient.

Licit and illicit coca market data are patchy, however, the data available indicate coca represents a significant agricultural market that impacts a sizeable population. The United Nations Office on Drugs and Crime reported the 2017 coca crop in the Andean region covered 245,500 hectares [120]. On the basis of Colombian and Peruvian data [121], lot sizes per coca-growing household are estimated at roughly one hectare. This means that perhaps a quarter of a million households across the Andean region are engaged in coca farming. The UNODC estimated that the total 2017 Andean coca crop yielded about one million metric tons of leaf. With average leaf prices per kilo of about USD 2, the coca harvest in the Andean region generated some USD 2 billion in revenue (UNODC 2019) [120]. This is significant for the region's agricultural economies. In Bolivia alone, for instance, the coca harvest is estimated at USD 375 to 461 million and may represent 8% to 10% of its agricultural gross domestic product [122].

Much coca leaf today is processed into illicit cocaine. In Perú, it is estimated that over 90% of coca harvested is directed into the illicit market [12]. In Colombia, the share of the illicit market is likely even higher, as its traditional coca consuming population is thought to be vastly smaller than either Perú's or Bolivia's. In contrast, the data available for Bolivia indicate a smaller share of the illicit cocaine market there, as 19,000 tons of Bolivia's coca leaf is said to be used for traditional consumption out of a total 35,500 to 44,200 metric tons produced [122].

Once the coca leaf from across the Andean region is processed into cocaine, it yields nearly 2000 metric tons [120], estimated to reach a global black market value of USD 94 to 143 billion once it is shipped around the world [123]. This represents an enormous source of illicit profits linked to crime, violence, and environmental degradation in the Andean region and beyond.

Increasing the research and innovation of coca's applications could, therefore, constitute a high-impact social, economic, and environmental opportunity. For instance, if the evidence of coca's safety could be scientifically established, it would be viable to strengthen and extend legal supply chains for coca products both in the Andean region and internationally. Indeed, scientific research and innovation on nutritional, medicinal, and agricultural coca products could help coca compete as a less harmful alternative to current illicit stimulants, while increasing the size of coca's legal market opportunity. Overall, this would help divert money away from the illicit drug trade, while generating legal economic options for coca farmers.

5. Inclusive and Equitable Research and Commercialization of *Erythroxylum* Species

To advance the coca research agenda, it is important to note that the main coca growing countries, Bolivia, Colombia, and Perú, are all party to the 2010 Nagoya Protocol. This international legal framework sets out to prevent undue appropriation and exploitation of cultural and genetic resources, while attempting to ensure benefits are fairly distributed among stakeholders, particularly, indigenous and traditional small farmer communities from which they are derived [124]. Each country has laid out its own approaches to comply with the Nagoya Protocol commitments, including community consultation mechanisms, collective branding, and appellation of origin, among others. In addition to legal compliance, there are ethical considerations in ensuring indigenous and small farmer communities stand to gain significantly from coca research activities. Not only have these communities experienced a disproportionate amount of the burden created by the policies against coca cultivation [118], but they have also safeguarded coca cultural knowledge and practices [76], making it possible for science to continue conducting research on these plants. It is, therefore, both a legal and ethical priority for research and commercialization models involving species in the genus *Erythroxylum* to enable the active participation, leadership, and fair benefit sharing of indigenous and farmer communities.

6. Tropane Alkaloid Biosynthesis in *E. coca*

Early research into the pharmaceutically active components of the coca leaf began in the mid 1800s with the first description and crystallization of cocaine [125]. The original pioneering research in tropane alkaloid biosynthesis was performed by the chemist Edward Leete, starting in the early 1960s. During this early period, the main methods used to elucidate intermediates in the biosynthetic pathway relied upon the use of feeding radiolabeled potential precursors to whole plants, followed by chemical degradation analyses [126,127]. In a variety of tropane producing plants, [2-^{14}C] ornithine feeding has produced conflicting results. A symmetrical incorporation of ornithine is reported for *Erythroxylum coca*, whereas unsymmetrical incorporation is evident in solanaceous plants [128–132]. Ornithine and arginine are converted into putrescine directly by either ornithine decarboxylase or indirectly by arginine decarboxylase, agmatine iminohydrolase, and N-carbamoylputrescine amidohydrolase, respectively [133]. Remote isotope labelling of N-methylputrescine shows stereoselective incorporation into the first ring in both *E. coca* and multiple species from the Solanaceae [134,135]. The committed step in tropane alkaloid biosynthesis in solanaceous plants is the formation of N-methylputrescine catalyzed by an S-adenosyl-L-methionine (SAM) dependent methyltransferase. The responsible enzyme was first isolated from tobacco [136] and other orthologs have been isolated from both the Solanaceae and the Convolvulaceae [137,138]. The [6-^{14}C] spermidine feeding to solanaceous plants led to the symmetrical distribution of radioactivity of the first ring, however, no further experiments were performed that investigated spermidine as the main polyamine involved [139]. The first ring closure occurs spontaneously from 4-methylaminobutanal to form the N-methyl-Δ^1-pyrrolinium cation [140]. This ring structure was shown to be incorporated into the final bicyclic alkaloid cocaine by feeding labeled [2-^{14}C]-1-methyl-Δ^1-pyrrolinium chloride and [1-^{13}C, ^{14}C, ^{15}N]-4methylaminobutanal diethyl acetate to intact *E. coca* plants [141].

Many hypotheses have been formed as to the origins of the second ring closure in tropane alkaloids. For many years, the compound hygrine was thought to be a direct intermediate based on feeding studies, but more recent studies using stable isotopes demonstrate that previous results are artifactual [142–144]. In solanaceous plants the best incorporation into the second ring has been achieved from racemic ethyl [2,3-^{13}C$_2$]-4-(N-methyl-2-pyrrolidinyl)-3-oxobutaboate [142,145]. Further evidence is demonstrated by the feeding of methyl (RS)-[1,2-^{13}C$_2$,1-^{14}C]-4-(1-methyl-2-pyrrolidinyl)-3-oxobutanoate to the leaves of *Erythroxylum coca* [146]. This strongly implicates the involvement of acetate derived metabolites in the formation of the second ring in tropane alkaloids.

Historically, the sole sources of data regarding enzymes involved in tropane alkaloid biosynthesis were derived from studies of members in the Solanaceae, however, a recent report has identified and characterized ornithine and arginine decarboxylases in *Erythroxylum coca*. The catalytic activity of ODC was confirmed through a yeast ODC deficient spe1Δ mutant complementation with EcODC. The spe1Δ mutant transformed with EcODC showed 80 times more spermidine than the untransformed spe1Δ mutant [50]. The committed step in tropane alkaloid biosynthesis is thought to be the formation of N-methylputrescine catalyzed by an S-adenosyl-L-methionine (SAM) dependent putrescine methyltransferase (PMT). Oxidative deamination of N-methylputrescine by methylputrescine oxidase (MPO) gives rise to a reactive intermediate (4-methylaminobutanal) which is thought to spontaneously cyclize, generating a five-membered ring, the N-methyl-Δ^1-pyrrolinium cation. In solanaceous species, the MPO belongs to a copper-dependent class of diamine oxidases [147,148].

To date, there have not been any reported ring closure enzymes characterized for tropane alkaloids in *Erythroxylum coca*, however, in *Atropa belladonna*, the formation of the tropane ring is catalyzed by two enzymes. First, a non-canonical type III polyketide synthase (AbPYKS) utilizes the N-methyl-Δ^1-pyrrolinium cation as a starter substrate and undergoes two rounds of malonyl-CoA-mediated chain elongation to yield 4-(1-methyl-2-pyrrolidinyl)-3-oxobutanoic acid. Then the 4-(1-methyl-2-pyrrolidinyl)-2-oxobutanoic acid undergoes a cyclization reaction mediated by tropinone synthase (AbCYP82M3), a cytochrome p450 enzyme to form tropinone [149]. The tropane biosynthetic pathway in coca differs from the pathway in solanaceous plants in that the decarboxylation at the 2-position does not occur and instead the carboxy group is methyl esterified to form 2-carboxymethyl-3-tropinone (methylecgonone). No information regarding the protection and retention of this function is available, however, the discovery of methyl salicylate in the essential oil of coca leaves suggests that carboxymethyl transferases are active in this tissue [150]. It is clear, however, that formation of this second ring results in the production of a bicyclic alkaloid containing an α-keto group at position C-3. While the biosynthetic pathway of tropane alkaloids in *E. coca* has varied from *A. belladonna* it would be reasonable for homologous enzymatic reactions to be shared in the formation of the tropane alkaloid backbone.

Reduction of the keto group is catalyzed by a member of the aldo-keto reductase family in *E. coca* which is in contrast with the use of a short chain dehydrogenase/reductase enzyme used by members of the Solanaceae [138,151]. This finding supports the theory that the ability to produce tropane alkaloids has evolved more than once during the evolution of the angiosperms [127]. Methylecgonone reductase (MecgoR) transcript levels and enzyme activity were analyzed and found to be highest in the young leaves. Immunolocalization experiments show that MecgoR is mainly localized in the palisade and spongy mesophyll tissue of leaves and sepals [151]. Methylecgonone is reduced at the C-3 position to yield methylecgonine. MecgoR is believed to be stereospecific in its reduction of the ketone, yielding exclusively the β-hydroxy isomer. In fact, attempts to use tropine (containing the α-OH) as a substrate in the reverse reaction were unsuccessful. The free β-hydroxy moiety is esterified via a BAHD acyltranferase known as cocaine synthase. This enzyme uses benzoyl CoA as the acyl donor and results in the formation of a benzoyl ester at the C-3 position yielding the final product benzoylmethylecgonine [51]. Cocaine synthase is also capable of using a multitude of alternate acyl-CoA donors, providing an explanation for the presence of alternative tropane alkaloid esters in coca leaves [152,153]. This includes the use of cinnamoyl-CoA to produce the compound cinnamoyl cocaine, a metabolite that can be present at higher levels than cocaine under certain developmental conditions [154]. Immunolocalization of cocaine synthase and cocaine were found to have the highest levels in the palisade layer, however, enzyme and product were also detected at lower levels in the spongy mesophyll and in the upper and lower epidermis [51]. The theoretical tropane alkaloid pathway is presented in Figure 8.

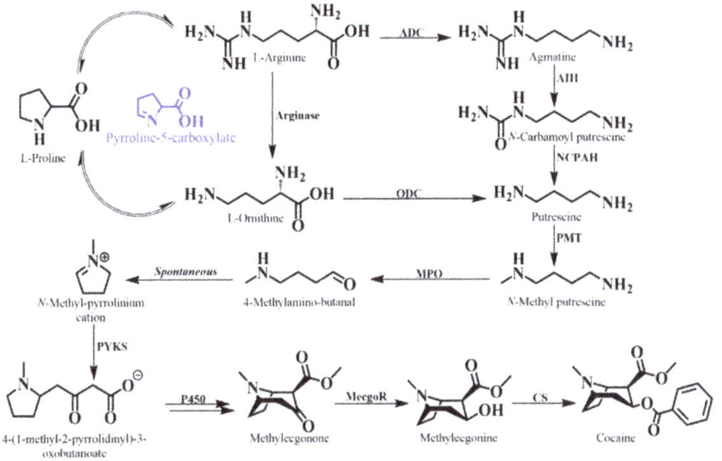

Figure 8. The theoretical tropane alkaloid biosynthetic pathway in *E. coca*. The name of each enzyme, along with their respective acronyms, and corresponding GenBank accession numbers are described. Enzymes with GenBank accession numbers have been reported and characterized. Enzymes without GenBank accession numbers have not yet been described in *E. coca*. The following enzymes are depicted in the figure above: Arginase, arginine decarboxylase (ADC) (accession no. JF909553), ornithine decarboxylase (ODC) (accession no. JF909554), agmatine iminohydrolase AIH, N-carbamoylputrescine amidohydrolase (NCPAH), putrescine methyltransferase (PMT), N-methylputrescine oxidase (MPO), pyrrolidine ketide synthase (PYKS), cytochrome p450 (p450), methylecgonone reductase (MecgoR) (accession no. GU562618), and cocaine synthase (CS) (accession no. KC140149).

Current molecular data on tropane alkaloid biosynthesis in *Erythroxylum coca* is limited as compared with other known tropane alkaloid producing species [155]. In *Erythroxylum coca*, cocaine and cinnamoylcocaine are stored in the vacuoles of the plants and are complexed with hydroxycinnamoyl quinate esters (HQAs). Chlorogenic acid is the main hydroxycinnamoyl quinate ester responsible for complexing with cocaine and cinnamoylcocaine in the vacuole. A BAHD acyltransferase enzyme (EcHQT) was characterized as the final enzymatic step of hydroxycinnamoyl quinate ester biosynthesis [156].

Plant tissue cultures are useful for biotechnological applications to investigate specialized metabolite pathways due to their facile and scalable nature. Calli tissue cultures are advantageous because, once properly established, they can be maintained indefinitely on solid gel medium by regularly transferring the calli to fresh medium [157]. *E. coca* calli cultures are important to study compounds that can influence and elicit any changes in tropane alkaloid biosynthesis. It has been demonstrated that *E. coca* calli cultures produce cocaine and can be influenced by the type of media the calli tissues are cultivated on, however, known chemical elicitors such as salicylic acid or coronalon had no significant effect on increasing the amount of tropane alkaloids. *E. coca* calli tissue cultures are useful tools to aid in gene discovery and identify unknown enzymatic reactions via stable isotope feeding of known precursors [158].

7. Perspectives

This new look at the *Erythroxylum* genus and its phytochemicals reveals a mostly untapped, potentially vast interdisciplinary research opportunity that could result in transformative social and economic outcomes. To begin with, *Erythroxylum* species could benefit from the rapid pace of technology development in omics research. This may clarify the evolutionary history and domestication process of species with high cultural significance, while assisting the development of new pharmaceutical, phytotherapeutic, nutritional, and industrial products. For instance, ongoing molecular studies using *Erythroxylum coca* and other relatives are yielding novel genes and enzymes that differ from the previously characterized solanaceous sequences. The potential to modularize these enzymes for metabolic engineering projects shows great promise. Already, studies incorporating both *E. coca* and solanaceous tropane pathway enzymes have been used together in yeast and bacteria to produce the simple tropanes tropine and pseudotropine [159]. Another study also combined several structural genes from both coca and solanaceous species to produce the compound cinnamoyltropine [160]. Indeed, key intermediates such as the N-methyl-Δ^1-pyrrolinium cation have been made in microorganisms suggesting a new system for the manipulation and combination of novel sequences for the purposes of drug design and rapid screening of novel alkaloids [161]. The discovery of convergent evolution in tropane biosynthetic pathways between the Erythroxylaceae and Solanaceae can provide insights into the building blocks of specialized metabolic pathways and how evolutionary pressures have harnessed these blocks to expand chemical diversity in living organisms.

Omics and molecular investigations could be complemented with applied research regarding the safety and value of nutritional, medical, and industrial applications based on coca and other *Erythroxylum* species. A main priority for this research should be the establishment and publicly available release of whole and diverse genomic data from members of the genus, as well as more detailed metabolomic databases both untargeted and targeted towards critical classes of compounds. These resources would then provide a basis for clinical research on coca-derived nutritional, phytotherapeutic and pharmacological metabolites and could help generate novel tools to address pressing public health challenges, such as stimulant addiction, depression, obesity, and malnutrition. Furthermore, these innovations could help strengthen the case for establishing (or strengthening) legal markets for controlled plants like *E. coca* and *E. novogranatense*. This could eventually help shrink the illicit drug trade and its negative effects, while providing licit economic opportunities for populations that are still experiencing the consequences of both illicit markets and harmful drug policies.

Author Contributions: Conceptualization, D.A.R., E.S., and J.C.D'A.; evolution and history, O.A.J.-M. and I.F.C.-B.; bio-prospecting and pharmacology, E.S. and J.A.S.; medical, nutritional and agricultural uses of coca plant, D.A.R., P.Z., and S.R.-S.; making and editing of the figures, B.G.C., J.C.D'A., and E.S.; writing—original draft preparation, D.A.R., E.S., O.A.J.-M., I.F.C.-B., S.R.-S, P.Z., J.A.S., B.G.C, and J.C.D'A.; writing—review and editing, D.A.R., E.S., and J.C.D'A.

Funding: This research was funded by startup funds to J.C.D. by the Leibniz Institute of Plant Genetics and Crop Plant Research (IPK), Gatersleben. We want to give a special thanks to Centro de Estudios sobre Seguridad y Drogas, University of Los Andes, for the funds for financing the project "Genómica poblacional de la domesticación de *Erythroxylum coca* y *E. novogranatense*" and to the Vice President of Research and Creation, University of Los Andes for the financial help with "Coca genomics: towards deciphering *Erythroxylum coca* genome in Colombia".

Acknowledgments: We thank agricultural engineer Miguel Tunjano for his logistic support.

Conflicts of Interest: The authors declare no conflict of interest.

References

1. Mishra, B.B.; Tiwari, V.K. Natural Products: An Evolving Role In Future Drug Discovery. *Eur. J. Med. Chem.* **2011**, *46*, 4769–4807. [CrossRef] [PubMed]
2. Veeresham, C. Natural Products Derived From Plants As A Source Of Drugs. *J. Adv Pharm. Technol. Res.* **2012**, *3*, 200–201. [CrossRef] [PubMed]

3. Davalos, E. New Answers To An Old Problem: Social Investment And Coca Crops In Colombia. *Int. J. Drug Policy.* **2016**, *31*, 121–130. [CrossRef] [PubMed]
4. Metaal, P. Coca in Debate: The Contradiction and Conflict Between the UN Drug Conventions and the Real World. In *Prohibition, Religious Freedom, and Human Rights: Regulating Traditional Drug Use*; Labate, B.C., Cavnar, C., Eds.; Springer: Berlin/Heidelberg, Germany, 2014; ISBN 978-3-642-40957-8.
5. Grisaffi, T. Social Control in Bolivia: A Humane Alternative to the Forced Eradication of Coca Crops. In *Drug Policies and the Politics of Drugs in the Americas*; Springer: New York, NY, USA, 2016; pp. 149–166.
6. Plowman, T.; Hensold, N. Names, Types, And Distribution Of Neotropical Species Of *Erythroxylum* (Erythroxylaceae). *Brittonia* **2004**, *56*, 1–53. [CrossRef]
7. Plowman, T. Coca Chewing And The Botanical Origins Of Coca (*Erythroxylum* spp.). In Proceedings of the Coca and Cocaine: Effects on People and Policy in Latin America; Stark, J., Pacini, D., Franquemont, C., Eds.; Cultural Survival, Inc. and LASP (Cornell University): Cambridge, MA, USA, 1986; Volume 30, p. 235.
8. Dillehay, T.D.; Rossen, J.; Ugent, D.; Karathanasis, A.; Vásquez, V.; Netherly, P.J. Early Holocene Coca Chewing In Northern Peru. *Antiquity* **2010**, *84*, 939–953. [CrossRef]
9. Plowman, T. The Ethnobotany Of Coca (*Erythroxylum* spp., Erythroxylaceae). *Repos. Inst. CEDRO* **1984**.
10. Ministerio de Gobierno de Bolivia - Consejo Nacional de Lucha contra el Tráfico Ilícito de Drogas (CONALTID). Estudio integral de la demanda de la hoja de coca en Bolivia. In Proceedings of the Quincuagésimo Quinto Periodo Ordinario de Sesiones. Symposium conducted at the meeting of Comisión Interamericana para el Control del Abuso de Drogas (CICAD), Washington, DC, USA, 28 May 2014; Washington, DC, USA.
11. Instituto Nacional de Estadística e Informática (INEI). *Análisis de los Resultados de la Encuesta Hogares Sobre Demanda de la Hoja de Coca 2013*; INEI: Lima, Peru, 2015.
12. Garcia-Yi, J. Social Control And As Supply-Side Harm Reduction Strategies. The Case Of An Indigenous Community In Peru. *Rev. Iberoam. Estud. Desarro. Iberoam. J. Dev. Stud.* **2014**, *3*, 58–82. [CrossRef]
13. Johnson, E.L. Alkaloid Content In *Erythroxylum Coca* Tissue During Reproductive Development. *Phytochemistry* **1996**, *42*, 35–38. [CrossRef]
14. Plowman, T.; Rivier, L. Cocaine and Cinnamoylcocaine Content of *Erythroxylum* Species. *Ann. Bot.* **1983**, *51*, 641–659. [CrossRef]
15. Acock, M.C.; Lydon, J.; Johnson, E.; Collins, R. Effects Of Temperature And Light Levels On Leaf Yield And Cocaine Content In Two *Erythroxylum* Species. *Ann. Bot.* **1996**, *78*, 49–53. [CrossRef]
16. Henman, A. *Mamacoca (Un Studio Complete De La Coca)*; Juan Gutenborg: Lima, Peru, 2005.
17. Schultes, R. Coca In The Northwest Amazon. In *Botanical Museum Leaflets*; Harvard University Herbaria: Cambridge, MA, USA, 1980; Volume 28, pp. 47–60.
18. Burchard, R. Chewing C: A New Perspective. *Cannabis Cult.* **1975**, 463–484.
19. Allen, C.J. To Be Quechua: The Symbolism Of Coca Chewing In Highland Peru. *Am. Ethnol.* **1981**, *8*, 157–171. [CrossRef]
20. Echeverri, J.A.; Pereira, E. Amazônica. In *O uso ritual das plantas de poder*; Labate, B., Goulart, S., Eds.; Mercado de Letras/FAPESP: Campinas, Brasil, 2005; pp. 117–185.
21. Allen, C.J. *The Hold Life Has: Coca And Cultural Identity In An. Andean Community*; Smithsonian Institution: Lima, Peru, 2002; ISBN 1-58834-359-6.
22. Weil, A.T. The Therapeutic Value Of Coca In Contemporary Medicine. *J. Ethnopharmacol.* **1981**, *3*, 367–376. [CrossRef]
23. The Angiosperm Phylogeny Group* An Update Of The Angiosperm Phylogeny Group Classification For The Orders And Families Of Flowering Plants: APG II. *Bot. J. Linn. Soc.* **2003**, *141*, 399–436. [CrossRef]
24. Matthews, M.L.; Endress, P.K. Comparative Floral Structure And Systematics In Rhizophoraceae, Erythroxylaceae And The Potentially Related Ctenolophonaceae, Linaceae, Irvingiaceae And Caryocaraceae (Malpighiales). *Bot. J. Linn. Soc.* **2011**, *166*, 331–416. [CrossRef]
25. Dahlgren, R.M.T. Rhizophoraceae and Anisophylleaceae: Summary Statement, Relationships. *Ann. Mo. Bot. Gard.* **1988**, *75*, 1259–1277. [CrossRef]
26. Schwarzbach, A.E.; Ricklefs, R.E. Systematic Affinities Of Rhizophoraceae And Anisophylleaceae, And Intergeneric Relationships Within Rhizophoraceae, Based On Chloroplast DNA, Nuclear Ribosomal DNA, And Morphology. *Am. J. Bot.* **2000**, *87*, 547–564. [CrossRef]
27. Islam, M. Tracing The Evolutionary History Of Coca (Erythroxylum). Ph.D. Thesis, University of Colorado, Boulder, CO, USA, 2011.

28. White, D.M.; Islam, M.B.; Mason-Gamer, R.J. Phylogenetic Inference In Section Archerythroxylum Informs Taxonomy, Biogeography, And The Domestication Of Coca (*Erythroxylum* Species). *Am. J. Bot.* **2019**, *106*, 154–165. [CrossRef]
29. Schulz, O.E. *Erythroxylaceae*; Engelmann: Wiesloch, Germany, 1907; Volume 29.
30. Jara Muñoz, O.A. El Complejo Erythroxylum macrophyllum (Erythroxylaceae): Delimitación Taxonómica Y Posición Filogenética. Universidad Nacional de Colombia: Bogota, Colombia, 2011.
31. Loiola, M.I.B. *Revisão Taxonômica De Erythroxylum, P. Browne Sect. Rhabdophyllum, O.E. Schulz (Erythroxylaceae Kunth)*; Herbarium Senckenbergianum: Frankfurt am Main, Germany, 2006.
32. Rury, P.M. Systematic Anatomy Of *Erythroxylum*, P. Browne: Practical And Evolutionary Implications For The Cultivated Cocas. *J. Ethnopharmacol.* **1981**, *3*, 229–263. [CrossRef]
33. Bohm, B.A.; Ganders, F.R.; Plowman, T. Biosystematics and Evolution of Cultivated Coca (Erythroxylaceae). *Syst. Bot.* **1982**, *7*, 121–133. [CrossRef]
34. Darwin, C. *The Different Forms Of Flowers On Plants Of The Same Species*; John Murray: London, UK, 1877.
35. Ganders, F.R. Heterostyly in *Erythroxylum coca* (Erythroxylaceae). *Bot. J. Linn. Soc.* **1979**, *78*, 11–20. [CrossRef]
36. Ruiz-zapata, T.; Kalin-Arroyo, M. Plant Reproductive Ecology of a Secondary Deciduous Tropical Forest in. *Biotropica* **1978**, *10*, 221–230. [CrossRef]
37. Kalin-Arroyo, M.; Cabrera, E. Preliminary Self Incompatibility Tests For Some Tropical Cloud Forest Species In Venezuela. *Incompat. Newsl.* **1977**, *8*.
38. Cuevas, E.; Molina-Freaner, F.; Eguiarte, L.E.; Domínguez, C.A. Patterns Of Male Sterility Within And Among Populations Of The Distylous Shrub *Erythroxylum havanense* (Erythroxylaceae). *Plant. Ecol.* **2005**, *176*, 165–172. [CrossRef]
39. Dominguez, C.A.; Avila-Sakar, G.; Vázquez-Santana, S.; Márquez-GuzmáN, J. Morph-Biased Male Sterility In The Tropical Distylous Shrub *Erythroxylum havanense* (Erythroxylaceae). *Am. J. Bot.* **1997**, *84*, 626–632. [CrossRef] [PubMed]
40. Rosas, F.; Domínguez, C.A. Male Sterility, Fitness Gain Curves And The Evolution Of Gender Specialization From Distyly In *Erythroxylum havanense*. *J. Evol. Biol.* **2009**, *22*, 50–59. [CrossRef]
41. Berry, P.E.; Tober, H.; Gomez, J. Agamospermy And The Loss Of Distyly In *Erythroxylum undulatum* (Erythroxylaceae) From Northern Venezuela. *Am. J. Bot.* **1991**, *78*, 595–600. [CrossRef]
42. Emche, S.D.; Zhang, D.; Islam, M.B.; Bailey, B.A.; Meinhardt, L.W. AFLP Phylogeny of 36 *Erythroxylum* Species. *Trop. Plant. Biol.* **2011**, *4*, 126–133. [CrossRef]
43. Johnson, E.L.; Zhang, D.; Emche, S.D. Inter- and Intra-specific Variation among Five *Erythroxylum* Taxa Assessed by AFLP. *Ann. Bot.* **2005**, *95*, 601–608. [CrossRef]
44. Plowman, T. The Identity Of Amazonian And Trujillo Coca. *Bot. Mus. Leafl. Harv. Univ.* **1979**, *27*, 45–68.
45. Plowman, T. The Identification Of Coca (*Erythroxylum* Species): 1860–1910. *Bot. J. Linn. Soc.* **1982**, *84*, 329–353. [CrossRef]
46. Johnson, E.L.; Schmidt, W.F.; Emche, S.D.; Mossoba, M.M.; Musser, S.M. Kaempferol (Rhamnosyl) Glucoside, A New Flavonol From *Erythroxylum coca* var. *ipadu*. *Biochem. Syst. Ecol.* **2003**, *31*, 59–67. [CrossRef]
47. Johnson, E.L.; Emche, S.D. Variation of Alkaloid Content in *Erythroxylum coca* Leaves from Leaf Bud to Leaf Drop. *Ann. Bot.* **1994**, *73*, 645–650. [CrossRef]
48. Johnson, E.L.; Schmidt, W.F.; Norman, H.A. Leaf Flavonoids as Chemotaxonomic Markers for Two *Erythroxylum* Taxa. *Z. Für Naturforschung C* **1997**, *52*, 577–585. [CrossRef]
49. Johnson, E.L.; Schmidt, W.F.; Norman, H.A. Flavonoids As Markers For *Erythroxylum* Taxa: *E. coca* var. *ipadu* and *E. novogranatense* var. *truxillense*. *Biochem. Syst. Ecol.* **1998**, *26*, 743–759. [CrossRef]
50. Docimo, T.; Reichelt, M.; Schneider, B.; Kai, M.; Kunert, G.; Gershenzon, J.; D'Auria, J.C. The First Step In The Biosynthesis Of Cocaine In *Erythroxylum coca*: The Characterization Of Arginine And Ornithine Decarboxylases. *Plant. Mol. Biol.* **2012**, *78*, 599–615. [CrossRef]
51. Schmidt, G.W.; Jirschitzka, J.; Porta, T.; Reichelt, M.; Luck, K.; Torre, J.C.P.; Dolke, F.; Varesio, E.; Hopfgartner, G.; Gershenzon, J.; et al. The Last Step in Cocaine Biosynthesis Is Catalyzed by a BAHD Acyltransferase. *Plant. Physiol.* **2015**, *167*, 89–101. [CrossRef]
52. Davey, J.W.; Blaxter, M.L. RADseq: Next-Generation Population Genetics. *Brief. Funct. Genomics* **2010**, *9*, 416–423. [CrossRef]

53. Davey, J.W.; Hohenlohe, P.A.; Etter, P.D.; Boone, J.Q.; Catchen, J.M.; Blaxter, M.L. Genome-Wide Genetic Marker Discovery And Genotyping Using Next-Generation Sequencing. *Nat. Rev. Genet.* **2011**, *12*, 499–510. [CrossRef]
54. Andrews, K.R.; Luikart, G. Recent Novel Approaches For Population Genomics Data Analysis. *Mol. Ecol.* **2014**, *23*, 1661–1667. [CrossRef]
55. Van Bakel, H.; Stout, J.M.; Cote, A.G.; Tallon, C.M.; Sharpe, A.G.; Hughes, T.R.; Page, J.E. The Draft Genome And Transcriptome Of *Cannabis sativa*. *Genome Biol.* **2011**, *12*, R102. [CrossRef] [PubMed]
56. Laverty, K.U.; Stout, J.M.; Sullivan, M.J.; Shah, H.; Gill, N.; Holbrook, L.; Deikus, G.; Sebra, R.; Hughes, T.R.; Page, J.E.; et al. A Physical And Genetic Map Of *Cannabis sativa* Identifies Extensive Rearrangements At The THC/CBD acid Synthase Loci. *Genome Res.* **2019**, *29*, 146–156. [CrossRef] [PubMed]
57. Zanolari, B.; Guilet, D.; Marston, A.; Queiroz, E.F.; de, Q.; Paulo, M.; Hostettmann, K. Tropane Alkaloids From The Bark Of *Erythroxylum vacciniifolium*. *J. Nat. Prod.* **2003**, *66*, 497–502. [CrossRef] [PubMed]
58. Graf, E.; Lude, W. Alkaloide aus *Erythroxylum vacciniifolium* Martius, 2. Mitt. Strukturaufklärung von Catuabin, A., B und C. *Arch. Pharm.* **1978**, *311*, 139–152. [CrossRef] [PubMed]
59. Manabe, H.; Sakagami, H.; Ishizone, H.; Kusano, H.; Fujimaki, M.; Wada, C.; Komatsu, N.; Nakashima, H.; Murakami, T.; Yamamoto, N. Effects Of Catuaba Extracts On Microbial and HIV Infection. *Vivo Athens Greece* **1992**, *6*, 161–165.
60. Satoh, M.; Satoh, Y.; Fujimoto, Y. Cytotoxic Constituents From *Erythroxylum catuaba* Isolation And Cytotoxic Activities Of Cinchonain. *Nat. Med.* **2000**, *54*, 97–100.
61. Coriolano de Oliveira, E.; Alves Soares Cruz, R.; de Mello Amorim, N.; Guerra Santos, M.; Carlos Simas Pereira Junior, L.; Flores Sanchez, E.; Pinho Fernandes, C.; Garrett, R.; Machado Rocha, L.; Lopes Fuly, A. Protective Effect Of The Plant Extracts Of *Erythroxylum* Sp. Against Toxic Effects Induced By The Venom Of Lachesis Muta Snake. *Molecules* **2016**, *21*, 1350. [CrossRef]
62. Chin, Y.-W.; Jones, W.P.; Waybright, T.J.; McCloud, T.G.; Rasoanaivo, P.; Cragg, G.M.; Cassady, J.M.; Kinghorn, A.D. Tropane Aromatic Ester Alkaloids From A Large-Scale Re-Collection Of *Erythroxylum pervillei* Stem Bark Obtained In Madagascar. *J. Nat. Prod.* **2006**, *69*, 414–417. [CrossRef]
63. Aguiar, J.S.; Araújo, R.O.; do Desterro Rodrigues, M.; Sena, K.X.; Batista, A.M.; Guerra, M.M.; Oliveira, S.L.; Tavares, J.F.; Silva, M.S.; Nascimento, S.C. Antimicrobial, Antiproliferative And Proapoptotic Activities Of Extract, Fractions And Isolated Compounds From The Stem Of *Erythroxylum caatingae* Plowman. *Int. J. Mol. Sci.* **2012**, *13*, 4124–4140. [CrossRef]
64. Silva, G.L.; Cui, B.; Chávez, D.; You, M.; Chai, H.-B.; Rasoanaivo, P.; Lynn, S.M.; O'Neill, M.J.; Lewis, J.A.; Besterman, J.M. Modulation of the Multidrug-Resistance Phenotype by New Tropane Alkaloid Aromatic Esters from *Erythroxylum pervillei*. *J. Nat. Prod.* **2001**, *64*, 1514–1520. [CrossRef]
65. Mahomoodally, M.F.; Gurib-Fakim, A.; Subratty, A.H. Antimicrobial Activities And Phytochemical Profiles Of Endemic Medicinal Plants Of Mauritius. *Pharm. Biol.* **2005**, *43*, 237–242. [CrossRef]
66. Mahomoodally, M.F.; Fakim, A.-G.; Subratty, A.H. Effects Of *Erythroxylum macrocarpum* (Erythroxylaceae), An Endemic Medicinal Plant Of Mauritius, On The Transport Of Monosaccharide, Amino Acid And Fluid Across Rat Everted Intestinal Sacs *in vitro*. *J. Cell Mol. Biol.* **2005**, *4*, 93–98.
67. Al-said, M.S.; Evans, W.C.; Grout, R.J. Alkaloids of *Erythroxylum macrocarpum* and *E. sideroxyloides*. *Phytochemistry* **1986**, *25*, 851–853. [CrossRef]
68. De Oliveira, S.L.; Tavares, J.F.; Branco, M.V.S.C.; Lucena, H.F.S.; Barbosa-Filho, J.M.; de Agra, M.F.; do Nascimento, S.C.; dos Aguiar, J.S.; da Silva, T.G.; de Simone, C.A.; et al. Tropane Alkaloids from *Erythroxylum caatingae* Plowman. *Chem. Biodivers.* **2011**, *8*, 155–165. [CrossRef]
69. Ribeiro, G.; de Amorim, L.L.; Guimarães, S.S. Antioxidant Activity and Phytochemical Screening of Extracts of *Erythroxylum suberosum* A. St.-Hil (Erythroxylaceae). *Res. J. Phytochem.* **2015**, *9*, 68–78.
70. De Barros, I.M.C.; Leite, B.H.; Leite, C.F.; Fagg, C.W.; Gomes, S.M.; Resck, I.S.; Fonseca-Bazzo, Y.M.; Magalhães, P.O.; Silveira, D. Chemical Composition And Antioxidant Activity Of Extracts From *Erythroxylum suberosum* A. St. Hil. leaves. *J. Appl. Pharm. Sci.* **2017**, *7*, 088–094.
71. Macedo, T.B.; Elias, S.T.; Torres, H.M.; Yamamoto-Silva, F.P.; Silveira, D.; Magalhães, P.O.; Lofrano-Porto, A.; Guerra, E.N.; Silva, M.A.G. Cytotoxic Effect Of *Erythroxylum suberosum* combined With Radiotherapy In Head And Neck Cancer Cell Lines. *Braz. Dent. J.* **2016**, *27*, 108–112. [CrossRef]

72. Picot, C.; Subratty, A.H.; Mahomoodally, M.F. Inhibitory Potential Of Five Traditionally Used Native Antidiabetic Medicinal Plants On A-Amylase, A-Glucosidase, Glucose Entrapment, And Amylolysis Kinetics in vitro. *Adv. Pharmacol. Sci.* **2014**, *2014*.
73. Hansen, K.; Adsersen, A.; Smitt, U.W.; Nyman, U.; Christensen, S.B.; Schwartner, C.; Wagner, H. Angiotensin Converting Enzyme (ACE) Inhibitory Flavonoids From *Erythroxylum laurifolium*. *Phytomedicine* **1996**, *2*, 313–317. [CrossRef]
74. Lohezic, F.; Amoros, M.; Boustie, J.; Girre, L. In-vitro Antiherpetic Activity of *Erythroxylon laurifolium* (Erythroxylaceae). *Pharm. Pharmacol. Commun.* **1999**, *5*, 249–253. [CrossRef]
75. Jelager, L.; Gurib-Fakim, A.; Adsersen, A. Antibacterial And Antifungal Activity Of Medicinal Plants Of Mauritius. *Pharm. Biol.* **1998**, *36*, 153–161. [CrossRef]
76. Gootenberg, P. *Andean Cocaine: The Making of a Global Drug*; Univ of North Carolina Press: Chapel Hill, NC, USA, 2008; ISBN 978-0-8078-3229-5.
77. Muro, A.; Aguirre, P.; Parra, D.; Piza, M. *Usos, Impactos y Derechos: Posibilidades, Políticas y Jurídicas para la Investigación de la Hoja de Coca en Colombia*; Elementa: Bogota, DC, Colombia, 2018.
78. Troyano, D.L.; Restrepo, D. *Coca Industrialization: A Path to Innovation, Development and Peace in Colombia*; Open Society Foundations: New York, NY, USA, 2018; ISBN 978-1-940983-80-6.
79. Biondich, A.S.; Joslin, J.D. Coca: The History And Medical Significance Of An Ancient Andean Tradition. *Emerg. Med. Int.* **2016**. [CrossRef] [PubMed]
80. Rivier, L. Analysis Of Alkaloids In Leaves Of Cultivated *Erythroxylum* And Characterization Of Alkaline Substances Used During Coca Chewing. *J. Ethnopharmacol.* **1981**, *3*, 313–335. [CrossRef]
81. Jenkins, A.J.; Llosa, T.; Montoya, I.; Cone, E.J. Identification And Quantitation Of Alkaloids In Coca Tea. *Forensic Sci. Int.* **1996**, *77*, 179–189. [CrossRef]
82. Novák, M.; Salemink, C.A.; Khan, I. Biological activity Of The Alkaloids Of *Erythroxylum coca* and *Erythroxylum novogranatense*. *J. Ethnopharmacol.* **1984**, *10*, 261–274. [CrossRef]
83. Rubio, N.C.; Hastedt, M.; Gonzalez, J.; Pragst, F. Possibilities For Discrimination Between Chewing Of Coca Leaves And Abuse Of Cocaine By Hair Analysis Including Hygrine, Cuscohygrine, Cinnamoylcocaine And Cocaine Metabolite/Cocaine Ratios. *Int. J. Legal Med.* **2015**, *129*, 69–84. [CrossRef]
84. Nersesyan, A.; Kundi, M.; Krupitza, G.; Barcelos, G.; Mišík, M.; Wultsch, G.; Carrion, J.; Carrion-Carrera, G.; Knasmueller, S. Induction Of Nuclear Anomalies In Exfoliated Buccal Cells Of Coca Chewers: Results Of A Field Study. *Arch. Toxicol.* **2013**, *87*, 529–534. [CrossRef]
85. WHO/UNICRI Cocaine Project. Available online: https://www.brucekalexander.com/articles-speeches/cocaine/188-whounicri-cocaine-project (accessed on 30 August 2019).
86. WHO: "Six Horsemen ride out". Available online: https://www.tni.org/es/node/17310 (accessed on 29 August 2019).
87. Galarza, M.; Peñaloza, R.; Echalar, L.; Aguilar, M.; Souvain, M.; Spielvogel, H. Efectos Del Acullico De Coca En La Prueba De Tolerancia A La Glucosa. *Biofarbo* **1997**, *57*, 57–60.
88. Brutsaert, T.; Milotich, M.; Frisancho, A.R.; Spielvogel, H. Coca Chewing Among High Altitude Natives: Work And Muscular Efficiencies Of Nonhabitual Chewers. *Am. J. Hum. Biol.* **1995**, *7*, 607–616. [CrossRef]
89. Favier, R.; Caceres, E.; Guillon, L.; Sempore, B.; Sauvain, M.; Koubi, H.; Spielvogel, H. Coca Chewing For Exercise: Hormonal And Metabolic Responses Of Nonhabitual Chewers. *J. Appl. Physiol.* **1996**, *81*, 1901–1907. [CrossRef]
90. Favier, R.; Caceres, E.; Sempore, B.; Cottet-Emard, J.M.; Gauquelin, G.; Gharib, C.; Spielvogel, H. Fluid Regulatory Hormone Response To Exercise After Coca-Induced Body Fluid Shifts. *J. Appl. Physiol.* **1997**, *83*, 376–382. [CrossRef] [PubMed]
91. Spielvogel, H.; Caceres, E.; Koubi, H.; Sempore, B.; Sauvain, M.; Favier, R. Effects Of Coca Chewing On Metabolic And Hormonal Changes During Graded Incremental Exercise To Maximum. *J. Appl. Physiol.* **1996**, *80*, 643–649. [CrossRef] [PubMed]
92. Hurtado Sánchez, C.A.; Cartagena Triveño, D.; Erostegui Revilla, C.P. Evaluación De La Respuesta Glucemica Post-Ingesta De La Hoja De Coca (Erythroxylum Coca) En Personas Sin Antecedente Patológico Metabólico. *Rev. Científica Cienc. Médica* **2013**, *16*, 20–24.
93. Casikar, V.; Mujica, E.; Mongelli, M.; Aliaga, J.; Lopez, N.; Smith, C.; Bartholomew, F. Does Chewing Coca Leaves Influence Physiology At High Altitude? *Indian. J. Clin. Biochem.* **2010**, *25*, 311–314. [CrossRef]

94. Hanna, J.M. Responses Of Quechua Indians To Coca Ingestion During Cold Exposure. *Am. J. Phys. Anthropol.* **1971**, *34*, 273–277. [CrossRef] [PubMed]
95. Little, M.A. Effects Of Alcohol And Coca On Foot Temperature Responses Of Highland Peruvians During A Localized Cold Exposure. *Am. J. Phys. Anthropol.* **1970**, *32*, 233–242. [CrossRef]
96. Rodríguez, A.; Guillon, L.; de Chavez, M. *Uso De La Hoja De Coca Y Hematología*; Instituto Boliviano de Biologia de Altura: La Paz, Bolivia, 1997.
97. Fuchs, A.; Burchard, R.E.; Curtain, C.C.; De Azeredo, P.R.; Frisancho, A.R.; Gagliano, J.A.; Katz, S.H.; Little, M.A.; Mazess, R.B.; Picón-Reátegui, E.; et al. Coca Chewing and High-Altitude Stress: Possible Effects of Coca Alkaloids on Erythropoiesis. *Curr. Anthropol.* **1978**, *19*, 277–291. [CrossRef]
98. Biondich, A.S.; Joslin, J.D. Coca: High Altitude Remedy Of The Ancient Incas. *Wilderness Environ. Med.* **2015**, *26*, 567–571. [CrossRef]
99. Montesinos, F. Metabolism Of Cocaine. *Bull. Narc.* **1965**, *17*, 11–17.
100. Langsjoen, O.M. Dental Effects Of Diet And Coca-Leaf Chewing On Two Prehistoric Cultures Of Northern Chile. *Am. J. Phys. Anthropol.* **1996**, *101*, 475–489. [CrossRef]
101. Ramos, A.W. Actividad Antibacteriana Del Extracto De Erythroxylum coca sobre Porphyromonas Gingivalis, estudio in vitro. Undergraduate Thesis, Universidad Nacional Mayor de San Marcos, Lima, Peru, 2012.
102. Seki, K.; Nishi, Y. *Coca, un Biobanco: Investigación Científica Sobre Alimentación, Curación y Regeneración*, 1st ed.; t'ika & teko: La Paz, Bolivia, 2012; ISBN 978-99954-824-8-0.
103. Mantegazza, P. Sulle virtù igieniche e medicinali della coca e sugli alimenti nervosi in generale. *Soc. Per Gli Annali Delle Scienze E Dell'Industria* **1859**.
104. Carter, W.E.; Mamani, M. *Coca en Bolivia*; Librería Editorial "Juventud": La Paz, Bolivia, 1986.
105. Sharma, A.; Couture, J. A Review Of The Pathophysiology, Etiology, And Treatment Of Attention-Deficit Hyperactivity Disorder (ADHD). *Ann. Pharmacother.* **2014**, *48*, 209–225. [CrossRef] [PubMed]
106. Storebø, O.J.; Ramstad, E.; Krogh, H.B.; Nilausen, T.D.; Skoog, M.; Holmskov, M.; Rosendal, S.; Groth, C.; Magnusson, F.L.; Moreira-Maia, C.R. Methylphenidate For Children And Adolescents With Attention Deficit Hyperactivity Disorder (ADHD). *Cochrane Database Syst. Rev.* **2015**. [CrossRef] [PubMed]
107. Gumucio, J.H. *Cocaine, the Legend About Coca and Cocaine*; Accion Andina, ICORI: La Paz, Bolivia, 1995.
108. Collazos, C.; Urquieta, R.; Alvistur, E. Nutrición Y Coqueo. *Rev. Viernes Méd.* **1965**, *16*, 36–44.
109. Duke, J.A.; Aulik, D.; Plowman, T. Nutritional Value Of Coca. *Bot. Mus. Leafl. Harv. Univ.* **1975**, *24*, 113–119.
110. Olivier, J.; Symington, E.A.; Jonker, C.Z.; Rampedi, I.T.; van Eeden, T.S. Comparison Of The Mineral Composition Of Leaves And Infusions Of Traditional And Herbal Teas. *South. Afr. J. Sci.* **2012**, *108*, 01–07. [CrossRef]
111. Penny, M.E.; Zavaleta, A.; Lemay, M.; Liria, M.R.; Huaylinas, M.L.; Alminger, M.; McChesney, J.; Alcaraz, F.; Reddy, M.B. Can Coca Leaves Contribute to Improving the Nutritional Status of the Andean Population? *Food Nutr. Bull.* **2009**, *30*, 205–216. [CrossRef]
112. Hallberg, L.; Hulthén, L. Prediction Of Dietary Iron Absorption: An Algorithm For Calculating Absorption And Bioavailability Of Dietary Iron. *Am. J. Clin. Nutr.* **2000**, *71*, 1147–1160. [CrossRef]
113. Del Anaya, M.S.; Troyano, D.L. *Guía: Producción Tecnificada De Abonos Orgánicos, Sólidos Y Líquidos A Partir De La Hoja De Coca Para Fertilización De Cultivos Transitorios*; Servicio Nacional de Aprendizaje: La Paz, Bolivia, 2017.
114. Cordero, T.; TeÓfila, A. Evaluación nutricional de la proteína de la hoja de Coca (*Erythroxylum coca* Lamarck var. *coca*). Undergrad. Thesis, Chem. Dep. UNMSM, Lima, Peru, 2002.
115. Nathanson, J.A.; Hunnicutt, E.J.; Kantham, L.; Scavone, C. Cocaine As A Naturally Occurring Insecticide. *Proc. Natl. Acad. Sci.* **1993**, *90*, 9645–9648. [CrossRef]
116. Blanco, E.C.; González, J.C.M. El Uso De La Hoja De Coca Como Manifestación Cultural Inmaterial. *Revistas* **2014**, *6*, 11.
117. Aguilar, A.; Chulver, P. *Análisis Para La Factibilidad De Exportación De La Hoja De Coca*; Fundación Acción Semilla: La Paz, Bolivia, 2019.
118. Martínez, T.; Castro, E. *¿Es Eficaz La Erradicacion Forzosa De Cultivos De Coca?* Centro de Estudios sobre Seguridad y Drogas: Bogota, DC, Colombia, 2018.
119. Glave, M.; Rosemberg, C. *La Comercialización De Hoja De Coca En El Perú; Análisis Del Mercado Formal (Grade)*: Lima, Peru, 2005.

120. United Nations Office on Drugs and Crime (UNODC) Colombia. *Monitoreo de Territorios Afectados por Cultivos Ilícitos 2018*; UNODC: Bogota, DC, Colombia, 2019.
121. United Nations Office on Drugs and Crime (UNODC) Perú. *Monitoreo de Cultivos de Coca, 2013*; UNODC: Lima, Peru, 2014.
122. United Nations Office on Drugs and Crime (UNODC) Estado Plurinacional de Bolivia. *Monitoreo de Cultivos de Coca 2018*; UNODC: La Paz, Bolivia, 2019.
123. Channing, G. *May Transnational Crime and the Developing World*; Global Financial Integrity: Washington, DC, USA, 2017.
124. Ruiz, M. *Las Relaciones entre las Herramientas de la Propiedad Intelectual, los Conocimientos Tradicionales y Recursos Genéticos, en el Contexto de la Aplicación del Protocolo de Nagoya: Alcances y Aproximaciones*; Deutsche Gesellschaft für Internationale Zusammenarbeit (GIZ) GmbH: San Salvador, El Salvador, 2016.
125. Niemann, A. Ueber eine neue organische Base in den Cocablättern. *Arch. Pharm.* **1860**, *153*, 291–308. [CrossRef]
126. Humphrey, A.J.; O'Hagan, D. Tropane alkaloid biosynthesis. A century old problem unresolved. *Nat. Prod. Rep.* **2001**, *18*, 494–502. [CrossRef] [PubMed]
127. Jirschitzka, J.; Mattern, D.J.; Gershenzon, J.; D'Auria, J.C. Learning From Nature: New Approaches To The Metabolic Engineering Of Plant Defense Pathways. *Curr. Opin. Biotechnol.* **2013**, *24*, 320–328. [CrossRef] [PubMed]
128. Hashimoto, T.; Yukimune, Y.; Yamada, Y. Putrescine and putrescine N-methyltransferase In The Biosynthesis Of Tropane Alkaloids In Cultured Roots Of *Hyoscyamus albus*.2. Incorporation of labeled precursors. *Planta* **1989**, *178*, 131–137. [CrossRef] [PubMed]
129. Leete, E. Stereospecific Incorporation Of Ornithine Into Tropine Moiety Of Hyoscyamine. *J. Am. Chem. Soc.* **1962**, *84*, 55–57. [CrossRef]
130. Leete, E. Biosynthesis Of Hyoscyamine: Proof That Ornithine-2-C^{14} Yields Tropine Labelled at C-1. *Tetrahedron Lett.* **1964**, 1619–1622. [CrossRef]
131. Leete, E. Biosynthesis Of The Pyrrolidine Rings Of Cocaine And Cuscohygrine From [5-^{14}C]-Labeled Ornithine Via A Symmetrical Intermediate. *J. Am. Chem. Soc.* **1982**, *104*, 1403–1408. [CrossRef]
132. Liebisch, H.W.; Ramin, H.; Schoffin, I.; Schütte, H.R. Zur Biosynthese der Tropanalkaloide. *Z. Naturforschung Part. B-Chem. Biochem. Biophys. Biol. Verwandten Geb.* **1965**, *20*, 1183–1185.
133. Alcazar, R.; Altabella, T.; Marco, F.; Bortolotti, C.; Reymond, M.; Koncz, C.; Carrasco, P.; Tiburcio, A.F. Polyamines: Molecules With Regulatory Functions In Plant Abiotic Stress Tolerance. *Planta* **2010**, *231*, 1237–1249. [CrossRef]
134. Hoye, T.R.; Bjorklund, J.A.; Koltun, D.O.; Renner, M.K. Methylputrescine Oxidation During Cocaine Biosynthesis: Study Of Prochiral Methylene Hydrogen Discrimination Using The Remote Isotope Method. *Org. Lett.* **2000**, *2*, 3–5. [CrossRef]
135. Wigle, I.D.; Mestichelli, L.J.J.; Spenser, I.D. ^{2}H NMR-spectroscopy as A Probe Of The Stereochemistry Of Biosynthetic Reactions - The Biosynthesis Of Nicotine. *J. Chem. Soc. Chem. Commun.* **1982**, 662–664. [CrossRef]
136. Hibi, N.; Higashiguchi, S.; Hashimoto, T.; Yamada, Y. Gene Expression In Tobacco Low-Nicotine Mutants. *Plant. Cell* **1994**, *6*, 723–735. [PubMed]
137. Kai, G.; Zhang, Y.; Chen, J.; Li, L.; Yan, X.; Zhang, R.; Liao, P.; Lu, X.; Wang, W.; Zhou, G. Molecular Characterization And Expression Analysis Of Two Distinct Putrescine N-Methyltransferases From Roots Of *Anisodus acutangulus*. *Physiol. Plant.* **2009**, *135*, 121–129. [CrossRef] [PubMed]
138. Teuber, M.; Azemi, M.E.; Namjoyan, F.; Meier, A.C.; Wodak, A.; Brandt, W.; Drager, B. Putrescine N-methyltransferases–A Structure-Function Analysis. *Plant. Mol. Biol.* **2007**, *63*, 787–801. [CrossRef]
139. Leete, E. Spermidine: An Indirect Precursor Of The Pyrrolidine Rings Of Nicotine And Nornicotine in *Nicotiana glutinosa*. *Phytochemistry* **1985**, *24*, 957–960. [CrossRef]
140. Leete, E. Recent Developments In The Biosynthesis Of The Tropane Alkaloids. *Planta Med.* **1990**, *56*, 339–352. [CrossRef]
141. Leete, E.; Kim, S.H.; Rana, J. Chemistry Of The Tropane Alkaloids And Related-Compounds.38. The Incorporation Of [2-^{13}C,^{14}C,^{15}N]-1-Methyl-D^1-Pyrrolinium Chloride Into Cuscohygrine in *Erythroxylum coca*. *Phytochemistry* **1988**, *27*, 401–406. [CrossRef]

142. Abraham, T.W.; Leete, E. New Intermediate In The Biosynthesis Of The Tropane Alkaloids in *Datura innoxia*. *J. Am. Chem. Soc.* **1995**, *117*, 8100–8105. [CrossRef]
143. Kaczkowski, J.; Schütte, H.R.; Mothes, K. Die Rolle des Acetats in der Biosynthese der Tropanalkaloide. *Biochim. Biophys. Acta* **1961**, *46*, 588–594. [CrossRef]
144. Liebisch, H.W.; Peisker, K.; Radwan, A.S.; Schütte, H.R. Zur Biosynthese der Tropanalkaloide.XI. Die Bildung der C_3-Brücke des Tropins. *Z. Pflanzenphysiol.* **1972**, *67*, 1–9. [CrossRef]
145. Robins, R.J.; Abraham, T.W.; Parr, A.J.; Eagles, J.; Walton, N.J. The Biosynthesis Of Tropane Alkaloids In *Datura stramonium*: The Identity Of The Intermediates Between *N*-Methylpyrrolinium Salt And Tropinone. *J. Am. Chem. Soc.* **1997**, *119*, 10929–10934. [CrossRef]
146. Leete, E.; Bjorklund, J.A.; Couladis, M.M.; Kim, S.H. Late Intermediates In The Biosynthesis Of Cocaine: 4-(1-Methyl-2-Pyrrolidinyl)-3-Oxobutanoate And Methylecgonine. *J. Am. Chem. Soc.* **1991**, *113*, 9286–9292. [CrossRef]
147. Heim, W.G.; Sykes, K.A.; Hildreth, S.B.; Sun, J.; Lu, R.H.; Jelesko, J.G. Cloning And Characterization Of A *Nicotiana tabacum* Methylputrescine Oxidase Transcript. *Phytochemistry* **2007**, *68*, 454–463. [CrossRef] [PubMed]
148. Katoh, A.; Shoji, T.; Hashimoto, T. Molecular Cloning Of *N*-Methylputrescine Oxidase From Tobacco. *Plant. Cell Physiol.* **2007**, *48*, 550–554. [CrossRef]
149. Bedewitz, M.A.; Jones, A.D.; D'Auria, J.C.; Barry, C.S. Tropinone Synthesis Via An Atypical Polyketide Synthase And P450-Mediated Cyclization. *Nat. Commun.* **2018**, *9*. [CrossRef]
150. Novák, M.; Salemink, C.A. The Essential Oil of *Erythroxylum coca*. *Planta Med.* **1987**, *53*, 113. [CrossRef]
151. Jirschitzka, J.; Schmidt, G.W.; Reichelt, M.; Schneider, B.; Gershenzon, J.; D'Auria, J.C. Plant Tropane Alkaloid Biosynthesis Evolved Independently In The Solanaceae and Erythroxylaceae. *Proc. Natl. Acad. Sci.* **2012**, *109*, 10304–10309. [CrossRef]
152. Casale, J.F.; Moore, J.M. Lesser Alkaloids Of Cocaine-Bearing Plants.2. 3-Oxo-Substituted Tropane Esters: Detection And Mass Spectral Characterization Of Minor Alkaloids Found In South American *Erythroxylum coca* var coca. *J. Chromatogr. A* **1996**, *749*, 173–180. [CrossRef]
153. Casale, J.F.; Moore, J.M. Lesser Alkaloids Of Cocaine-Bearing Plants.3. 2-Carbomethoxy-3-Oxo Substituted Tropane Esters: Detection And Gas Chromatographic Mass Spectrometric Characterization Of New Minor Alkaloids Found In South American Erythroxylum coca var coca. *J. Chromatogr. A* **1996**, *756*, 185–192. [CrossRef]
154. Casale, J.F.; Toske, S.G.; Colley, V.L. Alkaloid Content Of The Seeds From *Erythroxylum coca* var. coca. *J. Forensic Sci.* **2005**, *50*, 1402–1406.
155. Kim, N.; Estrada, O.; Chavez, B.; Stewart, C.; D'Auria, J.C. Tropane and Granatane Alkaloid Biosynthesis: A Systematic Analysis. *Molecules* **2016**, *21*. [CrossRef] [PubMed]
156. Torre, J.C.P.; Schmidt, G.W.; Paetz, C.; Reichelt, M.; Schneider, B.; Gershenzon, J.; D'Auria, J.C. The Biosynthesis Of Hydroxycinnamoyl Quinate Esters And Their Role In The Storage Of Cocaine In *Erythroxylum coca*. *Phytochemistry* **2013**, *91*, 177–186. [CrossRef] [PubMed]
157. Efferth, T. Biotechnology Applications of Plant Callus Cultures. *Engineering* **2019**, *5*, 50–59. [CrossRef]
158. Docimo, T.; Davis, A.J.; Luck, K.; Fellenberg, C.; Reichelt, M.; Phillips, M.; Gershenzon, J.; D'Auria, J.C. Influence Of Medium And Elicitors On The Production Of Cocaine, Amino Acids And Phytohormones By *Erythroxylum coca* calli. *Plant. Cell Tissue Organ. Cult.* **2015**, *120*, 1061–1075. [CrossRef]
159. Ping, Y.; Li, X.D.; Xu, B.F.; Wei, W.; Wei, W.P.; Kai, G.Y.; Zhou, Z.H.; Xiao, Y.L. Building Microbial Hosts for Heterologous Production of *N*-Methylpyrrolinium. *Acs Synth. Biol.* **2019**, *8*, 257–263. [CrossRef]
160. Srinivasan, P.; Smolke, C.D. Engineering A Microbial Biosynthesis Platform For De Novo Production Of Tropane Alkaloids. *Nat. Commun.* **2019**, *10*. [CrossRef]
161. Ping, Y.; Li, X.D.; You, W.J.; Li, G.Q.; Yang, M.Q.; Wei, W.P.; Zhou, Z.H.; Xiao, Y.L. De Novo Production of the Plant-Derived Tropine and Pseudotropine in Yeast. *Acs Synth. Biol.* **2019**, *8*, 1257–1262. [CrossRef]

Sample Availability: Samples of the compounds are not available from the authors.

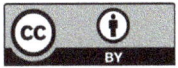

© 2019 by the authors. Licensee MDPI, Basel, Switzerland. This article is an open access article distributed under the terms and conditions of the Creative Commons Attribution (CC BY) license (http://creativecommons.org/licenses/by/4.0/).

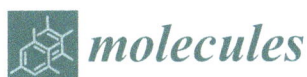

Article

Huberine, a New Canthin-6-One Alkaloid from the Bark of *Picrolemma huberi*

Carlos López [1], Manuel Pastrana [2], Alexandra Ríos [2], Alvaro Cogollo [3] and Adriana Pabón [2,*]

1. Instituto de Química, Universidad de Antioquia, Medellín 050010, Colombia; carlopez.udea@gmail.com
2. Grupo Malaria, Facultad de Medicina, Universidad de Antioquia, Medellín 050010, Colombia; manuel.pastrana@udea.edu.co (M.P.); alexrioso@hotmail.com (A.R.)
3. Jardín Botánico Joaquín Antonio Uribe, Medellín 050010, Colombia; cogolloi@yahoo.com
* Correspondence: adriana.pabon@udea.edu.co

Received: 6 February 2018; Accepted: 14 March 2018; Published: 17 April 2018

Abstract: A new alkaloid, Canthin-6-one, Huberine (**1**), together with three known compounds including 1-Hydroxy-canthin-6-one (**2**), Canthin-6-one (**3**) and stigma sterol (**4**), were isolated from the stem bark of *Picrolemma huberi*. The isolation was achieved by chromatographic techniques and the purification was performed on a C18 column using acetonitrile/water (90:10, v/v) with 0.1% formic acid as the mobile phase. The structural elucidation was performed via spectroscopic methods, notably 1D- and 2D-NMR, UV, IR, MS and HRMS. The antiplasmodial activity of the compounds was studied.

Keywords: canthin-6-one; *Picrolemma huberi*; Simaroubaceae; antiplasmodial activity

1. Introduction

Plants of the family Simaroubaceae are widely used in traditional medicine for the treatment of diseases in different countries around the world. Species belonging to the genus *Picrolemma* (Simaroubaceae) have long been used in traditional medicine for their antitumoral and antimalarial properties [1]. Previous phytochemical investigations of *Picrolema huberi* revealed the presence of terpenoids and alkaloids. Among these compounds, quassinoids and canthin-6-ones are principal constituents of the *Picrolemma* species [2–5]. Canthin-6-ones are a subclass of tryptophan-derived β-carboline alkaloids, and are characterized by an additional ring, D, giving the 6H-Indolo(3,2,1-de) (1,5) naphthyridin backbone. A general biosynthetic pathway of canthin-6-one alkaloids starts from tryptophan as a precursor and produces tryptamine which condense with acetic or ketoglutarate units, giving rise to a series of β-carboline intermediates, each time more oxidized. Except canthin-6-one itself, which has a simple structure, all the canthin-6-one alkaloids isolated from plants are oxidized at any position from C-1 to C-11 of the skeleton to form hydroxy and/or methoxy derivatives [1,6–9]. Meanwhile, more than 60 canthin-6-one alkaloids have been isolated from natural sources, mainly plants from the Rutaceae and Simaroubaceae families [10]. A broad range of biological activities has been reported for canthin-6-ones, such as antitumor, antibacterial, antifungal, antiparasitic, antiviral, anti-inflammatory, antiproliferative, and aphrodisiacal properties [11]. In this paper, we report the results of an investigation of the stem barks of *Picrolemma huberi*. Three canthinone alkaloids have been isolated; one of which is new, Figure 1. All of these alkaloids are reported for the first time from the genus *Picrolemma*.

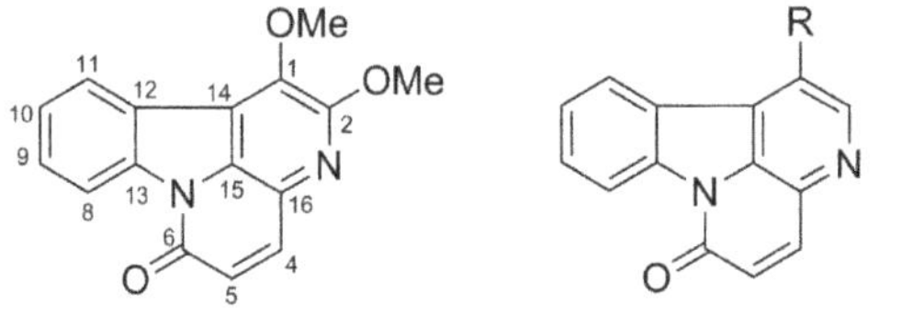

Figure 1. Canthin-6-one alkaloids isolated from *Picrolemma huberi* bark.

2. Results and Discussion

2.1. Identification of Isolated Compounds

Identification of compound 1 from the *Picrolemma huberi* bark. Compound **1**, named Huberine, was isolated as an amorphous, pale-yellow solid. The HR LCMS spectrum of **1** showed a pseudomolecular ion peak, [M + H] at *m/z* 281.0926, corresponding to a molecular formula $C_{16}H_{12}N_2O_3$. A positive Dragendorff test was obtained, suggesting that **1** was an alkaloid. IR absorption bands of conjugated carbonyl group were observed at 1664 cm^{-1} and unsaturation 1630 and 1598 cm^{-1}. The UV spectrum of **1** displayed absorption maxima at 227, 296, 356, and 376 nm, which were similar to those reported for canthin-6-one alkaloids [12]. The ^{13}C-NMR and DEPT-NMR spectra for **1** indicated the presence of 16 carbon signals, including two methoxyls, six methines and eight quaternary carbon signals. All the proton and protonated carbon signals of **1** were assigned unambiguously by an 2D-HSQC (Heteronuclear Single-Quantum Correlation) experiment. In the ^{1}H-NMR spectrum (Table 1), four mutually coupled aromatic protons at δ 8.67 (1H, d, *J* = 8.1 Hz, H-8), δ 7.66 (1H, t, *J* = 7.6 Hz, H-9), δ 7.51 (1H, t, *J* = 7.7 Hz, H-10) and δ 8.22 (1H, d, *J* = 7.6 Hz, H-11) were observed in the ^{1}H-^{1}H COSY spectrum, meaning that the ring A of compound **1** is not substituted.

Table 1. ^{1}H-NMR (600 MHz) and ^{13}C-NMR (125 MHz) spectral data of compound **1** in CDCl$_3$ (δ, in ppm, *J* in Hz).

Position	^{1}H (ppm), *J* (Hz)	^{13}C (ppm)	COSY Coupling	HMBC Coupling(^{2,3}*J*)
1		141.3		OCH$_3$
2		155.1		OCH$_3$
4	7.83(d, 9.6)	138.2	H-5	H-5
5	6.82(d, 9.6)	125.6	H-4	
6		160.1		H-4
8	8.67(d, 8.1)	117.4	H-9	H-9
9	7.66 (t, 7.6)	130.4	H-8, H-10	H-11
10	7.51 (t, 7.7)	125.8	H-9, H-11	
11	8.22(d, 7.6)	124.9	H-10	H-9
12		123.5		H-10
13		140.1		H-9, H-11
14		130.3		
15		130.3		H-4
16		126.4		H-5
OCH$_3$	4.15 (s)	54.7		
OCH$_3$	4.20 (s)	61.3		

Isolated vicinal doublets at δ 7.83 (1H, *J* = 9.6 Hz, H-4) and δ 6.82 (1H, *J* = 9.6 Hz, H-5) were characteristic of *cis*-coupled protons on the conjugated lactam ring of a canthin-6-one. A 2D-HMBC (Heteronuclear Multiple Bond Correlation) experiment further confirmed the structure of alkaloid **1**. In the spectrum, cross-peaks were found for H-4 (δ 7.83) with C-6 (δ 160.1) and C-15 (δ 130.3),

H-5 (δ 6.82) with C-16 (δ 126.4), showing that these are the quaternary carbons that join the C and D rings.

The placement of the methoxy groups was deduced from the HMBC experiments. The methoxy signals showed clear HMBC correlations with the C at 141.1 and 154.9, assigned as C-1 and C-2. The assignment of quaternary carbons was established by HSQC and HMBC spectral data. Thus, the structure of Huberine **1** was established as 1,2-dimethoxycanthin-6-one, which is reported here for the first time. The new compound **1** showed no effective antiplasmodial activity at concentrations evaluated (from 100 µg/mL to 1.56 µg/mL) in *Plasmodium falciparum* strain FCR-3.

Identification of compound **2** and **3** from the *Picrolemma huberi* bark. The structures of the known compounds **2** and **3** were identified as 1 hydroxycanthin-6-one (**2**) [13,14] and canthin-6-one (**3**) [15], by spectroscopic data (^{1}H-NMR, ^{13}C-NMR, 2D-NMR, and MS) and by comparison with published values. Although 1-hydroxycanthin-6-one (**3**) was isolated from the Simaroubaceae family, it has not been reported from *P. huberi*. Stigmasterol (**4**) was also isolated.

2.2. Antiplasmodial Activity In Vitro

The antiplasmodial activity of compounds **1**, **2** and **3** was evaluated in vitro against the multi-resistant strain of FCR-3 of *P. falciparum*. In the concentrations evaluated (from 100 µg/mL to 1.5 µg/mL), they did not show any activity.

3. Materials and Methods

3.1. General Procedures

Spectra were recorded on the following instruments: UV: Shimadzu UV-250 UV-Visible spectrophotometer (Canby, OR, USA); IR: Perkin Elmer 1600 (Waltham, MA, USA); NMR: BRUKER 600 MHz (Silberstreifen, Rheinstetten, DE); HRMS to compound (**1**) were measured on a Xevo Q-Tof Waters® spectrometer (Milford, MA, USA) and MS of compounds **2**, **3** and **4** were measured on a Nermag-Sidar R10-10C spectrometer (Argenteuil, FR) with a quadrupolar filter. All solvents, except those used for bulk extraction, were AR grade. Silica gel 60 F254 was used for column chromatography. Glass and aluminum-supported silica gel 60 F254 plates were used for preparative TLC. TLC spots were visualized under UV light (254 and 365 nm) after spraying with Dragendorff's reagent for alkaloid detection.

3.2. Plant Material

The stem bark of *P. huberi* was collected from the village, La Guada Reserve, [coordinates: 06°52'006" N to 75°08'49.9" W, (1.662 msnm)], close to Amalfi, Antioquia, Colombia, in January 2017. A voucher specimen (Tobón Juan Pablo 2392) has been deposited in the Herbarium JAUM (Joaquín Antonio Uribe Botanic Garden of Medellín, Antioquia, Colombia).

3.3. Extraction and Isolation

Dried stem bark (1.5 kg) of *P. huberi* was defatted with n-hexane (3 L). The marc was extracted with MeOH-H_2O (90:10) (6 L) by percolation for 72 h and the same material was re-extracted in the same manner. The extract was filtered and concentrated up to 1 L under reduced pressure, and then partitioned with EtOAc (2 L). The EtOAc layer was dried over anhydrous Na_2SO_4 and then concentrated under reduced pressure (0.5 L). This extract (30 g) was initially subjected to an acid-base extraction [11] to give $CHCl_3$ alkaloid (2.0 g).

The crude alkaloid (2.0 g) was subjected to column chromatography over silica gel using CH_2Cl_2 gradually enriched with methanol as eluent to yield ten fractions (A–J).

Fraction A (102 mg) was chromatographed on a silica gel column and eluted with DCM-AcOEt (1:1) to give six subfractions, A1–A6. Fraction A1 (75 mg) was chromatographed by preparative TLC with CH_2Cl_2-MeOH (95:5) and further purified by preparative RP-HPLC using the mobile phase

CH$_3$CN/H$_2$O (90:10), 0.1% formic acid to yield compound **1** (10 mg). Similar HPLC of fraction A2 (15.0 mg) yielded compound **2** (1.3 mg) eluting at 13.2 min, and HPLC of fraction A3 (38.0 mg) yielded compound **3** (1.0 mg) eluting at 9.5 min.

Antiplasmodial in vitro activity assay of each compound (from 100 µg/mL to 1.5 µg/mL) was evaluated in FCR3 strain. The diphosphate salt of chloroquine ($\geq$98%, SIGMA C6628), evaluated in a range of 2000 nM to 2.3 nM, was used as a treatment control in each assay [16].

3.4. Spectral Data

Huberine: 1,2-Dimethoxy-canthin-6-one (**1**). Yellow amorphous powder; UV (MeOH, max, nm): 207, 266, 294, 354, 369. IR (KBr, n, cm^{-1}): 1664, 1550, 1439, 1214, 1086, 753; ^{1}H- and ^{13}C-NMR data, see Table 1; MS: Waters LCT Premier (ESI-TOF) spectrometer at m/z 281.0926 [M + H]$^+$; calcd. for C$_{16}$H$_{12}$N$_2$O$_3$, 281.0926.

1-Hydroxy-canthin-6-one (**2**). Yellow amorphous powder. UV (MeOH, nm): 210, 249, 256,288, 341, 415. IR (KBr, cm^{-1}): 3276, 1567, 1600, 1629. ^{1}H-NMR (600 MHz, MeOD-d_4, δ in ppm, *J*), 8.60 (d, 1H, 8.4Hz), 8.35 (s, 1H), 8.27 (d, 1H, 7.7Hz), 8.02 (d, 1H, 9.7Hz), 7.69 (t, 1H, 8.4Hz), 7.58 (t, 1H, 8.0Hz), 6.80 (d, 1H, 9.7Hz). ^{13}C-NMR (150 MHz, DMSO-d_6, δ in ppm): 151.39 (C-1), 135.55 (C-2), 139.48 (C-4), 123.38 (C-5), 159.66 (C-6), 123.60 (C-8), 125.79 (C-9), 129.16 (C-10), 116.22 (C-11), 137.61 (C-12), 137.5 (C-13), 114.31(C-14), 133.32 (C-15), 128.11 (C-16). MS TOF ES$^+$ spectrometer at m/z 237.0708 [M + H]$^+$.

Canthin-6-one (**3**). Yellow amorphous powder. UV (MeOH, nm): 210, 249, 256,288, 341, 415. IR (KBr, cm^{-1}): 3276, 1567, 1600, 1629. ^{1}H-NMR (600 MHz, DMSO-d_6, δ, ppm, *J*/Hz): 8.35 (1H, d, *J* = 4.8 Hz, H-1), 8.86 (1H, d, *J* = 4.8 Hz, H-2), 8.7 (1H, d, *J* = 9.7 Hz, H-4), 7.02 (1H, d, *J* = 9.7 Hz, H-5), 8.55 (1H, d, *J* = 8.1 Hz, H-8), 7.79 (1H, t, *J* = 7.6 Hz, H-9), 7.62 (1H, t, *J* = 7.6 Hz, H-10), 8.42 (1H, d, *J* = 7.8 Hz, H-11). MS TOF ES$^+$ spectrometer at m/z 221.0715 [M + H]$^+$. Supplementary material is available online.

4. Conclusions

Huberine, a new canthin-6-one alkaloid (**1**) and 3 known compounds (**2**, **3** and **4**) were isolated from the stem bark of *P. huberi*. The structure of the new compound (**1**) was elucidated by spectroscopic data Huberine (**1**); it was isolated from this plant for the first time. The isolates were screened for inhibitory activity against *Plasmodium falciparum* strains. Compounds **1**, and **2** showed no effective antiplasmodial activity.

Supplementary Materials: The following are available online. Figure S1: Huberine: 1,2-Dimethoxy-canthin-6-one (**1**). ^{1}H-NMR (CDCl$_3$, 600 MHz); Huberine: 1,2-Dimethoxy-canthin-6-one (**1**). ^{13}C-NMR (CDCl$_3$, 150 MHz); Huberine: 1,2-Dimethoxy-canthin-6-one (**1**). COSY H-H (CDCl$_3$); Huberine: 1,2-Dimethoxy-canthin-6-one (**1**). HSQC (CDCl$_3$); Huberine: 1,2-Dimethoxy-canthin-6-one (**1**). HMBC (CDCl$_3$); Huberine: 1,2-Dimethoxy-canthin-6-one (**1**). HRMS; Huberine: 1,2-Dimethoxy-canthin-6-one (**1**). FT-IR, 1-Hydroxy-canthin-6-one (**2**). ^{1}H-NMR (MeOD-d4, 600 MHz); 1-Hydroxy-canthin-6-one (**2**). ^{13}C-NMR (DMSO-d_6, 150 MHz); 1-Hydroxy-canthin-6-one (**2**). COSY H-H (MeOD-d_4); 1-Hydroxy-canthin-6-one (**2**). HSQC (MeOD-d_4); 1-Hydroxy-canthin-6-one (**2**). HRMS; Canthin-6-one (**3**). ^{1}H-NMR (DMOS-d_6, 600 MHz); Canthin-6-one (**3**). HRMS.

Acknowledgments: This work was funded by General system of Royalties of Colombia (SGR), contract RC:20702305-8399DZZZZ.The authors would like to give special thanks to Silvia Blair for being the manager of this project and obtaining their funding. Also, to Jairo Saez for the advice on identification of the compounds from *P. huberi* and to Juan Pablo Tobón Agudelo who very kindly accompanied us to the collection of plant material. The authors are also very grateful to Bruno Figadere of l'UMR 8076 Bio CIS-Laboratoire Pharmacognosie, Faculté de Pharmacie—Université Paris-Sud for the high-resolution mass spectra.

Author Contributions: C.L.: Identification of the compounds from *P. huberi* and writing of the manuscript; M.P.: Preparation of extracts, isolation and purification of the compounds; A.R.: Conducting biological tests; A.C.: Identification, classification, collection and knowledge of the plant; A.P.: Conception, design, analysis and interpretation of results, and writing of the manuscript

Conflicts of Interest: The authors declare no conflict of interest.

References

1. Ohmoto, T.; Koike, K. *The Alkaloids*; Brossi, A., Ed.; Academic: New York, NY, USA, 1989; Volume 36, pp. 135–170.
2. Tischler, M.; Cardellina, J.H., II; Boyd, M.R.; Cragg, G.M. Cytotoxic quassinoids from *Cedronia granatensis*. *J. Nat. Prod.* **1992**, *55*, 667–671. [CrossRef] [PubMed]
3. Fo, E.R.; Fernandes, J.B.; Vieira, P.C.; da Silva, M.F.G.F. Canthin-6-one alkaloids from *Picrolemma granatensis*. *Phytochemistry* **1992**, *31*, 2499–2501. [CrossRef]
4. Rodrigues-Filho, E.; Fernandes, J.B.; Vieira, P.C.; Silva, M.F.G.F. Quassinoids and tetranortriterpenoids from *Picrolemma granatensis*. *Phytochemistry* **1993**, *34*, 501–504. [CrossRef]
5. Fo, E.R.; Fernandes, J.B.; Vieira, P.C.; da Silva, M.F.G.F.; Zukerman-Schpector, J.; Corrêa de Lima, R.M.O.; Nascimento, S.C.; Thomas, W. Protolimonoids and quassinoids from *Picrolemma granatensis*. *Phytochemistry* **1996**, *43*, 857–862. [CrossRef]
6. Haynes, H.F.; Nelson, E.R.; Price, J.R. Alkaloids of the Australian Rutaceae: *Pentaceras australis* Hook. FI Isolation of the alkaloids and identification of canthin-6-one. *Aust. J. Chem.* **1952**, *5*, 387–400. [CrossRef]
7. Crespi-Perellino, N.; Guicciardi, A.; Malyszko, G.; Minghetti, A. Biosynthetic relationship between indole alkaloids produced by cell cultures of *Ailanthus altissima*. *J. Nat. Prod.* **1986**, *49*, 814–822. [CrossRef]
8. Aragozzini, F.; Maconi, E.; Gualandris, R. Evidence for involvement of ketoglutarate in the biosynthesis of canthin-6-one from cell cultures of *Ailanthus altissima*. *Plant Cell Rep.* **1988**, *7*, 213–215. [CrossRef] [PubMed]
9. Anderson, L.A.; Hay, C.A.; Roberts, M.F.; Phillipson, J.D. Studies on *Ailanthus altissima* cell suspension cultures. *Plant Cell Rep.* **1986**, *5*, 387–390. [CrossRef] [PubMed]
10. Showalter, H.D.H. Progress in the synthesis of canthine alkaloids and ring-truncated congeners. *J. Nat. Prod.* **2013**, *76*, 455–467. [CrossRef] [PubMed]
11. Dai, J.; Li, N.; Wang, J.; Schneider, U. Fruitful Decades for Canthin-6-ones from 1952 to 2015: Biosynthesis, Chemistry, and Biological Activities. *Molecules* **2016**, *21*, 493. [CrossRef] [PubMed]
12. Ohmoto, T.; Koike, K.; Sakamoto, Y. Studies on the constituents of *Ailanthus altissima* Swingle. II. Alkaloidal constituents. *Chem. Pharm. Bull.* **1981**, *29*, 390–395. [CrossRef]
13. Suroor, A.K.; Shamsuddin, K.M. 1-Hydroxycanthin-6-one, an alkaloid from *Ailanthus giraldii*. *Phytochemistry* **1981**, *20*, 2062–2063.
14. Ohmoto, T.; Koike, K. Studies on the Constituents of *Ailanthus altissima* SWINGLE.III. The Alkaloidal Constituents. *Chem. Pharm. Bull.* **1984**, *32*, 170–173. [CrossRef]
15. Nafiah, M.A.; Mukhtar, M.R.; Omar, H.; Ahmad, K.; Morita, H.; Litaudon, M.; Awang, K.; Hadi, A.H. N-Cyanomethylnorboldine: A New Aporphine Isolated from Alseodaphneperakensis (Lauraceae). *Molecules* **2011**, *16*, 3402–3409. [CrossRef] [PubMed]
16. Pabón, A.; Ramirez, O.; Rios, A.; López, E.; De Las Salas, B.; Cardona, F.; Blair, S. Antiplasmodial and Cytotoxic Activity of Raw Plant extracts as reported by knowledgeable indigenous people of the amazon region (Vaupés Medio in Colombia). *Plant Med.* **2016**, *82*, 717–722. [CrossRef] [PubMed]

Sample Availability: Samples of the compounds **1**, **2** and **3** are available from the authors.

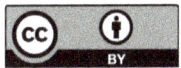

© 2018 by the authors. Licensee MDPI, Basel, Switzerland. This article is an open access article distributed under the terms and conditions of the Creative Commons Attribution (CC BY) license (http://creativecommons.org/licenses/by/4.0/).

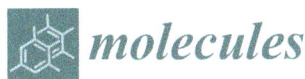

Article

Three New Cytotoxic Steroidal Alkaloids from *Sarcococca hookeriana*

Kang He [1,†], Jinxi Wang [2,†], Juan Zou [1], Jichun Wu [1], Shaojie Huo [1] and Jiang Du [1,*]

[1] The Key Laboratory of Miao Medicine of Guizhou Province, Guiyang College of Traditional Chinese Medicine, Guiyang 550025, Guizhou, China; hekang0851@163.com (K.H.); zoujuan@hotmail.com (J.Z.); wujichun2018@sina.com (J.W.); 15038115764@163.com (S.H.)
[2] The Ethnical Medicine Research Institute of Qian Dong Nan Miao and Dong Autonomous Prefecture, Kaili 556000, Guizhou, China; 15185660328@163.com
* Correspondence: dujang.gz@163.com; Tel.: +86-871-8830-8060
† These authors contributed equally to this work and are co-first authors.

Received: 13 April 2018; Accepted: 10 May 2018; Published: 15 May 2018

Abstract: Three new steroidal alkaloids with an unusual 3α tigloylamide group, named sarchookloides A–C (**1–3**), were isolated along with four known compounds (**4–7**) from the roots of *Sarcococca hookeriana*. Their structures and relative configuration were elucidated on the basis of spectroscopic methods including MS, UV, IR, 1D, and 2D NMR data. The isolated compounds were evaluated for their cytotoxicity against five human cancer cell lines: Hela, A549, MCF-7, SW480, and CEM in vitro. All three amide substituted steroidal alkaloids exhibited significant cytotoxic activities with IC_{50} values of 1.05–31.83 μM.

Keywords: *Sarcococca hookeriana*; sarchookloides A–C; steroidal alkaloid; cytotoxicity

1. Introduction

The genus *Sarcococca* (Buxaceae) includes about 20 species, eight of which are found in China [1]. Some of them are used in TCM and traditional folk medicine to treat stomach pain, rheumatism, swollen sore throat, and bruises [2–4]. Previous studies on this genus revealed that the steroidal alkaloids were the main chemical components, and possessed a range of bioactivities (e.g., cholinesterase inhibiting, antitumor, antibacterial, antiulcer, antiplasmodial, and antidiabetic) [5–20]. For the search of bioactive metabolites from this genus, our previous investigation on *Sarcococca ruscifolia* resulted in the discovery of two new steroidal alkaloids [16]. As part of our continuous exploration of active alkaloids, three new steroidal alkaloids, namely sarchookloides A–C (**1–3**) along with four known compounds, pachysamine G (**4**), pachysamine H (**5**), sarcovagine B (**6**), and pachyaximine A (**7**) (Figure 1), were isolated from the roots of *Sarcococca hookeriana*. The new compounds, sarchookloides A–C (**1–3**), were shown to possess a 3α substituent, which has rarely been reported [17]. The cytotoxicity assay on human cancer cell lines Hela, A549, MCF-7, SW480, and CEM in vitro demonstrated that these steroidal alkaloids exhibited potent antitumor activities. This paper describes the isolation, structure elucidation, and cytotoxicity activities of the isolates.

2. Results and Discussion

2.1. Structure Elucidation of Compounds

Compound **1** showed a quasi-molecular ion peak $[M + H]^+$ at m/z 461.3731 (calculated to be 461.3738) in the HR-ESI-MS (spectrum showed in Supplementary material), which corresponds to the molecular formula $C_{28}H_{48}N_2O_3$. The IR spectrum showed absorption bands at 3424 (hydroxyl group), 1662 (amide carbonyl group), and 1623 (double bond) cm^{-1}. The ^{1}H and ^{13}C NMR (DEPT) spectra (Table 1) displayed 28 carbon resonances due to four quaternary carbons, 10 methines, seven methylenes, and seven methyl groups, which revealed one amide carbonyl group and one double bond. The presence of five methyl signals [δ_H 0.67 (3H, s, H-18), 1.21 (3H, s, Me-19), 0.92 (3H, d, J = 6.4 Hz, Me-21), 2.23 (6H, s, N,N-dimethyl)] and one nitric proton signal [δ_H 6.09 (1H, d, J = 5.1 Hz, NH-3)] in the ^{1}H NMR (CDCl$_3$) spectrum in combination with 2D NMR data suggested that compound **1** belongs to the 20α-dimethylamino-3-amino-5α-pregnane type steroidal alkaloids [21].

Table 1. ^{1}H (600 MHz) and ^{13}C (150 MHz) NMR data of compounds **1**–**3** in CDCl$_3$.

Position	1		2		3	
	δ_H (J in Hz)	δ_C	δ_H (J in Hz)	δ_C	δ_H (J in Hz)	δ_C
1	1.67, 1.69, m	44.2	1.16, 1.87, m	40.6	0.95, 1.56, m	33.6
2	3.88, ddd (13.4, 6.7, 6.8)	69.0	3.97, brs (W$_{1/2}$ 14.8)	69.6	1.64, 1.71, m	26.2
3	3.99, ddd (7.8, 6.8, 5.1)	58.4	4.03, m	50.8	4.14, m	44.8
4	3.78, dd, (7.8, 3.9)	76.3	1.23, 2.04, m	28.8	1.39, 1.55, m	33.0
5	1.26, m	45.5	1.07, m	41.8	1.11, m	41.5
6	1.41, 1.79, m	24.4	1.48, 1.85, m	27.9	1.48, 1.87, m	27.8
7	1.01, 1.77, m	32.2	0.91, 1.68, m	32.1	0.88, 1.68, m	32.1
8	1.37, m	35.3	1.39, m	34.9	1.36, m	35.5
9	0.71, m	57.0	1.05, m	56.8	0.68, m	54.7
10	-	36.0	-	35.9	-	36.2
11	1.35, 1.44, m	21.0	1.30, 1.50, m	21.0	1.22, 1.51, m	20.9
12	1.12, 1.90, m	39.9	1.09, 1.90, m	40.0	1.08, 1.88, m	40.0
13	-	42.1	-	41.8	-	41.5
14	1.03, m	56.8	0.66, m	55.6	1.04, m	56.8
15	1.10, 1.60, m	24.2	1.06, 1.58, m	24.2	1.03, 1.57, m	24.2
16	1.50, 1.84, m	27.9	1.35, 1.44, m	28.4	1.19, m	28.6
17	1.34, m	54.8	1.32, m	54.8	1.33, m	54.7
18	0.67, s	12.6	0.64, s	12.6	0.63, s	12.5
19	1.21, s	19.3	1.02, s	14.5	0.79, s	11.6
20	2.50, m	61.6	2.45, m	61.6	2.45, m	61.6
21	0.92, d, (6.4)	10.2	0.89, d, (6.4)	10.2	0.88, d, (6.4)	10.3
NMe2	2.23, s	39.8	2.20, s	39.9	2.20, s	39.9
C=O	-	170.6	-	169.2	-	168.8
2′	-	131.4	-	132.2	-	132.6
3′	6.45, q, (6.9)	132.1	6.37, q, (6.9)	130.8	6.36, q, (6.9)	130.2
4′	1.76, d, (6.9)	14.3	1.75, d, (6.9)	14.2	1.73, d, (6.9)	14.1
5′	1.84, s	12.6	1.84, s	12.7	1.83, s	12.7
NH	6.09, d, (5.1)	-	5.82, d, (7.4)	-	5.93, d, (6.6)	-
2-OH	2.84, d, (7.2)	-	-	-	-	-
4-OH	4.40, d, (3.0)	-	-	-	-	-

The presence of two methyl [δ_H 1.76 (3H, d, J = 6.9 Hz, H-4′), 1.84 (3H, s, H-5′)] and an olefinic proton [δ_H 6.45 (1H, q, J = 6.9 Hz, H-3′)] signals in the ^{1}H NMR spectrum together with two methyl [δ_C 14.3 (C-4′), 12.6 (C-5′)], one double bond [δ_C 131.4 (C-2′), 132.1 (C-3′)], and one carbonyl [δ_C 170.6 (C-1′)] signals in the ^{13}C NMR spectrum led to the deduction of a tigloyl moiety, which was supported by the ^{1}H–^{1}H COSY-correlated signal of H-4′/H-3′ and the HMBC correlations of H-5′/C-3′, C-1′ and H-3′/C-1′ (Figure 2). Furthermore, the HMBC correlations of NH/C-2′ (Figure 2) proposed that the location of the tigloyl group was at N-3. In addition, the two hydroxyl groups assigned at the C-2 (δ_C 69.0) and C-4 (δ_C 76.3) positions were deduced from the ^{1}H NMR [δ_H 2.84 (1H, d, J = 7.2 Hz, OH-2), 4.40 (1H, d, J = 3.0 Hz, OH-4)] and ^{13}C NMR [δ_C 69.0 (C-2), 76.3 (C-4)] data in combination with the ^{1}H–^{1}H COSY [OH-2 /H-2 (δ_H 3.88) and OH-4 /H-4 (δ_H 3.78)] and HMBC [OH-2/C-1 (δ_C 44.2), C-3 (δ_C 58.4) and OH-4/C-3, C-5 (δ_C 45.5)] experiments. Therefore, the planar structure of compound **1** was constructed.

The ^{13}C NMR data of the ring A, coupling constants of H-2, H-3 and H-4 and NOESY data clearly indicated that compound **1** differs from the previously reported compounds of hookerianamide M [10] and sarcovagine A [18] with respect to the stereochemistry at C-2, C-3, and C-4 positions. In the ROESY spectrum (Figure 2), the correlations of H-19 [δ_H 1.21 (3H, s)] with OH-2 and OH-4 indicated the β orientations of the two hydroxyl groups. Furthermore, the obvious ROESY correlations (Figure 2) of HN with H-2, H-4 and H-5 [δ_H 1.26 (1H, m)] implied the α orientation of the tigloylamide group. The ring A of compound **1** may exist mainly as a stable boat conformation due to the substitution of 3α tigloylamide group [17]. Consequently, the structure and relative configuration of compound **1** was determined as (20S)-20-N,N-dimethylamino-2β,4β-dihydroxyl-3α-tigloylamino-5α-pregnane, which was named sarchookloide A (Figure 1).

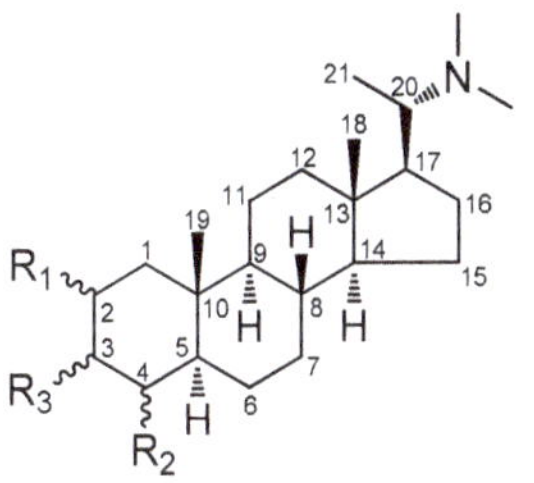

	R_1	R_2	R_3	Unsaturation
1	β OH	β OH	α NH-Tigloyl	
2	β OH	H	α NH-Tigloyl	
3	H	H	α NH-Tigloyl	
4	H	H	β NH-Tigloyl	
5	H	H	α NMe-Benzoyl	
6	α OH	β OAc	β NH-Tigloyl	
7	H	H	β OMe	$\Delta^{5,6}$

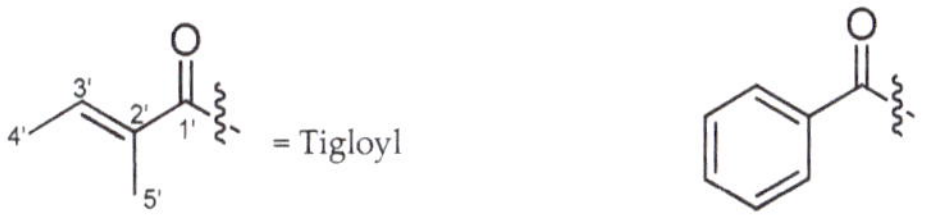

Figure 1. Structures of compounds 1–7.

Compound **2** had a molecular formula of $C_{28}H_{48}N_2O_2$, which was determined by HR-ESI-MS (m/z 445.3775 [M + H]$^+$), suggesting six degrees of unsaturation. The IR spectrum displayed absorptions indicating a hydroxyl group (3443 cm^{-1}), amide carbonyl group (1664 cm^{-1}) and double bond (1629 cm^{-1}). In the ^{13}C NMR and DEPT spectra (Table 1), 28 carbon signals were observed, including 23 carbon resonances assigned to a 20α-dimethylamino-3-amino-5α-pregnane type steroidal alkaloid skeleton and 5 carbon resonances for a tigloyl group [21]. The ^{1}H–^{1}H COSY correlated signal of H-4' [δ_H 1.75 (3H, d, J = 6.9 Hz)]/H-3' [δ_H 6.37 (1H, q, J = 6.9 Hz)] and the HMBC correlations of H-5' [δ_H 1.84 (1H, s)]/C-3' [δ_C 130.8], C-1' [δ_C 169.2], H-3'/C-1' and HN [δ_H 5.82 (1H, d, J = 7.4 Hz)]/C-1' (Figure 2) suggested that the tigloyl group were attached to N-3. The COSY correlations of H-2 [δ_H 3.97 (1H, brs)]/H-1 [δ_H 1.16, 1.87 (2H, m)], H-3 [δ_H 4.03 (1H, m)] proposed that the location of the hydroxyl group was at C-2.

The similarity of the NMR data of compounds **2** and 20α-dimethylamino-2α-hydroxyl-3β-tigloylamino-5α-pregnane [16] suggested that they possessed the same planar structure. The ROESY correlations (Figure 2) of HN with H-2 and H-5 [δ_H 1.07 (1H, m)] implied the α orientation of the tigloylamide group and the β orientation of the hydroxyl group. This was also supported by the discrepant $W_{1/2}$ (14.8) of H-2 [10] and the ^{13}C NMR data of the ring A in **2** compared with the data of reported compounds [16]. The substitution of 3α tigloylamide group led to the main boat conformation of the ring A in compound **2**. Consequently, the structure and relative configuration of compound **2** was determined as (20S)-20-N,N-dimethylamino-2β-hydroxyl-3α-tigloylamino-5α-pregnane, which was named sarchookloide B (Figure 1).

Compound **3** was given the molecular formula $C_{28}H_{48}N_2O$ according to its HR-ESI-MS data at m/z 429.3829 [M + H]$^+$ (calculated as 429.3839), corresponding to six degrees of unsaturation. The IR spectrum of compound **3** included the absorption bands for amide carbonyl group (1665 cm^{-1}) and double bond (1625 cm^{-1}). The ^{13}C NMR and DEPT spectra (Table 1) of compound **3** exhibited 28 carbon signals corresponding to four quaternary carbons, eight methines, nine methylene, and seven methyl groups, of which 23 carbon resonances were ascribed to 20α-dimethylamino-3-amino-5α-pregnane type steroidal alkaloid skeleton and five carbon resonances were attributed to a tigloyl group [21].

Compound **3** and pachysamine G [19] exhibited the same planar structure, which was supported by the similar NMR data found for both of them. The α-orientations of the tigloylamide group was assigned by the ROESY correlations (Figure 2) of HN [δ_H 5.93 (1H, d, J = 6.6 Hz)] with H-5 [δ_H 1.11 (1H, m)] in combination with the different shift of the ring A in compound **3** compared with the data of pachysamine G in ^{13}C NMR spectrum. Similar to compounds **1** and **2**, the boat conformation of the ring A in compound **3** was the main conformation [17]. Therefore, the structure and relative configuration of compound **3** was determined as (20S)-20-N,N-dimethylamino-3α-tigloylamino-5α-pregnane, which was named sarchookloide C (Figure 1).

The known compounds **4**–**7** were identified as pachysamine G (**4**) [19], pachysamine H (**5**) [19], sarcovagine B (**6**) [18], and pachyaximine A (**7**) [20] through a comparison of their spectroscopic data with those reported in the literature.

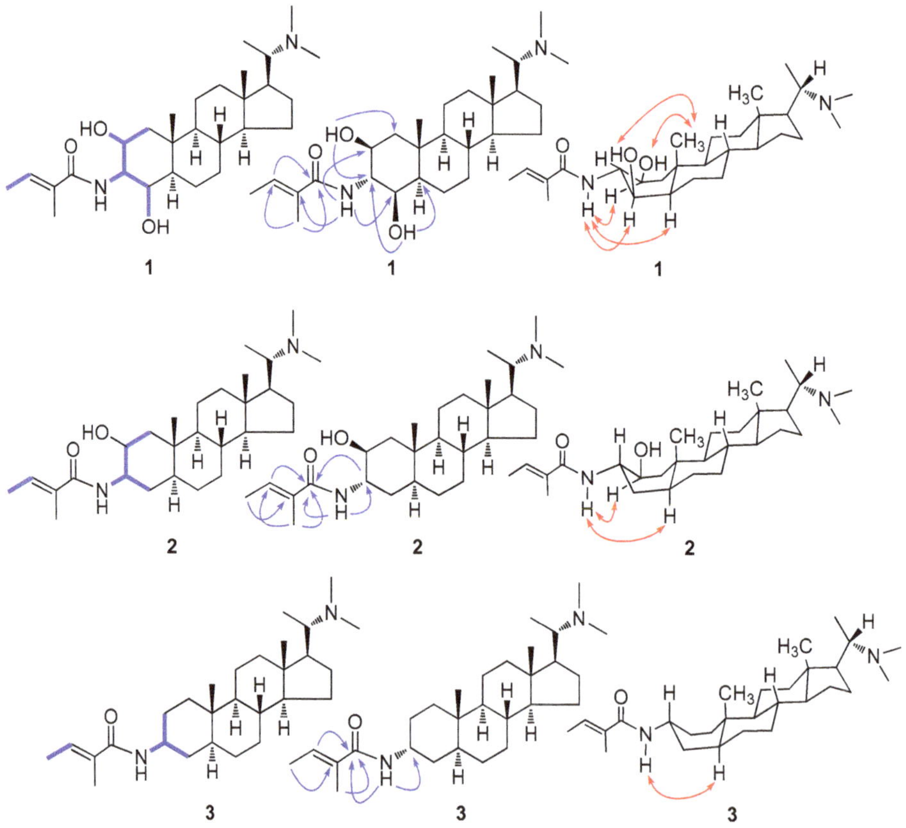

Figure 2. Key 1H–1H COSY (-), HMBC (→) and ROESY (↔) correlations of compounds **1**–**3**.

2.2. Results of the Cytotoxicity Test

All compounds were evaluated using a MTT cytotoxicity assay against human cervical cancer cell line Hela, lung adenocarcinoma cell line A549, breast cancer cell line MCF-7, colon cancer cell line SW480, and leukemia CEM cells (adriamycin was used as the positive control). The IC$_{50}$ values of all compounds against the indicated cancer cells are summarized in Table 2. Compound **5** had the greatest cytotoxicity to all cells, as its range of IC$_{50}$ values was approximately 1.05–2.23 µM. All three amide-substituted compounds, except for pachyaximine A, exhibited significant cytotoxic activity on all cells, which suggests that the amide group of these compounds was the necessary group for the cytotoxicity. In addition, Hela and A549 were the more sensitive cell lines to these types of compounds compared to all tested cancer cells because the IC$_{50}$ values of all compounds were less than 10 µM. Furthermore, all active compounds showed effects that were comparable to the chemotherapeutic drug adriamycin in inhibiting the growth of all cancer cells, which suggests that three amide-substituted pregnane-type steroidal alkaloids might have the potential to be anticancer agents.

Table 2. Cytotoxicity of compounds **1–7** [a] against Hela, A549, MCF-7, SW480, and CEM cells in vitro (IC$_{50}$ [b], µM).

Compounds	Cell Lines				
	Hela	A549	MCF-7	SW480	CEM
1	4.13 ± 0.14	2.53 ± 0.15	4.47 ± 0.06	6.42 ± 0.10	4.26 ± 0.11
2	7.93 ± 0.09	8.73 ± 0.16	28.53 ± 0.17	8.97 ± 0.10	31.83 ± 0.25
3	1.24 ± 0.10	2.87 ± 0.14	2.53 ± 0.12	3.08 ± 0.14	3.43 ± 0.13
4	2.43 ± 0.11	2.98 ± 0.17	3.70 ± 0.26	26.04 ± 0.21	3.05 ± 0.13
5	1.06 ± 0.14	1.18 ± 0.11	2.23 ± 0.15	1.49 ± 0.10	1.05 ± 0.06
6	1.38 ± 0.09	4.96 ± 0.12	1.65 ± 0.09	3.76 ± 0.14	6.06 ± 0.16
7	>100	>100	>100	>100	>100
Adriamycin [c]	0.62 ± 0.08	0.77 ± 0.06	1.26 ± 0.05	1.19 ± 0.11	0.98 ± 0.08

[a] All results are expressed as mean ± SD; n = 3 for all groups. [b] IC$_{50}$: 50% inhibitory concentration. [c] Adriamycin was the positive control.

3. Materials and Methods

3.1. General Experimental Procedures

Optical rotations were obtained on a JASCO model 1020 polarimeter (Horiba, Tokyo, Japan). UV spectra were measured on a Shimadzu UV-2401PC spectrophotometer (Shimadzu, Kyoto, Japan). IR (KBr) spectra were measured on a Bio-Rad FTS-135 spectrometer (Bio-Rad, Hercules, CA, USA). The 1D and 2D NMR spectra were recorded on Bruker AVANCE III-600 spectrometers with TMS used as an internal standard (Bruker, Bremerhaven, Germany). The mass spectra were obtained on a Waters AutoSpec Premier P776 (Waters, NY, USA). The silica gel (200–300 mesh) for column chromatography and the TLC plates (GF$_{254}$) were obtained from Qingdao Marine Chemical Factory (Qingdao, Shandong, China). The Sephadex LH-20 (20–150 µm) used for chromatography was purchased from Pharmacia Fine Chemical Co. Ltd. (Pharmacia, Uppsala, Sweden). Fractions were visualized by heating silica gel plates sprayed with Dragendorff's reagent. The cell lines Hela, A549, MCF-7, SW480, and CEM were obtained from the Cell Bank of the Chinese Academy of Sciences (Shanghai, China), while MTT were obtained from Sigma Company.

3.2. Plant Material

The plants of *Sarcococca hookeriana* Baill. were collected in Hezhang County, Guizhou Province, China, in April 2012 and identified by Prof. Qingwen Sun, Guiyang College of Traditional Chinese Medicine. A voucher specimen (No. 20120401401) was deposited at the Key Laboratory of Miao Medicine of Guizhou Province, Guiyang College of Traditional Chinese Medicine.

3.3. Extraction and Isolation

The air-dried and powdered roots of *S. hookeriana* Baill. (2.5 kg) were extracted with 95% (25 L) EtOH under reflux three times, with an extraction time of 2 h. The combined extracts (443 g) were concentrated and suspended in H$_2$O (3 L). The suspension was extracted with CHCl$_3$ to obtain the CHCl$_3$ fraction (94 g). The CHCl$_3$ fraction was subjected to silica gel column chromatography (Si CC) and eluted with petroleum ether-diethylamine (100:1, 95:5, 9:1, 8:2) to yield four fractions (Fractions A–D). Fraction B (1.6 g) was subjected to Si CC and eluted with petroleum ether-diethylamine (100:2, 9:1) to yield the fractions B1–B3. Fraction B2 (330 mg) was chromatographed using Si CC and was developed with petroleum ether-diethylamine (100:2) to yield compounds **3** (21 mg) and **4** (35 mg). Si CC was performed on Fraction C (12.3 g) with a gradient eluent of petroleum ether-diethylamine (100:5, 9:1, 8:2) to yield four fractions (fractions C1–C4). Fraction C2 (1.4 g) was first subjected to Si CC (petroleum ether-diethylamine, 100:5), before being purified on Sephadex LH-20. This yielded compounds **2** (26 mg), **5** (30 mg) and **7** (31 mg). Fraction C4 (985 mg) was purified on Sephadex LH-20, before Si CC was used (petroleum ether-diethylamine, 9:1) to separate compounds **1** (33 mg) and **6** (19 mg).

3.3.1. Sarchookloide A (**1**)

This was a white amorphous powder with a HR-ESI-MS m/z of 461.3731 [M + H]$^+$ (calculated for $C_{28}H_{49}N_2O_3$, 461.3738). The $[\alpha]_D^{22}$ was +52.99 (c 0.58, MeOH); UV (MeOH) had a λ_{max} of 209.4 nm; and IR (KBr) had a ν_{max} of 3424, 2931, 2867, 1662 and 1623 cm^{-1}. The ^{1}H and ^{13}C NMR data are shown in Table 1.

3.3.2. Sarchookloide B (**2**)

This was a white amorphous powder with a HR-ESI-MS m/z of 445.3775 [M +H]$^+$ (calculated for $C_{28}H_{49}N_2O_2$, 445.3789). The $[\alpha]_D^{22}$ was +30.18 (c 0.57, MeOH); UV (MeOH) had a λ_{max} of 205.8 nm; and IR (KBr) had a ν_{max} of 3442, 2930, 2966, 1664 and 1629 cm^{-1}. The ^{1}H and ^{13}C NMR data are shown in Table 1.

3.3.3. Sarchookloide C (**3**)

This was a white amorphous powder with a HR-ESI-MS m/z of 429.3829 [M + H]$^+$ (calculated for $C_{28}H_{49}N_2O$, 429.3839). The $[\alpha]_D^{22}$ was +7.10 (c 0.62, MeOH); UV (MeOH) had a λ_{max} of 207.2 nm; and IR (KBr) had a ν_{max} of 3454, 2930, 2853, 1665 and 1625 cm^{-1}. The ^{1}H and ^{13}C NMR data are shown in Table 1.

3.4. Cytotoxicity Assay

The cytotoxicity of compounds **1–7** was tested on the human cervical cancer cell line Hela, lung adenocarcinoma cell line A549, breast cancer cell line MCF-7, colon cancer cell line SW480 and leukemia CEM cells. All cells were cultured in a RPMI-1640 or DMEM medium (Hyclone, Logan, UT, USA), which was supplemented with 10% fetal bovine serum (Hyclone) in 5% CO_2 at 37 °C. The cytotoxicity assay was performed using the MTT method in 96-well microplates [22]. Briefly, the adherent cells (100 µL) were seeded into each well of 96-well cell culture plates and allowed to adhere for 12 h before the addition of the drug. The suspended cells were seeded just before the addition of the drug at an initial density of 1×10^5 cells/mL. Each tumor cell line was exposed to the tested compound at different concentrations for 48 h. The experiments were performed in triplicate. Adriamycin (Sigma, St. Louis, MO, USA) was used as a positive control. After treatment, cell viability was measured and the cell growth curve was plotted. The IC_{50} values were calculated by the Reed and Muench method [23].

4. Conclusions

We obtained three new pregnane-type steroidal alkaloids, sarchookloides A–C (**1–3**), along with four known compounds, pachysamine G (**4**), pachysamine H (**5**), sarcovagine B (**6**), and pachyaxime A (**7**), from the roots of *Sarcococca hookeriana*. The new compounds, sarchookloides A–C (**1–3**), were shown to possess a 3α substituent, which has rarely been reported. By performing a cytotoxic assay on Hela, A549, MCF-7, SW480 and CEM cell lines in vitro, all three amide substituted compounds exhibited significant cytotoxic activities on all cells, which suggests that the three amide group of these compounds was the necessary group for the cytotoxicity. The most active compound, pachysamine H (**5**), inhibited all cancer cells with IC$_{50}$ values in the range of approximately 1.05–2.23 µM. The results suggested that these types of steroidal alkaloids merit further biological evaluation of their cytotoxic activities and might have the potential to be studied for anticancer activity.

Supplementary Materials: The following ^{1}H NMR, ^{13}C NMR, 2D NMR, HR-ESI-MS spectra and the RAW data of the new compounds are available as supporting data. Supplementary materials are available online.

Author Contributions: K.H. and J.D. designed the experiments and revised the paper; K.H. and J.W. performed the experiments, analyzed the data, and wrote the paper; J.W. and J.Z. contributed to bioassay reagents and materials and analyzed the data; J.W., S.H. and J.D. revised the paper. All authors read and approved the final manuscript.

Acknowledgments: This research work was financially supported by the Science and Technology Foundation of Guizhou Province [grant number J (2013) 2071], the Science and Technology Cooperation Program of Guizhou Province [grant number LH (2015) 7277], the Youth Science and Technology Talent Project of Guizhou Province [grant number (2017) 5618], and the Open Project of the Key Laboratory of Miao Medicine of Guizhou Province [grant number K (2017) 004].

Conflicts of Interest: We wish to confirm that there are no known conflicts of interest associated with this publication and that there has been no significant financial support for this work that could have influenced its outcome.

References

1. Editorial Committee of Flora of China. *Flora Reipublicae Popularis Sinicae*; Science Press: Beijing, China, 2004; Volume 45, pp. 41–56.
2. Editorial Committee of Zhong Hua Ben Cao. *Zhong Hua Ben Cao*; Shanghai Scientific and Technological Press: Shanghai, China, 1999; Volume 13, pp. 224–227.
3. Zhang, Y.Y.; Li, T.Y.; Tang, F.; Yang, L.N. Parmacodynamics study in Li medicine plants *Sarcococca vagans* Stapf. *Chin. J. Ethnomed. Ethnopharm.* **2016**, *26*, 46–48.
4. Li, H.C.; Yang, J.; Yuan, D.P.; Liu, Y. Advances in studies on chemical constituents in plants of *Sarcococca hookeriana* and their biological activities. *Lishizhen Med. Mater. Med. Res.* **2016**, *27*, 1711–1713.
5. Ullah Jan, N.; Ali, A.; Ahmad, B.; Iqbal, N.; Adhikari, A.; Inayat Ur, R.; Musharraf, S.G. Evaluation of antidiabetic potential of steroidal alkaloid of *Sarcococca saligna*. *Biomed. Pharmacoth.* **2018**, *100*, 461–466.
6. Zhang, P.; Shao, L.; Shi, Z.; Zhang, Y.; Du, J.; Cheng, K.; Yu, P. Pregnane alkaloids from *Sarcococca ruscifolia* and their cytotoxic activity. *Phytochem. Lett.* **2015**, *14*, 31–34. [CrossRef]
7. Adhikari, A.; Vohra, M.I.; Jabeen, A.; Dastagir, N.; Choudhary, M.I. Antiinflammatory steroidal alkaloids from *Sarcococca wallichii* of Nepalese origin. *Nat. Prod. Commun.* **2015**, *10*, 1533–1536.
8. Zhang, P.Z.; Wang, F.; Yang, L.J.; Zhang, G.L. Pregnane alkaloids from *Sarcococca hookeriana* var. digyna. *Fitoterapia* **2013**, *89*, 143–148. [PubMed]
9. Yan, Y.X.; Sun, Y.; Chen, J.C.; Wang, Y.Y.; Li, Y.; Qiu, M.H. Cytotoxic steroids from *Sarcococca saligna*. *Planta Med.* **2011**, *77*, 1725–1729. [CrossRef] [PubMed]
10. Devkota, K.P.; Wansi, J.D.; Lenta, B.N.; Khan, S.; Choudhary, M.I.; Sewald, N. Bioactive steroidal alkaloids from *Sarcococca hookeriana*. *Planta Med.* **2010**, *76*, 1022–1025. [CrossRef] [PubMed]
11. Choudhary, M.I.; Adhikari, A.; Samreen; Atta Ur, R. Antileishmanial steroidal alkaloids from roots of *Sarcococca coriacea*. *J. Chem. Soc. Pakistan* **2010**, *32*, 799–802.
12. Devkota, K.P.; Lento, B.N.; Wansi, J.D.; Choudhary, M.I.; Sewald, N. Cholinesterase inhibiting, antileishmanial and antiplasmodial steroidal alkaloids from *Sarcococca hookeriana* of Nepalese origin. *Planta Med.* **2008**, *74*, 979. [CrossRef]
13. Devkota, K.P.; Lenta, B.N.; Wansi, J.D.; Choudhary, M.I.; Kisangau, D.P.; Naz, Q.; Sewald, N. Bioactive 5 alpha-pregnane-type steroidal alkaloids from *Sarcococca hookeriana*. *J. Nat. Prod.* **2008**, *71*, 1481–1484. [CrossRef] [PubMed]
14. Devkota, K.P.; Lenta, B.N.; Choudhary, M.I.; Naz, Q.; Fekam, F.B.; Rosenthal, P.J.; Sewald, N. Cholinesterase inhibiting and antiplasmodial steroidal alkaloids from *Sarcococca hookeriana*. *Chem. Pharm. Bull.* **2007**, *55*, 1397–1401. [CrossRef] [PubMed]

15. Devkota, K.P.; Choudhary, M.I.; Ranjit, R.; Samreen; Sewald, N. Structure activity relationship studies on antileishmanial steroidal alkaloids from *Sarcococca hookeriana*. *Nat. Prod. Res.* **2007**, *21*, 292–297. [CrossRef] [PubMed]
16. He, K.; Du, J. Two new steroidal alkaloids from the roots of *Sarcococca ruscifolia*. *J. Asian Nat. Prod. Res.* **2010**, *12*, 233–238. [CrossRef] [PubMed]
17. Qiu, M.H.; Nie, R.L.; Li, Z.R. Chemical structure and activity screening of pachysandra alkaloids. *Acta Bot. Yunnanica* **1994**, *16*, 296–300.
18. Yu, S.S.; Zou, Z.M.; Zen, J.; Yu, D.Q.; Cong, P.Z. Four new steroidal alkaloids from the roots of *Sarcococca vagans*. *Chin. Chem. Lett.* **1997**, *8*, 511–514.
19. Qiu, M.H.; Nie, R.L.; Li, Z.R.; Zhou, J. Three new steroidal alkaloids from *Pachysandra axillaris*. *Acta Bot. Sin.* **1990**, *32*, 626–630.
20. Naeem, I.; Khan, N.; Choudhary, M.I.; Rahman, A. Alkaloids of *Sarcococca saligna*. *Phytochemistry* **1996**, *43*, 903–906. [CrossRef]
21. Qiu, M.H.; Wang, D.Z.; Nie, R.L. Study on ^{13}C NMR of pachysandra alkaloids. *Chin. J. Magn. Reson.* **1995**, *12*, 155–165.
22. Mosmann, T. Rapid colorimetric assay for cellular growth and survival: Application to proliferation and cytotoxicity assays. *J. Immunol. Methods* **1983**, *65*, 55–63. [CrossRef]
23. Reed, L.J.; Muench, H. A simple method of estimating fifty percent endpoint. *Am. J. Hyg.* **1938**, *27*, 493–497.

Sample Availability: Samples of the compounds **1–7** are available from the authors.

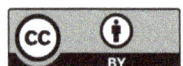

© 2018 by the authors. Licensee MDPI, Basel, Switzerland. This article is an open access article distributed under the terms and conditions of the Creative Commons Attribution (CC BY) license (http://creativecommons.org/licenses/by/4.0/).

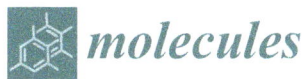

Article

Cholinesterase Inhibition Activity, Alkaloid Profiling and Molecular Docking of Chilean *Rhodophiala* (Amaryllidaceae)

Luciana R. Tallini [1], Jaume Bastida [1], Natalie Cortes [2], Edison H. Osorio [3], Cristina Theoduloz [4] and Guillermo Schmeda-Hirschmann [5,6,*]

1. Grup de Productes Naturals, Departament de Biologia, Sanitat i Medi Ambient, Facultat de Farmàcia, Universitat de Barcelona, 08028 Barcelona, Spain; lucianatallini@gmail.com (L.R.T.); jaumebastida@ub.edu (J.B.)
2. Grupo de Investigación en Sustancias Bioactivas, Facultad de Ciencias Farmacéuticas y Alimentarias, Universidad de Antioquia UdeA, Calle 70 No, 52-21, Medellín 050010, Colombia; natalie.cortes@udea.edu.co
3. Departamento de Ciencias Básicas, Universidad Católica Luis Amigó, SISCO, Transversal 51A No. 67B-90, Medellín 050034, Colombia; edison.osorio@gmail.com
4. Laboratorio de Cultivo Celular, Facultad de Ciencias de la Salud, Universidad de Talca, Talca 3460000, Chile; ctheodul@utalca.cl
5. Laboratorio de Química de Productos Naturales, Instituto de Química de Recursos Naturales, Universidad de Talca, Talca 3460000, Chile
6. Programa de Investigación de Excelencia Interdisciplinaria en Química y Bio-orgánica de Recursos Naturales (PIEI-QUIM-BIO), Universidad de Talca, Talca 3460000, Chile
* Correspondence: schmeda@utalca.cl; Tel.: +56-975-211-106

Academic Editor: John C. D'Auria
Received: 5 June 2018; Accepted: 19 June 2018; Published: 26 June 2018

Abstract: Amaryllidaceae plants are the commercial source of galanthamine, an alkaloid approved for the clinical treatment of Alzheimer's disease. The chemistry and bioactivity of Chilean representatives of *Rhodophiala* genus from the family of Amaryllidaceae have not been widely studied so far. Ten collections of five different Chilean *Rhodophiala* were analyzed in vitro for activity against enzymes such as acetylcholinesterase (AChE) and butyrylcholinesterase (BuChE) as well as for their alkaloid composition by GC-MS. To obtain an insight into the potential AChE and BuChE inhibitory activity of the alkaloids identified in the most active samples, docking experiments were carried out. Although galanthamine was found neither in aerial parts nor in bulbs of *R. splendens*, these plant materials were the most active inhibitors of AChE (IC_{50}: 5.78 and 3.62 µg/mL, respectively) and BuChE (IC_{50}: 16.26 and 14.37 µg/mL, respectively). Some 37 known alkaloids and 40 still unidentified compounds were detected in the samples, suggesting high potential in the Chilean Amaryllidaceae plants as sources of both novel bioactive agents and new alkaloids.

Keywords: *Rhodophiala*; alkaloids; molecular docking; AChE; BuChE; GC-MS

1. Introduction

The vast structural and chemical diversity of natural products gives them a significant role in drug discovery [1]. Alkaloids are of particular interest in biomedicine and drug discovery research [2] due to their structural diversity and specific biological potential [3]. The Amaryllidaceae is a plant family that contains an exclusive, large and still expanding alkaloid group known as the Amaryllidaceae alkaloids, which are characterized by unique skeleton arrangements and a broad spectrum of biological activities [4,5]. Amaryllidaceae plants have been used in folk medicine for their therapeutic and toxic properties [6]. Hippocrates of Kos (460–370 BP), considered the father of modern medicine, recommended the oil of *Narcissus* (Amaryllidaceae) species for the treatment of symptoms that today would be recognized as cancer [7].

The Amaryllidaceae alkaloids are classified mainly into nine skeleton types: norbelladine, lycorine, homolycorine, crinine, haemanthamine, narciclasine, tazettine, montanine and galanthamine (Figure 1) [4]. The most important Amaryllidaceae alkaloid is galanthamine, which was isolated for the first time from *Galanthus woronowii* in the 1950s and was approved for the clinical treatment of mild to moderate Alzheimer's disease (AD) by the Food and Drug Administration (FDA) at the beginning of this century [8,9]. Alzheimer's disease (AD), characterized by severe and progressive memory loss, is the most common form of dementia and is becoming increasingly prevalent in people older than 65 years [10,11]. It is estimated that 47 million people live with dementia in the world today, with an economic impact estimated at 818 billion dollars [12]. Known factors involved in the development of AD include a reduced cholinergic neurotransmission level, oxidative stress, amyloid-β-peptide (Aβ) and tau protein aggregation [13].

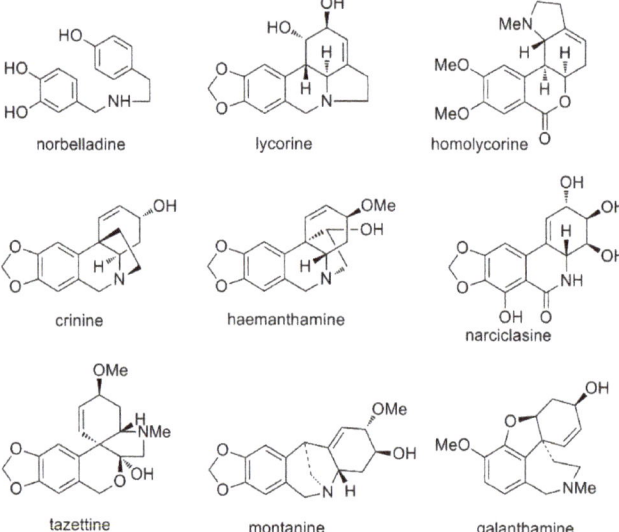

Figure 1. Amaryllidaceae alkaloid types.

Acetylcholinesterase (AChE) and butyrylcholinesterase (BuChE) are involved in the hydrolysis of the neurotransmitter acetylcholine (ACh) [14]. Acetylcholinesterase is highly selective for ACh hydrolysis, and BuChE can metabolize different substrates [15]. In the brain of AD patients, AChE activity tends to decrease while that of BuChE increases [16]. Consequently, cholinesterase inhibitors that suppress both AChE and BuChE may provide a better therapeutic response rather than AChE-selective agents [17].

Little is known on the chemistry and bioactivity of the South American endemic Amaryllidaceae genus *Rhodophiala*. The *Rhodophiala* species have high ornamental potential due to its attractive red, yellow, white or orange flowers [18–22]. The approximately 40 species described at present occur in Argentina, Bolivia, southern Brazil, Chile and Uruguay [22]. *Rhodophiala* plants have a tunicate bulb of 4–6 cm diameter, which is set 20–30 cm underground, a single umbel holding up to six flowers, each flower being 4–6 cm wide and a flower stem 35 to 50 cm long [18].

Rhodophiala species are well known ornamental plants. Propagation of the Chilean species was reported [19] as well as phylogenetic [20] and morphological studies [21,22]. The renewed interest on galanthamine sources including the search for additional alkaloids with inhibitory activity towards the enzymes AChE and BuChE has prompted research work on the South American species of this family. Brazilian [23] and Argentinean wild Amaryllidaceae [24] showed high structural diversity in the alkaloid patterns and encouraged work on the Chilean species of this family. The knowledge of the chemical composition and anti-cholinesterase activity of the Chilean species belonging to genus *Rhodophiala* is limited. The comparative studies of their chemical composition are needed to identify the best potential sources of bioactive alkaloids in the South American species.

The aim of this work was to disclose the potential of Chilean *Rhodophiala* species as inhibitors of the enzymes AChE and BuChE as well as to analyze the alkaloid content and composition of native species by gas chromatography coupled to mass spectrometry (GC-MS) looking for galanthamine sources and searching for other compounds with effect of AChE and BuChE. Molecular docking studies were also carried out to investigate the affinity of the alkaloids identified in the most promising sample at the active sites of AChE and BuChE.

2. Results and Discussion

Twenty alkaloid extracts from five different Chilean *Rhodophiala* species (Figures 2 and 3) were assessed for inhibitory activity towards the enzymes AChE and BuChE. The alkaloid composition of the extracts was analyzed by GC-MS and the single alkaloid content was quantified and reported as mg GAL/g alkaloid extract (AE). The extracts have been obtained as described in Section 2.2. Briefly, the (fresh) plant material was lyophilized to obtain the dry tissues content (values included in the Table) of the different plant parts investigated. The extraction yields are calculated and reported from the lyophilized plant material.

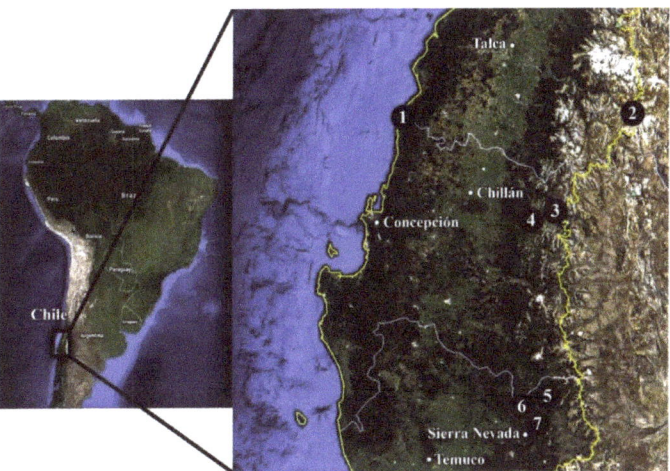

Figure 2. Map of Chile showing the collection sites of the *Rhodophiala* species. 1: Arcos de Calán; 2: Laguna del Maule; 3: Nevado de Chillán; 4: Las Trancas; 5: Volcán Lonquimay; 6: Malalcahuello; 7: Sierra Nevada. Map source: Google Earth.

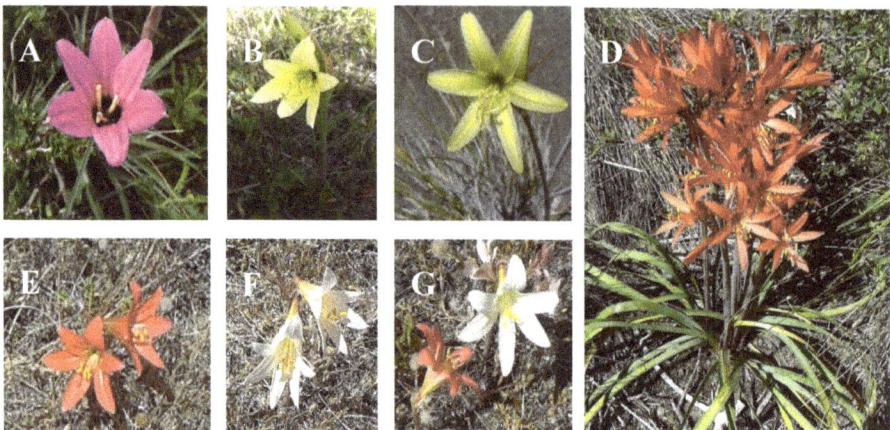

Figure 3. Flowering *Rhodophiala* species from central-southern Chile. (**A**) *R. andicola* (Poepp.) Traub; (**B**) *R. araucana* (Phil.) Traub; (**C**) *R. montana* (Phil.) Traub; (**D**) *R. splendens* (Renjifo) Traub; (**E**) *R. pratensis* (Poepp.) Traub.; (**F**) *R. pratensis* white flowers and (**G**) *R. pratensis* plants with red and white flowers.

2.1. AChE and BuChE Inhibitory Activities

The crude alkaloid samples from the different Chilean *Rhodophiala* were tested in vitro for AChE and BuChE-inhibitory activity. The percent dry weight of the samples, w/w extraction yields, and cholinesterase inhibition are summarized in Table 1. Galanthamine was used as a control and presented AChE and BuChE inhibition with IC_{50} values of 0.48 ± 0.07 and 3.70 ± 0.24 µg/mL, respectively. All the alkaloid extracts tested were active against AChE. The highest AChE inhibitory potential was found in bulbs of *R. pratensis* (sample Q) followed by *R. splendens* (sample S) with IC_{50} values of 3.32 ± 0.26 and 3.62 ± 0.02 µg/mL, respectively. Lowest activity was measured for the aerial part of *R. pratensis* (sample N) (IC_{50} value: 102.27 ± 6.61 µg/mL). Nearly 50% of the samples showed some activity against BuChE, with better effect for the bulbs of *R. splendens* (sample S) (IC_{50} 14.37 ± 1.94 µg/mL).

The bulb (I) and leaf (J) extracts of *R. montana* presented moderate activity against both enzymes with better effect of (I) against AChE and (J) towards BuChE. The differences in the chemical profiles of I and J could explain these results. However, the high number of unknown alkaloids in the extracts precludes further discussion. The bulb (Q) and leaf (R) extracts of white flowering *R. pratensis* were active towards AChE, with IC_{50} of 3.32 and 8.39 µg/mL, respectively but with mild to low effect against BuChE (Table 1), reducing the pharmacological interest of this species. The high AChE and BuChE inhibitory activity of *R. splendens* bulb (S) and aerial parts/leaves (T) renders this plant as the most promising species in the search for active molecules for AD therapy (Table 1).

Table 1. Percent dry weight, w/w extraction yields from dry starting material, percent alkaloid extract (from the crude extract), acetyl-(AChE) and butyryl- (BuChE) cholinesterase inhibitory activity of alkaloid-enriched extracts from Chilean *Rhodophiala*.

Scientific Names, Abbreviated Collection Place and Reference Letter	% Dry Weight [a]	w/w Extraction Yield [b]	% Alkaloid Extract [c]	AChE IC_{50} (µg/mL) [d]	BuChE IC_{50} (µg/mL) [d]
Aerial parts					
R. andicola, SN (B)	15.46	30.63	3.16	18.16 ± 2.94	138.27 ± 6.83
R. andicola, NC (D)	18.70	22.10	2.86	12.30 ± 0.74	43.41 ± 2.64
R. andicola, VL (F)	20.00	17.50	2.07	74.44 ± 5.53	>200
R. araucana, M, (H)	17.70	25.30	3.78	*e	*e
R. montana, LM (J)	21.40	9.40	1.14	33.57 ± 2.16	16.38 ± 0.78
R. pratensis, AC, RF, nl, sand dunes (L)	14.84	27.08	1.93	72.59 ± 4.26	>200
R. pratensis, AC, RF, L (N)	14.53	10.10	3.72	102.27 ± 6.61	>200
R. pratensis, AC, RF, nl (P)	11.68	32.39	2.87	31.97 ± 3.24	>200
R. pratensis, AC, WF (R)	10.67	16.47	1.15	8.39 ± 0.27	>200
R. splendens, LT, (T)	14.81	44.26	1.53	5.78 ± 0.93	16.26 ± 3.34
Bulbs					
R. andicola, SN (A)	25.41	7.53	2.15	13.29 ± 1.01	45.76 ± 9.72
R. andicola, NC (C)	28.90	6.00	2.23	7.26 ± 0.16	47.38 ± 4.08
R. andicola, VL (E)	23.50	7.40	2.37	22.77 ± 1.57	113.24 ± 2.77
R. araucana, M, (G)	19.80	7.90	2.73	6.23 ± 0.24	45.71 ± 3.51
R. montana, LM, (I)	28.00	3.26	1.50	18.13 ± 0.51	40.05 ± 9.03
R. pratensis, AC, RF, nl, sand dunes (K)	18.87	19.73	1.50	11.81 ± 0.17	>200
R. pratensis, AC, RF, L (M)	20.98	11.73	2.84	44.23 ± 4.08	>200
R. pratensis, AC, RF, nl (O)	18.76	7.36	2.33	47.66 ± 1.78	>200
R. pratensis, AC, WF (Q)	19.64	4.84	2.29	3.32 ± 0.26	52.16 ± 0.57
R. splendens, LT, (S)	21.35	35.05	1.60	3.62 ± 0.02	14.37 ± 1.94

[a] after lyophilization; [b] from lyophilized material; [c] from the crude extract; [d] all IC_{50} were calculated using $R^2 \geq 0.99$; [e] insufficient sample; WF: white flowers; RF: red flowers; L: with leaves; nl: no leaves; Collection place: AC: Arcos de Calán, Región del Maule; LM: Laguna del Maule; LT: Las Trancas; M: Malalcahuello, Región de la Araucanía; NC: Nevado de Chillán; SN: Sierra Nevada; VL: volcan Lonquimay.

2.2. Alkaloid Identification by GC-MS

The activity of the Chilean *Rhodophiala* towards acetylcholinesterase is a consequence of the chemical composition of the extracts. Therefore, the alkaloid composition is a key point to understand the chemical diversity of these plants as a source of potential therapies for AD. The alkaloids occurring in the different extracts were identified by comparing their GC-MS spectra and Kovats Retention Index (RI) values with those of authentic samples. Thirty-seven known alkaloids were identified in these samples (Figure 4). About 50% of them belong to three different alkaloid types, namely: lycorine, haemanthamine and crinine. The others belong to six different alkaloid types: tazettine, homolycorine, galanthamine, montanine, mesembrenone and narciclasine. Two unusual alkaloids known as ismine and galanthindole were also found. The occurrence and quantification of the alkaloids in the samples is summarized in Table 2: (**A**) (aerial parts) and (**B**) (bulbs). The number of alkaloids detected varied among extracts, ranging from 8 in the aerial parts of *R. andicola* collected in Sierra Nevada (B) to 23 in the bulb of *R. pratensis* (K). Forty structures found in these samples could not be identified, suggesting high potential of Chilean *Rhodophiala* species in the search for new alkaloids. The number of unidentified compounds ranged from 3 in aerial parts of *R. andicola* (A, B and D), *R. pratensis* (P) and *R. splendens* (T) to 12 in aerial parts of *R. montana* (J). Representative chromatograms of the samples are shown in Figures 5–9.

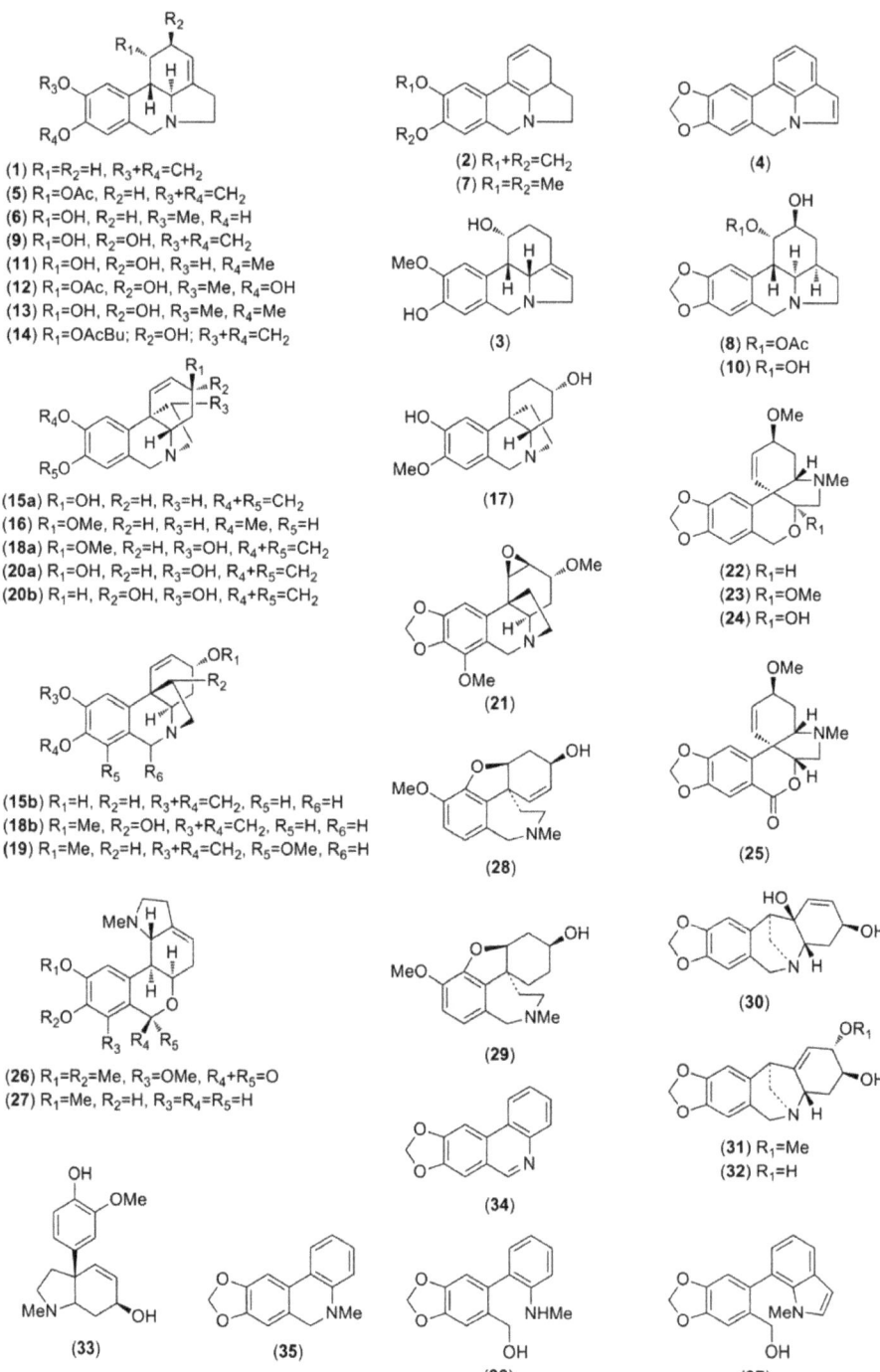

Figure 4. Alkaloids identified in Chilean *Rhodophiala* species by GC-MS.

Table 2. (**A**) Identification of alkaloids occurring in the aerial parts of Chilean *Rhodophiala* species by GC-MS. Values are expressed as mg GAL/g AE; (**B**) Identification of alkaloids occurring in the bulbs of Chilean *Rhodophiala* species by GC-MS. Values are expressed as mg GAL/g AE.

(A)

Alkaloid	M+	BP	RI	B	D	F	H	J	L	N	P	R	T
Lycorine-type													
lycorene (1)	255	254	2346.8	8.6	7.5	25.1	46.0	46.9	35.5	37.3	35.4	60.8	13.1
anhydrolycorine (2)	251	250	2543.1	-	-	-	-	9.4	5.1	7.2	T	-	-
kirkine (3)	253	252	2588.2	-	T	5.9	11.2	9.6	9.9	8.3	11.8	13.2	-
11,12-dehydroanhydrolycorine (4)	249	248	2646.4	8.6	-	-	-	7.2	5.3	-	6.0	7.2	-
1-O-acetylcaranine (5)	313	226	2653.1	-	7.5	13.5	8.4	15.6	8.1	21.8	7.5	9.4	7.8
norpluviine (6)	273	228	2683.6	-	-	-	-	-	-	-	-	-	-
assoanine (7)	267	266	2708.9	-	T	-	-	-	-	-	-	6.2	-
3,4-dihydro 1-acetyllycorine (8)	331	330	2723.3	-	-	-	-	-	-	-	-	-	-
lycorine (9)	287	226	2791.7	-	T	5.7	14.7	5.1	7.1	-	10.1	24.8	5.3
dihydrolycorine (10)	289	288	2833.9	-	-	-	-	-	-	-	T	T	-
pseudolycorine (11)	289	228	2856.4	-	-	-	-	-	-	-	-	-	-
sternbergine (12)	331	228	2838.8	-	-	-	6.4	-	-	-	T	-	-
methylpseudolycorine (13)	303	242	2911.2	-	-	-	-	-	-	-	-	-	-
1-O-(3′acetoxybutanoyl)lycorine (14)	415	226	3248.8	-	-	-	5.3	-	-	-	-	-	-
Haemanthamine/crinine type													
vittatine (15a)/crinine (15b)	271	271	2512.4	-	11.6	53.1	34.4	14.8	17.2	21.4	38.7	35.7	48.0
8-O-demethylmaritidine (16)	273	273	2540.0	-	T	7.7	-	-	-	-	6.2	5.6	-
deacetylcantabricine (17)	275	275	2573.1	-	-	-	-	-	-	-	T	-	6.4
haemanthamine (18a)/crinamine (18b)	301	272	2673.4	-	11.6	45.4	34.4	7.7	17.2	21.4	32.5	30.1	25.0
buphanidrine (19)	315	315	2748.3	-	-	-	-	-	-	-	-	-	-
11-hydroxyvittatine (20a)/hamayne (20b)	287	258	2750.5	-	-	-	-	-	-	-	-	-	16.6
undulatine (21)	331	331	2892.5	-	-	-	-	7.1	-	-	-	-	-
Tazettine-type													
deoxytazettine (22)	315	231	2575.6	60.7	59.1	95.8	22.3	-	11.2	16.3	16.0	29.9	55.6
O-methyltazettine (23)	345	261	2641.1	6.1	5.5	6.7	5.0	-	T	5.2	-	5.2	-
tazettine (24)	331	247	2685.1	54.6	36.0	66.2	10.3	-	11.2	11.1	10.1	14.9	30.7
epimacronine (25)	329	245	2848.0	-	12.5	17.0	7.0	-	-	-	5.9	9.8	24.9
					5.1	5.9	T	-	T	-	-	T	T

Table 2. Cont.

Alkaloid	M+	BP	RI	(A)									
				B	D	F	H	J	L	N	P	R	T
Homolycorine-type													
nerinine (26)	347	109	2513.5	-	-	9.1	-	-	8.6	22.4	6.5	19.5	-
8-O-demethylhomolycorine (27)	301	109	2856.4	-	-	-	-	-	8.6	22.4	6.5	19.5	-
Galanthamine-type													
galanthamine (28)	287	286	2519.9	-	5.1	14.1	7.1	5.8	-	-	-	-	-
lycoramine (29)	289	288	2544.6	-	-	8.6	7.1	5.8	-	-	-	-	-
					5.1	5.5	-						
Montanine-type													
pancratinine C (30)	287	176	2623.5	-	-	-	-	8.1	28.3	19.7	15.2	26.7	-
montanine (31)	301	301	2663.1	-	-	-	-	-	-	-	-	-	-
pancracine (32)	287	287	2737.4	-	-	-	-	8.1	28.3	19.7	15.2	26.7	-
Mesembrenone-type													
demethylmesembrenol (33)	275	205	2343.2	-	-	-	-	-	T	-	T	T	-
Narciclasine-type													
trisphaeridine (34)	223	223	2322.9	12.7	11.2	13.5	5.8	6.2	5.5	44.5	-	10.4	32.2
dihydrobicolorine (35)	239	238	2366.1	12.7	5.1	6.0	5.8	6.2	5.5	39.4	T	5.2	22.7
				T	6.1	7.5	T	-	T	5.1	T	5.2	9.5
Other-type													
ismine (36)	257	238	2304.6	5.2	32.9	62.1	8.5	-	5.9	-	5.7	17.7	34.5
galanthindole (37)	281	281	2534.8	-	7.6	17.0	T	-	T	-	T	6.0	14.3
				5.2	25.3	45.1	8.5	-	5.9	-	5.7	11.7	20.2
Not identified				46.0	26.8	46.1	42.0	126.9	35.9	78.5	20.6	73.4	21.8
unknown (ismine-derivate) *	227	226	2232.2	-	-	-	-	-	-	8.8	-	-	-
unknown (ismine-derivate) *	227	225	2232.2	-	5.6	6.8	5.6	-	-	8.9	-	-	6.2
unknown	269	238	2258.9	-	5.1	6.9	-	-	-	-	-	-	6.4
unknown (mesembrenone-type) *	245	175	2280.8	-	-	-	-	-	6.0	-	-	10.5	-
unknown	269	268	2285.5	-	-	-	-	-	-	9.7	-	-	-
unknown	253	252	2313.1	5.9	T	-	-	5.9	-	13.7	T	-	-
unknown	251	251	2335.2	-	-	-	-	6.2	-	9.9	-	-	-

Table 2. Cont.

(A)

Alkaloid	M+	BP	RI	B	D	F	H	J	L	N	P	R	T
unknown (lycorine-type) *	257	256	2379.0	-	-	-	-	-	-	-	-	-	-
unknown	253	252	2405.0	-	-	-	-	8.9	6.2	10.3	-	5.5	-
unknown (lycorine-type) *	269	211	2480.5	-	-	-	T	28.1	-	6.1	T	7.1	-
unknown	271	238	2492.7	-	-	-	-	-	-	-	-	-	-
unknown (homolycorine-type) *	331	109	2557.5	-	-	-	-	-	5.3	5.7	7.0	33.0	-
unknown (crinine/haemanthamine-type) *	329	329	2564.1	-	-	-	-	-	5.3	-	T	7.3	-
unknown	257	225	2579.2	-	-	-	-	-	-	5.4	-	-	-
unknown	299	238	2584.0	-	-	-	T	-	-	-	-	-	-
unknown (crinine/haemanthamine-type) *	315	254	2616.4	-	-	-	-	17.5	6.0	-	5.7	-	-
unknown (tazettine-type) *	315	231	2616.9	-	-	-	-	-	-	-	-	-	-
unknown (lycorine-type) *	329	268	2646.1	-	-	-	-	5.1	-	-	-	-	-
unknown	297	297	2655.7	-	-	-	-	5.4	-	-	-	-	-
unknown (tazettine-type) *	345	261	2662.6	17.9	16.1	24.6	5.6	-	-	-	-	-	9.2
unknown (crinine/haemanthamine-type) *	345	272	2671.8	22.2	-	-	-	-	-	-	-	-	-
unknown (crinine/haemanthamine-type) *	283	283	2692.5	-	-	-	-	6.9	-	-	-	-	-
unknown	303	302	2703.2	-	-	-	-	-	7.1	-	-	-	-
unknown (crinine/haemanthamine-type) *	315	315	2724.2	-	-	-	-	16.8	-	-	-	-	-
unknown (lycorine-type) *	253	252	2735.3	-	-	-	-	-	-	-	-	-	-
unknown (homolycorine-type) *	345	109	2735.6	-	-	-	-	5.9	-	-	-	-	-
unknown (crinine/haemanthamine-type) *	347	331	2795.5	-	-	-	-	6.5	-	-	-	-	-
unknown (crinine/haemanthamine-type) *	345	331	2795.7	-	-	-	5.6	-	-	-	-	-	-
unknown (crinine/haemanthamine-type) *	347	331	2795.8	-	-	-	-	-	-	-	-	-	-
unknown (lycorine-type) *	251	250	2846.6	-	-	7.8	-	-	-	-	-	-	-
unknown	335	335	2860.6	-	-	-	-	-	-	-	-	-	-
unknown (lycorine-type) *	345	242	2868.8	-	-	-	5.3	-	-	-	-	-	-
unknown	373	372	2881.9	-	-	-	-	-	-	-	-	-	-
unknown (lycorine-type) *	357	356	2942.1	-	-	-	-	-	-	-	7.9	10.0	-
unknown (lycorine-type) *	279	278	3016.0	-	-	-	-	13.7	-	-	-	-	-
unknown (galanthamine-type) *	375	330	3027.5	-	-	-	-	-	-	-	-	-	-

Table 2. Cont.

(A)

Alkaloid	M⁺	BP	RI	A	B	C	D	E	F	G	H	I	J	K	L	M	N	O	P	Q	R	S	T
unknown (lycorine-type) *	267	266	3032.9	-	-	-	-	-	-	-	-	-	-	-	-	-	-	-	-	-	-	-	-
unknown (lycorine-type) *	375	374	3049.2	-	-	-	-	-	-	-	-	-	-	-	-	-	-	-	-	-	-	-	-
unknown (lycorine-type) *	355	226	3066.6	-	-	-	-	-	-	-	-	6.1	-	-	-	-	-	-	-	-	-	-	-
unknown (lycorine-type) *	373	226	3161.0	-	-	-	-	-	-	-	-	13.8	-	-	-	-	-	-	-	-	-	-	-
Total					133.2		154.2		311.1		166.1		208.7		148.1		240.1		138.1		274.1		205.3

(B)

Alkaloid	M⁺	BP	RI	A	B	C	D	E	F	G	H	I	J	K	L	M	N	O	P	Q	R	S	T
Lycorine-type																							
lycorene (1)	255	254	2346.8	44.1	-	58.2	-	43.2	-	79.0	-	78.6	7.6	-	42.6	-	26.1	T	33.8	-	41.2	-	38.5
anhydrolycorine (2)	251	250	2543.1	-	18.1	-	15.4	-	25.0	-	27.3	24.6	T	9.4	-	T	10.1	-	13.3	14.9	-	7.7	-
kirkine (3)	253	252	2588.2	-	5.0	-	6.0	-	-	-	5.1	T	-	6.1	-	-	-	-	-	-	-	T	-
11,12-dehydroanhydrolycorine (4)	249	248	2646.4	-	11.0	-	8.6	-	8.1	-	8.5	19.0	-	6.6	-	-	6.4	-	7.3	6.6	-	8.5	-
1-O-acetylcaranine (5)	313	248	2653.1	-	-	-	-	-	-	-	-	17.4	-	-	-	-	-	-	-	-	-	-	-
norpluviine (6)	273	228	2683.6	-	-	-	-	-	-	-	-	-	-	-	-	-	-	-	-	-	-	-	-
assoanine (7)	267	266	2708.9	-	-	-	-	-	-	-	T	-	-	-	-	-	-	-	-	-	-	-	T
3,4-dihydro 1-acetyllycorine (8)	331	330	2723.3	-	-	-	-	-	-	-	-	-	-	-	-	-	-	-	-	-	-	-	-
lycorine (9)	287	226	2791.7	-	10.0	-	21.8	-	10.1	-	27.5	10.0	-	15.4	-	T	T	-	7.4	19.7	T	-	16.3
dihydrolycorine (10)	289	288	2833.9	-	-	-	-	-	-	-	-	-	-	T	-	-	9.6	-	T	T	-	-	T
pseudolycorine (11)	289	228	2856.4	-	-	-	6.4	-	-	-	10.6	-	-	5.1	-	-	-	-	-	-	-	6.0	-
sternbergine (12)	331	228	2838.8	-	-	-	-	-	-	-	-	-	-	-	-	-	-	5.8	-	-	-	-	-
methylpseudolycorine (13)	303	242	2911.2	-	-	-	-	-	-	-	T	-	-	-	-	-	-	-	-	-	-	-	-
1-O-(3′acetoxybutanoyl)lycorine (14)	415	226	3248.8	-	-	-	-	-	-	-	-	-	-	-	-	-	-	-	-	-	-	-	-
Haemanthamine/crinine type																							
vittatine (15a)/crinine (15b)	271	271	2512.4	60.0	-	49.5	10.8	31.7	-	43.7	7.1	17.4	T	28.6	5.6	-	33.8	6.2	45.5	7.3	44.9	7.3	36.9	6.3
8-O-demethylmaritidine (16)	273	273	2540.0	-	-	-	T	-	-	-	-	-	-	-	-	-	-	-	-	-	-	-	6.0
deacetylcantabricine (17)	275	275	2573.1	-	-	-	-	-	-	-	-	-	-	-	-	-	-	-	-	-	-	-	-

Table 2. Cont.

(B)

Alkaloid	M+	BP	RI	A	C	E	G	I	K	M	O	Q	S
haemanthamine (18a)/crinamine (18b)	301	272	2673.4	60.0	31.7	31.7	36.6	5.8	23.0	27.6	38.2	31.0	16.4
buphanidrine (19)	315	315	2748.3	-	-	-	-	5.9	-	-	-	-	-
11-hydroxyvittatine (20a)/hamayne (20b)	287	258	2750.5	-	7.00	-	T	-	-	-	-	6.6	8.2
undulatine (21)	331	331	2892.5	-	-	-	-	5.7	-	-	-	-	-
Tazettine-type													
deoxytazettine (22)	315	231	2575.6	**74.8**	**56.1**	**85.9**	**33.1**	-	**21.8**	**18.0**	**8.9**	**17.9**	**21.9**
O-methyltazettine (23)	345	261	2641.1	8.3	10.7	13.1	9.6	-	-	-	-	-	T
tazettine (24)	331	247	2685.1	58.7	23.0	61.7	14.8	-	10.9	12.7	8.9	9.9	14.3
epimacronine (25)	329	245	2848.0	7.8	22.4	11.1	8.7	-	10.9	5.3	T	8.0	7.6
				-	T	T	T	-	-	-	-	-	-
Homolycorine-type													
nerinine (26)	347	109	2513.5	**9.4**	-	**10.6**	-	-	**13.9**	**14.1**	**10.1**	**28.5**	**9.8**
8-O-demethylhomolycorine (27)	301	109	2856.4	9.4	-	10.6	-	-	13.9	14.1	10.1	21.1	-
				-	-	-	-	-	-	-	-	7.4	9.8
Galanthamine-type													
galanthamine (28)	287	286	2519.9	-	**19.0**	**11.9**	**12.3**	T	-	-	-	-	-
lycoramine (29)	289	288	2544.6	-	5.1	6.8	5.4	-	-	-	-	-	-
				-	13.9	5.1	6.9	-	-	-	-	-	-
Montanine-type													
pancratinine C (30)	287	176	2623.5	-	-	-	**5.2**	**7.8**	**41.7**	**23.1**	**12.5**	**24.7**	**6.4**
montanine (31)	301	301	2663.1	-	-	-	-	T	5.3	T	-	-	-
pancracine (32)	287	287	2737.4	-	-	-	5.2	7.8	29.8	23.1	12.5	24.7	-
				-	-	-	-	-	6.6	-	-	-	6.4
Mesembrenone-type													
demethylmesembrenol (33)	275	205	2343.2	-	-	-	-	-	**7.2**	**5.2**	-	**5.1**	-
				-	-	-	-	-	7.2	5.2	T	5.1	-
Narciclasine-type													
trisphaeridine (34)	223	223	2322.9	**12.9**	**12.7**	**13.3**	**5.8**	**5.7**	-	-	-	-	**5.1**
dihydrobicolorine (35)	239	238	2366.1	5.5	6.3	5.3	T	5.7	T	T	T	T	5.1
				7.4	6.4	8.0	5.8	T	T	T	T	T	T
Other-type													
ismine (36)	257	238	2304.6	**19.2**	**35.6**	**28.2**	**21.8**	-	**7.9**	**7.8**	**5.3**	**8.0**	**7.3**
				6.6	9.9	9.5	6.6	-	T	T	T	T	T

Table 2. Cont.

(B)

Alkaloid	M⁺	BP	RI	A	C	E	G	I	K	M	O	Q	S
galanthindole (37)	281	281	2534.8	12.6	25.7	18.7	15.2	-	7.9	7.8	5.3	8.0	7.3
Not identified				29.9	41.4	41.2	79.8	76.8	92.6	50.5	32.0	76.0	36.0
unknown (ismine-derivate) *	227	226	2232.2	-	-	-	-	-	-	-	-	-	-
unknown (ismine-derivate) *	227	225	2232.2	-	T	6.2	5.1	-	-	-	T	-	-
unknown	269	238	2258.9	-	T	-	-	-	-	-	-	-	-
unknown (mesembrenone-type) *	245	175	2280.8	-	-	-	-	-	15.3	11.8	6.1	11.4	-
unknown	269	268	2285.5	-	-	-	-	-	-	-	-	-	-
unknown	253	252	2313.1	5.4	-	-	-	6.7	-	-	5.1	-	-
unknown	251	251	2335.2	-	-	-	-	6.2	-	-	-	-	-
unknown (lycorine-type) *	257	256	2379.0	-	-	-	8.0	-	-	-	-	-	-
unknown	253	252	2405.0	-	6.4	-	5.1	6.9	8.3	8.0	6.0	5.4	5.5
unknown (lycorine-type) *	269	211	2480.5	-	-	-	T	34.5	5.3	5.1	-	-	-
unknown	271	238	2492.7	5.7	-	-	-	-	-	-	-	-	-
unknown (homolycorine-type) *	331	109	2557.5	-	-	-	-	-	19.7	18.5	8.7	46.7	-
unknown (crinine/haemanthamine-type) *	329	329	2564.1	-	-	-	-	-	6.2	7.1	6.1	7.2	-
unknown	257	225	2579.2	-	-	-	-	-	-	-	-	-	-
unknown	299	238	2584.0	-	-	T	-	-	-	-	-	-	-
unknown (crinine/haemanthamine-type) *	315	254	2616.4	-	-	-	-	5.4	8.6	-	-	-	-
unknown (tazettine-type) *	315	231	2616.9	-	-	5.2	-	-	-	-	-	-	-
unknown (lycorine-type) *	329	268	2646.1	-	-	-	-	-	7.9	-	-	5.3	-
unknown	297	297	2655.7	-	-	-	-	-	-	-	-	-	-
unknown (tazettine-type) *	345	261	2662.6	18.8	11.2	23.0	-	-	-	-	-	-	7.3
unknown (crinine/haemanthamine-type) *	345	272	2671.8	-	-	-	-	-	-	-	-	-	-
unknown (crinine/haemanthamine-type) *	283	283	2692.5	-	-	-	-	-	-	-	-	-	-
unknown	303	302	2703.2	-	-	-	-	-	21.3	-	-	-	-
unknown (crinine/haemanthamine-type) *	315	315	2724.2	-	-	-	-	-	-	-	-	-	-
unknown (lycorine-type) *	253	252	2735.3	-	-	-	17.1	-	-	-	-	-	-
unknown (homolycorine-type) *	345	109	2735.6	-	-	-	-	-	-	-	-	-	-
unknown (crinine/haemanthamine-type) *	347	331	2795.5	-	-	-	-	-	-	-	-	-	-
unknown (crinine/haemanthamine-type) *	345	331	2795.7	-	-	-	-	-	-	-	-	-	-

Table 2. Cont.

(B)

Alkaloid	M+	BP	RI	A	C	E	G	I	K	M	O	Q	S
unknown (crinine/haemanthamine-type) *	347	331	2795.8	-	-	-	-	6.9	-	-	-	-	-
unknown (lycorine-type) *	251	250	2846.6	-	-	6.8	9.9	-	-	-	-	-	-
unknown	335	335	2860.6	-	7.6	-	-	-	-	-	-	-	-
unknown (lycorine-type) *	345	242	2868.8	-	-	-	-	-	-	-	-	-	-
unknown	373	372	2881.9	-	-	-	-	-	-	-	-	-	7.8
unknown (lycorine-type) *	357	356	2942.1	-	-	-	-	-	-	-	-	-	7.0
unknown (lycorine-type) *	279	278	3016.0	-	-	-	-	10.2	-	-	-	-	-
unknown (galanthamine-type) *	375	330	3027.5	-	7.0	-	-	-	-	-	-	-	-
unknown (lycorine-type) *	267	266	3032.9	-	9.2	-	7.3	-	-	-	-	-	-
unknown (lycorine-type) *	375	374	3049.2	-	-	-	-	-	-	-	-	-	8.4
unknown (lycorine-type) *	355	226	3066.6	-	-	-	5.8	-	-	-	-	-	-
unknown (lycorine-type) *	373	226	3161.0	-	-	-	21.5	-	-	-	-	-	-
Total				250.3	272.5	265.9	280.4	186.0	256.3	178.6	148.1	246.3	161.9

BP: Base Peak; T: Traces; **B**: *R. andicola*, SN; **D**: *R. andicola*, NC; **F**: *R. andicola*, VL; **H**: *R. araucana*; **J**: *R. montana*; **L**: *R. pratensis*, RF, nl, dunes; **N**: *R. pratensis*, AP, RF, L; **P**: *R. pratensis*, RF, nl; **R**: *R. pratensis*, WF; **T**: *R. splendens*; **A**: *R. andicola*, SN; **C**: *R. andicola*, NC; **E**: *R. andicola*, VL; **G**: *R. araucana*; **I**: *R. montana*; **K**: *R. pratensis*, RF, nl, dunes; **M**: *R. pratensis*, RF, L; **O**: *R. pratensis*, RF, nl; **Q**: *R. pratensis*, WF; **S**: *R. splendens*; -: not detected; * proposed structure-type according to the fragmentation pattern.

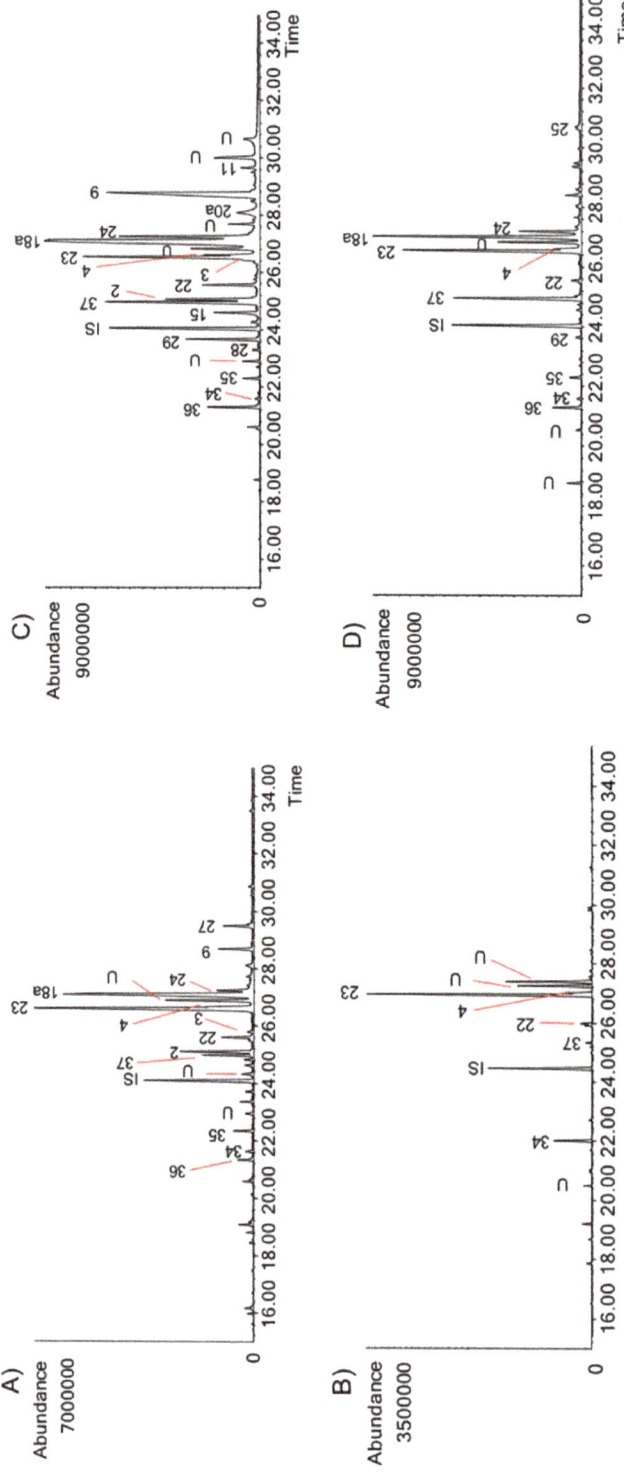

Figure 5. GC chromatograms of the alkaloids from Chilean *Rhodophiala* species. Numbers refer to Table 2. (**A**) Bulbs of *R. andicola* (Sierra Nevada); (**B**) Aerial parts of *R. andicola* (Sierra Nevada); (**C**) Bulbs of *R. andicola* (Nevado de Chillán); (**D**) Aerial parts of *R. andicola* (Nevado de Chillán). IS: internal standard; U: unknown.

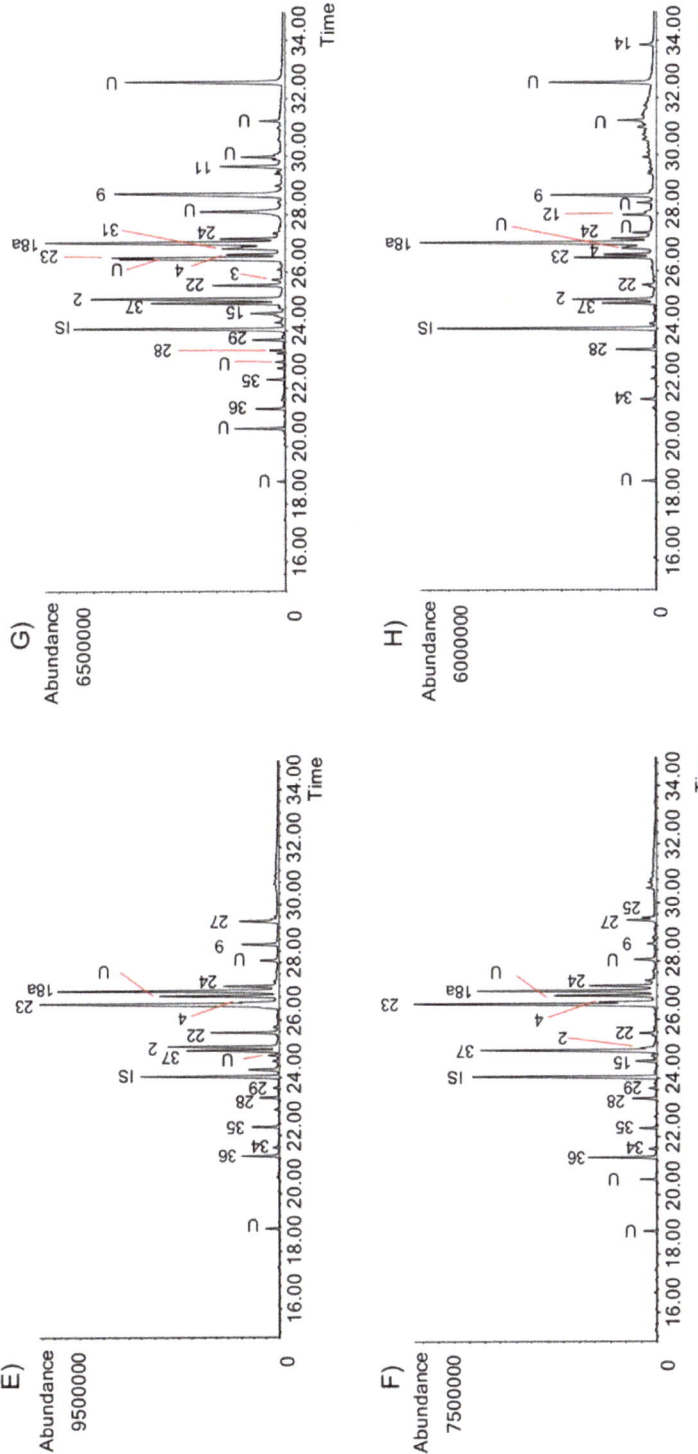

Figure 6. GC chromatograms of the alkaloids from Chilean *Rhodophiala* species. Numbers refer to Table 2. (**E**) Bulbs of *R. andicola* (Volcán Lonquimay); (**F**) Aerial parts of *R. andicola* (Volcán Lonquimay); (**G**) Bulbs of *R. araucana*; (**H**) Aerial parts of *R. araucana*. IS: internal standard; U: unknown.

Molecules **2018**, *23*, 1532

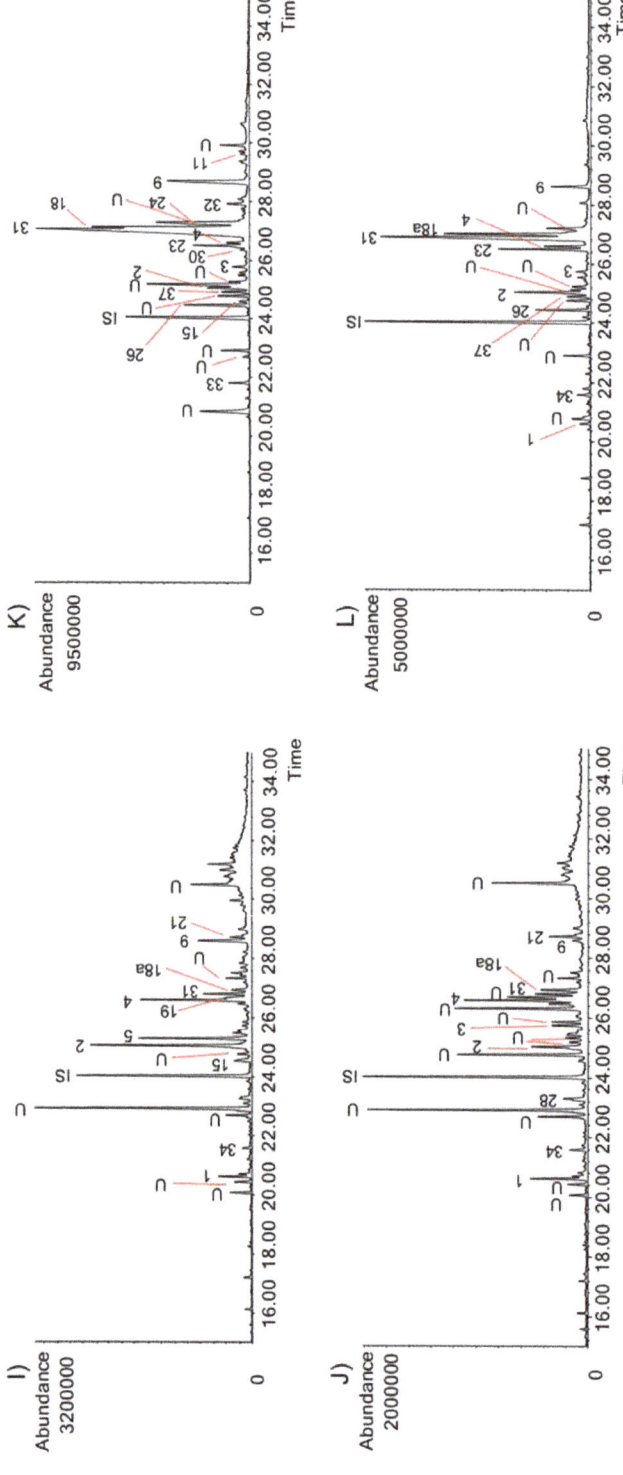

Figure 7. GC chromatograms of the alkaloids from Chilean *Rhodophiala* species. Numbers refer to Table 2. (**I**) Bulbs of *R. montana*; (**J**) Aerial parts of *R. montana*; (**K**) Bulbs of *R. pratensis* (red flowers, without leaves, growing on sand dunes); (**L**) Aerial parts of *R. pratensis* (red flowers, without leaves, growing on sand dunes). IS: internal standard; U: unknown.

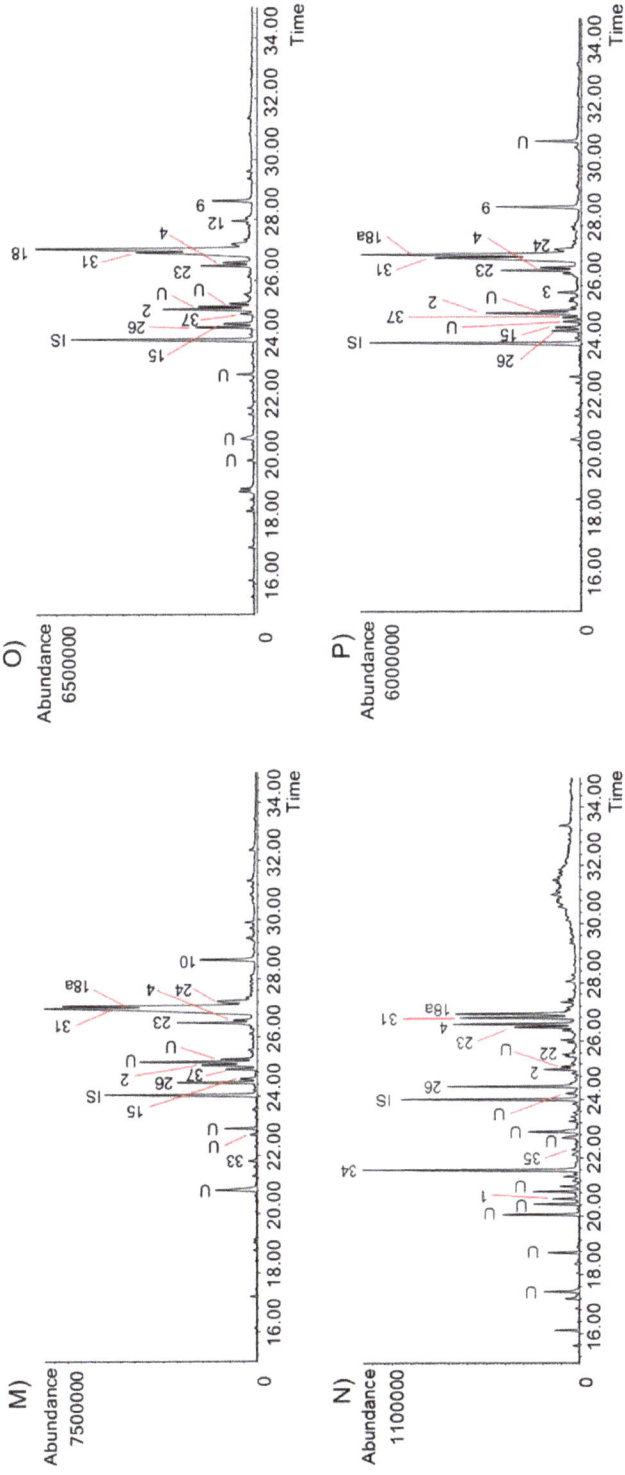

Figure 8. GC chromatograms of the alkaloids from Chilean *Rhodophiala* species. Numbers refer to Table 2. (**M**) Bulbs of *R. pratensis* (red flowers, with leaves); (**N**) Aerial parts of *R. pratensis* (red flowers, with leaves); (**O**) Bulbs of *R. pratensis* (red flowers, without leaves); (**P**) Aerial parts of *R. pratensis* (red flowers, without leaves). IS: internal standard; U: unknown.

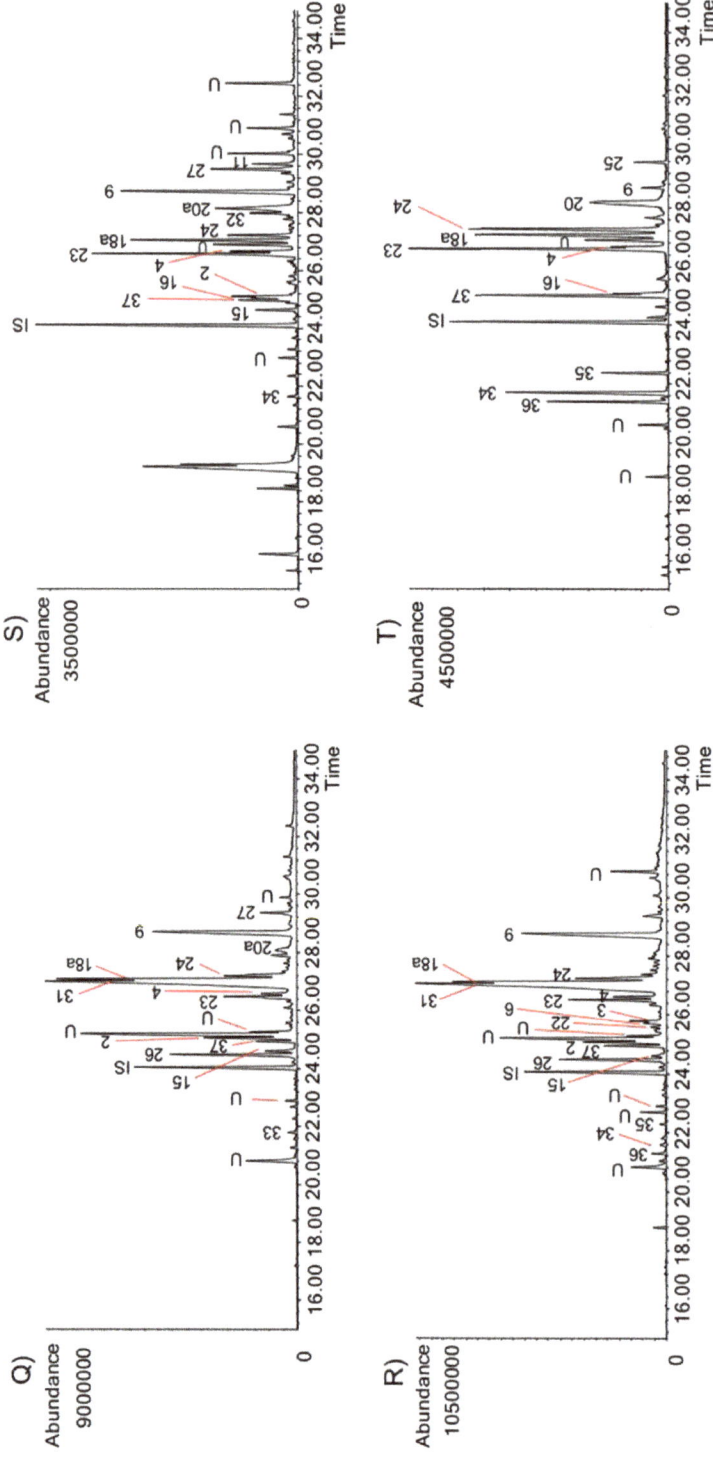

Figure 9. GC chromatograms of the alkaloids from Chilean *Rhodophiala* species. Numbers refer to Table 2. (**Q**) Bulbs of *R. pratensis* (white flowers); (**R**) Aerial parts of *R. pratensis* (white flowers); (**S**) Bulbs of *R. splendens*; (**T**) Aerial parts of *R. splendens*. IS: internal standard; U: unknown.

The highest alkaloid concentration was detected in the aerial parts of *R. andicola* (F) and in the aerial parts of *R. pratensis* (R) (311.1 and 274.1 mg GAL/g AE, respectively). Lowest content was found in the aerial parts of *R. andicola* (B) and in the aerial parts of *R. pratensis* (P) (133.2 and 138.1 mg GAL/g AE, respectively). In 70% of the samples, lycorine-, haemanthamine/crinine- and tazettine-type alkaloids were predominant. Lycorine-type alkaloids were present in all species with higher content in *R. araucana* (G) and *R. montana* bulbs (I) (79.0 and 78.6 mg GAL/g AE, respectively) and lowest values in the aerial parts of *R. andicola* (B) and (D) (8.6 and 7.5 mg GAL/g AE, respectively).

Haemanthamine/crinine-alkaloids occur in all samples except the aerial parts of *R. andicola* (B). However, the higher content was found in the bulbs of *R. andicola* from the same collection place (A) and in the aerial parts of the plant collected at Volcan Lonquimay (F). Compounds from the tazettine-type were not detected in the aerial parts and bulbs of *R. montana* (I and J). From the different Amaryllidaceae alkaloids groups, tazettine-type alkaloids were the main compounds in several samples, occurring in highest concentration in *R. andicola* (E, F) with values of 85.9 and 95.8 mg GAL/g AE of tazettine-type alkaloids in bulbs and aerial parts, respectively.

Galanthamine-type alkaloids were detected in low quantities in three species, namely *R. andicola*, *R. araucana* and *R. montana* (samples C, D, E, F, G, H and J) ranging between 5.1 to 19.0 mg GAL/g AE. Montanine-type alkaloids were present in all species, except *R. andicola*. The highest level of montanine-type compounds was detected in *R. pratensis* (K) (41.7 mg GAL/g AE), which presented three different alkaloids: pancratinine C, montanine and pancracine (5.3, 29.8 and 6.6 mg GAL/g AE, respectively). Mesembrenone-type was the least representative alkaloid-type. It was represented by demethylmesembrenol, detected in low quantities in three different samples of *R. pratensis* (K, M and Q) (7.2, 5.2 and 5.1 mg GAL/g AE, respectively). Narciclasine-type occurs in most samples in a range between 5.1 mg GAL/g AE in bulbs of *R. splendens* (S) to 44.5 and 32.2 mg GAL/g AE in aerial parts of *R. pratensis* with red flowers and leaves (N) and aerial parts of *R. splendens* (T), respectively. All species investigated presented ismine and/or galanthindole alkaloids, except *R. montana*. Forty structures occurring in the extracts could not be identified using the available databases. Three of the unidentified compounds were highly representative among the samples.

The compound with m/z 252 [M^+ = 253] (RI 2405.0) occurs in 60% of the samples. The m/z 109 with [M^+ = 331] (RI 2557.5), which probably belongs to the homolycorine-type alkaloids, was detected in 40% of the samples and in high amounts in bulbs of *R. pratensis* with white flowers (46.7 mg GAL/g AE). Finally, m/z 261 with [M^+ = 345] (RI 2662.6) was detected in 45% of the samples and in high quantity in aerial parts of *R. andicola* collected at Volcan Lonquimay (24.6 mg GAL/g AE).

The highest content of non-identified alkaloids was detected in the aerial parts of *R. montana* (J) and in the bulbs of *R. pratensis* (red flowers and without leaves) collected in the sand dunes at the sea shore (K) (126.9 and 92.6 mg GAL/g AE, respectively). The lowest content was detected in aerial parts of *R. pratensis* with red flowers and without leaves (P) and in aerial parts of *R. splendens* (T) (20.6 and 21.8 mg GAL/g AE, respectively).

2.3. Molecular Docking

In this study, *R. splendens* was the most active inhibitor of AChE and BuChE. Alkaloid analysis by GC-MS allowed the identification of 17 compounds in the leaf extract of *R. splendens* (T) including two unidentified constituents (Table 2). The 15 alkaloids identified in the extract were evaluated for their theoretical AChE and BuChE inhibitory potential by molecular docking (Tables 3 and 4). As expected, no alkaloid identified in sample T presented better theoretical AChE inhibitory activity than galanthamine. Molecular simulation of six alkaloids identified in sample T on the 4BDS structure theoretically showed higher enzymatic inhibition against BuChE than galanthamine by 0.80 kcal/mol.

Table 3. AChE and BuChE inhibitory activities of some alkaloids identified in the aerial parts of R. splendens (T) and the reference compound galanthamine. Values are expressed as IC_{50} (µg/mL).

Alkaloid	AChE	BuChE
11-hydroxyvittatine (20a)	122.17 ± 22.03	>200
lycorine (9)	101.70 ± 23.79	>200
8-O-demethylmaritidine (16)	113.21 ± 8.21	127.87 ± 2.45
hamayne (20b)	135.09 ± 15.33	48.40 ± 1.13
deacetylcantabricine (17)	>200	>200
haemanthamine (18a)	184.68 ± 11.58	>200
galanthamine (28)	0.48 ± 0.07	3.70 ± 0.24

Table 4. Estimated free energy binding of molecular docking between alkaloids identified in aerial parts of R. splendens and cholinesterases (AChE and BuChE). Values are expressed in kcal/mol.

Alkaloid	AChE [*a]	BuChE [*b]
11-hydroxyvittatine (20a)	−8.43	−9.03
lycorine (9)	−8.82 [*c]	−8.94
8-O-demethylmaritidine (16)	−8.74 [*d]	−8.93
hamayne (20b)	−8.28	−8.54
deacetylcantabricine (17)	−7.90	−8.43
haemanthamine (18a)	−8.80	−8.34
galanthamine (28)	−9.55 [*c]	−8.23 [*c]
epimacronine (25)	−9.36 [*c]	−7.63
tazettine (24)	−8.66 [*c]	−7.87
O-methyltazettine (23)	−8.54	−7.87
11,12-dehydroanhydrolycorine (4)	−8.41	−7.44
galanthindole (37)	−7.81	−7.41
trisphaeridine (34)	−7.38	−7.27
dihydrobicolorine (35)	−7.33	−7.38
ismine (36)	−6.78	−7.08

[*a] PBD code: 1DX6; [*b] PBD code: 4BDS; [*c] Cortes et al., 2015; [*d] Cortes et al., 2017.

To gain further insight into the molecular docking results, an experiment was carried out to check the AChE and BuChE inhibitory activities of 11-hydroxyvittatine (20), lycorine (9), 8-O-demethylmaritidine (16), hamayne (20b), deacetylcantabricine (17) and haemanthamine (18a) (Table 3). The best AChE and BuChE inhibitory activities were obtained for lycorine (9) (IC_{50} 101.70 ± 23.79 µg/mL) and hamayne (20b) (IC_{50} 48.40 ± 1.13 µg/mL), respectively. However, their theoretical BuChE inhibition was not supported by the experimental assays. The difference in origin of the BuChE structure used in the molecular docking (human) and experimental assays (equine serum), as well as the inability of these compounds to arrive at the BuChE active site of the enzyme could help to explain the difference between theoretical and practical results.

Two important regions in the active sites of the hBuChE enzymes have been located: the first corresponding to the catalytic triad composed by the residues His438, Ser198, and Glu325 [25], while the second corresponds to a choline binding site (α-anionic site), composed principally by the residues Trp82 and Phe329 [25]. A graphical representation of molecular binding of 11-hydroxyvittatine (20a) and hamayne (20b) alkaloids with the hBuChE protein is presented in Figure 10. The alkaloid 11-hydroxyvittatine (20a) shows two strong interactions, hydrogen bonds, with the residues Trp82 and Trp430; however, this molecule does not present any interactions close to the catalytic triad His438, Ser198, and Glu325. On the other hand, hamayne (20b) shows one hydrogen bond interaction with the residue Gly115, an amino acid located close to the catalytic triad His438, Ser198, and Glu325. In the case of the interactions at the choline binding site (α-anionic site), both alkaloids show the same π–π stacking interaction with the residue Trp82. These molecular interactions suggest that the β-orientation of the hydroxyl group at C-3 in 11-hydroxyvittatine (20a) could theoretically increase the BuChE inhibition on the 4BDS structure by 0.49 kcal/mol, compared to the α-orientation of the hydroxyl group at the C-3 position in hamayne (**20b**). However, in the experimental assays, hamayne (**20b**) showed BuChE inhibitory activity (48.40 ± 1.13 µg/mL). It can be hypothesized that the β-orientation of the hydroxyl group at C-3 in 11-hydroxyvittatine (**20a**) probably makes it difficult for the compound to arrive at the catalytic triad in the active site of the BuChE.

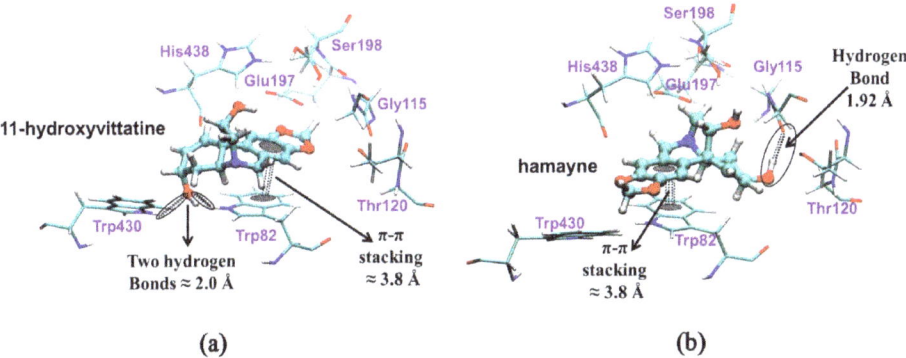

Figure 10. Graphical representations of the binding of (**a**) 11-hydroxivittatine (**20a**) and (**b**) hamayne (**20b**) in the gorge of the active site of *h*BuChE.

Studies on alkaloid composition associated with cholinesterase inhibition and binding-mode prediction have been reported [26,27]. A work on Argentinean Amaryllidaceae [24] reported the composition and acetylcholinesterase inhibition of four wild growing species, including *Rhodophiala mendocina*. Two *R. mendocina* samples collected in different locations presented similar activity towards AChE with IC_{50} values of 2.0 µg/mL but with relevant differences in the qualitative and quantitative alkaloid composition. The sample from the Provincia de San Juan showed high content of haemanthamine/crinamine (31.2%), tazettine (32.9%) and lycorine (13.3%) while the plant collected in the Provincia de Neuquen presented 6.8% haemanthamine/crinamine and 20.4% of lycorine, respectively. Galanthamine was found in both samples with 0.6 and 0.8% for the San Juan and Neuquen plants, respectively. In a report from acetylcholinesterase inhibitory alkaloids from Brazilian Amaryllidaceae [23] the bulbs of *Rhodophiala bifida* (Herb.) Traub were investigated. The activity on AChE was moderate with an IC_{50} value of 8.45 µg/mL, being lower than that from *R. mendocina* [24]. The alkaloid extract of *R. bifida* bulbs contained high amounts of montanine (91.94%). The alkaloid composition of the Chilean *Rhodophiala ananuca* (formerly: *Hippeastrum ananuca*) was described [28,29]. The bulbs contained phenantridine alkaloids, including hippeastidine and epi-homolycorine.

The alkaloid montanine isolated from *R. bifida* showed activity towards a panel of eight human cancer cell lines. According to [30], montanine at 2.5 µg/mL was more active than doxorubicine on the multi-drug resistant breast cell line NCLADR. Montanine also showed antimicrobial effect with MIC of 5 µg/mL against *S. aureus* ATCC 6538 and *E. coli* ATCC 24922 and 20 µg/mL against *P. aeruginosa* ATCC 27853, respectively [31]. In a screening towards *Trichomonas vaginalis*, dichloromethane and n-butanol extracts from Brazilian *Hippeastrum* species and *Rhodophiala bifida* showed activity against the protozoa [32]. The most active fractions contained the alkaloids lycorine and lycosinine.

In a study on the alkaloids of *Zephyranthes robusta* (Amaryllidaceae), the compounds isolated were evaluated as inhibitors of human cholinesterases [33]. The authors used human erythrocye AChE and serum BuChE. The compounds were tested in a range of 0.5–500 µg/mL and the inhibition was reported as IC_{50} values in µMolar concentration. While the activity of the reference compound galanthamine was similar in both studies, 11-hydroxyvittattine, lycorine and haemanthamine were not active on the human AChE and BuChE. 8-*O*-demethylmaritidine and hamayne were inactive on human BuChE but presented activity on erythrocyte AChE. The differences in the results can be explained by the biological source of the enzymes (human cholinesterases for [33] and electric eel AChE and horse (equine serum) BuChE in this work. For a better comparison of results, the use of enzymes from the same biological source should be recommended.

In summary, the AChE and BuChE inhibitory activity of the Chilean *Rhodophiala* species investigated led to an interesting source of inhibitors that do not contain the alkaloid galanthamine. Our results suggest that Chilean *Rhodophiala* could be a promising source of new alkaloids with effect towards cholinesterases. The difficulty in finding a species with high activity against AChE and BuChE, the similarity of the AChE and BuChE inhibitory values, the low complexity of the alkaloid profile of aerial parts of *R. splendens*, together with the absence of galanthamine-type alkaloids in this sample, prompted us to further explore the results.

3. Materials and Methods

3.1. Plant Material

The samples were collected in central-southern Chile and were identified following the reference [19,34]. *Rhodophiala andicola* (Poepp.) Traub, was collected at Sierra Nevada (Región de la Araucanía, 27 January 2016), the slopes of Volcán Lonquimay (Región de la Araucanía, Provincia del Malleco, 19 December 2016) and the slopes of Nevado de Chillán (Región del Bio-Bio, 30 December 2016). *Rhodophiala araucana* (Phil.) Traub was collected at Malalcahuello, Región de la Araucanía (19 December 2016), and *Rhodophiala montana* (Phil.) Traub at the roadside to Laguna del Maule, Región del Maule (2 January 2017). Samples from *Rhodophiala pratensis* (Poepp.) Traub were collected at Arcos de Calán, Región del Maule (12 December 2016) including plants growing on sand dunes and grasslands close to the sea. Plants with red and white flowers were collected separately. According to [34], the plant with red flowers fits the description of *R. pratensis*. *Rhodophiala splendens* (Renjifo) Traub was collected at Las Trancas, Región del Bio-Bio (2 January 2016). The plants were identified by Dr. Patricio Peñailillo, Herbario de la Universidad de Talca. Voucher herbarium specimens have been deposited at the Universidad de Talca as follows: *R. andicola* (N° 4081); *R. araucana* (N° 4083); *R. montana* (N° 4080); *R. pratensis* (N° 4084); *R. pratensis* (white flower) (N° 8085); *R. splendens* (N° 4082). A map with the collection places is shown in Figure 2. Pictures of the species investigated are illustrated in Figure 3.

3.2. Extraction

The freshly collected plant material was cleaned and separated into bulbs and aerial parts, frozen and lyophilized before extraction. The dry weight percentage was determined. The lyophilized plant material was extracted with MeOH under sonication for 10 min (3×) changing the solvent each time. The plant to solvent ratio ranged from 1:10 to 1:60 and was selected according to the volume of plant material for extraction. The combined MeOH solubles were taken to dryness under reduced pressure to afford the crude extracts. The crude extracts were then acidified to pH 3 with diluted H_2SO_4 (2%, v/v) and the neutral material was removed with Et_2O. The aqueous solutions were basified up to pH 9–10 with NH_4OH (25%, v/v) and extracted with EtOAc to provide the alkaloid extracts which were used for all experiments (enzyme inhibition assays and chemical analysis by GC-MS).

3.3. Acetylcholinesterase (AChE) and Butyrylcholinesterase (BuChE) Inhibitory Activity

Cholinesterase inhibitory activities were determined according to [35] with some modifications [36]. Stock solutions with 518U of AchE from *Electrophorus electricus* (Merck, Darmstadt, Germany) and BuChE from equine serum (Merck, Darmstadt, Germany), respectively, were prepared and kept at −20 °C. Acetylthiocholine iodide (ATCI), *S*-butyrylthiocholine iodide (BTCI) and 5,5′-dithiobis (2-nitrobenzoic acid) (DTNB) were obtained from Merck (Darmstadt, Germany). Fifty microliters of AChE or BuChE (both enzymes used at 6.24 U) in phosphate buffer

(8 mM K_2HPO_4, 2.3 mM NaH_2PO_4, 0.15 NaCl, pH 7.5) and 50 µL of the sample dissolved in the same buffer were added to the wells. The plates were incubated for 30 min at room temperature. Then, 100 µL of the substrate solution (0.1 M Na_2HPO_4, 0.5 M DTNB, and 0.6 mM ATCI or 0.24 mM BTCI in Millipore water, pH 7.5) was added. After 10 min, the absorbance was read at 405 nm in a Labsystem microplate reader (Thermo Fischer, Waltham, MA, USA). Enzyme activity was calculated as percent compared to a control using buffer without any inhibitor. Galanthamine served as positive control. In a first step, samples were assessed at 10, 100 and 200 µg/mL towards both enzymes. Samples with an IC_{50} > 200 µg/mL were considered inactive. Samples with an IC_{50} < 200 µg/mL were further analyzed to determine the IC_{50} values. The cholinesterase inhibitory data were analyzed with the software Microsoft Office Excel 2010 (Microsoft, Redmond, WA, USA).

3.4. Alkaloids Identification and Quantification

3.4.1. Equipment

The equipment used for the identification and quantification of the alkaloids was a GC-MS 6890N apparatus (Agilent Technologies, Santa Clara, CA, USA) coupled with MSD5975 inert XL operating in the electron ionization (EI) mode at 70 eV. A Sapiens-X5 MS column (30 m × 0.25 mm i.d., film thickness 0.25 µm) was used. The temperature gradient was as follows: 12 min at 100 °C, 100–180 °C at 15 °C/min, 180–300 °C at 5 °C/min and 10 min hold at 300 °C. The injector and detector temperatures were 250 and 280 °C, respectively, and the flow-rate of carrier gas (He) was 1 mL/min. Two mg of each alkaloid extract was dissolved in 1 mL of $MeOH:CHCl_3$ (1:1, v/v) and 1 µL was injected using the splitless mode. Codeine (0.05 mg/mL) was used as an internal standard in all the samples.

3.4.2. Alkaloids Identification

Amaryllidaceae alkaloids occurring in the samples were identified by comparison of the Rt, fragmentation patterns and data interpretation of the spectra. The database used was built using single alkaloids previously isolated and identified by spectroscopic and spectrometric methods (NMR, UV, CD, IR, MS) in the Natural Products Laboratory, Universidad de Barcelona, the NIST 05 Database and literature data [37–42].

3.4.3. Alkaloid Quantification

To quantify the single constituents, a calibration curve of galanthamine (10, 20, 40, 60, 80 and 100 µg/mL) was used. The same amount of codeine (0.05 mg/mL) was added to each solution sample as an internal standard. The peak areas were manually obtained considering selected ions for each compound (usually the base peak of their MS, i.e., m/z at 286 for galanthamine, at 299 for codeine). The ratio between the values obtained for galanthamine and codeine in each solution was plotted against the corresponding concentration of galanthamine to obtain the calibration curve and its equation (y = 0.0224x − 0.2037; R^2 = 0.9977). All data were standardized to the area of the internal standard (codeine) and the equation obtained for the calibration curve of galanthamine was used to calculate the amount of each alkaloid. Results are expressed as mg GAL, which was finally related to the alkaloid extract weight. As the peak area does not only depend on the corresponding alkaloid concentration but also on the intensity of the mass spectra fragmentation, the quantification is not absolute. However, the methodology is considered suitable to compare the specific alkaloid amount between samples [39,42].

3.5. Molecular Docking

The molecular docking simulations for the alkaloids identified in *Rhodophiala splendens*, the most promising species found in this study, were performed to investigate the binding mode into the active site of two different enzymes, namely *Torpedo californica* AChE (TcAChE) and *h*BuChE: proteins with PDB codes 1DX6 [43] and 4BDS [44], respectively. The 3D-structures of the alkaloids were drawn using the Chemcraft program [45], and then submitted to a geometrical optimization procedure at PBE0 [46]/6-311+g* [47] level of theory using the Gaussian 09 program [48]. All optimized alkaloids were confirmed as a minimum on the potential energy surface. The docking simulations for the set of optimized ligands were performed using the AutoDock v.4.2 program [49]. AutoDock combines a rapid energy evaluation through pre-calculated grids of affinity potentials with a variety of search algorithms to find suitable binding positions for a ligand on a given macromolecule. To compare the results from the docking simulations, the water molecules, cofactors, and ions were excluded from each X-ray crystallographic structure. Likewise, the polar hydrogen atoms of the enzymes were added, and the non-polar hydrogen atoms were merged. Finally, the enzyme was treated as a rigid body. The grid maps of interaction energy for various atom types with each macromolecule were calculated by the auxiliary program AutoGrid, choosing a grid box with dimensions of 70 × 70 × 70 Å around the active site, which was sufficiently large to include the most important residues of each enzyme. The docking searches for the best orientations of the ligands binding to the active site of each protein were performed using the Lamarckian Genetic Algorithm (LGA) [50]. The LGA protocol applied a population size of 2000 individuals, while 2,500,000 energy evaluations were used for the 50 LGA runs. The best conformations were chosen from the lowest docked energy solutions in the cluster populated by the highest number of conformations. The best docking complex solutions (poses) were analyzed according to the potential intermolecular interactions (ligand/enzyme), such as hydrogen bonding and the cation–π, π–π stacking.

Author Contributions: G.S.-H. and J.B. conceived and designed the experiments; L.R.T., N.C., E.H.O. and C.T. performed the experiments; L.R.T., J.B. and G.S.-H. analyzed the data; C.T. and G.S.-H. collected and processed the samples; G.S.-H., J.B., L.R.T. and E.H.O. wrote the paper.

Funding: This research was funded by PIEI-QUIM-BIO, Universidad de Talca, CCiTUB and Programa CYTED (416RT0511). L.R.T. and J.B. are members of the Research Group 2017-SGR-604 at the University of Barcelona.

Acknowledgments: L.R.T. is thankful to CAPES (Coordenação de Pessoal de Nível Superior-Bolsista CAPES, Processo 13553135) for a doctoral fellowship.

Conflicts of Interest: The authors declare no conflict of interest. The founding sponsors had no role in the design of the study; in the collection, analyses, or interpretation of data; in the writing of the manuscript, and in the decision to publish the results.

References

1. Newman, D.J.; Cragg, G.M. Natural products as sources of new drugs from 1981 to 2014. *J. Nat. Prod.* **2016**, *79*, 629–661. [CrossRef] [PubMed]
2. Lu, J.-J.; Bao, J.-L.; Chen, X.-P.; Huang, M.; Wang, Y.-T. Alkaloids isolated from natural herbs as the anticancer agents. *Evid.-Based Complement. Altern. Med.* **2012**, *2012*, 485042. [CrossRef] [PubMed]
3. Feher, M.; Schmidt, J.M. Property Distributions: Differences between drugs, natural products, and molecules from combinatorial chemistry. *J. Chem. Inf. Comput. Sci.* **2003**, *43*, 218–227. [CrossRef] [PubMed]
4. Bastida, J.; Lavilla, R.; Viladomat, F. Chemical and biological aspects of *Narcissus* alkaloids. In *The Alkaloids: Chemistry and Physiology*; Cordell, G.A., Ed.; Elsevier: Amsterdam, The Netherlands, 2006; Volume 63, pp. 87–179, eBook ISBN 9780080466552; Hardcover ISBN 9780124695634.
5. Bastida, J.; Berkov, S.; Torras, L.; Pigni, N.B.; de Andrade, J.P.; Martínez, V.; Codina, C.; Viladomat, F. Chemical and biological aspects of Amaryllidaceae alkaloids. In *Recent Advances in Pharmaceutical Sciences*; Muñoz-Torrero, D., Ed.; Transworld Research Network: Kerala, India, 2011; pp. 65–100, ISBN 978-81-7895-528-5.
6. Ingrassia, L.; Lefranc, F.; Mathieu, V.; Darro, F.; Kiss, R. Amaryllidaceae isocarbostyril alkaloids and their derivatives as promising antitumor agents. *Transl. Oncol.* **2008**, *1*, 1–13. [CrossRef] [PubMed]
7. Van Goiestsenoven, G.; Mathieu, V.; Lefranc, F.; Kornienko, A.; Evidente, A.; Kiss, R. Narciclasine as well as other Amaryllidaceae isocarnostyrils are promising GTP-ase targeting agents against brain cancers. *Med. Res. Rev.* **2013**, *33*, 439–455. [CrossRef] [PubMed]

8. Heinrich, M.; Teoh, H.L. Galanthamine from showdrop—The development of a modern drug against Alzheimer's disease from local Caucasian knowledge. *J. Ethnopharmacol.* **2004**, *9*, 147–162. [CrossRef] [PubMed]
9. Maelicke, A.; Samochocki, M.; Jostock, R.; Fehrenbacher, A.; Ludwig, J.; Albuquerque, E.X.; Zerlin, M. Allosteric sensitization of nicotinic receptors by galanthamine, a new treatment strategy for Alzheimer's disease. *Biol. Psychiatry* **2001**, *49*, 279–288. [CrossRef]
10. Craig, L.A.; Hong, N.S.; McDonald, R.J. Revisiting the cholinergic hypothesis in the development of Alzheimer's disease. *Neurosci. Biobehav. Rev.* **2011**, *35*, 1397–1409. [CrossRef] [PubMed]
11. Querfurth, H.W.; LaFerla, F.M. Alzheimer's disease. *N. Engl. J. Med.* **2010**, *362*, 329–344. [CrossRef] [PubMed]
12. Alzheimer's Disease International. Available online: https://www.alz.co.uk/research/WorldAlzheimerReport2016.pdf (accessed on 13 October 2017).
13. Selkoe, D.J. Alzheimer's disease: Genes, proteins, and therapy. *Physiol. Rev.* **2001**, *81*, 741–766. [CrossRef] [PubMed]
14. Basiri, A.; Murugaiyah, V.; Osman, H.; Kumar, R.S.; Kia, Y.; Awang, K.B.; Ali, M.A. An expedient, ionic liquid mediated multi-component synthesis of novel piperidone grafted cholinesterase enzymes inhibitors and their molecular modeling study. *Eur. J. Med. Chem.* **2013**, *67*, 221–229. [CrossRef] [PubMed]
15. Greig, N.H.; Lahiri, D.K.; Sambamurti, K. Butyrylcholinesterase: An important new target in Alzheimer's disease therapy. *Int. Psychogeriatr.* **2002**, *14*, 77–91. [CrossRef] [PubMed]
16. Giacobini, E. Cholinesterase inhibitors: New roles and therapeutic alternatives. *Pharmacol. Res.* **2004**, *50*, 433–440. [CrossRef] [PubMed]
17. Ballard, C.G. Advances in the treatment of Alzheimer's disease: Benefits of dual cholinesterase inhibition. *Eur. Neurol.* **2002**, *47*, 64–70. [CrossRef] [PubMed]
18. Olate, E.; Bridgen, M. Techniques for the in vitro propagation of *Rhodophiala* and *Leucocoryne* spp. *Acta Hortic.* **2005**, *673*, 335–342. [CrossRef]
19. Schiappacasse, F.; Peñailillo, P.; Yáñez, P. *Propagación de Bulbosas Chilenas Ornamentals*; Editorial Universidad de Talca: Talca, Chile, 2002; ISBN 956-7059-50-0.
20. Muñoz, M.; Riegel, R.; Seemann, P.; Penailillo, P.; Schiappacasse, F.; Nunez, J. Phylogenetic relationships of *Rhodolirium montanum* Phil. and related species based on nucleotide sequences from ITS region and karyotype analysis. *Gayana Bot.* **2011**, *68*, 40–48. [CrossRef]
21. Schiappacasse, F.; Peñailillo, P.; Basoalto, A.; Seemann, P.; Riegel, R.; Muñoz, M.; Jara, G.; Durán, C. Biotechnological applications on plant breeding of Chilean *Rhodophiala* species: Morphological and physiological studies. *Agro Sur* **2007**, *35*, 65–67. [CrossRef]
22. Baeza, C.; Almendras, F.; Ruiz, E.; Peñailillo, P. Comparative karyotype studies in species of *Miltinea* Ravenna, *Phycella* Lindl. and *Rhodophiala* C. Presl (Amaryllidaceae) from Chile. *Rev. Fac. Cienc. Agrar.* **2012**, *44*, 197–209, ISSN printed 0370-4661, ISSN online 1853-8665.
23. De Andrade, J.P.; Giordani, R.B.; Torras-Claveria, L.; Pigni, N.B.; Berkov, S.; Font-Bardia, M.; Calvet, T.; Konrath, E.; Bueno, K.; Sachett, L.G.; et al. The Brazilian Amaryllidaceae as a source of acetylcholinesterase inhibitory alkaloids. *Phytochem. Rev.* **2016**, *15*, 147–160. [CrossRef]
24. Ortiz, J.E.; Berkov, S.; Pigni, N.B.; Theoduloz, C.; Roitman, G.; Tapia, A.; Bastida, J.; Feresin, G.E. Wild Argentinian Amaryllidaceae, a new renewable source of the acetylcholinesterase inhibitor galanthamine and other alkaloids. *Molecules* **2012**, *17*, 13473–13482. [CrossRef] [PubMed]
25. Nicolet, Y.; Lockridge, O.; Masson, P.; Fontecilla-Camps, J.C.; Nachon, F. Crystal structure of human butyrylcholinesterase and of its complexes with substrate and products. *J. Biol. Chem.* **2003**, *278*, 41141–41147. [CrossRef] [PubMed]
26. Cortes, N.; Alvarez, R.; Osorio, E.H.; Alzate, F.; Berkov, S.; Osorio, E. Alkaloid metabolite profiles by GC/MS and acetylcholinesterase inhibitory activities with binding-mode predictions of five Amaryllidaceae plants. *J. Pharmaceut. Biomed. Anal.* **2015**, *102*, 222–228. [CrossRef] [PubMed]
27. Cortes, N.; Sierra, K.; Alzate, F.; Osorio, E.H.; Osorio, E. Alkaloids of Amaryllidaceae as inhibitors of cholinesterases (AChEs and BuChEs): An integrated bioguided study. *Phytochem. Anal.* **2017**, *29*, 217–227. [CrossRef] [PubMed]

28. Pacheco, P.; Silva, M.; Sammes, P.G.; Watson, W.H. Estudio químico de las Amaryllidaceae chilenas. Nuevos alcaloides de *Hippeastrum ananuca*. *Bol. Soc. Chil. Quim.* **1982**, *27*, 289.
29. Pacheco, P.; Silva, M.; Steglich, W.; Watson, W.H. Alkaloids of Chilean Amaryllidaceae I hippeastidine and epi-homolycorine two novel alkaloids. *Rev. Latinoam. Quim.* **1978**, *9*, 28–32.
30. Castilhos, T.S.; Giordani, R.; Dutilh, J.; Bastida, J.; de Carvalho, J.E.; Henriques, A.T.; Zuanazzi, J.A.S. Chemical and biological investigation of the alkaloids from *Rhodophiala bífida* (Herb.) Traub (Amaryllidaceae). In Proceedings of the 24° Reuniao Annual da Sociedade Brasileira de Química, Pocos de Caldas, Brazil, 28–31 May 2001.
31. Castilhos, T.S.; Giordani, R.; Henriques, A.T.; Menezes, F.S.; Zuanazzi, J.A.S. Availacao in vitro das atividades antiinflamatoria, antioxidante e antimicrobiana do alcaloide montanina. *Rev. Bras. Pharmacogn.* **2007**, *17*, 209–214. [CrossRef]
32. Vieira, P.; Giordani, R.; de Carli, G.; Tasca, T.; Zuanazzi, J. Screening and bioguided fractionation of Amaryllidaceae species with activity against *Trichomonas vaginalis*. *Planta Med.* **2010**, *76*, 470. [CrossRef]
33. Kulhánková, A.; Cahlíková, L.; Novák, Z.; Macáková, K.; Kuneš, J.; Opletal, L.P. Alkaloids from *Zephyranthes robusta* Baker and their acetylcholinesterase- and butyrylcholinesterase-inhibitory activity. *Chem. Biodivers.* **2013**, *10*, 1120–1127. [CrossRef] [PubMed]
34. Flora de Chile en su Habitat. Available online: www.floradechile.cl/monocoty/family/amaryllis.htm (accessed on 16 June 2018).
35. Ellman, G.L.; Courtney, K.D.; Andres, V., Jr.; Featherstone, R.M. A new and rapid colorimetric determination of acetylcholinesterase activity. *Biochem. Pharmacol.* **1961**, *7*, 88–95. [CrossRef]
36. López, S.; Bastida, J.; Viladomat, F.; Codina, C. Acetylcholinesterase inhibitory activity of some Amaryllidaceae alkaloids and *Narcissus* extracts. *Life Sci.* **2002**, *71*, 2521–2529. [CrossRef]
37. De Andrade, J.P.; Pigni, N.B.; Torras-Claveria, L.; Berkov, S.; Codina, C.; Viladomat, F.; Bastida, J. Bioactive alkaloid extracts from *Narcissus broussonetii*: Mass spectral studies. *J. Pharmaceut. Biomed.* **2012**, *70*, 13–25. [CrossRef] [PubMed]
38. De Andrade, J.P.; Guo, Y.; Font-Bardia, M.; Calvet, T.; Dutilh, J.; Viladomat, F.; Codina, C.; Nair, J.J.; Zuanazzi, J.A.S.; Bastida, J. Crinine-type alkaloids from *Hippeastrum aulicum* and *H. calyptratum*. *Phytochemistry* **2014**, *103*, 188–195. [CrossRef] [PubMed]
39. Torras-Claveria, L.; Berkov, S.; Codina, C.; Viladomat, F.; Bastida, J. Metabolomic analysis of bioactive Amaryllidaceae alkaloids of ornamental varieties of *Narcissus* by GC-MS combined with k-means cluster analysis. *Ind. Crop. Prod.* **2014**, *56*, 211–222. [CrossRef]
40. Tallini, L.R.; de Andrade, J.P.; Kaiser, M.; Viladomat, F.; Nair, J.J.; Zuanazzi, J.A.S.; Bastida, J. Alkaloid constituents of the Amaryllidaceae plant *Amaryllis belladonna* L. *Molecules* **2017**, *22*, 1437. [CrossRef] [PubMed]
41. Tallini, L.R.; Osorio, E.H.; dos Santos, V.D.; Borges, W.d.S.; Kaiser, M.; Viladomat, F.; Zuanazzi, J.A.S.; Bastida, J. *Hippeastrum reticulatum* (Amaryllidaceae): Alkaloids profiling, biological activities and molecular docking. *Molecules* **2017**, *22*, 2191. [CrossRef] [PubMed]
42. Guo, Y.; Pigni, N.B.; Zheng, Y.; de Andrade, J.P.; Torras-Claveria, L.; Borges, W.S.; Viladomat, F.; Codina, C.; Bastida, J. Analysis of bioactive Amaryllidaceae alkaloid profiles in *Lycoris* species by GC-MS. *Nat. Prod. Commun.* **2014**, *9*, 1081–1086. [PubMed]
43. Greenblatt, H.M.; Kryger, G.; Lewis, T.; Silman, I.; Sussman, J.L. Structure of acetylcholinesterase complexed with (−)-galanthamine at 2.3 Å resolution. *FEBS Lett.* **1999**, *463*, 321–326. [CrossRef]
44. Nachon, F.; Carletti, E.; Ronco, C.; Trovaslet, M.; Nicolet, Y.; Jean, L.; Renard, P.-Y. Crystal structures of human cholinesterases in complex with huprine W and tacrine: Elements of specificity for anti-Alzheimer's drugs targeting acetyl- and butyryl-cholinesterase. *Biochem. J.* **2013**, *453*, 393–399. [CrossRef] [PubMed]
45. ChemCraft. Available online: http://www.chemcraftprog.com/citation.html (accessed on 9 October 2017).
46. Adamo, C.; Barone, V. Toward reliable density functional methods without adjustable parameters: The PBE0 model. *J. Chem. Phys.* **1999**, *110*, 6158–6170. [CrossRef]
47. Petersson, G.A.; Bennett, A.; Tensfeldt, T.G.; Al-Laham, M.A.; Shirley, W.A.; Mantzaris, J.; Mantzaris, J. A complete basis set model chemistry. I. The total energies of closed-shell atoms and hydrides of the first-row elements. *J. Chem. Phys.* **1988**, *89*, 2193–2218. [CrossRef]
48. Frisch, M.J.; Trucks, G.W.; Schlegel, H.B.; Scuseria, G.E.; Robb, M.A.; Cheeseman, J.R.; Scalmani, G.; Barone, V.; Mennucci, B.; Petersson, G.A.; et al. *Gaussian 09, Revis. E.01*; Gaussian, Inc.: Wallingford, CT, USA, 2013.

49. Moris, G.M.; Huey, R.; Lindstrom, W.; Sanner, M.F.; Belew, R.K.; Goodsell, D.S.; Olson, A.J. Autodock4 and AutoDockTools4: Automated docking with selective receptor flexibility. *J. Comput. Chem.* **2009**, *16*, 2785–2791. [CrossRef] [PubMed]
50. Thomsen, R.; Christensen, M.H. MolDock: A new technique for high-accuracy molecular docking. *J. Med. Chem.* **2006**, *49*, 3315–3321. [CrossRef] [PubMed]

Sample Availability: Samples of the compounds are not available from the authors.

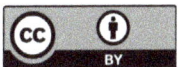

© 2018 by the authors. Licensee MDPI, Basel, Switzerland. This article is an open access article distributed under the terms and conditions of the Creative Commons Attribution (CC BY) license (http://creativecommons.org/licenses/by/4.0/).

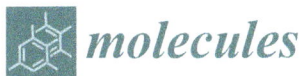

Article

Mahimbrine A, a Novel Isoquinoline Alkaloid Bearing a Benzotropolone Moiety from *Mahonia imbricata*

Mao-Sheng Zhang [1], Yan Deng [1], Shao-Bin Fu [1], Da-Le Guo [2] and Shi-Ji Xiao [1,*]

[1] School of Pharmacy, Zunyi Medical University, Zunyi 563006, China; maosheng.zhang@163.com (M.-S.Z.); 13658521539@163.com (Y.D.); fushb@126.com (S.-B.F.)
[2] School of Pharmacy, Chengdu University of Traditional Chinese Medicine, Chengdu 611137, China; guodale2008@163.com
* Correspondence: xiaoshiji84@163.com; Tel.: +86-0851-28643428

Received: 17 May 2018; Accepted: 22 June 2018; Published: 26 June 2018

Abstract: A novel isoquinoline alkaloid, mahimbrine A, possessing a rare benzotropolone framing scaffold, was isolated from the endemic plant of *Mahonia imbricata*. Its structure was established on the basis of extensive spectroscopic analysis. A plausible biosynthetic route of mahimbrine A was proposed. Mahimbrine A showed no antimicrobial activity at the concentration of 1 mg/mL.

Keywords: *Mahonia imbricata*; Berberidaceae; isoquinoline alkaloid; mahimbrine A

1. Introduction

Mahonia imbricata Ying *et* Boufford, as one of the endemics of seed plants in China, is a perennial shrub of the family Berberidaceae, distributed only in Guizhou and Yunan provinces of Southwest China [1]. Plants of the genus *Mahonia* have long been used as a traditional medicine to treat tuberculosis, periodontitis, dysentery, pharyngolaryngitis, eczema, and wounds [2]. Previous chemical investigations on this genus have involved a series of chemical constituents. Among these constituents, alkaloids are principal constituents of the genus *Mahonia* [3–5]. As part of an ongoing research program to isolate and determine structures of secondary metabolites from medicinal endemic plants of southwestern China [6,7], we performed a phytochemical study on *M. imbricate*. As a result, a novel isoquinoline alkaloid, possessing a rare benzotropolone substituent, was isolated (Figure 1). Its structure was established by means of spectroscopic analysis including one- and two-dimensional NMR spectroscopy. Moreover, the hypothetical biosynthetic route was proposed. Mahimbrine A was tested against four gram-positive bacterial strains and four gram-negative bacteria.

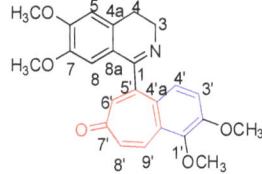

Figure 1. Structure of mahimbrine A.

2. Results and Discussion

2.1. Structure Elucidation of Mahimbrine A

Mahimbrine A was obtained as a brown gum. Its molecular formula was established as $C_{24}H_{23}NO_5$ on the basis of the HR-ESI-MS ([M + H]$^+$ at m/z 406.1632, calcd. 406.1649 and [2M + H]$^+$ at m/z 811.3226, calcd. 811.3225), which requires 14 degrees of unsaturation. The IR absorptions at 3434 and 1633 cm^{-1} suggested the presence of hydroxyl and carbonyl groups in the molecule. UV absorptions at λ_{max} 230 and 288 nm deduced the presence of an α, β-unsaturated carbonyl moiety [8]. The ^{1}H, ^{13}C NMR and HSQC spectra of mahimbrine A (Table 1) showed 24 carbon resonances due to a methine at δ_H 2.91 (2H, m), δ_C 25.8; four methoxyl groups at δ_H 3.60 (3H, s), 3.93 (6H, s), 3.94 (3H, s), δ_C 56.2, 56.2, 56.2, 61.8; a methine at δ_H 3.90 (1H, m), 4.03 (1H, m), δ_C 47.9; a 1,2,3,4-tetrasubstituted phenyl ring moiety at δ_H 7.04 (1H, d, J = 9.1 Hz), 7.28 (1H, d, J = 9.1 Hz), δ_C 153.7, 148.4, 1131.5, 129.2, 128.8, 114.5; a 1,2,4,5-tetrasubstituted phenyl ring moiety at δ_H 6.57 (1H, s), 6.78 (1H, s), δ_C 151.8, 147.9, 131.4, 121.9, 110.6, 110.6; a carbonyl at δ_C 188.4; and an unsaturated system at δ_H 8.20 (1H, d, J = 13.0 Hz), 6.87 (1H, dd, J = 13.0, 2.7 Hz), 6.74 (1H, d, J = 2.7 Hz), δ_C 168.4, 148.8, 134.9, 133.6, 133.5.

Table 1. ^{1}H and ^{13}C NMR data for mahimbrine A (400/100 MHz, in CDCl$_3$).

Position	δ_H	δ_C	Position	δ_H	δ_C
1		168.4	1'		148.4
3	4.03, 3.90, m	47.9	2'		153.7
4	2.91, m	25.8	3'	7.04, d (9.1)	114.5
4a		131.4	4'	7.28, d (9.1)	128.8
5	6.78, s	110.6	4'a		129.2
6		151.8	5'		148.8
7		147.9	6'	6.74, d (2.7)	133.5
8	6.57, s	110.6	7'		188.4
8a		121.9	8'	6.87, dd (13.0, 2.7)	134.9
6-OCH$_3$	3.94, s	56.2	9'	8.20, d (13.0)	133.6
7-OCH$_3$	3.60, s	56.2	9'a		131.5
1'-OCH$_3$	3.93, s	61.8			
2'-OCH$_3$	3.93, s	56.2			

The obvious HMBC correlations (Figure 2) from H-3 to C-1, C-4a, H-4 to C-5, C-4a, C-8a, H-5 to C-4, C-7, C-8a, H-8 to C-1, C-4a, C-6, OCH$_3$ to C-6 and OCH$_3$ to C-7 evidenced the presence of a dihydroisoquinoline unit with two methoxyl groups located at C-6 and C-7, respectively. The HMBC correlations of H-9' to C-7' (δ_C 188.4), C-4'a, H-8' to C-6', C-9'a (δ_C 131.5), and H-6' to C-4'a (δ_C 129.2), C-8'a, established the presence of a tropolone moiety, which was further verified by the vicinal coupling constants of H-8'/H-9' (J = 13.0 Hz) [9]. Moreover, the HMBC correlations of H-9' to C-1', C-4'a, H-4' to C-2', C-5', C-9'a confirmed the tropolone moiety and 1,2,3,4-tetrasubstituted phenyl ring moiety connected via a bridged bond at C-4'a and C-9'a. Similarly, two methoxyl groups at C-1' and C-2' were also assigned. The HMBC correlations of H-6' to C-1, C-4'a and H-4' to C-5 indicated that the dihydroisoquinoline unit and benzotropolone unit were connected to each other by C-1 and C-5'. Thus, the final structure of this compound was determined and named mahimbrine A.

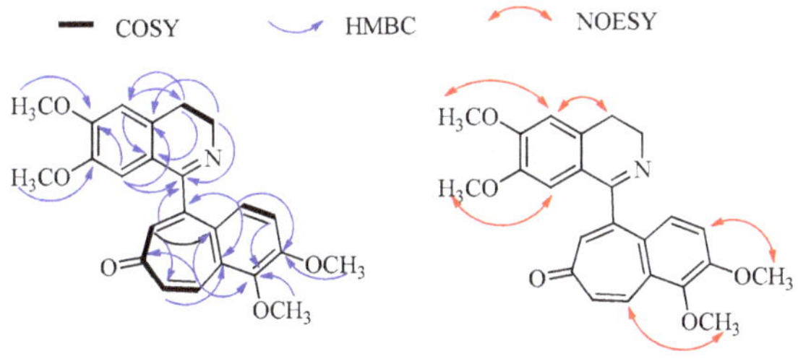

Figure 2. Key COSY, HMBC and NOESY correlations of mahimbrine A.

2.2. Plausible Biogenetic Pathway

A plausible biogenetic pathway for mahimbrine A was postulated (Scheme 1). As a precursor, naphthylacetic acid and dopamine via condensation reaction to give an amide intermediate **1** [10], which subsequently undergoes a Bischler-Napieralski reaction to generate intermediate **2** [11]. Intermediate **2** is then oxidized to yield intermediate **3** [12]. Intermediate **3** can spontaneously convert to its enol form. This enol intermediate then undergoes ring expansion rearrangement to give intermediate **4** [13], which is finally methylated to get mahimbrine A.

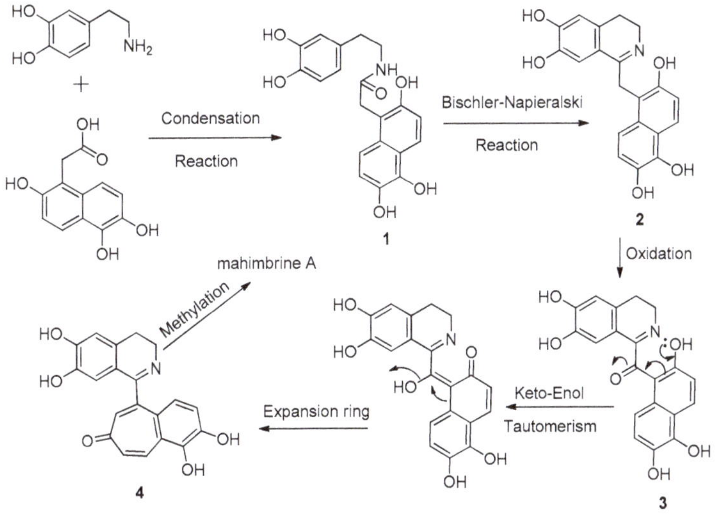

Scheme 1. Proposed Biogenetic Pathway of mahimbrine A.

2.3. Antimicrobial Activity

The antimicrobial activity of mahimbrine A was evaluated against four gram-positive bacterial strains *Staphylococcus aureus* ATCC 6538, *Micrococcus luteus* CMCC 28001, *Staphylococcus epidermidis* ATCC 12228, and *Bacillus subtilis* ATCC 21332; and four gram-negative bacteria *Pseudomonas aeruginosa* ATCC 27853, *Escherichia coli* ATCC 25922, *Salmonella typhimurium* ATCC 14028, and *Enterobacter aerogenes* ATCC 13048, by a microdilution titre technique; neither was active [14]. Gentamicin and streptomycin were used as positive controls. Discs containing 10 µL DMSO solutions were used as a negative control. All tests were performed in triplicate.

3. Experimental Section

3.1. General Procedures

UV spectra were recorded on a Perkin-Elmer Lambda 35 UV-VIS spectrophotometer (Perkin-Elmer, Waltham, MA, USA). IR spectra were measured on a PerkinElmer one FT-IR spectrometer (KBr) (Perkin-Elmer, Waltham, MA, USA). 1D and 2D-NMR spectra were recorded on a Bruker-Ascend-400 or an Agilent DD2400-MR instrument using TMS as the internal reference. HR-ESI-MS spectra were measured on a LTQ Orbitrap XL mass spectrometer (Thermo Scientific, Waltham, MA, USA). Column chromatography was performed using silica gel (300–400 mesh, Qingdao marine Chemical Ltd., Qingdao, China). Semi-preparative HPLC was performed on LC3000 system (Beijing ChuangXingTongHeng Science And Technology Co., Ltd., Beijing, China) equipped with an ODS column (5 μm, i.d. 10 mm × 250 mm, YMC). Original raw data of 1D, 2D NMR spectra and HR-ESI-MS of mahimbrine A are available in the supplementary materials.

3.2. Plant Material

The plant was collected from Loushanguan in Zunyi City, People's Republic of China, in October 2013, and identified as *Mahonia imbricata* by Prof. Jian-Wen Yang, Zunyi Medical University. A voucher specimen (20131020) was deposited with the Herbarium of the School of Pharmacy, Zunyi Medical University.

3.3. Extraction and Isolation

The air-dried and finely ground stems of *Mahonia imbricata* (30 kg) were extracted with 90% ethanol for three times at room temperature (5 days each). The ethanol extract was evaporated under reduced pressure to get a crude extract (2 kg), which was further suspended in acidic water (pH 3–4) and then filtered to obtain the filtrate. The filtrate was alkalized to pH 9–10 and extracted successively with $CHCl_3$ and n-BuOH (each 3 times), respectively. The $CHCl_3$ extract was subjected to silica gel column chromatography (80 mm × 600 mm, 1400 g, 300–400 mesh), eluted with a gradient of $CHCl_3$/MeOH (v/v = 100:1–1:100) to afford ten fractions (A–J). Fraction C was separated by Sephadex LH-20 column chromatography ($CHCl_3$/MeOH = 1:1) and divided into 15 subfractionses (fraction A.1–A.15). Mahimbrine A (3.8 mg) was obtained from fraction A.6 by sempipreparative HPLC (MeOH/H_2O = 55:45, flow rate 4 mL/min).

3.4. Spectral Data

Mahimbrine A: brown gum; UV (CH_3OH): 230 (2.68), 288 (2.43); IR (KBr): 3434, 2920, 1633, 1590, 1512, 1384, 1292, 1026, 810; ^1H and ^{13}C NMR data, Table 1. HR-ESI-MS: m/z 406.1632 [M + H]$^+$, $C_{24}H_{24}NO_5^+$, calcd. 406.1649; m/z 811.3226 [2M + H]$^+$, calcd. 811.3225.

4. Conclusions

In conclusion, mahimbrine A has been isolated from the endemic plant of *Mahonia imbricate* and its chemical structure has been elucidated. It displays an interesting structure with a dihydroisoquinoline moiety bound to a rare benzotropolone ring system. The structure of mahimbrine A was elucidated by HR-ESI-MS, 1D, 2D NMR and a biosynthetic pathway was proposed. Mahimbrine A did not show antimicrobial activity at the tested concentration of 1 mg/mL. The interesting structural architecture of this natural product might find further applications.

Supplementary Materials: 1D, 2D NMR spectra and HR-ESI-MS of mahimbrine A are available online.

Author Contributions: M.-S.Z. conceived and designed the experiments; Y.D. isolation and purification of mahimbrine A from *Mahonia imbricata*; S.-B.F. performed the biological activity tests. D.-L.G. characterization of 2D NMR spectra; S.-J.X. identification of mahimbrine A and writing of the manuscript.

Acknowledgments: This work was financially supported by the National Natural Sciences Foundation of China (No. 31560102), and the United Fund of Guizhou Province, Zunyi Medical University and Zunyi City (QKHJ-LKZ [2010] 26).

Conflicts of Interest: The authors declare no conflict of interest.

References

1. Ying, J.S.; Cheng, D.Z. *Flora of China*; Science Press: Beijing, China, 2001; Volume 20, p. 242.
2. He, J.M.; Mu, Q. The medicinal uses of the genus *Mahonia* in traditional Chinese medicine: An ethnopharmacological, phytochemical and pharmacological review. *J. Ethnopharmacol.* **2015**, *175*, 668–683. [CrossRef] [PubMed]
3. Müller, K.; Ziereis, K. The antipsoriatic *Mahonia aquifolium* and its active constituents; I. Pro- and antioxidant properties and inhibition of 5-lipoxygenase. *Planta Med.* **1994**, *60*, 421–424. [CrossRef] [PubMed]
4. Račková, L.; Májeková, M.; Košťálová, D.; Štefek, M. Antiradical and antioxidant activities of alkaloids isolated from *Mahonia aquifolium*. Structural aspects. *Bioorg. Med. Chem.* **2004**, *12*, 4709–4715. [CrossRef] [PubMed]
5. Hsieh, T.J.; Chia, Y.C.; Wu, Y.C.; Chen, Z.Y. Chemical Constituents from the Stems of *Mahonia japonica*. *J. Chin. Chem. Soc.* **2004**, *51*, 443–446. [CrossRef]
6. Xiao, S.J.; Lei, X.X.; Xia, B.; Xiao, H.P.; He, D.H.; Fang, D.M.; Qi, H.Y.; Chen, F.; Ding, L.S.; Zhou, Y. Two novel norlignans from *Gymnotheca chinensis*. *Tetrahedron Lett.* **2014**, *55*, 2869–2871. [CrossRef]
7. Xiao, S.J.; Lei, X.X.; Xia, B.; Xu, D.Q.; Xiao, H.P.; Xu, H.X.; Chen, F.; Ding, L.S.; Zhou, Y. Two novel polycyclic spiro lignans from *Gymnotheca involucrate*. *Tetrahedron Lett.* **2014**, *55*, 5949–5951. [CrossRef]
8. He, D.H.; Ding, L.S.; Xu, H.X.; Lei, X.X.; Xiao, H.P.; Zhou, Y. Gymnothelignans A–O: Conformation and absolute configuration analyses of lignans bearing tetrahydrofuran from *Gymnotheca chinensis*. *J. Org. Chem.* **2012**, *77*, 8435–8443. [CrossRef] [PubMed]
9. Kuroyanagi, M.; Shirota, O.; Sekita, S.; Nakane, T. Transannular cyclization of (4S,5S)-germacrone-4, 5-epoxide into guaiane and secoguaiane-type sesquiterpenes. *Nat. Prod. Comm.* **2012**, *7*, 441–446.
10. Tam, E.K.W.; Liu, L.Y.; Chen, A.Q. 2-Furanylboronic acid as an effective catalyst for the direct amidation of carboxylic acids at room temperature. *Eur. J. Org. Chem.* **2015**, *2015*, 1100–1107. [CrossRef]
11. Nimgirawath, S.; Lorpitthaya, R.; Wanbanjob, A.; Taechowisan, T.; Shen, Y.M. Total synthesis and the biological activities of (+/−)-norannuradhapurine. *Molecules* **2008**, *14*, 89–101. [CrossRef] [PubMed]
12. Daniel, L.C.; Paresh, M.T.; Matthew, F.B.; Badawi, M.M. Chiral auxiliary mediated pictet-spengler reactions: Asymmetric syntheses of (−)-laudanosine, (+)-glaucine and (−)-xylopinine. *Tetrahedron* **1997**, *53*, 16327–16340.
13. Xin, M.; Bugg, T.D.H. Biomimetic formation of 2-tropolones by dioxygenase-catalysed ring expansion of substituted 2,4-cyclohexadienones. *Chembiochem* **2010**, *11*, 272–276. [CrossRef] [PubMed]
14. Cheng, D.D.; Zhang, Y.Y.; Gao, D.M.; Zhang, H.M. Antibacterial and anti-inflammatory activities of extract and fractions from *Pyrrosia petiolosa* (Christ et Bar.) Ching. *J. Ethnopharmacol.* **2014**, *155*, 1300–1305. [CrossRef] [PubMed]

Sample Availability: Samples of the compound mahimbrine A are available from the authors.

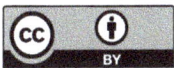

© 2018 by the authors. Licensee MDPI, Basel, Switzerland. This article is an open access article distributed under the terms and conditions of the Creative Commons Attribution (CC BY) license (http://creativecommons.org/licenses/by/4.0/).

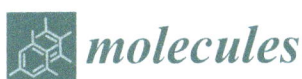

Article

Native *V. californicum* Alkaloid Combinations Induce Differential Inhibition of Sonic Hedgehog Signaling

Matthew W. Turner [1,2], Roberto Cruz [2], Jordan Elwell [2], John French [2], Jared Mattos [2] and Owen M. McDougal [2,*]

[1] Biomolecular Sciences Graduate Programs, Boise State University, 1910 University Drive, Boise, ID 83725, USA; matthewturner1@u.boisestate.edu
[2] Department of Chemistry and Biochemistry, Boise State University, 1910 University Drive, Boise, ID 83725, USA; rcruzromero@usbr.gov (R.C.); jordanelwell@u.boisestate.edu (J.E.); johnfrench@u.boisestate.edu (J.F.); jaredmattos@gmail.com (J.M.)
* Correspondence: owenmcdougal@boisestate.edu; Tel.: +1-208-426-3964

Received: 28 July 2018; Accepted: 30 August 2018; Published: 1 September 2018

Abstract: *Veratrum californicum* is a rich source of steroidal alkaloids such as cyclopamine, a known inhibitor of the Hedgehog (Hh) signaling pathway. Here we provide a detailed analysis of the alkaloid composition of *V. californicum* by plant part through quantitative analysis of cyclopamine, veratramine, muldamine and isorubijervine in the leaf, stem and root/rhizome of the plant. To determine whether additional alkaloids in the extracts contribute to Hh signaling inhibition, the concentrations of these four alkaloids present in extracts were replicated using commercially available standards, followed by comparison of extracts to alkaloid standard mixtures for inhibition of Hh signaling using Shh-Light II cells. Alkaloid combinations enhanced Hh signaling pathway antagonism compared to cyclopamine alone, and significant differences were observed in the Hh pathway inhibition between the stem and root/rhizome extracts and their corresponding alkaloid standard mixtures, indicating that additional alkaloids present in these extracts are capable of inhibiting Hh signaling.

Keywords: hedgehog signaling; *Veratrum californicum*; cyclopamine; HPLC-MS; Shh-Light II cells

---

1. Introduction

The Hedgehog (Hh) signaling pathway plays a vital role in embryonic development [1,2]. In mammals, the Hh signaling pathway consists of the secreted ligands Sonic hedgehog (Shh), Desert hedgehog (Dhh) and Indian hedgehog (Ihh); the transmembrane receptor proteins Patched (Ptch1 and Ptch2), the transmembrane signal transducer Smoothened (Smo), and the Gli transcription factors (Gli1, Gli2, Gli3) [3]. In the absence of Hh ligands, Ptch1 prevents the translocation of Smo to the primary cilia, thereby inhibiting the nuclear localization of Gli and suppressing transcriptional activity. Upon binding of Hh ligands to Ptch1, Smo suppression is abolished and downstream pathway activity proceeds, resulting in nuclear translocation and activation of Gli. Although the Hh ligand proteins all act as morphogens and have similar physiological effects, each Hh ligand performs specialized functions due to the spatial and temporal differences in their expression [4]. The Shh signaling pathway is a major regulator of various processes, including cell differentiation and proliferation, and tissue polarity [2,5]. Inhibition of Shh signaling is widely researched because aberrant Shh signaling is a hallmark of many cancers [6–8], including prostate, gallbladder, pancreatic, and basal cell carcinoma [9–12]. Basal cell carcinoma (BCC) is the most common human cancer and is driven predominantly by the hyperactivation of the Hh pathway [13–15]. For this reason, a significant number of BCC patients experience a clinical benefit from vismodegib (Erivedge®), a Smo inhibitor approved by the US Food and Drug Administration (FDA) to treat metastatic or reoccurring BCC [16]. In phase 2 trials in BCC patients, a majority experienced clinical benefit with vismodegib treatment that included

30% of metastatic BCC patients demonstrating a 30% decrease in visible tumor dimension, and 64% experiencing stable tumor size. In patients with locally advanced BCC, 43% showed a 30% decrease in visible tumor dimension, and 38% demonstrating stable tumor size. However, development of resistance to vismodegib in up to 20% of advanced BCC patients within one year of treatment represents a significant limitation [15,17]. Various studies have implicated amino acid mutations in the vismodegib binding-site in Smo as a mechanism underlying acquired resistance [15,18,19]. Due to adverse side effects and the potential for acquired resistance to vismodegib there is a continued need to investigate novel compounds that target the Hh signaling pathway, and identification of natural products that act as Hh signaling inhibitors continues to be investigated [20–23].

Veratrum californicum (V. californicum) is native to the western United States and is rich in steroidal alkaloids, including cyclopamine, veratramine, isorubijervine and muldamine [6,24]. Of these alkaloids, the most notorious is cyclopamine, a teratogen antagonist of the Shh signaling pathway [25]. Interest in V. californicum arose in the 1950s when unsettling high incidences of craniofacial birth defects in lambs were observed by shepherds in Idaho. Numerous review articles have recounted the history of scientific interest in V. californicum, the efforts undertaken by researchers at the Poisonous Plant Research Laboratory in Logan, UT to identify and validate the causative agents of the observed birth defects, and the chronological order of the isolation and structural elucidation of individual steroidal alkaloids [6,26,27]. However, few reports in the literature have used modern, highly sensitive analytical techniques to examine the full array of steroidal alkaloids in V. californicum [28]. Our lab has implemented extraction techniques of the root and rhizome of V. californicum aimed at isolating these steroidal alkaloids and characterizing their bioactivity towards Hh signaling using Shh-Light II cell assays [28,29]. In the current study, we used ethanol extraction of the leaves, stems and roots of V. californicum to determine if alkaloid ratios in the extract yield synergistic amplification of Hh signaling suppression as compared to traditional single alkaloid activity. The extracts were characterized using liquid chromatography and high resolution electrospray ionization time of flight tandem mass spectrometry, and their biological activity was tested using Shh-Light II cells. The concentrations of cyclopamine, veratramine, isorubijervine and muldamine were determined, and mixtures of commercially available standards were prepared in the same ratios as found in the extracts derived from the leaf, stem and root/rhizome of V. californicum. We sought to test whether well-characterized steroidal alkaloids, at ratios consistent with native plant content, exhibited a synergistic effect to inhibit Hh pathway signaling commensurate with plant extract. Additionally, we sought to determine if additional alkaloids present in the V. californicum contribute to Hh signaling inhibition. Earlier investigations of V. californicum alkaloids may have failed to identify less abundant alkaloids that are biologically significant and potentially valuable novel Hh pathway signaling antagonists.

2. Results

2.1. Qualitative Comparison of V. californicum Alkaloids by Plant Part

Qualitative variation is observed in the alkaloid composition of V. californicum by plant part. The alkaloid profiles of the extracts from the leaf, stem and root/rhizome of V. californicum are shown in Figure 1a–c. Identification of each alkaloid peak was achieved by high resolution mass spectrometry and verified by elution time compared to commercially available standards. Data for the most prominent peaks labelled in Figure 1a–c including retention time, m/z, molecular formula (MF) and alkaloid identity are summarized in Table 1. Mass spectra showing the m/z for each alkaloid used to estimate molecular formulas listed in Table 1 are shown in Supplemental Figure S1.

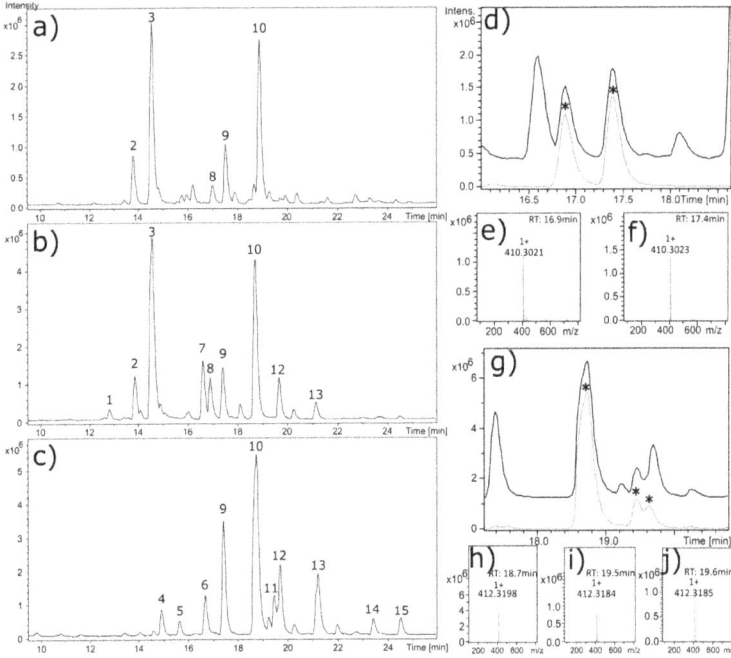

Figure 1. Alkaloid chromatograms for biomass extracts from the (**a**) leaf, (**b**) stem, and (**c**) root/rhizome of *V. californicum*. Common and unique alkaloids identified by MS are observed in each extract. Labelled peaks correspond to the data summarized in Table 1. Additional observed peaks that are not labelled did not have molecular formulas consistent with jervine-type alkaloids. Extracted ion chromatograms (EIC) are shown in (**d**,**g**) demonstrating the presence of veratramine and cyclopamine isomers in stem and root/rhizome extracts, respectively. The total ion chromatogram is shown in (**d**) for the stem extract (black) and EIC (grey) generated using the m/z window 410.3023 ± 0.01. The mass spectra for the peaks indicated by * in (**d**) are shown in (**e**,**f**). The total ion chromatogram is shown in (**g**) for the root extract (black) and the EIC (grey) generated m/z window 412.3186 ± 0.02. The mass spectra for the peaks indicated by * in (**g**) are shown in (**h**–**j**).

Table 1. Summary of the data corresponding to peaks identified in Figure 1a–c. N/A is used to designate alkaloids with identity not available; N/A[1] may be etioline or another isomer of isorubijervine; N/A[2] may be an isomer of veratramine, and N/A[3] may be an isomer of cyclopamine.

Peak	Retention Time (min)	m/z	Molecular Formula	Alkaloid
1	12.8	576.3836	$C_{33}H_{53}NO_7$	N/A
2	13.9	572.3530	$C_{33}H_{49}NO_7$	Veratrosine
3	14.6	574.3699	$C_{33}H_{51}NO_7$	Cycloposine
4	14.9	414.3337	$C_{27}H_{43}NO_2$	N/A [1]
5	15.7	430.3282	$C_{27}H_{43}NO_3$	N/A
6	16.6	428.3136	$C_{27}H_{41}NO_3$	N/A
7	16.7	576.3846	$C_{33}H_{53}NO_7$	N/A
8	16.9	410.3021	$C_{27}H_{39}NO_2$	Veratramine
9	17.4	410.3023	$C_{27}H_{39}NO_2$	N/A [2]
10	18.7	412.3186	$C_{27}H_{41}NO_2$	Cyclopamine
11	19.5	412.3184	$C_{27}H_{41}NO_2$	N/A [3]
12	19.7	414.3342	$C_{27}H_{43}NO_2$	Isorubijervine
13	21.1	458.3587	$C_{29}H_{47}NO_3$	Muldamine
14	23.4	400.3550	$C_{27}H_{45}NO$	N/A
15	24.5	456.3446	$C_{29}H_{45}NO_3$	N/A

Cyclopamine (Peak 10, m/z 412.3186) and veratramine (Peak 9, m/z 410.3023) were observed in each of the three plant part extracts. Alkaloids present in both the stem and leaf extracts include cycloposine (Peak 3, m/z 574.3699) and veratrosine (Peak 4, m/z 572.3530), which are glycosylated cyclopamine and veratramine, respectively. Peak 1 is a glycosylated alkaloid observed only in stem extract, with an m/z of 576.3836, corresponding to molecular formula $C_{33}H_{53}NO_7$. In the stem and root/rhizome extracts, isorubijervine (Peak 12, m/z 414.3342) and muldamine (Peak 13, m/z 458.3587) are both observed.

Peaks 4, 5, 6, 14 and 15 in Figure 1c correspond to unique alkaloids present only in the root/rhizome extract. These alkaloids have m/z of 414.3337, 430.3282, 428.3136, 400.3550 and 456.3446 and correspond to the estimated molecular formulas of $C_{27}H_{43}NO_2$, $C_{27}H_{43}NO_3$, $C_{27}H_{41}NO_3$, $C_{27}H_{45}NO$ and $C_{29}H_{45}NO_3$, respectively. Potential cyclopamine isomers were observed in the root extract, with a m/z consistent with cyclopamine observed to elute with three distinct retention times. Figure 1g shows the extracted ion chromatogram (EIC) for cyclopamine generated using the m/z window 412.3186 ± 0.02, and the corresponding mass spectra are shown in Figure 1h–j. Figure 1d shows the EIC for veratramine using the m/z window 410.3023 ± 0.01, and the corresponding mass spectra are shown in Figure 1e,f.

2.2. Quantitative Analysis of V. californicum Alkaloids

Quantification of cyclopamine, veratramine, isorubijervine and muldamine in alkaloid extracts were determined using charged aerosol detection and calibration curves generated from commercially available standards, with values of R^2 greater than 0.99. Extractions were preformed three times, and alkaloid concentrations are shown by plant part in Table 2 as mg of each alkaloid extracted per g of initial biomass ± the standard deviation of the concentration observed in triplicate quantities. The quantity of cyclopamine was determined to be 0.21 ± 0.02 mg/g, 3.23 ± 0.16 mg/g, and 7.38 ± 0.08 mg/g for the leaf, stem and root/rhizome, respectively.

Table 2. Quantification of cyclopamine, veratramine, muldamine and isorubijervine by plant part. Alkaloid quantities are reported as mg of alkaloid per g of plant biomass.

Plant Part	Cyclopamine	Veratramine	Muldamine	Isorubijervine
Leaf	0.21 ± 0.02	0.09 ± 0.01	Not Detected	Not Detected
Stem	3.23 ± 0.16	1.33 ± 0.13	0.36 ± 0.06	1.00 ± 0.08
Root/Rhizome	7.38 ± 0.08	3.07 ± 0.14	3.47 ± 0.23	2.92 ± 0.09

2.3. Bioactivity Evaluation of Combined Standards and Plant Extracts

Alkaloid standard mixtures were created using commercially available standards in the same ratios as observed in the three plant parts. HPLC was used to validate that the alkaloid standard mixtures matched the concentrations of the ethanolic extract, as is shown for the root/rhizome extract and root standard mixture in Supplemental Figure S2. The bioactivity of these alkaloid standard mixtures were quantified using Shh-Light II cells, and compared to cyclopamine alone at the same concentration, and to V. californicum extracts derived from leaf, stem, and root/rhizome of the plant. The treatment conditions evaluating Hh signaling inhibition in Shh-Light II cells are summarized in Supplemental Table S1 with extracts and alkaloid standard mixtures normalized to cyclopamine concentrations of 0.5 and 0.1 µM, referred to as "high concentration" and "low concentration" treatments herein. The results of the biological assays are shown in Figure 2. There is no significant difference between cyclopamine, the alkaloid standard mixtures, and the plant extracts at high concentration treatments shown in Figure 2a. In the low concentration treatments shown in Figure 2b, there is no significant difference observed between cyclopamine standard, and the leaf standard mixture or the leaf extract, indicating that the addition of 0.04 µM veratramine in the standard mixture did not enhance Hh signaling inhibition. No difference is observed between the leaf extract at low concentration and the corresponding combined standard cocktail.

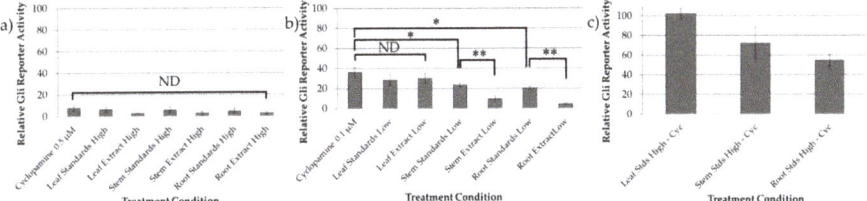

Figure 2. Bioactivity data for cyclopamine alone, the alkaloid standard mixtures, and the plant extracts at (**a**) high concentration (0.5 µM) and (**b**) low concentration (0.1 µM). No significant difference was observed between treatment conditions at high concentration. Statistically noteworthy differences were observed in the low concentration treatments, and * indicates $p < 0.05$, and ** indicates $p < 0.01$. The inhibitory activity of veratramine, isorubijervine and muldamine in the absence of cyclopamine in the same concentrations as the high concentration treatment conditions is shown in (**c**).

The alkaloid standard mixtures of the stem and root/rhizome samples were significantly different ($p < 0.05$) than cyclopamine alone at the same concentration, with relative Gli-reporter activity determined to 23.56 ± 1.86% and 20.59 ± 1.50% for the stem and root/rhizome, respectively, compared to 36.31 ± 5.13% for 0.1 µM cyclopamine. The inhibitory activity of these compounds was tested in the absence of cyclopamine in the same concentrations as the high concentration treatment conditions, and the results are shown Figure 2c. No Hh inhibition was shown for the leaf standards mixture minus cyclopamine (0.2 µM veratramine), indicating that veratramine does not inhibit the Hh signaling pathway. Modest Hh inhibition was demonstrated for the stem and root/rhizome standard mixtures minus cyclopamine, indicating that isorubijervine and muldamine exhibit Hh antagonism. There is a significant difference ($p < 0.01$) between the stem and root/rhizome extracts and their corresponding alkaloid standard mixtures, signifying that additional alkaloids present in the extracts are capable of inhibiting Hh signaling.

3. Discussion

The current investigation sought to achieve three objectives. The first was to provide a detailed analysis of the alkaloid composition of *V. californicum* based on plant part by performing a quantitative comparison of the alkaloids present in the leaf, stem and root/rhizome of the plant. The second was to evaluate the potential synergistic activity of cyclopamine, veratramine, isorubijervine and muldamine at ratios consistent with alkaloids present in three plant parts, and determine if the alkaloid combinations resulted in more effective Hh pathway antagonism than cyclopamine alone. The third was to determine if additional alkaloids present in the extracts contribute to Hh signaling inhibition by comparing the inhibitory potential of the plant extracts to alkaloid standard mixtures with identical concentrations of cyclopamine, veratramine, isorubijervine and muldamine.

Qualitative differences were observed in the alkaloid composition of *V. californicum* by plant part. Using high resolution mass spectrometry, we identified alkaloids that have previously been unreported for *V. californicum*. The molecular formula and mass of Peak 1 is consistent with that expected for glycosylated isorubijervine or etioline. Glycosylate etioline has previously been reported in the root of *Solanum spirale* [30]. Additional investigation beyond the scope of the current project is required to definitely determine the identify of this alkaloid in *V. californicum*. Etioline is an intermediary in the biosynthetic pathway of cyclopamine, and its presence in the extract may be expected [6]. Peak 4, observed solely in the root/rhizome extract has an m/z and predicted molecular formula consistent with etioline. In this study, potential cyclopamine isomers (see Figure 1g) were observed in the root/rhizome extract analyzed by LC-MS. One of these potential cyclopamine isomers may be dihydroveratramine, which has previously been identified in *Veratrum album* by Wilson, et al. [31]. However, the relative retention time between dihydroveratramine and cyclopamine, observed by Wilson, et al., does not support this conclusion, because dihydroveratramine (RT: 13.66 min) was observed to elute prior to cyclopamine (RT: 15.09 min), whereas the purported cyclopamine isomer observed in this study elutes after cyclopamine (see Table 1) under similar HPLC conditions. No naturally occurring isomers of cyclopamine have been previously observed in *V. californicum*.

In Shh-Light II cells using the Dual-Glo® Luciferase Assay System, we evaluated the inhibition of Hh signaling of cyclopamine alone, combinations of alkaloid standards, and the inhibitory potential of extracts from each plant part. As shown in Figure 2a, there is no significant difference between cyclopamine, the alkaloid standard mixtures, and the plant extracts at high concentration treatments. There are trends that indicate enhanced inhibition of alkaloid standard mixtures and extracts compared to cyclopamine alone, but these do not amount to statistically significant differences. The reason for this result may be due to low levels of Gli reporter activity observed in each treatment. However, as demonstrated in Figure 2b, it was determined that addition of 0.1 µM muldamine, veratramine and isorubijervine enhance Hh signaling inhibition significantly when compared to cyclopamine alone, as demonstrated by the stem and root/rhizome standard mixtures compared to cyclopamine alone. Addition of veratramine to cyclopamine does not enhance Hh signaling inhibition as demonstrated by the leaf standard mixture compared to solely cyclopamine. By replicating concentrations of cyclopamine, veratramine, isorubijervine and muldamine observed in plant extracts using commercially available standards and comparing the inhibitory potential of the plant extracts to alkaloid standard mixtures, we determined that additional alkaloids present in the crude stem and root/rhizome extracts inhibit Hh signaling. The alkaloids present in the leaf extract include cycloposine, veratrosine, cyclopamine, veratramine, and the potential veratramine isomer labeled Peak 8 in Figure 1. No difference is observed between the leaf extract at low concentration and the corresponding combined standard mixture. This result indicates that cycloposine, veratrosine and Peak 8 do not contribute to Hh signaling inhibition in this model system. However, it has been proposed that hydrolysis of the glycosidic linkage in glycosylated alkaloids during digestion contributed to the teratogenic effects of *V. californicum* alkaloids when consumed by foraging sheep [32]. Furthermore, no significant difference is observed between cyclopamine alone, the leaf standard mixture or the leaf extract, indicating that the addition of 0.04 µM veratramine in the standard mixture, or the additional alkaloids present in the leaf extract did not enhance Hh signaling inhibition. We observed a significant difference between the alkaloid standard mixtures of the stem and root/rhizome samples and cyclopamine alone. This indicates the addition of veratramine, isorubijervine and muldamine enhance Hh inhibition. However, the modest enhancement of Hh inhibition seems to be additive rather than synergistic, with the addition of these alkaloids providing additional, albeit more weakly inhibitory compounds. No Hh inhibition was demonstrated for 0.2 µM veratramine in the leaf standard minus cyclopamine treatment, indicating veratramine does not inhibit the Hh signaling pathway. This corroborates feeding trials in which veratramine was shown to cause teratogenic malformations in sheep distinct from cyclopia, such as hypermobility of the knee joints leading to bow-legged lambs unable to stand [33]. The stem and root/rhizome standard mixtures containing veratramine, isorubijervine and muldamine indicate that muldamine and/or isorubijervine inhibit the Hh pathway. Muldamine has been shown to result in craniofacial defects in hamsters in feeding studies that may be attributed to interruption of normal Hh signaling [34]. Further investigation to isolate, characterize, and assess the bioactivity of individual, less abundant alkaloids present in the stem and root/rhizome extracts is underway.

4. Materials and Methods

4.1. Chemicals and Solvents

Cyclopamine (>99% purity) was purchased from Alfa Aesar (Ward Hill, MA, USA), veratramine (>98% purity) was purchased from Abcam Biotechnology Company (Cambridge, UK), and isorubijervine (99% purity) and muldamine (99% purity) were purchased from Logan Natural Products (Plano, TX, USA). The purity of the reference standards was verified in house by HPLC-MS. Extraction and purification solvents, 95% ethanol, ammonium hydroxide and chloroform were purchased from Fisher Scientific (Pittsburgh, PA, USA). High pressure liquid chromatography (HPLC) mobile phases included 0.1% formic acid and HPLC grade acetonitrile (>99% purity, Fisher Scientific).

4.2. Sample Extraction and Preparation

A complete specimen of *V. californicum* was harvested in the Boise National Forest, Idaho at an elevation of 2134 m. The leaf, stem and roots/rhizomes of the plant were separated, and all plant parts were cut into smaller pieces to fit into quart size sealable bags. The specimens were placed in a cooler on a bed of ice for transportation. The biomass was collected at a late stage in the plant's life cycle; the plant had noticeable brown edges along its leaves and top indicating annual deterioration of above ground material in preparation for winter. Within two hours and upon arrival in the lab, the plant material was chopped into 2 cm segments and dried for 14 h using a LabConco Freezone 4.5 freeze drying unit (Labconco Corporation, Kansas City, MO, USA), followed by storage at −20 °C. The biomass was flash frozen in liquid nitrogen, and pulverized into a fine powder using a mortar and pestle. Approximately 2.0 g of powdered biomass was added to a 250 mL round bottom flask followed by 100 mL of 95% ethanol. The resultant slurry was sonicated for 1 h and then agitated for 24 h on a stir plate. The biomass was removed by vacuum filtration (Whatman filter paper, 0.45 μm), and solvent removed by rotary evaporation. The dried crude extract was dissolved in 10 mL of ethanol, and the solution was warmed to 40 °C and sonicated to achieve complete dissolution. Addition of 35% aqueous ammonia achieved alkaline solvent conditions (pH ≥ 10). The aqueous alkaline solution was added directly to a supported liquid extraction (SLE) column (Chem Elut, Agilent, Santa Clara, CA, USA) and allowed to adsorb for 10 min, followed by elution of alkaloids with chloroform (3 × 10 mL) using a vacuum manifold set to a pressure of 2 mbar. The chloroform fractions were combined, filtered, and evaporated to dryness. All samples were dissolved in 1 mL ethanol as a mixture of alkaloids.

4.3. Alkaloid Quantification

The concentrations of cyclopamine, veratramine, isorubijervine and muldamine in alkaloid extracts were determined using an UltiMate 3000 HPLC (Thermo Scientific, Waltham, MA, USA) equipped with a Corona Veo RS charge aerosol detector (CAD) and MSQ Plus mass spectrometer (MS). HPLC separation of alkaloids was achieved using a Thermo Acclaim 120 C_{18} column (2.1 × 150 mm, 3 μm), and mobile phases consisting of 0.1% formic acid (*v/v*) in water (Buffer A) and 0.1% formic acid (*v/v*) in acetonitrile (Buffer B) with a flow rate of 0.3 mL/min. A linear gradient method beginning at 95% Buffer A and 5% Buffer B, up to 60% Buffer B over a 25 min run time achieved desired separation of alkaloids from the extracts. Cyclopamine, veratramine, isorubijervine and muldamine standards were used to create a calibration curve at concentrations of 0.1, 0.5, 1.0, 5.0 and 10.0 mM with detection recorded by a CAD with the power function set to pA 1.70. Calibration curves were generated in triplicate for each alkaloid at each of the five alkaloid concentrations. The quantity of these alkaloids were determined from the alkaloid mixtures obtained from the leaf, stem and root extracts in triplicate.

4.4. Alkaloid Identification

In order to identify the steroidal alkaloids in *V. californicum* leaf, stem and root/rhizome extracts, samples were analyzed by HPLC-MS, where the mass spectrometer was an ultra-high resolution Quadrupole Time of Flight (QTOF) instrument (Bruker maXis, Billerica, MA, USA). The electrospray ionization (ESI) source was operated under the following conditions: positive ion mode, 1.2 bar nebulizer pressure, 8 L/min flow of N_2 drying gas heated to a temperature of 200 °C, 3000 V to −500 V voltage between HV capillary and HV end-plate offset, mass range set from 80 to 800 *m/z*, and the quadrupole ion energy at 4.0 eV. Sodium formate was used to calibrate the system in this mass range of 80 to 800 *m/z*. HPLC separation was achieved using a XTerra MS C_{18} column, 3.5 μm, 2.1 × 150 mm

(Waters, Milford, MA, USA). The flow rate was 250 µL/min. The mobile phases were 5% acetonitrile and 0.1% formic acid in water (Buffer A) and acetonitrile and 0.1% formic acid (Buffer B). The linear gradient method was used to separate analytes starting at 5% Buffer B and increasing to 60% Buffer B over 25 min. A 1 µL sample injection was used. Data were analyzed with the Compass Data Analysis software package (Bruker Corporation).

4.5. Cell Culture

Shh-Light II cells (JHU-068) were maintained in Dulbecco's Modified Eagle Medium (DMEM) (Gibco, Carlsbad, CA, USA) supplemented with 0.4 mg/mL geneticin, 0.15 mg/mL Zeocin™ (Invitrogen, Carlsbad, CA, USA), and 10% bovine calf serum. The cells were grown at 37 °C in an atmosphere of 5% CO_2 in air and 100% relative humidity. This mouse embryonal NIH 3T3 cell line contains a stably transfected luciferase reporter with eight copies of the consensus Gli binding site [35]. Alkaloid treatment conditions were dissolved in ethanol and added to DMEM media containing 0.5% bovine calf serum.

4.6. Biological Assays

Cell density was determined using Trypan Blue (Stemcell Technologies, Vancouver, BC, Canada) and a hemocytometer. Shh-Light II cells were seeded in a 96-well plate with 10,000 cells per well, and grown to complete confluence in the media described above. When cells were confluent, the media was replaced with DMEM supplemented with 0.5% bovine calf serum, and treated with 0.1 ng of N-terminal mouse recombinant Shh (R&D Systems, Minneapolis, MN, USA) dissolved in DMEM, and select alkaloid treatment. In each experiment, the controls and treatment wells contained all vehicles, with a final ethanol concentration of 0.05%. Gli activity in the Shh-Light II cell line was assayed 48 h after treatment with Shh protein and select compounds using the Dual-Luciferase Reporter Assay System (Promega, Madison, WI, USA). The Gli-activity was measured by luminescence emitted from cells using a Synergy H1m Microplate reader (BioTek, Winooski, VT, USA). The Gli-activity determined in the biological assay is presented as a relative response ratio (RRR) as described in the Dual-Luciferase Reporter Assay System manual. Each experiment was performed three times.

Supplementary Materials: The following are available online; Supplementary S1–S2, Table S1.

Author Contributions: Conceptualization, O.M.M., M.W.T.; Biomass Acquisition, J.M., R.C., J.E.; Alkaloid Extractions, M.W.T., R.C., J.E.; LC-MS Analysis, M.W.T.; Bioactivity Assay, M.W.T., J.F.; Methodology, O.M.M., M.W.T.; Resources, O.M.M.; Data Curation, M.W.T.; Writing—Original Draft Preparation, M.W.T.; Writing—Review & Editing, O.M.M., M.W.T.; Supervision, O.M.M.; Funding Acquisition, O.M.M.

Funding: This research was funded by Institutional Development Awards (IDeA) from the National Institute of General Medical Sciences of the National Institutes of Health under Grants #P20GM103408 (INBRE) and P20GM109095 (COBRE in Matrix Biology), the National Science Foundation, Grants # 0619793 and #0923535; the MJ Murdock Charitable Trust, Idaho State Board of Education, and Research Corporation. Contents are solely the responsibility of the authors and do not necessarily represent the official views of NIH.

Acknowledgments: We also acknowledge support from the Biomolecular Research Centre at Boise State University.

Conflicts of Interest: The authors declare no conflict of interest.

References

1. Ingham, P.W. Hedgehog signaling in animal development: Paradigms and principles. *Gene Dev.* **2001**, *15*, 3059–3087. [CrossRef] [PubMed]
2. Rimkus, T.; Carpenter, R.; Qasem, S.; Chan, M.; Lo, H.W. Targeting the Sonic Hedgehog Signaling Pathway: Review of Smoothened and GLI Inhibitors. *Cancers* **2016**, *8*, 22. [CrossRef] [PubMed]
3. Finco, I.; Lapensee, C.R.; Krill, K.T.; Hammer, G.D. Hedgehog Signaling and Steroidogenesis. *Annu. Rev. Physiol.* **2015**, *77*, 105–129. [CrossRef] [PubMed]

4. Varjosalo, M.; Taipale, J. Hedgehog: Functions and mechanisms. *Gene Dev.* **2008**, *22*, 2454–2472. [CrossRef] [PubMed]
5. Pathi, S.; Pagan-Westphal, S.; Baker, D.P.; Garber, E.A.; Rayhorn, P.; Bumcrot, D.; Tabin, C.J.; Blake Pepinsky, R.; Williams, K.P. Comparative biological responses to human Sonic, Indian, and Desert hedgehog. *Mech. Dev.* **2001**, *106*, 107–117. [CrossRef]
6. Chandler, C.M.; Mcdougal, O.M. Medicinal history of North American. *Veratrum. Phytochem. Rev.* **2013**, *13*, 671–694. [CrossRef] [PubMed]
7. Onishi, H.; Katano, M. Hedgehog signaling pathway as a therapeutic target in various types of cancer. *Can. Sci.* **2011**, *102*, 1756–1760. [CrossRef] [PubMed]
8. Ok, C.Y.; Singh, R.R.; Vega, F. Aberrant Activation of the Hedgehog Signaling Pathway in Malignant Hematological Neoplasms. *Am. J. Pathol.* **2012**, *180*, 2–11. [CrossRef] [PubMed]
9. Wilkinson, S.E.; Furic, L.; Buchanan, G.; Larsson, O.; Pedersen, J.; Frydenberg, M.; Risbridger, G.P.; Taylor, R.A. Hedgehog signaling is active in human prostate cancer stroma and regulates proliferation and differentiation of adjacent epithelium. *Prostate* **2013**, *73*, 1810–1823. [CrossRef] [PubMed]
10. Matsushita, S.; Onishi, H.; Nakano, K.; Nagamatsu, I.; Imaizumi, A.; Hattori, M.; Oda, Y.; Tanaka, M.; Katano, M. Hedgehog pathway as a therapeutic target for gallbladder cancer. Immunohistochemical staining for Gli1 in gallbladder cancer. *Can. Sci.* **2014**, *105*. [CrossRef]
11. Onishi, H.; Kai, M.; Odate, S.; Iwasaki, H.; Morifuji, Y.; Ogino, T.; Morisaki, T.; Nakashima, Y.; Katano, M. Hypoxia activates the hedgehog signaling pathway in a ligand-independent manner by upregulation of Smo transcription in pancreatic cancer. *Can. Sci.* **2011**, *102*, 1144–1150. [CrossRef] [PubMed]
12. Wong, C.S.M.; Strange, R.C.; Lear, J.T. Basal cell carcinoma. *BMJ* **2003**, *327*, 794–798. [CrossRef] [PubMed]
13. Oro, A.E.; Higgins, K.M.; Hu, Z.; Bonifas, J.M.; Epstein, E.H.; Scott, M.P. Basal Cell Carcinomas in Mice Overexpressing Sonic Hedgehog. *Science* **1997**, *276*, 817–821. [CrossRef] [PubMed]
14. Xie, J.; Murone, M.; Luoh, S.M.; Ryan, A.; Gu, Q.; Zhang, C.; Bonifas, J.M.; Lam, C.W.; Hynes, M.; Goddard, A.; et al. Activating Smoothened mutations in sporadic basal-cell carcinoma. *Nature* **1998**, *391*, 90–92. [CrossRef] [PubMed]
15. Sharpe, H.J.; Pau, G.; Dijkgraaf, G.J.; Basset-Seguin, N.; Modrusan, Z.; Januario, T.; Tsui, V.; Durham, A.M.; Dlugosz, A.A.; Haverty, P.M.; et al. Genomic Analysis of Smoothened Inhibitor Resistance in Basal Cell Carcinoma. *Cancer Cell* **2015**, *27*, 327–341. [CrossRef] [PubMed]
16. Lyons, T.G.; O'Kane, G.M.; Kelly, C.M. Efficacy and safety of vismodegib: A new therapeutic agent in the treatment of basal cell carcinoma. *Expert Opin. Drug Saf.* **2014**, *13*, 1125–1132. [CrossRef] [PubMed]
17. Chang, A.L.S.; Oro, A.E. Initial Assessment of Tumor Regrowth after Vismodegib in Advanced Basal Cell Carcinoma. *Arch. Dermatol.* **2012**, *148*, 1324–1325. [CrossRef] [PubMed]
18. Pricl, S.; Cortelazzi, B.; Col, V.D.; Marson, D.; Laurini, E.; Fermeglia, M.; Licitra, L.; Pilotti, S.; Bossi, P.; Perrone, F. Smoothened (SMO) receptor mutations dictate resistance to vismodegib in basal cell carcinoma. *Mol. Oncol.* **2014**, *9*, 389–397. [CrossRef] [PubMed]
19. Yauch, R.L.; Dijkgraaf, G.J.P.; Alicke, B.; Januario, T.; Ahn, C.P.; Holcomb, T.; Pujara, K.; Stinson, J.; Callahan, C.A.; Tang, T.; et al. Smoothened Mutation Confers Resistance to a Hedgehog Pathway Inhibitor in Medulloblastoma. *Science* **2009**, *326*, 572–574. [CrossRef] [PubMed]
20. Gao, L.; Chen, F.; Li, X.; Xu, S.; Huang, W.; Ye, Y. Three new alkaloids from Veratrum grandiflorum Loes with inhibition activities on Hedgehog pathway. *Bioorg. Med. Chem. Lett.* **2016**, *26*, 4735–4738. [CrossRef] [PubMed]
21. Khanfar, M.A.; Sayed, K.A.E. The Veratrum alkaloids jervine, veratramine, and their analogues as prostate cancer migration and proliferation inhibitors: Biological evaluation and pharmacophore modeling. *Med. Chem. Res.* **2013**, *22*, 4775–4786. [CrossRef]
22. Ma, H.; Li, H.Q.; Zhang, X. Cyclopamine, a Naturally Occurring Alkaloid, and Its Analogues May Find Wide Applications in Cancer Therapy. *Curr. Top. Med. Chem.* **2013**, *13*, 2208–2215. [CrossRef] [PubMed]
23. Wilson, S.R.; Strand, M.F.; Krapp, A.; Rise, F.; Petersen, D.; Krauss, S. Hedgehog antagonist cyclopamine isomerizes to less potent forms when acidified. *J. Pharm. Biomed. Anal.* **2010**, *52*, 707–713. [CrossRef] [PubMed]
24. McNeal, D.W.; Shaw, S.D. Veratrum. In *Flora of North America North of Mexico*; Flora of North America Editorial Committee, Ed.; Oxford University Press: New York, NY, USA; Oxford, UK, 2002; Volume 26, pp. 72–76.

25. Cooper, M.K.; Porter, J.A.; Young, K.E.; Beachy, P.A. Teratogen-Mediated Inhibition of Target Tissue Response to Shh Signaling. *Science* **1998**, *280*, 1603–1607. [CrossRef] [PubMed]
26. Chen, J.K. I only have eye for ewe: The discovery of cyclopamine and development of Hedgehog pathway-targeting drugs. *Nat. Prod. Rep.* **2016**, *33*, 595–601. [CrossRef] [PubMed]
27. Heretsch, P.; Tzagkaroulaki, L.; Giannis, A. Cyclopamine and Hedgehog signaling: Chemistry, Biology, Medical Perspectives. *Angew. Chem. Int. Ed.* **2010**, *49*, 3418–3427. [CrossRef] [PubMed]
28. Chandler, C.M.; Habig, J.W.; Fisher, A.A.; Ambrose, K.V.; Jimenez, S.T.; McDougal, O.M. Improved extraction and complete mass spectral characterization of steroidal alkaloids from Veratrum californicum. *Nat. Prod. Commun.* **2013**, *8*, 1059–1064. [PubMed]
29. Turner, M.W.; Cruz, R.; Mattos, J.; Baughman, N.; Elwell, J.; Fothergill, J.; Nielsen, A.; Brookhouse, J.; Bartlett, A.; Malek, P.; et al. Cyclopamine bioactivity by extraction method from Veratrum californicum. *Bioorg. Med. Chem.* **2016**, *24*, 3752–3757. [CrossRef] [PubMed]
30. Ripperger, H. Steroidal alkaloids from roots of Solanum spirale. *Phytochemistry* **1996**, *43*, 705–707. [CrossRef]
31. Wilson, S.R.; Strand, M.F.; Krapp, A.; Rise, F.; Herstad, G.; Malterud, K.E.; Krauss, S. Hedgehog antagonists cyclopamine and dihydroveratramine can be mistaken for each other in Veratrum album. *J. Pharm. Biomed. Anal.* **2010**, *53*, 497–502. [CrossRef] [PubMed]
32. Keeler, R.F. Teratogenic compounds of Veratrum californicum (Durand) VII. The structure of the glycosidic alkaloid cycloposine. *Steroids* **1969**, *13*, 579–588. [CrossRef]
33. Keeler, R.; Binns, W. Teratogenic compounds of Veratrum californicum (Durand) III. Malformations of the veratramine-induced type from ingestion of plant or roots. *Proc. Soc. Exp. Biol. Med.* **1967**, *126*, 452–454. [CrossRef] [PubMed]
34. Keeler, R.F. Teratogenic effects of cyclopamine and jervine in rats, mice and hamsters. *Proc. Soc. Exp. Biol.* **1975**, *149*, 302–306. [CrossRef] [PubMed]
35. Taipale, J.; Chen, J.K.; Cooper, M.K.; Wang, B.; Mann, R.K.; Milenkovic, L.; Scott, M.P.; Beachy, P.A. Effects of oncogenic mutations in Smoothened and Patched can be reversed by cyclopamine. *Nature* **2000**, *406*, 1005–1009. [CrossRef] [PubMed]

Sample Availability: Samples of the compounds are not available from the authors.

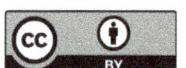

© 2018 by the authors. Licensee MDPI, Basel, Switzerland. This article is an open access article distributed under the terms and conditions of the Creative Commons Attribution (CC BY) license (http://creativecommons.org/licenses/by/4.0/).

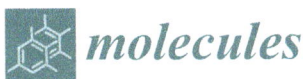

Article

Attempted Synthesis of *Vinca* Alkaloids Condensed with Three-Membered Rings

András Keglevich [1], Szabolcs Mayer [1], Réka Pápai [2], Áron Szigetvári [3], Zsuzsanna Sánta [3], Miklós Dékány [3], Csaba Szántay Jr. [3], Péter Keglevich [1,*] and László Hazai [1]

[1] Department of Organic Chemistry and Technology, University of Technology and Economics, Budapest, Hungary, H-1111 Budapest, Gellért tér 4., Hungary; keglevich.andras@mail.bme.hu (A.K.); mayer.szabolcs.g@gmail.com (S.M.); hazai@mail.bme.hu (L.H.)
[2] ComInnex, Inc., Graphisoft Park (Building D), H-1031 Budapest, Záhony u. 7., Hungary; reka134@gmail.com
[3] Spectroscopic Research Department, Gedeon Richter Plc., H-1475 Budapest 10, P. O. Box 27, Hungary; szigetvaria@richter.hu (Á.S.); Zs.Santa@richter.hu (Z.S.); m.dekany@richter.hu (M.D.); cs.szantay@richter.hu (C.S.J.)
* Correspondence: pkeglevich@mail.bme.hu; Tel.: +36-1-463-1195

Received: 30 August 2018; Accepted: 2 October 2018; Published: 9 October 2018

Abstract: Our successful work for the synthesis of cyclopropanated vinblastine and its derivatives by the Simmons–Smith reaction was followed to build up further three-membered rings into the 14,15-position of the vindoline part of the dimer alkaloid. Halogenated 14,15-cyclopropanovindoline was prepared by reactions with iodoform and bromoform, respectively, in the presence of diethylzinc. Reactions of dichlorocarbene with vindoline resulted in the 10-formyl derivative. Unexpectedly, in the case of the dimer alkaloids vinblastine and vincristine, the rearranged products containing an oxirane ring in the catharanthine part were isolated from the reactions. The attempted epoxidation of vindoline and catharanthine also led to anomalous rearranged products. In the epoxidation reaction of vindoline, an *o*-quinonoid derivative was obtained, in the course of the epoxidation of catharanthine, a hydroxyindolenine type product and a spiro derivative formed by ring contraction reaction, were isolated. The coupling reaction of vindoline and the spiro derivative obtained in the epoxidation of catharanthine did not result in a bisindole alkaloid. Instead, two surprising vindoline trimers were discovered and characterized by NMR spectroscopy and mass spectrometry.

Keywords: halogencyclopropane; dichlorocarbene; epoxidation; vindoline; catharanthine; dimer alkaloids; vindoline trimer

1. Introduction

The "dimer alkaloids" vinblastine (vincaleukoblastine, VLB, **1**) and vincristine (VCR, **2**) (Figure 1), isolated from the Madagascar periwinkle *Catharanthus roseus*, belong to the family of the so-called "bisindole" alkaloids [1–5]. Their structure comprises two indole-related "monomers": derivatives of catharanthine (**3**) and vindoline (**4**). VLB (**1**), VCR (**2**) and some of their analogs are anti-microtubule drugs that have been playing an important role in cancer chemotherapy for decades [6–10], and there are still many ongoing medicinal chemistry projects targeted at synthesizing new derivatives to improve the therapeutic effect of this family of drugs by increasing their selectivity or reducing their toxicity [11,12].

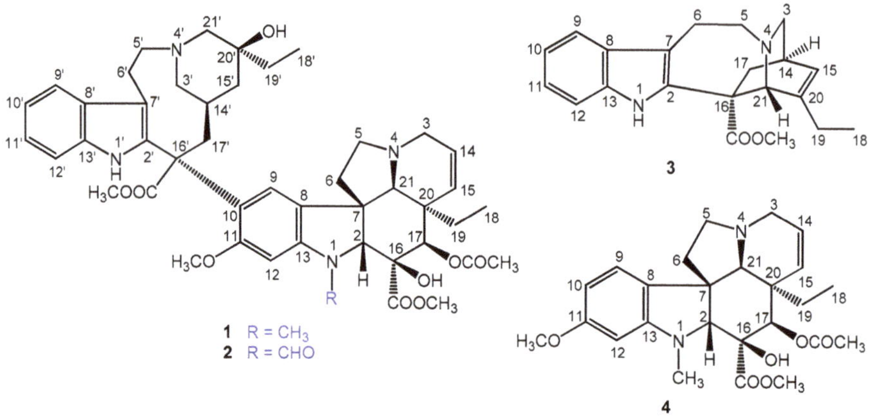

Figure 1. The alkaloids vinblastine (1), vincristine (2), catharanthine (3) and vindoline (4).

It is interesting to note that relatively minor changes in the bisindole structure can result in major changes in the biological activity. For example, one of the simplest such modification is the catalytic hydrogenation of the olefinic bond in the vindoline part of VLB (1), leading to 14,15-dihydrovinblastine (5), whose antitumor activity is significantly lower than that of VLB (1) (Figure 2) [13]. On the other hand, if instead of only being saturated, there is also a methylene bridge connecting C-14 and C-15, the resulting compound's bioactivity changes dramatically. In our previous work [14–16] we synthesized different kinds of bisindole alkaloids condensed with a cyclopropane ring at position 14,15 of the vindoline part, namely cyclopropanovinblastine (6), cyclopropanovincristine, cyclopropanovinorelbin, and other derivatives. We reported their significant tumor cell inhibiting activity on different tumor types and tumor cell lines.

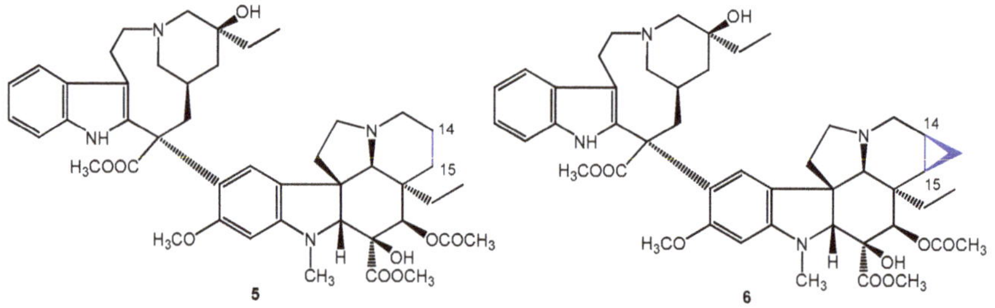

Figure 2. The alkaloids 14,15-dihydrovinblastine (5) and 14,15-cyclopropanovinblastine (6).

As a continuation of that work, our objective is the synthesis of further derivatives of potentially cytotoxic dimer alkaloids condensed with, e.g., a halogen substituted cyclopropane or oxirane ring. In our research group, these molecules have been a missing link in the analysis of the structure-activity relationship of the *Vinca* alkaloids. Synthetic studies were not only performed on the dimer alkaloids, but also on their building blocks, i.e., catharanthine (3) and vindoline (4).

2. Results and Discussion

2.1. Generation of Halogencyclopropane Ring with the Simmons–Smith Reaction

Our first purpose was to build up the halogencyclopropane ring in place of the C(14)=C(15) carbon-carbon double bond of the vindoline ring (4). Based on the work of Beaulieu et al. [17], vindoline (4) was reacted with bromoform and iodoform in the presence of diethylzinc in dichloromethane (Scheme 1). The Simmons–Smith reaction resulted stereospecifically in **8** 14,15-bromocyclopropanovindoline (31% yield) and **10** 14,15-iodocyclopropanovindoline (9% yield). By achieving the reaction with 10-bromovindoline (**7**) [18], the **9** bromocyclopropane and **11** iodocyclopropane derivatives were obtained in yields of 40% and 22%. The configurations of the 14, 15, and 22 carbon atoms were determined by NMR spectroscopy (14:(S), 15:(R), and 22:(S)).

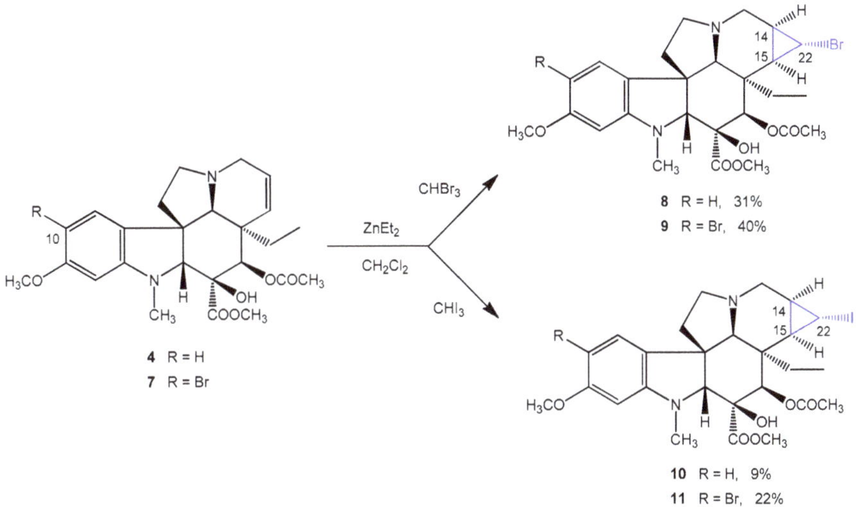

Scheme 1. The formation of the bromo- and iodocyclopropane ring.

2.2. Reactions with Dichlorocarbene

The following step of our current work was the investigation of the reactions of *Vinca* alkaloids with dichlorocarbene. Dichlorocyclopropano derivatives of monomeric and dimeric alkaloids were aimed at as an extension of our previous work.

First, the classical method of the reaction of dichlorocarbene with alkenes [19] was tried on vindoline (**4**) as a model compound (Scheme 2). A chloroform solution of vindoline (**4**) was treated with an aqueous solution of sodium hydroxide at room temperature in the presence of the phase transfer catalyst benzyltriethylammonium chloride (TEBAC). Unexpectedly, the dichlorocyclopropano derivative (**12**) could not be detected in the reaction. However, a formyl group was built in at position 10, resulting in 10-formylvindoline (**13**), a compound that is already known in the literature [20–22].

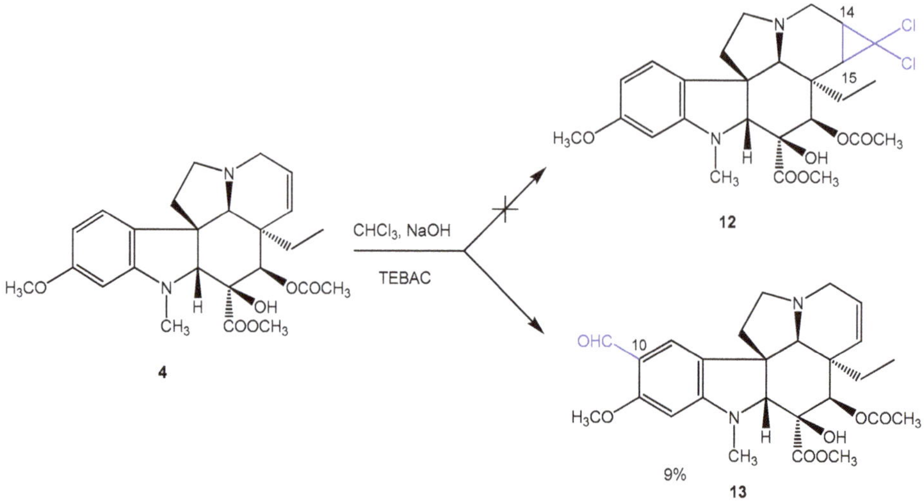

Scheme 2. The classical method of the dichlorocarbene reaction was tried on vindoline (**4**) first.

The above-mentioned dichlorocarbene reaction on the dimeric alkaloids vinblastine (**1**) and vincristine (**2**) was also investigated. In these reactions, instead of the expected dichlorocarbene adducts **14** and **16**, interesting ring-opened oxirane derivatives (**15** and **17**) were isolated in various yields (Scheme 3).

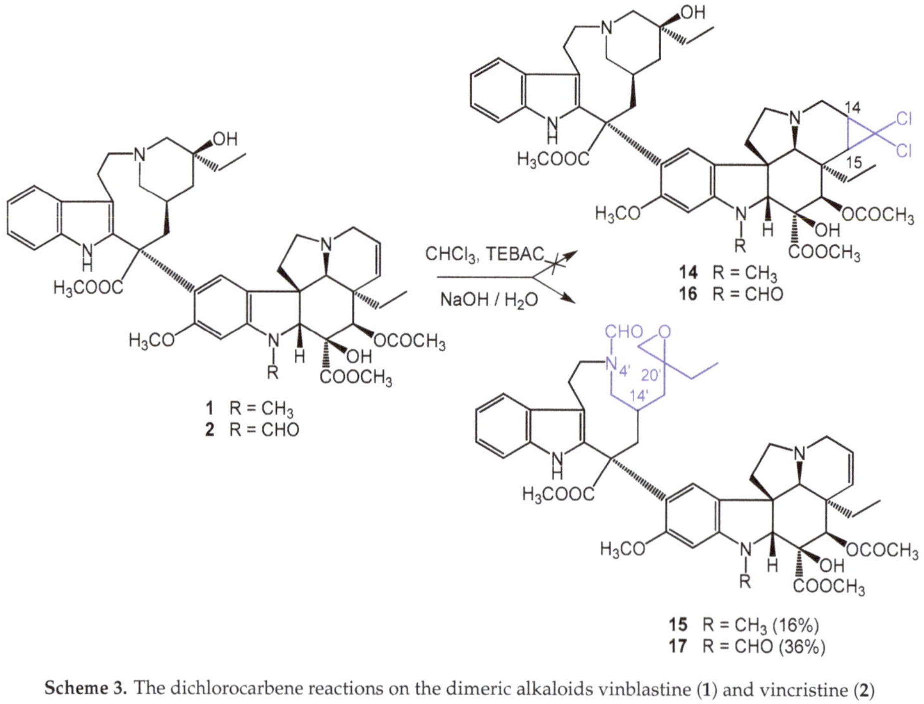

Scheme 3. The dichlorocarbene reactions on the dimeric alkaloids vinblastine (**1**) and vincristine (**2**) led to ring-opened oxirane derivatives (**15** and **17**).

A plausible interpretation of the oxirane formation is outlined in Scheme 4 (where **V** can represent non-modified and different kinds of modified "vindoline" units as well). First, electrophilic dichlorocarbene attacks the nucleophilic tertiary amine nitrogen at position 4', leading to an ammonium compound as the intermediate. Then the hydroxyl group at C-20' might become deprotonated under basic reaction conditions, the anionic moiety attacks C-21', and N-4' is neutralized during a heterolytic cleavage of a carbon-nitrogen bond. Finally, one of the chloro groups may undergo substitution with OH, and a formyl group forms by the elimination of hydrogen chloride.

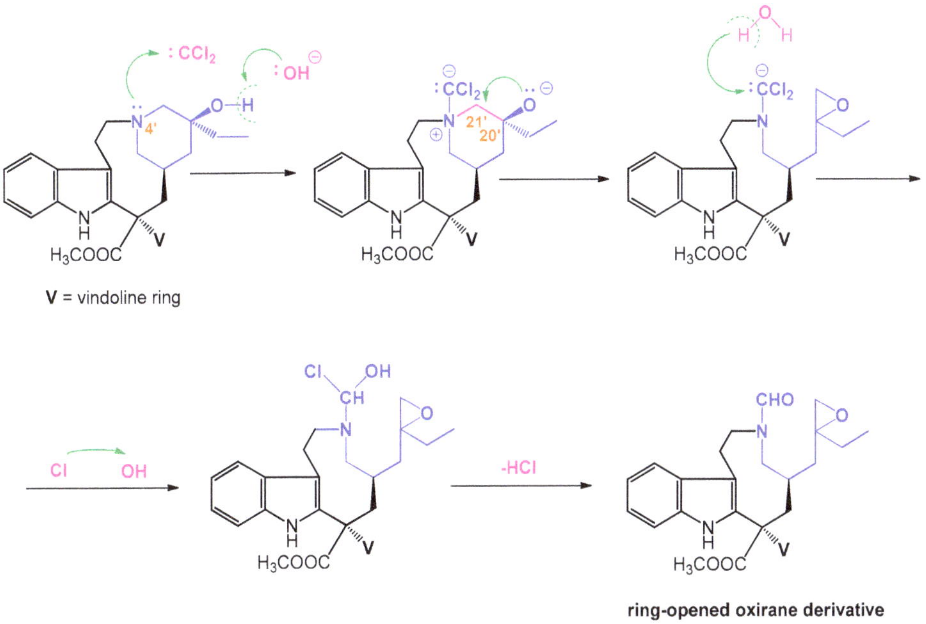

Scheme 4. The proposed mechanism for oxirane formation.

2.3. Attempted Epoxidation of Vinca Alkaloid Building Blocks

Another objective of our research was the exploration of the reactivity of "monomeric" alkaloids (e.g., vindoline, catharanthine) towards epoxidizing agents. In the literature, only few oxirane derivatives of *Vinca* alkaloids are known. For instance, the 3-oxo derivative of catharanthine could be epoxidized with *m*-chloroperoxybenzoic acid [23]. Another example, mehranine, the 14,15-epoxi derivative of aspidospermidine, was isolated from *Tabernaemontana bovina* and its total synthesis was recently presented [24].

The vindoline and catharanthine derivatives bearing an oxirane ring were also tried to be obtained in similar reactions, and they it was attempted to use them in coupling reactions to afford epoxidized bisindole alkaloids.

First, the oxidation of 10-bromovindoline (**7**) with *m*-chloroperoxybenzoic acid (*m*-CPBA) was studied. The reaction could be performed either in the presence or absence of perchloric acid, which may influence the outcome of the oxidation [25]. When carrying out the reaction in methanol without HClO$_4$, none of the oxidated products could be isolated. Surprisingly, when HClO$_4$ was used in the reaction, the debromination and demethylation at the aromatic ring occurred. An *o*-quinoidal compound (**19**) was isolated in 27% yield, but the desired oxirane **18** could not be obtained (Scheme 5). Starting from compound **19**, the reaction has been described in a short article published last year by us [26].

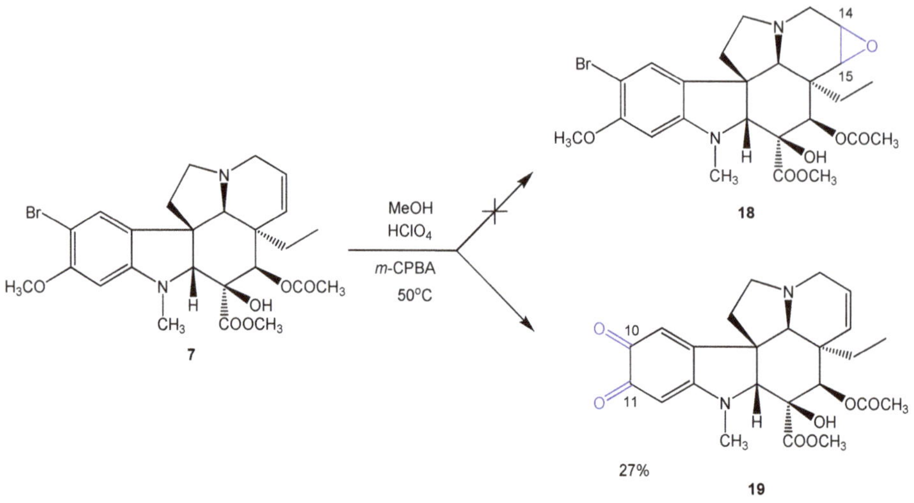

Scheme 5. The attempted epoxidation of 10-bromovindoline (**7**) in the presence of perchloric acid.

Hereafter the above-mentioned two methods of oxidation with *m*-CPBA were also tried on catharanthine (**3**). In the absence of perchloric acid, the oxidation led to a mixture of two products: catharanthine N^4-oxide (**20**) in 34% yield (a similar preparation of **20** is known from the literature [18]), and a new compound (N^4-oxide of 7-hydroxyindolenine catharanthine, **21**) in 35% yield (Scheme 6).

N-Oxide **20** is known to be unstable, it easily undergoes a [2,3]-sigmatropic rearrangement, leading to isoxazolidine **22** [27,28]. This kind of rearrangement during the NMR measurements (room temperature, CDCl$_3$ as solvent) was also observed. Although Langlois et al. provided ^{1}H and ^{13}C NMR spectral data for **22** [19], they could not give an unequivocal assignment of the NMR peaks. In this paper, we report the unambiguous ^{1}H and ^{13}C-NMR assignments for **22**, which has become achievable because of the advancements in NMR instrumentation and measurement techniques since 1976.

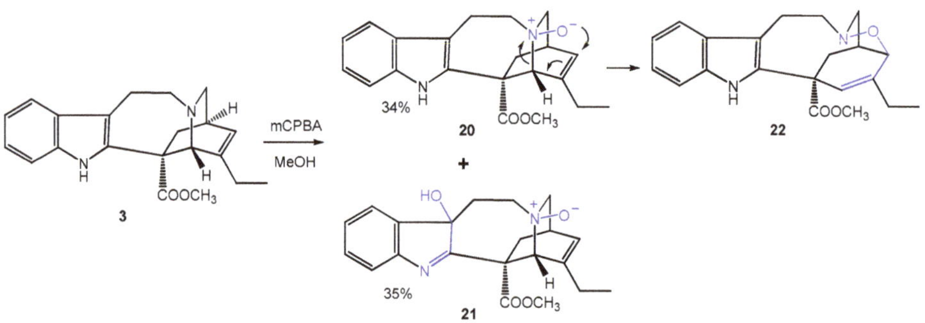

Scheme 6. The oxidation with *m*-chloroperoxybenzoic acid was tried on catharanthine (**3**) without perchloric acid for the first time.

On the other hand, when perchloric acid is applied during the oxidation of catharanthine (**3**) with *m*-CPBA, two anomalous products were obtained. The major product (58% yield) was 7β-hydroxyindolenine catharanthine (**23**), the minor product (12% yield) was the spiro derivative **24** (Scheme 7).

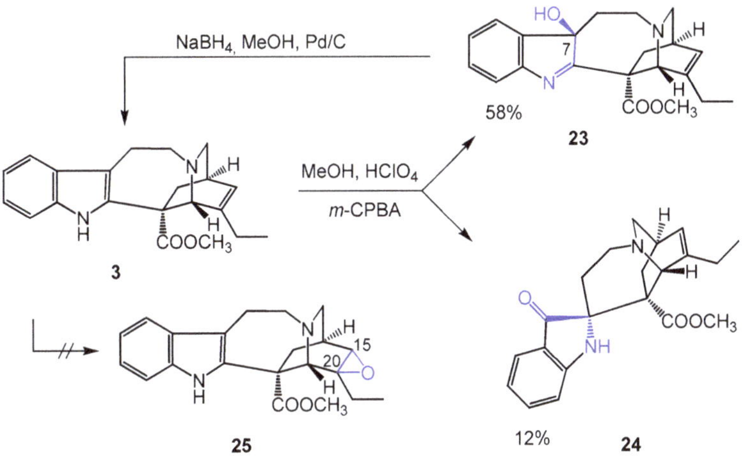

Scheme 7. The oxidation with *m*-chloroperoxybenzoic acid was tried on catharanthine (**3**) in the presence of perchloric acid as well.

The synthesis of 7β-hydroxyindolenine catharanthine (**23**) is already known [29]. The authors used singlet oxygen to oxidize catharanthine (**3**). They determined the configuration of compound **23** at C-7 by NMR spectroscopy using nuclear Overhauser effect (NOE) measurements. Our independent NMR assignments, including the determination of the relative stereochemistry of our product, were in full agreement with those reported in Reference [29]. Hydroxyindolenines are also natural products, e.g., the 15,20-dihydro derivative of **23** is known as coronaridine hydroxyindolenine and was isolated from *Ervatamia coronaria* var. *plena* [30].

To utilize **23** in an oxidative coupling reaction [22] with vindoline (**4**) with the purpose of obtaining new bisindole alkaloids, the double bond at N-1–C-2 has to be saturated, supposing that the coupling reaction requires a secondary amino group (i.e., R^1R^2NH) on the catharanthine site. Thus, a reduction of **23** was aimed at with sodium borohydride to obtain its 1,2-dihydro derivative, but the reaction resulted in the elimination of the hydroxyl group, returning it to catharanthine (**3**).

Rosamine, a natural product isolated from *Catharanthus roseus*, was reported by Atta-ur-Rahman et al. with the same constitution as **24** [31], although they did not specify the configuration of any of the stereogenic centers. We determined the relative configuration of **24** based on NOE measurements (Figure 3), but we could not decide if **24** was rosamine. The reason for that was the unavailability of reliable spectral data for rosamine (in Reference [31], only the ^{1}H NMR chemical shifts and coupling constants for the methyl groups and H-21 were given), so a reliable comparison of the spectral data of **24** with those of rosamine was not possible.

The stereogenic centers of **24** are C-2, N-4, C-14, C-16 and C-21 (Figure 3). Since **24** has a rigid cage structure (2-azabicyclo[2.2.2]octane) condensed with a six-membered ring, the relative configurations of N-4, C-14, C-16, and C-21 are fixed (the configuration at C-21 can be arbitrarily established as *R*, then N-4, C-14, and C-16 must be *R*,*R*,*R*). With this in mind, the configuration of C-2 was determined as follows. The NOESY correlation between NH-1 (6.60 ppm) and one of the protons at C-17 (1.95 ppm) implies that the configuration of C-2 is *R* (otherwise we would expect correlations between NH-1 and the protons at C-5), and the actual three-dimensional structure is supported by several other NOESY correlations (Figure 3).

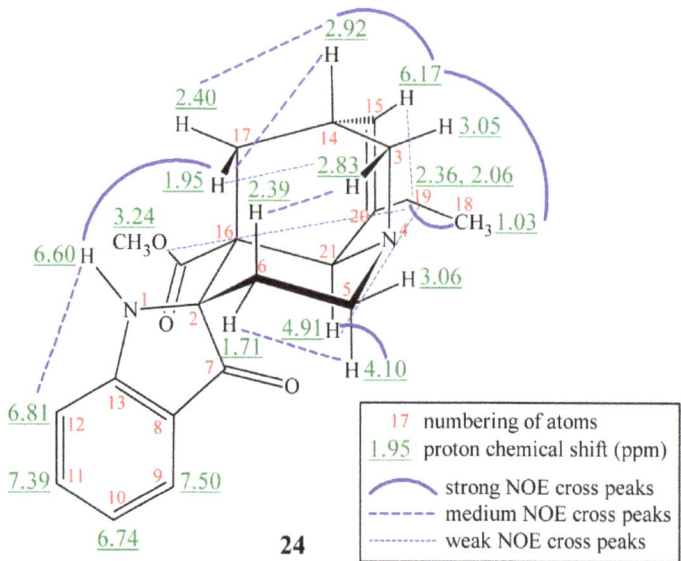

Figure 3. The three-dimensional structure of the spiro derivative of catharanthine (**24**).

2.4. Coupling Reaction of the Spiro Derivative of Catharanthine and Vindoline

The coupling reaction of **24** with vindoline (**4**) was carried out according to a general procedure formerly used by our research group in the course of synthesizing VLB derivatives [14,15], which is an oxidation in the presence of trifluoroethanol and FeCl$_3$ in acidic medium, followed by the reduction of the intermediate with sodium borohydride (Scheme 8).

Instead of the desired bisindole **26**, only unexpected products were found in the reaction mixture. We encountered that vindoline coupled to itself: a cationic trimeric vindoline (**27**) and a trimeric vindoline ketone (**28**) were isolated. The presence of a third product, *N*-methyl quaternary salt of a spiro derivative **29** suggests that the role of the spiro derivative **24** in the reaction might be the demethylation of the mesomer **27**. To support our assumption, the reaction was repeated without adding the spiro derivative of catharanthine (**24**). This way, only *O*-methylated trimeric vindoline (**27**) could be isolated and ketone **28** was not found in the reaction mixture, which substantiates our hypothesis.

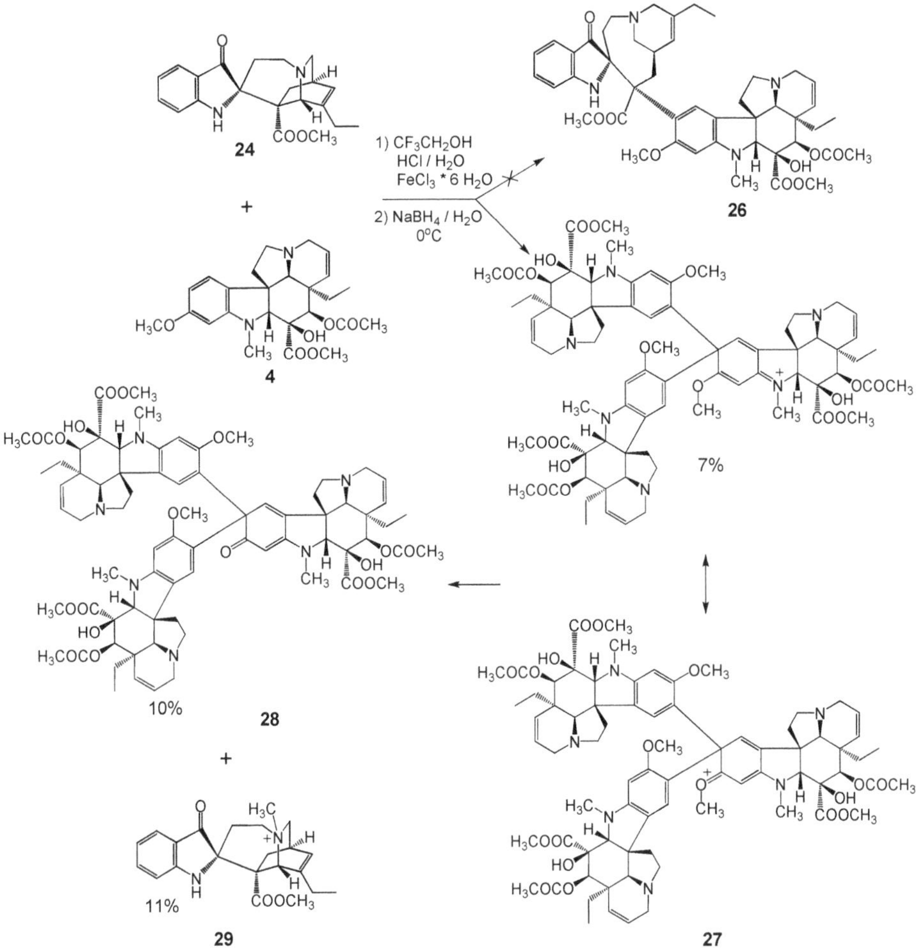

Scheme 8. The coupling reaction of the spiro derivative of catharanthine (**24**) and vindoline (**4**) led to similar trimeric vindoline derivatives.

3. Experimental Section

3.1. General

Vinblastine, vincristine, and catharanthine were derived from the corresponding sulfate salts; the bases were released directly before using them in the reactions. m-Chloroperoxybenzoic acid (m-CPBA) of 77% assay was purchased from Sigma-Aldrich (Budapest, Hungary) and was used as received. Melting points were measured on a VEB Analytik Dresden PHMK-77/1328 apparatus (Dresden, Germany) and are uncorrected. IR spectra were recorded on the Zeiss IR 75 and 80 instruments (Thornwood, NY, USA). NMR measurements were performed on a Varian VNMRS 800 MHz NMR spectrometer equipped with a ^{1}H{^{13}C/^{15}N} Triple Resonance ^{13}C Enhanced Salt Tolerant Cold Probe, a Varian VNMRS 500 MHz NMR spectrometer equipped with a ^{1}H {^{13}C/^{15}N} 5 mm PFG Triple Resonance ^{13}C Enhanced Cold Probe (Varian, Inc., Palo Alto, CA, USA), and a Bruker Avance III HDX 500 MHz NMR spectrometer equipped with a ^{1}H {^{13}C/^{15}N} 5 mm TCI CryoProbe (Bruker Corporation, Billerica, MA, USA). ^{1}H And ^{13}C chemical shifts are given on the delta scale as parts per million (ppm) with tetramethylsilane (TMS) (^{1}H, ^{13}C) or dimethylsulfoxide-d_6 (^{13}C) as the internal standard (0.00 ppm and 39.4 ppm, respectively). ^{1}H-^{1}H, direct ^{1}H-^{13}C, and long-range ^{1}H-^{13}C scalar spin-spin connectivites were established from 2D COSY, TOCSY, HSQC, and HMBC experiments. ^{1}H-^{1}H spatial proximities were determined using either two-dimensional NOESY/ROESY experiments or their selective 1D counterparts. All pulse sequences were applied by using the standard spectrometer software package. All experiments were performed at 298 K. NMR spectra were processed using VnmrJ 2.2 Revision C (Varian, Inc. Palo Alto, CA, USA), Bruker TopSpin 3.5 pl 6 (Bruker Corporation, Billerica, MA, USA) and ACD/Spectrus Processor version 2017.1.3 (Advanced Chemistry Development, Inc., Toronto, ON, Canada). HRMS and MS analyses were performed on an LTQ FT Ultra as well as an LTQ XL (Thermo Fisher Scientific, Bremen, Germany) system. The ionization method was ESI operated in the positive ion mode. For the CID (collision-induced dissociation) experiment, helium was used as the collision gas, and the normalized collision energy (expressed in percentage), which is a measure of the amplitude of the resonance excitation RF voltage applied to the endcaps of the linear ion trap, was used to induce fragmentation. The protonated molecular ion peaks were fragmented by CID at a normalized collision energy of 35–55%. The samples were dissolved in methanol. Data acquisition and analysis were accomplished with Xcalibur software version 2.0 (Thermo Fisher Scientific, Bremen, Germany). TLC was carried out using Kieselgel 60F$_{254}$ (Merck, Budapest, Hungary) glass plates.

3.2. Bromocyclopropanation of Vindoline (4)

Vindoline (**4**) (228 mg, 0.50 mmol) was dissolved in dichloromethane (5 mL) and under Ar with 1.28 mL (1.28 mmol in 1 M hexane solution) of diethylzinc and then 88 µL (1.00 mmol) bromoform was injected to the solution. After stirring for 2 h at room temperature the reaction mixture was filtered and the filtrate was diluted with dichloromethane (50 mL) and washed with water (100 mL). The aqueous phase was extracted with dichloromethane (4 × 50 mL) and the combined organic phase was dried over magnesium sulfate, filtered, and the filtrate was evaporated to dryness. The crude product was separated by preparative TLC (dichloromethane-methanol 19:1) and 86 mg (31%) of product (**8**) was isolated. Mp 118–119 °C.

TLC (dichloromethane-methanol 20:1); R_f = 0.71.

IR (KBr) 2963, 1744, 1617, 1502, 1230, 1039 cm^{-1}.

^{1}H NMR (499.9 MHz, CDCl$_3$) δ (ppm) 0.68 (t, J = 7.3 Hz, 3H, H$_3$-18), 0.97 (dd, J = 9.7, 3.8 Hz, 1H, H-15), 1.00 (dq, J = 14.4, 7.3 Hz, 1H, H$_x$-19), 1.62 (dddd J = 9.7, 3.8, 3.5, 0.7 Hz, 1H, H-14), 1.91 (dq, J = 14.4, 7.3 Hz, 1H, H$_y$-19), 2.21 (s, 3H, C(17)-OC(O)CH$_3$), 2.22–2.40 (m, 5H, H$_2$-6, H-21, H$_x$-3, H$_x$-5), 2.63 (s, 3H, N(1)-CH$_3$), 3.23–3.33 (br m, 1H, H$_y$-5), 3.44 (br d, J = 11.4 Hz, 1H, H$_y$-3), 3.52 (t, J = 3.8 Hz, 1H, H-22), 3.57 (s, 1H, H-2), 3.78 (s, 3H, C(11)-OCH$_3$), 3.81 (s, 3H, C(16)-COOCH$_3$), 5.53 (s, 1H, H-17), 6.07 (d, J = 2.2 Hz, 1H, H-12), 6.30 (dd, J = 8.2, 2.2 Hz, 1H, H-10), 6.84 (d, J = 8.2 Hz, 1H, H-9), 7.96 (br s, 1H, C(16)-OH).

^{13}C NMR (125.7 MHz, CDCl$_3$) δ (ppm) 8.2 (C-18), 21.6 (C(17)-OC(O)CH$_3$), 23.3 (C-14), 23.5 (C-22), 28.0 (C-15), 34.4 (C-19), 38.7 (N(1)-CH$_3$), 41.8 (C-20), 44.6 (C-6), 51.9 (C-3), 52.2 (C-7), 52.7 (C(16)-COOCH$_3$), 53.5 (C-5), 55.6 (C(11)-OCH$_3$), 69.6 (C-21), 76.3 (C-17), 78.9 (C-16), 83.7 (C-2), 95.9 (C-12), 105.1 (C-10), 122.7 (C-9), 125.6 (C-8), 153.7 (C-13), 161.2 (C-11), 171.2 (C(17)-OC(O)CH$_3$), 171.9 (C(16)-COOCH$_3$).

HRMS: M + H = 549.15965 (C$_{26}$H$_{34}$O$_6$N$_2$Br, Δ = 0.3 ppm). HR-ESI-MS-MS (CID = 35%, rel. int. %): 489(100); 457(1); 429(1); 314(1).

3.3. Bromocyclopropanation of 10-Bromovindoline (7)

The compound 10-Bromovindoline (**7**) (268 mg, 0.50 mmol) was dissolved in dichloromethane (5 mL) and under Ar with 1.28 mL (1.28 mmol in 1 M hexane solution) of diethylzinc and then 88 µL (1.00 mmol), the bromoform was injected to the solution. After stirring for 3 h at room temperature the reaction mixture was diluted with dichloromethane (40 mL) and washed with water (100 mL). The aqueous phase was extracted with dichloromethane (2 × 50 mL) and the combined organic phase was dried over magnesium sulfate, filtered and the filtrate was evaporated to dryness. The crude product was purified by preparative TLC (dichloromethane-methanol 30:1) and 126 mg (40%) of product (**9**) was isolated. Mp 144–146 °C.

TLC (dichloromethane-methanol 30:1); R_f = 0.54.

IR (KBr) 2965, 1743, 1604, 1498, 1232, 1041 cm^{-1}.

^{1}H NMR (799.7 MHz, CDCl$_3$) δ (ppm) 0.73 (t, J = 7.3 Hz, 3H, H$_3$-18), 0.96–1.01 (m, 2H, H-15, H$_x$-19), 1.66 (dt, J = 9.7, 3.5 Hz, 1H, H-14), 1.93 (dq, J = 14.4, 7.3 Hz, 1H, H$_y$-19), 2.22–2.33 (m, 7H, C(17)-OC(O)CH$_3$, H-21, H$_2$-6, H$_x$-3), 2.35–2.40 (m, 1H, H$_x$-5), 2.66 (s, 3H, N(1)-CH$_3$), 3.26–3.38 (br m, 1H, H$_y$-5), 3.44–3.50 (br m, 1H, H$_y$-3), 3.51 (br t, J = 3.5 Hz, 1H, H-22), 3.59 (s, 1H, H-2), 3.83 (s, 3H, C(16)-COOCH$_3$), 3.90 (s, 3H, C(11)-OCH$_3$), 5.53 (s, 1H, H-17), 6.10 (s, 1H, H-12), 7.07 (s, 1H, H-9), 7.98 (br, 1H, C(16)-OH).

^{13}C NMR (201.1 MHz, CDCl$_3$) δ (ppm) 8.1 (C-18), 21.7 (C(17)-OC(O)CH$_3$), 23.2 br (C-14), 23.3 br (C-22), 27.9 (C-15), 34.5 (C-19), 38.7 (N(1)-CH$_3$), 41.8 (C-20), 44.4 (C-6), 51.9 (C-3), 52.1 (C-7), 52.5 (C(16)-COOCH$_3$), 53.4 (C-5), 56.3 (C(11)-OCH$_3$), 69.5 (C-21), 76.1 (C-17), 78.7 (C-16), 83.6 (C-2), 94.5 (C-12), 100.2 (C-10), 126.1 (C-9), 126.5 br (C-8), 152.9 (C-13), 156.8 (C-11), 171.1 (C(17)-OC(O)CH$_3$), 171.7 (C(16)-COOCH$_3$).

HRMS: M + H = 627.07035 (C$_{26}$H$_{33}$O$_6$N$_2$Br$_2$, Δ = 0.6 ppm), HR-ESI-MS-MS (CID = 35%; rel. int. %): 567(100); 507(2).

3.4. Iodocyclopropanation of Vindoline (4)

Vindoline (**4**) (228 mg, 0.50 mmol) was dissolved in dichloromethane (20 mL) and under an Ar at 0 °C 1.28 mL (1.28 mmol in 1 M hexane solution) of diethylzinc, it was injected to the solution. Then 394 mg (1.00 mmol) of iodoform was added and the reaction mixture was stirred for 30 min at 0 °C and then for 6 h at room temperature. After allowing the solution to stand overnight, the addition of diethylzinc (1.28 mL) and iodoform (394 mg) was repeated at 0 °C. After stirring for 7 h at room temperature, the reaction mixture was filtered and the filtrate was diluted with dichloromethane (30 mL) and washed with water (100 mL). The aqueous phase was extracted with dichloromethane (5 × 60 mL) and the combined organic phase was dried over magnesium sulfate, filtered, and the filtrate was evaporated to dryness. The crude product was separated by preparative TLC (dichloromethane-methanol 19:1) and 28 mg (9%) of product (**10**) was isolated. Mp 116–117 °C.

TLC (dichloromethane-methanol 20:1); R_f = 0.75.

IR (KBr) 2963, 1742, 1615, 1502, 1231, 1039 cm^{-1}.

^{1}H NMR (499,9 MHz, CDCl$_3$) δ (ppm) 0.68 (t, J = 7.3 Hz, 3H, H$_3$-18), 0.93 (dd, J = 9.2, 4.3 Hz, 1H, H-15), 0.99 (dq, J = 14.3, 7.3 Hz, 1H, H$_x$-19), 1.52–1.57 (m, 1H, H-14), 1.89 (dq, J = 14.3, 7.3 Hz, 1H, H$_y$-19), 2.21–2.31 (m, 7H, H$_x$-3, H$_2$-6, C(17)-OC(O)CH$_3$, H-21), 2.32–2.41 (m, 1H, H$_x$-5), 2.63 (s, 3H, N(1)-CH$_3$), 3.13 (dd, J = 4.3, 3.7 Hz, 1H, H-22), 3.23–3.35 (m, 1H, H$_y$-5), 3.42–3.50 (m, 1H, H$_y$-3), 3.56 (s, 1H, H-2), 3.78 (s, 3H, C(11)-OCH$_3$), 3.81 (s, 3H, C(16)-COOCH$_3$), 5.53 (s, 1H, H-17), 6.07 (d, J = 2.3 Hz, 1H, H-12), 6.30 (dd, J = 8.2, 2.3 Hz, 1H, H-10), 6.83 (d, J = 8.2 Hz, 1H, H-9), 8.03 (br, 1H, C(16)-OH).

^{13}C NMR (125.7 MHz, CDCl$_3$) δ (ppm) -9.5 (C-22), 8.1 (C-18), 22.4 (C(17)-OC(O)CH$_3$), 24.3 (C-14), 29.0 (C-15), 34.5 (C-19), 38.6 (N(1)-CH$_3$), 42.1 (C-20), 44.6 (C-6), 52.2 (C-3), 52.3 (C-7), 52.4 (C(16)-COOCH$_3$), 53.3 (C-5), 55.4 (C(11)-OCH$_3$), 69.7 (C-21), 76.5 (C-17), 78.9 (C-16), 83.8 (C-2), 95.9 (C-12), 105.0 (C-10), 122.5 (C-9), 125.5 (C-8), 153.6 (C-13), 161.2 (C-11), 171.2 (C(17)-OC(O)CH$_3$), 171.9 (C(16)-COOCH$_3$).

HRMS: M + H = 597.14664 (C$_{26}$H$_{34}$O$_6$N$_2$I, Δ = 1.7 ppm). HR-ESI-MS-MS (CID = 35%) (rel. int. %): 537(100); 505(1); 477(2); 441(1); 381(3); 362(2); 188(2).

3.5. Iodocyclopropanation of 10-Bromovindoline (7)

The compound 10-Bromovindoline (**7**) (268 mg, 0.50 mmol) was dissolved in dichloromethane (20 mL) and under Ar at 0 °C with 1.28 mL (1.28 mmol in 1 M hexane solution) of diethylzinc being injected into the solution. Then 394 mg (1.00 mmol) of iodoform was added and the reaction mixture was stirred for 30 min at 0 °C and then for 8 h at room temperature. After allowing the solution to stand overnight, the addition of diethylzinc (1.28 mL) and iodoform (394 mg) was repeated at 0 °C. After stirring for 6 h at room temperature, the reaction mixture was filtered and the filtrate was diluted with dichloromethane (30 mL) and washed with water (100 mL). The aqueous phase was extracted with dichloromethane (5 × 60 mL) and the combined organic phase was dried over magnesium sulfate, filtered and the filtrate was evaporated to dryness. The crude product was separated by preparative TLC (dichloromethane-methanol 19:1) and 74 mg (22%) of product (**11**) was isolated. Mp > 350 °C.

TLC (dichloromethane-methanol 20:1); R_f = 0.86.

IR (KBr) 3444, 2927, 1740, 1228, 742 cm^{-1}.

^{1}H NMR (499,9 MHz, CDCl$_3$) δ (ppm) 0.71 (t, 3H, J = 7.3 Hz, H$_3$-18), 0.93 (dd, J = 9.2, 4.3 Hz, 1H, H-15), 0.93–1.01 (m, 1H, H$_x$-19), 1.54–1.58 (m, 1H, H-14), 1.89 (dq, J = 14.6, 7.3 Hz, 1H, H$_y$-19), 2.22–2.27 (m, 4H, H$_x$-3, H$_2$-6, H-21), 2.27 (s, 3H, C(17)-OC(O)CH_3), 2.32–2.39 (m, 1H, H$_x$-5), 2.64 (s, 3H, N(1)-CH_3), 3.10 (t, J = 4.3 Hz, 1H, H-22), 3.24–3.30 (m, 1H, H$_y$-5), 3.43–3.47 (m, 1H, H$_y$-3), 3.57 (s, 1H, H-2), 3.81 (s, 3H, C(16)-COOCH_3), 3.88 (s, 3H, C(11)-OCH_3), 5.51 (s, 1H, H-17), 6.09 (s, 1H, H-12), 7.05 (s, 1H, H-9), 8.01 (br, 1H, C(16)-OH).

^{13}C NMR (125.7 MHz, CDCl$_3$) δ (ppm) -9.7 (C-22), 8.1 (C-18), 22.4 (C(17)-OC(O)CH$_3$), 24.2 (C-14), 28.9 (C-15), 34.7 (C-19), 38.7 (N(1)-CH$_3$), 42.1 (C-20), 44.5 (C-6), 52.17 (C-3), 52.22 (C-7), 52.5 (C(16)-COOCH$_3$), 53.1 (C-5), 56.3 (C(11)-OCH$_3$), 69.6 (C-21), 76.3 (C-17), 78.7 (C-16), 83.8 (C-2), 94.5 (C-12), 100.1 (C-10), 126.2 (C-9), 126.4 (C-8), 152.8 (C-13), 156.7 (C-11), 171.2 (C(17)-OC(O)CH$_3$), 171.7 (C(16)-COOCH$_3$).

HRMS: M + H = 675.05411 (C$_{26}$H$_{33}$O$_6$N$_2$BrI, Δ = −2.9 ppm). ESI-MS-MS (CID = 35%) (rel. int. %): 615(100); 555(2); 459(1).

*3.6. Attempted Dichlorocyclopropanation of Vindoline (**4**)*

Vindoline (**4**) (256 mg, 0.56 mmol) and TEBAC (9 mg, 0.04 mmol) were dissolved in chloroform (1.4 mL), then a solution of sodium hydroxide (0.6 g, 15.00 mmol) in water (0.6 mL) was added dropwise to the reaction mixture, and stirred at room temperature for 2 h. The pH of the reaction mixture was adjusted to 7 using 1 M hydrochloric acid. Water was added and the mixture was extracted with chloroform. The combined organic phase was washed with water, dried over magnesium sulfate, and evaporated under reduced pressure. The residue was purified by preparative TLC (dichloromethane-methanol 20:1) and 24 mg (9%) of product (**13**) [20–22] was obtained.

*3.7. Attempted Dichlorocyclopropanation of Vinblastine (**1**)*

Vinblastine (**1**) (120 mg, 0.15 mmol) was dissolved in chloroform (0.4 mL), TEBAC (3 mg, 0.013 mmol) was added, and 200 mg (5.00 mmol) of NaOH in water (0.2 mL) was added dropwise. After stirring at room temperature for 2 h, the pH of the reaction mixture was neutralized using 1 M hydrochloric acid. Water (20 mL) was added and the mixture was extracted with chloroform (2 × 10 mL). The combined organic phase was dried over magnesium sulfate and evaporated under reduced pressure. The residue was purified by preparative TLC (dichloromethane-methanol 10:1) and 20 mg (16%) of product (**15**) was obtained. Mp 205−207 °C.

TLC (dichloromethane-methanol 10:1); R_f = 0.60.

IR (KBr) 3470, 2964, 1740, 1669, 1614, 1501, 1461, 1371, 1227, 1040, 742 cm^{-1}.

^{1}H NMR (799.7 MHz, CDCl$_3$) δ (ppm) 0.39 (t, J = 7.5 Hz, 3H, H$_3$-18'), 0.82 (t, J = 7.4 Hz, 3H, H$_3$-18), 0.91 (dd, J = 13.8, 12.3 Hz, 1H, H$_x$-15'), 1.06 (dq, J = 14.7, 7.5 Hz, 1H, H$_x$-19'), 1.36 (dq, J = 14.4, 7.4 Hz, 1H, H$_x$-19), 1.46 (dd, J = 13.8, 3.4 Hz, 1H, H$_y$-15'), 1.66 (dq, J = 14.7, 7.5 Hz, 1H, H$_y$-19'), 1.83 (dq, J = 14.4, 7.4 Hz, 1H, H$_y$-19), 1.99–2.05 (m, 1H, H-14'), 2.11 (s, 3H, C(17)-OC(O)CH_3), 2.14 (ddd, J = 14.0, 8.7, 7.4 Hz, 1H, H$_x$-6'), 2.30 (br d, J = 16.5 Hz, 1H, H$_x$-17'), 2.43 (d, J = 4.9 Hz, 1H, H$_x$-21'), 2.44–2.47 (m, 1H, H$_x$-5), 2.48 (dd, J = 13.2, 11.2 Hz, 1H, H$_x$-3'), 2.55–2.56 (m, 1H, H$_y$-21'), 2.62–2.66 (m, 2H, H-21, H$_y$-6), 2.66 (s, 3H, N(1)-CH_3), 2.79–2.83 (m, 1H, H$_x$-3), 3.01–3.09 (br m, 1H, H$_y$-17'), 3.15–3.20 (m, 1H, H$_x$-6'), 3.31–3.35 (m, 1H, H$_y$-5), 3.37–3.42 (m, 2H, H$_x$-5', H$_y$-3), 3.50–3.61 (m, 2H, H$_y$-6', H$_y$-5') overlapped with 3.56 (br s, 3H, C(16′)-COOCH$_3$), 3.73 (s, 1H, H-2), 3.80 (s, 3H, C(16)-COOCH$_3$), 3.81 (s, 3H, C(11)-OCH$_3$), 3.84–3.87 (m, 1H, H$_y$-3′), 5.28–5.31 (m, 1H, H-15), 5.52 (s, 1H, H-17), 5.87 (ddd, J = 10.4, 4.8, 0.8 Hz, 1H, H-14), 6.11 (s, 1H, H-12), 6.65 (s, 1H, H-9), 7.10–7.14 (m, 2H, H-10′, H-12′), 7.16–7.19 (m, 1H, H-11′), 7.35 (br s, 1H, N(4′)-CHO), 7.51–7.53 (m, 1H, H-9′), 7.95 (br, 1H, NH-1′), 9.85 (br, 1H, C(16)-OH).

^{13}C NMR (201.1 MHz, CDCl$_3$) δ (ppm) 8.4 (C-18′), 8.5 (C-18), 21.2 (C(17)-OC(O)CH$_3$), 24.9 (C-19′), 25.1 (C-6′), 28.8 (br, C-14′), 30.9 (C-19), 38.5 (N(1)-CH$_3$), 39.1 (C-17′), 42.6 (C-15′), 42.7 (C-20), 43.6 (C-6), 49.5 (C-5′), 50.5 (C-3), 51.37 (C-5), 51.40 (C-3′), 52.2 (C(16)-COOCH$_3$), 52.4 (C(16′)-COOCH$_3$), 53.3 (C-7), 54.5 (C-21′), 55.7 (C(11)-OCH$_3$), 56.4 (br, C-16′), 58.7 (C-20′), 66.4 (C-21), 76.6 (C-17), 79.7 (C-16), 84.0 (C-2), 94.0 (br, C-12), 110.8 (C-12′), 111.1 (br, C-7′), 117.6 (C-9′), 119.3 (C-10′), 120.0 (br, C-10), 122.5 (C-11′), 123.8 (br, C-8), 124.6 (C-14), 125.3 (C-9), 128.3 (C-8′), 129.9 (C-15), 133.0 (br, C-2′), 135.3 (br, C-13′), 153.3 (C-13), 157.9 (C-11), 163.4 (N(4′)-CHO), 171.0 (C(17)-OC(O)CH$_3$), 171.8 (C(16)-COOCH$_3$), 174.4 (br, C(16′)-COOCH$_3$).

HRMS: M + Na = 839.41764 (C$_{45}$H$_{60}$O$_{10}$N$_4$Na, Δ = −3.0 ppm). ESI-MS-MS (CID = 35%, rel. int. %): 821(12), 779(100), 761(4), 747(4), 677(7), 570(45).

3.8. Attempt to Dichlorocyclopropanation of Vincristine (2)

Vincristine (**2**) (130 mg, 0.16 mmol) was dissolved in chloroform (1 mL) and TEBAC (7 mg, 0.031 mmol) was added. Then 230 mg (5.75 mmol) of NaOH in water (0.23 mL) was added dropwise. After stirring at room temperature for 2 h, the pH of the reaction mixture was neutralized with 1 M hydrochloric acid. Water (10 mL) was added and the mixture was extracted with dichloromethane (2 × 10 mL). The combined organic phase was dried over magnesium sulfate and evaporated under reduced pressure. The residue was purified by preparative TLC (dichloromethane-methanol 10:1) and 49 mg (36%) of product (**17**) was obtained. Mp 233–235 °C (decomp.).

TLC (dichloromethane-methanol 10:1); R_f = 0.53.

IR (KBr) 3469, 1738, 1668, 1460, 1232, 744 cm^{-1}.

NMR: two signal sets in a ratio of ca. 2:1 (conformational isomers due to hindered rotation of N-formyl group on the vindoline subunit of **2**).

Major signal set:

^{1}H NMR (499.9 MHz, CDCl$_3$) δ (ppm) 0.35–0.41 (m, 3H, H$_3$-18′), 0.77 (br t, J = 7.3 Hz, 3H, H$_3$-18), 0.97–1.06 (m, 2H, H$_x$-19′, H$_x$-15′), 1.26–1.43 (m, 3H, H$_x$-19, H$_y$-19′, H$_y$-15′), 1.59–1.69 (m, 1H, H$_y$-19), 1.88–1.98 (br m, 1H, H-14′), 2.01–2.08 (br m, 1H, H$_x$-6) overlapped with 2.07 (br s, 3H, C(17)-OC(O)CH$_3$), 2.33–2.44 (m, 2H, H$_x$-17′, H$_x$-21′), 2.45–2.54 (m, 2H, H$_y$-21′, H$_x$-3′), 2.54–2.70 (m, 2H, H$_y$-6, H$_x$-5), 2.84–2.93 (m, 2H, H$_x$-3, H-21), 3.00–3.10 (br m, 1H, H$_y$-17′), 3.17–3.22 (m, 1H, H$_x$-6′), 3.35–3.43 (m, 3H, H$_y$-3, H$_y$-5, H$_x$-5′), 3.46–3.53 (m, 1H, H$_y$-6′), 3.53–3.60 (m, 1H, H$_y$-5′), 3.62 (s, 3H, C(16′)-COOCH$_3$), 3.73 (s, 3H, C(16)-COOCH$_3$), 3.81 (br d, J = 13.7 Hz, 1H, H$_y$-3′), 3.89 (br s, 3H, C(11)-OCH$_3$), 4.76 (br s, 1H, H-2), 5.25 (br s, 1H, H-17), 5.42–5.46 (m, 1H, H-15), 5.91–5.95 (m, 1H, H-14), 6.80 (br s, 1H, H-12), 6.93 (br s, 1H, H-9), 7.09–7.15 (m, 1H, H-10′), 7.15–7.22 (m, 2H, H-12′, H-11′), 7.36 (br s, 1H, N(4′)-CHO), 7.51–7.55 (m, 1H, H-9′), 7.94 (br, 1H, NH-1′), 8.74 (s, 1H, N(1)-CHO), 9.23 (br, 1H, C(16)-OH).

^{13}C NMR (125.7 MHz, CDCl$_3$) δ (ppm) 8.1 (C-18, C-18′), 21.1 (C(17)-OC(O)CH$_3$), 24.9 (C-19′), 25.0 (C-6′), 28.7 (br, C-14′), 30.7 (C-19), 38.6 (br, C-17′), 40.3 (C-6), 42.3 (C-20), 42.5 (C-15′), 49.5 (C-5′), 49.7 (C-5), 49.9 (C-3), 51.6 (C-3′), 52.6 (C(16′)-COOCH$_3$), 52.9 (C(16)-COOCH$_3$), 53.5 (C-7), 53.8 (C-21′), 56.1 (C(11)-OCH$_3$), 56.7 (br, C-16′), 58.4 (C-20′), 65.0 (C-21), 72.6 (C-2), 77.0 (C-17), 79.8 (C-16), 94.8 (br, C-12), 111.1 (C-12′), 111.9 (C-7′), 117.7 (C-9′), 119.6 (C-10′), 122.8 (C-11′), 124.6 (C-8), 125.0 (C-14), 126.6 (br, C-10), 126.9 (C-9), 128.3 (C-8′), 129.6 (C-15), 132.1 (C-2′), 135.6 (C-13′), 141.7 (C-13), 157.7 (C-11), 160.1 (N(1)-CHO), 163.4 (N(4′)-CHO), 170.5 (C(17)-OC(O)CH$_3$), 170.7 (C(16)-COOCH$_3$), 173.6 (br, C(16′)-COOCH$_3$).

Minor signal set:

^{1}H NMR (499.9 MHz, CDCl$_3$) δ (ppm) 0.35–0.41 (m, 3H, H$_3$-18′), 0.64–0.70 (m, 3H, H$_3$-18), 0.97–1.06 (m, 2H, H$_x$-19′, H$_x$-15′), 1.26–1.43 (m, 3H, H$_x$-19, H$_y$-19′, H$_y$-15′), 1.59–1.69 (m, 1H, H$_y$-19), 1.88–1.98 (br m, 1H, H-14′), 2.01–2.08 (br m, 1H, H$_x$-6), 2.10 (br s, 3H, C(17)-OC(O)CH$_3$), 2.33–2.44 (m, 2H, H$_x$-17′, H$_x$-21′), 2.45–2.54 (m, 2H, H$_y$-21′, H$_x$-3′), 2.54–2.70 (m, 2H, H$_y$-6, H$_x$-5), 2.84–2.90 (m, 1H, H$_x$-3), 2.95 (br s, 1H, H-21), 3.00–3.10 (br m, 1H, H$_y$-17′), 3.17–3.22 (m, 1H, H$_x$-6′), 3.35–3.43 (m, 3H, H$_y$-3, H$_y$-5, H$_x$-5′), 3.46–3.53 (m, 1H, H$_y$-6′), 3.53–3.60 (m, 1H, H$_y$-5′), 3.62 (s, 3H, C(16′)-COOCH$_3$), 3.78 (s, 3H, C(16)-COOCH$_3$), 3.81 (br d, J = 13.7 Hz, 1H, H$_y$-3′), 3.90 (br s, 3H, C(11)-OCH$_3$), 4.52 (br s, 1H, H-2), 5.29 (br s, 1H, H-17), 5.42–5.46 (m, 1H, H-15), 5.92–5.96 (m, 1H, H-14), 6.86 (br s, 1H, H-9), 7.09–7.15 (m, 1H, H-10′), 7.15–7.22 (m, 2H, H-12′, H-11′), 7.36 (br s, 1H, N(4′)-CHO), 7.51–7.55 (m, 1H, H-9′), 7.80 (br s, 1H, H-12), 7.96 (br, 1H, NH-1′), 8.21 (s, 1H, N(1)-CHO), 9.23 (br, 1H, C(16)-OH).

^{13}C NMR (125.7 MHz, CDCl$_3$) δ (ppm) 7.9 (C-18), 8.1 (C-18′), 21.1 (C(17)-OC(O)CH$_3$), 25.0 (C-19′, C-6′), 28.7 (br, C-14′), 30.7 (C-19), 38.6 (br, C-17′), 40.0 (C-6), 42.3 (C-20), 42.4 (C-15′), 49.6 (C-5, C-5′), 50.0 (C-3), 51.7 (C-3′), 52.6 (C(16)-COOCH$_3$), 52.9 (C(16′)-COOCH$_3$), 53.1 (C-7), 53.8 (C-21′), 56.1 (C(11)-OCH$_3$), 56.7 (br, C-16′), 58.4 (C-20′), 64.3 (C-21), 74.4 (C-2), 76.0 (C-17), 81.5 (C-16), 101.7 (br, C-12), 111.1 (C-12′), 111.7 (C-7′), 117.6 (C-9′), 119.5 (C-10′), 122.7 (C-11′), 124.3 (C-8), 125.1 (C-14), 125.7 (C-9), 126.6 (br, C-10), 128.2 (C-8′), 129.6 (C-15), 132.5 (C-2′), 135.6 (C-13′), 141.6 (C-13), 157.2 (C-11), 160.5 (N(1)-CHO), 163.4 (N(4′)-CHO), 170.3 (C(16)-COOCH$_3$), 170.4 (C(17)-OC(O)CH$_3$), 173.7 (C(16′)-COOCH$_3$).

HRMS: M + Na = 853.39557 (C$_{45}$H$_{58}$O$_{11}$N$_4$Na, Δ = −4.5 ppm). ESI-MS-MS (CID = 35%, rel. int. %): 835(19), 811(7), 793(100), 775(4), 733(18), 705(3).

3.9. Epoxidation of 10-Bromovindoline (7)

To a solution of 10-bromovindoline (**7**) (300 mg, 0.56 mmol) in methanol (5 mL) and 72% perchloric acid (0.17 mL), *m*-CPBA (306 mg, 1.37 mmol) in methanol (2 mL) was added dropwise at 0 °C, and the reaction mixture was stirred at reflux for 5 h. Methanol was evaporated, 10% aqueous sodium carbonate solution (20 mL) was added to the residue, and the mixture was extracted with dichloromethane (3 × 20 mL). The combined organic phase was dried over magnesium sulfate and evaporated under reduced pressure. The residue was purified by preparative TLC (dichloromethane-methanol 15:1) and 70 mg (27%) of product (**19**) was obtained. Mp. 365 °C (decomp.).

TLC (dichloromethane-methanol 20:1); R_f = 0.30.

IR (KBr) 3445, 1745, 1677, 1589, 1414, 1254 cm^{-1}.

^{1}H NMR (499.9 MHz, CDCl$_3$) δ (ppm) 0.71 (t, J = 7.4 Hz, 3H, H$_3$-18), 1.47 (dq, J = 14.8, 7.4 Hz, 1H, H$_x$-19), 1.75 (dq, J = 14.8, 7.4 Hz, 1H, H$_y$-19), 2.08 (s, 3H, C(17)-OC(O)CH$_3$), 2.22 (ddd, J = 13.6, 11.2, 5.0 Hz, 1H, H$_x$-6), 2.46 (ddd, J = 13.6, 9.0, 6.2 Hz, 1H, H$_y$-6), 2.74 (ddd, J = 11.2, 9.8, 6.2 Hz, 1H, H$_x$-5), 2.92–2.98 (m, 5H, H-21, N(1)-CH$_3$, H$_x$-3), 3.48–3.54 (m, 2H, H$_y$-5, H$_y$-3), 3.82 (s, 3H, C(16)-COOCH$_3$), 4.18 (s, 1H, H-2), 5.16 (s, 1H, H-17), 5.35 (br d, J = 10.2 Hz, 1H, H-15), 5.51 (s, 1H, H-12), 5.96 (ddd, J = 10.2, 5,1, 1.3 Hz, 1H, H-14), 6.38 (s, 1H, H-9).

^{13}C NMR (125.7 MHz, CDCl$_3$) δ (ppm) 7.5 (C-18), 20.8 (C(17)-OC(O)CH$_3$), 31.1 (C-19), 35.3 (N(1)-CH$_3$), 42.2 (C-6), 42.8 (C-20), 50.3 (C-3), 50.7 (C-5), 51.5 (C-7), 52.9 (C(16)-COOCH$_3$), 66.8 (C-21), 74.7 (C-17), 79.2 (C-16), 82.1 (C-2), 94.7 (C-12), 123.8 (C-9), 124.7 (C-14), 129.4 (C-15), 157.6 (C-8), 157.9 (C-13), 170.1 (C(17)-OC(O)CH$_3$), 170.6 (C(16)-COOCH$_3$), 174.6 (C-11), 180.7 (C-10).

HRMS: M + H = 457.19636 (C$_{24}$H$_{29}$O$_7$N$_2$, Δ = −1.2 ppm). ESI-MS-MS (CID = 45%, rel. int. %): 439(23), 429(34), 415(34), 411(3), 397(100), 379(10), 369(9), 368(10), 347(6), 337(27), 295(15), 290(7), 190(7).

3.10. Epoxidation of Catharanthine (3)

Method A. Without perchloric acid. To a solution of catharanthine (**3**) (160 mg, 0.48 mmol) in dry methanol (10 mL), *m*-CPBA (184 mg, 0.82 mmol) was added, and the reaction mixture was stirred at room temperature for 1 h. The reaction mixture was diluted with 10% aqueous sodium carbonate (10 mL) and extracted with dichloromethane (3 × 10 mL). The combined organic phase was dried over magnesium sulfate and evaporated under reduced pressure. The residue was purified by preparative

TLC (dichloromethane-methanol 4:1) and products **20** (57 mg, 34%) and **21** (62 mg, 35%) were isolated. *N*-oxide **20** is prone to rearrangement and transforms into isoxazolidine **22**, which is a stable compound.

20 and **22**; mp 116–117 °C. TLC (dichloromethane-methanol 4:1); R_f (*N*-oxide form (**20**)) = 0.76 and R_f (neutral form (**22**)) = 0.90.

IR (KBr) 3378, 3185, 2960, 1735, 1460, 1435, 1237, 744 cm^{-1}.

NMR: (chemical shifts might vary slightly with concentration, pH and the exact ratio of **20** and **22**)

N-oxide **20**:

^{1}H NMR (499.9 MHz, CDCl$_3$) δ (ppm) 1.04 (t, J = 7.4 Hz, 3H, H$_3$-18), 1.58–1.62 (m, 1H, H$_x$-17), 2.12–2.19 (m, 1H, H$_x$-19), 2.44–2.50 (m, 1H, H$_y$-19), 2.83–2.88 (m, 1H, H$_y$-17), 2.92–2.96 (m, 1H, H-14), 2.96–3.02 (m, 1H, H$_x$-6), 3.40–3.48 (m, 2H, H$_x$-3, H$_y$-6), 3.67 (s, 3H, C(16)-COOCH_3), 3.74–3.79 (m, 1H, H$_y$-3), 3.92 (ddd, J = 13.2, 8.3, 1.6 Hz, 1H, H$_x$-5), 4.27–4.34 (m, 1H, H$_y$-5), 4.72–4.74 (m, 1H, H-21), 6.07–6.10 (m, 1H, H-15), 7.06–7.09 (m, 1H, H-10), 7.11–7.15 (m, 1H, H-11), 7.21–7.24 (m, 1H, H-12), 7.41–7.43 (m, 1H, H-9), 7.88 (br s, 1H, NH-1).

^{13}C NMR (125.7 MHz, CDCl$_3$) δ (ppm) 10.4 (C-18), 19.8 (C-6), 28.3 (C-19), 30.0 (C-14), 32.3 (C-17), 51.0 (C-16), 53.2 (C(16)-COOCH$_3$), 73.5 (C-3), 74.4 (C-21), 76.9 (C-5), 111.1 (C-12), 111.7 (C-7), 118.2 (C-9), 120.3 (C-10), 122.8 (C-11), 124.3 (C-15), 127.4 (C-8), 133.7 (C-2), 134.9 (C-13), 145.9 (C-20), 171.5 (C(16)-COOCH$_3$).

Isoxazolidine **22**:

^{1}H NMR (499.9 MHz, CDCl$_3$) δ (ppm) 1.14 (t, J = 7.5 Hz, 3H, H$_3$-18), 1.98 (dd, J = 14.2, 6.1 Hz, 1H, H$_x$-17), 2.18–2.26 (m, 1H, H$_x$-19), 2.26–2.30 (m, 1H, H$_y$-17), 2.36–2.45 (m, 1H, H$_y$-19), 2.58 (dd, J = 10.6, 5.2 Hz, 1H, H$_x$-3), 2.75–2.80 (m, 1H, H$_x$-6), 2.94–3.01 (m, 1H, H$_x$-5), 3.13–3.20 (m, 1H, H-14), 3.29–3.37 (m, 3H, H$_y$-3, H$_y$-5, H$_y$-6), 3.77 (s, 3H, C(16)-COOCH_3), 4.53 (d, J = 10.0 Hz, 1H, H-15), 6.19–6.20 (m, 1H, H-21), 7.00–7.04 (m, 1H, H-10), 7.10–7.13 (m, 1H, H-11), 7.24–7.26 (m, 1H, H-12), 7.39–7.42 (m, 1H, H-9), 8.67 (br s, 1H, NH-1).

^{13}C NMR (125.7 MHz, CDCl$_3$) δ (ppm) 11.3 (C-18), 23.7 (C-6), 27.4 (C-19), 32.5 (C-17), 39.9 (C-14), 46.7 (C-16), 53.1 (C(16)-COOCH$_3$), 55.5 (C-3), 55.8 (C-5), 76.6 (C-15), 110.8 (C-12), 113.6 (C-7), 118.4 (C-9), 119.5 (C-10), 121.9 (C-21), 122.7 (C-11), 127.9 (C-2), 128.0 (C-8), 135.2 (C-13), 141.5 (C-20), 174.9 (C(16)-COOCH$_3$).

HRMS:

N-oxide **20**:

M+H = 353.18559 (C$_{21}$H$_{25}$O$_3$N$_2$, Δ = −1.1 ppm). ESI-MS-MS (CID = 45%, rel. int. %): 336(100), 321(7), 303(6), 294(4), 293(3), 275(2), 266(6), 229(2), 189(2), 171(2), 144(12).

Isoxazolidine **22**:

M+H = 353.18567 (C$_{21}$H$_{25}$O$_3$N$_2$, Δ = −0.9 ppm). ESI-MS-MS (CID = 45%, rel. int. %): 335(100), 321(36), 303(36), 294(22), 293(15), 275(11), 266(38), 171(5), 144(4).

21; mp 146–147 °C. TLC (dichloromethane-methanol 4:1); R_f = 0.52.

IR (KBr) 3581, 3365, 2959, 1744, 1570, 1242, 774 cm^{-1}.

^{1}H NMR (499.9 MHz, DMSO-d_6:CDCl$_3$ = 1:1 + 5 v/v% CF$_3$COOH) δ (ppm) 1.07 (t, J = 7.4 Hz, 3H, H$_3$-18), 1.99–2.11 (m, 2H, H$_x$-17, H$_x$-19), 2.16–2.25 (m, 1H, H$_x$-6), 2.25–2.34 (m, 1H, H$_y$-19), 2.49–2.56 (m, 1H, H$_y$-6), 2.87–2.93 (m, 1H, H$_y$-17), 3.11–3.15 (m, 1H, H-14), 3.34–3.40 (m, 1H, H$_x$-3), 3.67 (s, 3H, C(16)-COOCH_3), 3.90–3.95 (m, 1H, H$_y$-3), 4.14–4.29 (m, 1H, H$_x$-5), 4.54–4.63 (m, 1H, H$_y$-5), 5.59 (d, J = 1.4 Hz, 1H, H-21), 6.24–6.27 (m, 1H, H-15), 7.28–7.32 (m, 1H, H-10), 7.36–7.40 (m, 1H, H-11), 7.44–7.46 (m, 1H, H-12), 7.47–7.49 (m, 1H, H-9).

^{13}C NMR (125.7 MHz, DMSO-d_6:CDCl$_3$ = 1:1 + 5 v/v% CF$_3$COOH) δ (ppm) 10.2 (C-18), 26.9 (C-19), 29.0 (C-14), 30.0 (C-6), 34.6 (C-17), 52.3 (C-16), 53.3 (C(16)-COOCH$_3$), 64.3 (br, C-3), 65.2 (br, C-5), 70.8 (C-21), 82.8 (C-7), 120.6 (C-12), 122.5 (C-9), 125.9 (C-15), 126.9 (C-10), 129.7 (C-11), 140.2 (br, C-8), 141.4 (C-20), 152.0 (C-13), 168.1 (C(16)-COOCH$_3$), 184.0 (C-2).

HRMS: M + H = 369.18063 (C$_{21}$H$_{25}$O$_4$N$_2$, Δ = −0.7 ppm). ESI-MS-MS (CID = 45%, rel. int. %): 351(16), 335(9), 324(29), 307(100), 292(5), 264(14), 205(3), 187(4), 160(6).

Method B. Using perchloric acid. To a solution of catharanthine (**3**) (247 mg, 0.73 mmol) in methanol (10 mL) and 72% perchloric acid (0.10 mL), *m*-CPBA (184 mg, 0.82 mmol) was added at 0 °C, and the reaction mixture was stirred at room temperature for 18 h. The reaction mixture was diluted with 10% aqueous sodium carbonate (10 mL) and extracted with dichloromethane (3×10 mL). The combined organic phase was dried over magnesium sulfate and evaporated under reduced pressure. The residue was purified by preparative TLC (dichloromethane-methanol 10:1) and products **23** (149 mg, 58%) and **24** (30 mg, 12%) were isolated.

Compound **23**; mp 87–89 °C. TLC (dichloromethane-methanol 10:1); R_f = 0.55.

IR (KBr) 3436, 2960, 1741, 1459, 1222, 1078, 757 cm^{-1}.

^{1}H NMR (499.9 MHz, DMSO-d_6) δ (ppm) 0.96 (t, J = 7.4 Hz, 3H, H$_3$-18), 1.73 (dd, J = 13.2, 2.3 Hz, 1H, H$_x$-17), 1.75–1.83 (m, 1H, H$_x$-6), 1.87–1.96 (m, 2H, H$_y$-6, H$_x$-19), 2.07 (dqd, J = 16.1, 7.4, 2.0 Hz, H$_y$-19), 2.52 (dt, J = 8.3, 2.6 Hz, 1H, H$_x$-3), 2.55–2.58 (br m, 1H, H-14), 2.59 (br d, J = 8.3 Hz, 1H, H$_y$-3), 2.73–2.78 (m, 1H, H$_y$-17), 2.79–2.84 (m, 1H, H$_x$-5), 3.50 (s, 3H, C(16)-COOCH_3), 3.61 (ddd, J = 14.3, 12.4, 2.3 Hz, 1H, H$_y$-5), 4.57 (~d, J = 1.1 Hz, 1H, H-21), 5.75–5.77 (m, 1H, H-15), 6.01 (d, J = 0.9 Hz, 1H, C(7)-O*H*), 7.18–7.22 (m, 1H, H-10), 7.28–7.32 (m, 1H, H-11), 7.33–7.36 (m, 1H, H-12), 7.36–7,39 (m, 1H, H-9).

^{13}C NMR (125.7 MHz, DMSO-d_6) δ (ppm) 11.2 (C-18), 25.9 (C-19), 30.7 (C-14), 32.9 (C-6), 39.2 (C-17), 46.7 (C-5), 47.6 (C-3), 52.0 (C(16)-COOCH$_3$), 57.4 (C-16), 57.8 (C-21), 87.1 (C-7), 119.9 (C-12), 121.9 (C-9), 122.4 (C-15), 126.1 (C-10), 128.8 (C-11), 143.0 (C-8), 148.1 (C-20), 152.4 (C-13), 171.6 (C(16)-COOCH$_3$), 190.3 (C-2).

HRMS: M + H = 353.18553 (C$_{21}$H$_{25}$O$_3$N$_2$, Δ = −1.2 ppm). ESI-MS-MS (CID = 35%, rel. int. %): 335(80), 321(100), 303(3), 189(4), 171(8).

Compound **24**; mp 99–101 °C (decomp.). TLC (dichloromethane-methanol 10:1); R_f = 0.13.

IR (KBr) 1730, 1693, 1618, 755 cm^{-1}.

^{1}H NMR (499.9 MHz, DMSO-d_6:CDCl$_3$ = 2:1 (v/v)) δ (ppm) 1.03 (t, J = 7.4 Hz, 3H, H-18), 1.71 (br d, J = 14.8 Hz, 1H, H$_x$-6), 1.95 (br d, J = 13.3 Hz, 1H, H$_x$-17), 2.06 (dqd, J = 16.4, 7.4, 1.6 Hz, H$_x$-19), 2.30–2.43 (m, 3H, H$_y$-19, H$_y$-6, H$_y$-17), 2.83 (br d, 1H, J = 10.8 Hz, H$_x$-3), 2.90–2.94 (m, 1H, H-14), 3.03–3.08 (m, 2H, H$_y$-3, H$_x$-5), 3.24 (s, 3H, C(16)-COOCH_3), 4.10 (td, J = 12.9, 3.2 Hz, 1H, H$_y$-5), 4.92 (br s, 1H, H-21), 6.17 (br d, J = 6.4 Hz, 1H, H-15), 6.55–6.64 (br, 1H, NH-1), 6.72–6.77 (m, 1H, H-10), 6.79–6.82 (m, 1H, H-12), 7.37–7.42 (m, 1H, H-11), 7.49–7.52 (m, 1H, H-9).

^{13}C NMR (125.7 MHz, DMSO-d_6:CDCl$_3$ = 2:1 (v/v)) δ (ppm) 10.7 (C-18), 23.4 (C-6), 26.5 (C-19), 28.9 (C-14), 30.3 (C-17), 44.7 (C-5), 50.3 (C-3), 51.9 (C-16), 52.0 (C(16)-COOCH$_3$), 54.0 (C-21), 65.0 (C-2), 112.1 (C-12), 118.5 (C-10), 119.4 (C-8), 124.2 (C-9), 128.0 (C-15), 137.3 (C-11), 144.2 (C-20), 159.9 (C-13), 171.2 (C(16)-COOCH$_3$), 202.2 (C-7).

HRMS: M + H = 353.18512 (C$_{21}$H$_{25}$O$_3$N$_2$, Δ = −2.4 ppm). ESI-MS-MS (CID = 45%, rel. int. %): 335(3), 321(2), 276(2), 189(100), 172(6), 160(38), 146(23).

3.11. Reduction of the 7-Hydroxy Derivative of Catharanthine (**23**)

To a solution of 7-hydroxyindolenine catharanthine (**23**) (300 mg, 0.85 mmol) in methanol (20 mL), 700 mg of 10% Pd/C and NaBH$_4$ (483 mg, 12.77 mmol) was added at 10 °C. The reaction mixture was stirred under an argon atmosphere for 30 min. After filtering the catalyst, a few drops of acetic acid was added, the filtrate was diluted with dichloromethane (50 mL) and washed with 10% aqueous sodium carbonate. The aqueous phase was extracted with dichloromethane (2 × 20 mL), the combined organic phase was washed with water (50 mL), dried over magnesium sulfate and evaporated under reduced pressure. The residue was purified by preparative TLC (dichloromethane-methanol 9:1) and catharanthine (**3**) was obtained (111 mg, 39%).

3.12. Coupling of the Catharanthine Derivative (**24**) *with Vindoline* (**4**)

Compound **24** (210 mg, 0.60 mmol) and vindoline (271 mg, 0.59 mmol) (**4**) were added to a mixture that consisted of water (21.3 mL), 1 *M* hydrochloric acid (1.1 mL) and 2,2,2-trifluoroethanol (2.2 mL).

Under an argon atmosphere, FeCl$_3$·6 H$_2$O (802 mg, 2.97 mmol) was added. The reaction mixture was stirred at room temperature for 2 h. At 0 °C, sodium borohydride (24 mg, 0.63 mmol) in water (1.9 mL) was added dropwise. After 30 min of stirring, the pH was adjusted to 8 with cc. ammonium hydroxide. The reaction mixture was extracted with dichloromethane (2 × 60 mL), the combined organic phase was washed with water (100 mL), dried over magnesium sulfate and evaporated under reduced pressure. The residue was purified by preparative TLC (dichloromethane-methanol 6:1). A cationic vindoline trimer (**27**) (18 mg, 7%), a vindoline trimer ketone (**28**) (26 mg, 10%), and the N-methyl-spiro derivative of catharanthine (**29**) (24 mg, 11%) were obtained.

Compound **27**:

TLC (dichloromethane-methanol 7:1), R_f = 0.27.

NMR: two signal sets in a ratio of ca. 3:2 (conformational isomers). Chemical shifts vary slightly with pH, temperature, and the composition of the NMR solvent. The three vindoline subunits of **27** are denoted as A, B, and B'. The two subunits that have the same constitution (vindoline-10-yl) are called B and B'.

Major signal set:

^{1}H NMR (799.7 MHz, CD$_3$OD:CD$_3$CN:D$_2$O = 1:1:1 (v/v)) δ (ppm) 0.35 (t, J = 7.4 Hz, 3H, H$_3$-18B), 0.52 (t, J = 7.4 Hz, 3H, H$_3$-18B'), 0.57 (t, J = 7.4 Hz, 3H, H$_3$-18A), 1.15–1.20 (m, 1H, H$_x$-19B'), 1.25–1.30 (m, 1H, H$_x$-19B), 1.47–1.53 (m, 1H, H$_x$-19A), 1.53–1.58 (m, 1H, H$_y$-19A), 1.55–1.61 (m, 1H, H$_y$-19B'), 1.58–1.63 (m, 1H, H$_y$-19B), 1.62–1.67 (m, 1H, H$_x$-6A), 2.02 (s, 6H, C(17B)-OC(O)CH$_3$, C(17B')-OC(O)CH$_3$), 2.06 (s, 3H, C(17A)-OC(O)CH$_3$), 2.15–2.20 (m, 1H, H$_x$-6B'), 2.20–2.24 (m, 2H, H$_y$-6A, H$_y$-6B'), 2.26–2.30 (m, 2H, H$_x$-6B, H-21B), 2.32–2.35 (m, 1H, H$_x$-5B), 2.37–2.41 (m, 1H, H$_y$-6B), 2.54–2.58 (m, 1H, H$_x$-5B'), 2.64 (s, 3H, N(1B)-CH$_3$), 2.65 (s, 1H, H-21B'), 2.67–2.71 (m, 1H, H$_x$-5A), 2.71 (s, 3H, N(1B')-CH$_3$), 2.73–2.77 (m, 1H, H$_x$-3B), 2.85–2.89 (m, 1H, H$_x$-3B'), 2.94–2.98 (m, 1H, H$_x$-3A), 3.12 (s, 1H, H-21A), 3.28 (s, 3H, N(1A)-CH$_3$), 3.30–3.34 (m, 1H, H$_y$-5A), 3.37–3.43 (m, 3H, H$_y$-5B', H$_y$-5B, H$_y$-3A), 3.45–3.53 (m, 2H, H$_y$-3B', H$_y$-3B), 3.66 (s, 1H, H-2B), 3.69 (s, 1H, H-2B'), 3.73 (s, 3H, C(11B')-OCH$_3$), 3.74 (s, 3H, C(11B)-OCH$_3$), 3.78 (s, 3H, C(16B')-COOCH$_3$), 3.79 (s, 3H, C(16B)-COOCH$_3$), 3.83 (s, 3H, C(16A)-COOCH$_3$), 3.97 (s, 3H, C(11A)-OCH$_3$), 4.39 (s, 1H, H-2A), 5.08 (s, 1H, H-17A), 5.08–5.11 (m, 1H, H-15B), 5.19–5.22 (m, 1H, H-15B'), 5.32 (s, 1H, H-17B'), 5.38–5.41 (s, 1H, H-15A), 5.43 (s, 1H, H-17B), 5.79–5.82 (m, 1H, H-14B), 5.87–5.90 (m, 1H, H-14B'), 5.94–5.97 (m, 1H, H-14A), 6.27 (s, 1H, H-12B), 6.36 (s, 1H, H-12B'), 6.39 (s, 1H, H-12A), 6.42 (s, 1H, H-9B'), 6.63 (s, 1H, H-9B), 7.29 (s, 1H, H-9A).

^{13}C NMR (201.1 MHz, CD$_3$OD:CD$_3$CN:D$_2$O = 1:1:1 (v/v)) δ (ppm) 7.6 (C-18A), 9.2 (C-18B), 9.5 (C-18B'), 21.0 (C(17B)-OC(O)CH$_3$, C(17A)-OC(O)CH$_3$, C(17B')-OC(O)CH$_3$), 30.8 (C-19A), 31.9 (C-19B'), 32.7 (C-19B), 37.3 (N(1A)-CH$_3$), 38.3 (N(1B')-CH$_3$), 38.7 (N(1B)-CH$_3$), 43.2 (C-6A), 43.3 (C-20A), 44.0 (C-6B, C-6B'), 44.1 (C-20B'), 44.4 (C-20B), 49.2 (C-5A), 50.6 (C-3A), 51.6 (C-3B'), 51.9 (C-3B, C-7A), 52.1 (C-5B'), 53.3 (C(16B')-COOCH$_3$), 53.4 (C(16B)-COOCH$_3$), 53.7 (C-7B), 53.8 (C-5B), 54.0 (C(16A)-COOCH$_3$), 54.1 (C-7B'), 56.5 (C(11B')-OCH$_3$), 57.2 (C(11B)-OCH$_3$), 59.3 (C(11A)-OCH$_3$), 59.4 (C-10A), 63.4 (C-21A), 67.8 (C-21B'), 69.2 (C-21B), 76.8 (C-17A), 76.9 (C-17B'), 77.0 (C-17B), 80.1 (C-16B, C-16A), 80.5 (C-16B'), 83.8 (C-2B'), 84.0 (C-2B), 84.6 (C-2A), 91.3 (C-12A), 95.1 (C-12B'), 95.5 (C-12B), 115.9 (C-10B), 116.9 (C-10B'), 124.0 (C-9B'), 126.0 (C-14B), 126.1 (C-9B), 126.2 (C-14B'), 126.4 (C-14A), 126.5 (C-8B'), 126.6 (C-8B), 130.2 (C-15A), 130.6 (C-15B, C-15B'), 132.3 (C-8A), 145.9 (C-9A), 155.3 (C-13B), 155.7 (C-13B'), 159.9 (C-11B), 160 (C-11B'), 169.9 (C-13A), 172.0 (C(16A)-COOCH$_3$), 172.2 (C(17A)-OC(O)CH$_3$), 172.8 (C(17B')-OC(O)CH$_3$), 173.0 (C(17B)-OC(O)CH$_3$), 173.4 (C(16B')-COOCH$_3$), 173.7 (C(16B)-COOCH$_3$), 190.6 (C-11A).

Minor signal set:

^{1}H NMR (799.7 MHz, CD$_3$OD:CD$_3$CN:D$_2$O = 1:1:1 (v/v)) δ (ppm) 0.29 (t, J = 7.4 Hz, 3H, H$_3$-18A), 0.46 (t, J = 7.4 Hz, 3H, H$_3$-18B'), 0.61 (t, J = 7.4 Hz, 3H, H$_3$-18B), 0.85–0.89 (m, 1H, H$_x$-19A), 1.09–1.14 (m, 2H, H$_x$-19B, H$_x$-19B'), 1.41–1.45 (m, 1H, H$_y$-19A), 1.50–1.54 (m, 1H, H$_y$-19B'), 1.57–1.61 (m, 1H, H$_y$-19B), 2.00 (s, 3H, C(17A)-OC(O)CH$_3$), 2.01 (s, 3H, C(17B)-OC(O)CH$_3$), 2.02 (s, 3H, C(17B')-OC(O)CH$_3$), 2.07–2.11 (m, 2H, H$_x$-6B', H$_x$-6B), 2.19–2.26 (m, 3H, H$_y$-6B, H$_x$-6A, H$_y$-6B'), 2.43–2.47 (m, 1H, H$_x$-5B'), 2.47–2.51 (m, 1H, H$_y$-6A), 2.57 (s, 1H, H-21B'), 2.63–2.66 (m, 1H, H$_x$-5B), 2.68 (s, 3H, N(1B')-CH$_3$), 2.72

(s, 3H, N(1B)-CH_3), 2.77–2.80 (m, 1H, H$_x$-5A), 2.79–2.83 (m, 1H, H$_x$-3B'), 2.87 (s, 1H, H-21B), 2.90–2.96 (m, 2H, H$_x$-3A, H$_x$-3B), 2.98 (s, 1H, H-21A), 3.23 (s, 3H, N(1A)-CH_3), 3.37–3.42 (m, 2H, H$_y$-5B', H$_y$-5B), 3.42–3.45 (m, 1H, H$_y$-5A), 3.44–3.49 (m, 3H, H$_y$-3A, H$_y$-3B, H$_y$-3B'), 3.62 (s, 3H, C(11B')-OCH_3), 3.65 (s, 1H, H-2B'), 3.67 (s, 1H, H-2B), 3.73 (s, 3H, C(11B)-OCH_3), 3.75 (s, 3H, C(16B)-COOCH_3), 3.76 (s, 3H, C(16B')-COOCH_3), 3.80 (s, 3H, C(16A)-COOCH_3), 4.01 (s, 3H, C(11A)-OCH_3), 4.50 (s, 1H, H-2A), 4.95 (s, 1H, H-17A), 5.19 (s, 1H, H-17B), 5.22–5.26 (m, 2H, H-15B', H-15A), 5.24 (s, 1H, H-17B'), 5.35–5.38 (m, 1H, H-15B), 5.87–5.90 (m, 1H, H-14B'), 5.90–5.93 (m, 2H, H-14A, H-14B), 6.20 (s, 1H, H-12A), 6.23 (s, 2H, H-12B, H-12B'), 6.52 (s, 1H, H-9B), 6.55 (s, 1H, H-9B'), 7.39 (br s, 1H, H-9A).

^{13}C NMR (201.1 MHz, CD$_3$OD:CD$_3$CN:D$_2$O = 1:1:1 (v/v)) δ (ppm) 7.6 (C-18A), 8.1 (C-18B), 8.7 (C-18B'), 20.8 (C(17A)-OC(O)CH$_3$), 21.0 (C(17B)-OC(O)CH$_3$), 21.1 (C(17B')-OC(O)CH$_3$), 31.4 (C-19B), 31.6 (C-19B'), 32.1 (C-19A), 37.2 (N(1A)-CH$_3$), 38.2 (N(1B)-CH$_3$), 38.3 (N(1B')-CH$_3$), 42.7 (C-6A), 43.4 (C-20A), 43.8 (C-20B), 43.9 (C-20B'), 44.3 (C-6B'), 44.9 (C-6B), 50.1 (C-5A), 50.7 (C-5B), 50.9 (C-3A), 51.2 (C-3B), 51.4 (C-7A), 51.6 (C-3B'), 51.9 (C-5B'), 53.2 (C(16B)-COOCH$_3$), 53.3 (C(16B')-COOCH$_3$), 53.9 (C(16A)-COOCH$_3$), 54.1 (C-7B'), 54.4 (C-7B), 56.5 (C(11B)-OCH$_3$), 56.7 (C(11B')-OCH$_3$), 58.0 (C-10A), 59.5 (C(11A)-OCH$_3$), 65.2 (C-21A), 66.1 (C-21B), 67.1 (C-21B'), 76.6 (C-17A), 76.9 (C-17B), 77.2 (C-17B'), 79.6 (C-16A), 80.8 (C-16B'), 81.2 (C-16B), 83.3 (C-2B), 83.4 (C-2B'), 84.9 (C-2A), 89.4 (C-12A), 94.7 (C-12B), 95.6 (C-12B'), 115.9 (C-10B), 117.3 (C-10B'), 124.3 (C-9B), 125.2 (C-8B), 125.3 (C-9B'), 125.4 (C-8B'), 125.7 (C-14B), 125.9 (C-14B'), 126.1 (C-14A), 130.1 (C-15A), 130.8 (C-15B'), 131.0 (C-15B), 132.5 (C-8A), 147.2 (br, C-9A), 154.6 (C-13B), 154.9 (C-13B'), 159.8 (C-11B), 160.7 (C-11B'), 169.9 (C-13A), 171.7 (C(17A)-OC(O)CH$_3$), 172.1 (C(16A)-COOCH$_3$), 172.5 (C(17B)-OC(O)CH$_3$), 172.9 (C(17B')-OC(O)CH$_3$), 173.0 (C(16B)-COOCH$_3$), 173.3 (C(16B')-COOCH$_3$), 191.8 (C-11A).

HRMS: M + H = 1365.65951 (C$_{75}$H$_{93}$O$_{18}$N$_6$, Δ = 3.97 ppm). ESI-MS-MS (CID = 35%, rel. int. %): 1347(17), 1305(73), 1245(9), 1203(10), 1096(100), 1036(17).

Compound **28**:

TLC (dichloromethane-methanol 10:1), R_f = 0.35.

IR (KBr) 3433, 1749, 1619, 1289, 1207, 1151, 1025, 821 cm^{-1}.

NMR: The three vindoline subunits of **28** are denoted as A, B, and B'. The two subunits that have the same constitution (vindoline-10-yl) are called B and B'. A minor signal set (ca. 10%) can also be detected due to conformational isomerism. The assignment of the major signal set is given below.

^{1}H NMR (799.7 MHz, DMSO-d_6:CD$_3$CN:D$_2$O = 3:1:1 (v/v)) δ (ppm) 0.30 (t, J = 7.3 Hz, 3H, H$_3$-18A), 0.43 (t, J = 7.3 Hz, 3H, H$_3$-18B), 0.50 (t, J = 7.3 Hz, 3H, H$_3$-18B'), 0.82–0.86 (m, 1H, H$_x$-19B'), 0.92–0.96 (m, 1H, H$_x$-19A), 1.21 (dq, J = 15.2, 7.3 Hz, 1H, H$_x$-19B), 1.39–1.43 (m, 1H, H$_y$-19A), 1.43–1.50 (m, 2H, H$_y$-19B' H$_y$-19B), 1.91 (s, 3H, C(17A)-OC(O)CH_3), 1.94 (s, 3H, C(17B')-OC(O)CH_3), 1.93–1.97 (m, 1H, H$_x$-6B), 1.96 (s, 3H, C(17B)-OC(O)CH_3), 2.08–2.16 (m, 3H, H$_y$-6B, H$_x$-6B', H$_y$-6B'), 2.16–2.20 (m, 2H, H$_x$-5B, H$_x$-6A), 2.31 (s, 1H, H-21B), 2.34–2.38 (m, 1H, H$_y$-6A), 2.55–2.59 (m, 2H, H$_x$-5A, H$_x$-5B'), 2.58 (s, 3H, N(1B)-CH_3), 2.61–2.65 (m, 8H, N(1B')-CH_3, H$_x$-3B, N(1A)-CH_3, H-21A), 2.73 (br s, 1H, H-21B'), 2.79 (br d, J = 16.4 Hz, 1H, H$_x$-3A), 2.85 (br d, J = 16.7 Hz, 1H, H$_x$-3B'), 3.23–3.27 (m, 1H, H$_y$-5B), 3.29–3.35 (m, 2H, H$_y$-5A, H$_y$-5B'), 3.37–3.42 (m, 3H, H$_y$-3B', H$_y$-3B, H$_y$-3A), 3.49 (s, 1H, H-2B), 3.53 (s, 3H, C(11B)-OCH_3), 3.55 (s, 1H, H-2B'), 3.58 (s, 3H, C(11B')-OCH_3), 3.65 (s, 3H, C(16A)-COOCH_3), 3.67 (s, 3H, C(16B')-COOCH_3), 3.68 (s, 3H, C(16B)-COOCH_3), 3.91 (s, 1H, H-2A), 4.97 (s, 1H, H-17A), 5.09 (s, 1H, H-12A), 5.10–5.12 (m, 2H, H-15A, H-17B'), 5.16 (br d, J = 9.6 Hz, 1H, H-15B), 5.20–5.23 (m, 2H, H-17B, H-15B'), 5.81–5.83 (m, 2H, H-14B, H-14A), 5.83–5.86 (m, 1H, H-14B'), 6.12 (s, 1H, H-12B), 6.18 (s, 1H, H-9B), 6.20 (s, 1H, H-12B'), 6.80 (s, 1H, H-9B'), 7.17 (s, 1H, H-9A).

^{13}C NMR (201.1 MHz, DMSO-d_6:CD$_3$CN:D$_2$O = 3:1:1 (v/v)) δ (ppm) 7.2 (C-18B'), 7.7 (C-18A), 8.1 (C-18B), 20.6 (C(17A)-OC(O)CH$_3$), 20.77 (C(17B')-OC(O)CH$_3$), 20.81 (C(17B)-OC(O)CH$_3$), 30.7 (C-19B'), 30.9 (C-19B), 31.2 (C-19A), 34.4 (N(1A)-CH$_3$), 38.2 (N(1B)-CH$_3$), 38.8 (N(1B')-CH$_3$), 42.6 (C-20A), 42.7 (C-20B'), 42.8 (C-6A), 43.0 (C-20B), 43.2 (C-6B), 44.4 (C-6B'), 50.3 (C-7A), 50.4 (C-3A), 50.5 (C-5B'), 50.6 (C-3B'), 50.9 (C-5A), 51.0 (C-3B), 51.8 (C-5B), 52.1 (C(16B')-COOCH$_3$), 52.3 (C(16B)-COOCH$_3$), 52.5 (C(16A)-COOCH$_3$), 52.9 (C-7B), 53.1 (C-7B'), 55.3 (C(11B)-OCH$_3$), 55.4 (C(11B')-OCH$_3$), 59.6 (C-10A), 65.6 (C-21B'), 67.1 (C-21B), 67.2 (C-21A), 75.7 (C-17A), 76.1 (C-17B'), 76.2 (C-17B), 78.7

(C-16A), 79.5 (C-16B), 79.7 (C-16B'), 81.7 (C-2A), 82.6 (C-2B), 83.4 (C-2B'), 92.1 (C-12A), 93.8 (C-12B), 94.3 (C-12B'), 118.5 (C-10B'), 123.0 (C-10B), 123.36 (C-8B), 123.42 (C-8B'), 124.56 (C-14A), 124.67 (C-14B'), 124.73 (C-9B'), 124.88 (C-9B), 124.89 (C-14B), 129.9 (C-15A), 130.3 (C-15B), 130.6 (C-15B'), 133.4 (C-8A), 140,0 (C-9A), 152.4 (C-13B), 152.6 (C-13B'), 158.3 (C-11B), 159.5 (C-11B'), 162.2 (C-13A), 170.1 (C(17A)-OC(O)CH$_3$), 170.5 (C(17B')-OC(O)CH$_3$), 171.1 (C(17B)-OC(O)CH$_3$), 171.79 (C(16A)-COOCH$_3$), 171.83 (C(16B')-COOCH$_3$), 172.1 (C(17B)-COOCH$_3$), 199.1 (C-11A).

HRMS: $[(M + 2H)/2]^{2+}$ = 676.32271 ($C_{74}H_{92}O_{18}N_6$, Δ = −0.2 ppm). ESI-MS-MS (CID = 45%, rel. int. %): 646(100), 637(14), 616(17), 595(45), 565(16), 542(39), 512(16), 457(16).

Compound **29**:

TLC (dichloromethane-methanol 7:1), R_f = 0.11.

^{1}H NMR (799.7 MHz, DMSO-d_6:CD$_3$CN:D$_2$O = 3:1:1 (v/v)) δ (ppm) 1.02 (t, J = 7.3 Hz, 3H, H$_3$-18), 1.93–1.97 (m, 1H, H$_x$-6), 2.04–2.09 (m, 1H, H$_x$-19), 2.07–2.10 (m, 1H, H$_x$-17), 2.18–2.24 (m, 1H, H$_y$-19), 2.27–2.31 (m, 1H, H$_y$-17), 2.55–2.60 (m, 1H, H$_y$-6), 2.92–2.95 (m, 1H, H$_x$-3), 3.04 (s, 3H, N(4)-CH$_3$), 3.14–3.16 (m, 1H, H-14), 3.23 (s, 3H, C(16)-COOCH$_3$), 3.58–3.61 (m, 1H, H$_x$-5), 3.65–3.68 (m, 1H, H$_y$-3), 4.10–4.14 (m, 1H, H$_y$-5), 4.94 (d, J = 1.6 Hz, 1H, H-21), 6.41–6.44 (m, 1H, H-15), 6.80–6.84 (m, 1H, H-10), 6.87–6.90 (m, 1H, H-12), 7.48–7.50 (m, 1H, H-9), 7.50–7.53 (m, 1H, H-11).

^{13}C NMR (201.1 MHz, DMSO-d_6:CD$_3$CN:D$_2$O = 3:1:1 (v/v)) δ (ppm) 10.5 (C-18), 25.0 (C-6), 27.1 (C-19), 28.2 (C-17), 29.1 (C-14), 52.6 (C-16), 52.9 (C(16)-COOCH$_3$), 55.6 (N(4)-CH$_3$), 56.8 (C-5), 60.5 (C-3), 63.5 (C-2), 63.7 (C-21), 112.8 (C-12), 118.9 (C-8), 119.2 (C-10), 124.6 (C-9), 130.7 (C-15), 138.9 (C-11), 140.8 (C-20), 160.8 (C-13), 169.9 (C(16)-COOCH$_3$), 213.1 (C-7).

HRMS: M + H = 367.20122 ($C_{22}H_{27}O_3N_2$, Δ = −1.1 ppm). ESI-MS-MS (CID = 55%, rel. int. %): 203(100), 160(7).

4. Conclusions

Halogenated 14,15-cyclopropanovindoline derivatives were prepared by Simmons–Smith reactions with iodoform and bromoform in the presence of diethylzinc. Reactions of dichlorocarbene and catharanthine (**3**), vindoline (**4**), vinblastine (**1**) and vincristine (**2**) resulted in unexpected products. In the case of VLB (**1**), an interesting ring-opened oxirane derivative (**15**) was obtained with two different methods. Our attempt to produce epoxidized monomeric alkaloids also led to anomalous derivatives without an oxirane ring. It could have been easily noticed that the presence or absence of perchloric acid had had a crucial role in the outcome of these reactions. Eventually, we were surprised to discover two similar vindoline trimers (**27,28**) in the coupling reaction of vindoline (**4**) and a spiro derivative of catharanthine (**24**). Only the O-methylated trimeric vindoline derivative (**27**) was managed to be obtained when vindoline (**4**) was put in itself into the conditions of the formerly mentioned coupling reaction attempt without a catharanthine derivative (**24**).

Author Contributions: A.K., S.M., R.P. and P.K. performed the experiments; P.K. and L.H. conceived and designed the experiments; Á.S., Z.S., M.D. and C.S.J. achieved the NMR, MS and HRMS analyses and analyzed the data; A.K., Á.S., C.S.J., P.K. and L.H. wrote the paper.

Funding: This research received no external funding.

Acknowledgments: The authors are grateful to Gedeon Richter Plc for providing *Vinca* alkaloids as a gift.

Conflicts of Interest: The authors declare no conflict of interest.

References

1. Noble, R.L.; Beer, C.T.; Cutts, J.H. Role of chance observations in chemotherapy: *Vinca rosea*. *Ann. N. Y. Acad. Sci.* **1958**, *76*, 882–894. [CrossRef]
2. Noble, R.L. *Catharanthus roseus* (*Vinca rosea*)—importance and value of a chance observation. *Lloydia* **1964**, *27*, 280–281.
3. Noble, R.L. The discovery of *Vinca* alkaloids—chemotherapeutic agents against cancer. *Biochem. Cell. Biol.* **1990**, *68*, 1344–1351. [CrossRef] [PubMed]

4. Svoboda, G.H.; Neuss, N.; Gorman, M. Alkaloids of *Vinca* rosea Linn. (*Catharanthus roseus* G. Don.) V.: Preparation and characterization of alkaloids. *J. Am. Pharm. Assoc. Sci. Ed.* **1959**, *48*, 659–666. [CrossRef]
5. Svoboda, G.H. Alkaloids of *Vinca rosea* (*Catharanthus rosea*). 9. Extraction and characterization of leurosidine and leurocristine. *Lloydia* **1961**, *24*, 173–178.
6. Brossi, A.; Suffness, M. Antitumor Bisindol Alkaloids from *Catharanthus roseus* (L.). In *The Alkaloids*; Academic Press Inc.: New York, NY, USA, 1990; Volume 37, pp. 1–240.
7. Sisodiya, P.S. Plant derived anticancer agents: A review. *Int. J. Res. Dev. Phar. Life Sci.* **2013**, *2*, 293–308.
8. Sears, J.E.; Boger, D.L. Total synthesis of vinblastine, related natural products, and key analogues and development of inspired methodology suitable for the systematic study of their structure–function properties. *Acc. Chem. Res.* **2015**, *48*, 653–662. [CrossRef] [PubMed]
9. Sri, A.S. Pharmacological activity of *Vinca* alkaloids. *J. Pharmacogn. Phytochem.* **2016**, *4*, 27–34.
10. Chi, S.; Xie, W.; Zhang, J.; Xu, S. Theoretical insight into the structural mechanism for the binding of vinblastine with tubulin. *J. Biomol. Struct. Dyn.* **2015**, *33*, 2234–2254. [CrossRef] [PubMed]
11. Bölcskei, H.; Szabó, L.; Szántay, Cs. Synthesis of vinblastine derivatives. *Front. Nat. Prod. Chem.* **2005**, *1*, 43–49. [CrossRef]
12. Keglevich, P.; Hazai, L.; Kalaus, Gy.; Szántay, Cs. Modifications on the basic skeletons of vinblastine and vincristine. *Molecules* **2012**, *17*, 5893–5914. [CrossRef] [PubMed]
13. Noble, R.L.; Beer, T.; McIntyre, R.W. Biological effects of dihydrovinblastine. *Cancer* **1967**, *20*, 885–890. [CrossRef]
14. Keglevich, P.; Hazai, L.; Dubrovay, Zs.; Dékány, M.; Szántay, Cs., Jr.; Kalaus, Gy.; Szántay, Cs. Bisindole alkaloids condensed with a cyclopropane ring. Part 1. 14,15-Cyclopropanovinblastine and -vincristine. *Heterocycles* **2014**, *89*, 653–668.
15. Keglevich, P.; Hazai, L.; Dubrovay, Zs.; Sánta, Zs.; Dékány, M.; Szántay, Cs., Jr.; Kalaus, Gy.; Szántay, Cs. Bisindole alkaloids condensed with a cyclopropane ring. Part 2. Cyclopropano-vinorelbine and its derivatives. *Heterocycles* **2015**, *90*, 316–326.
16. Keglevich, P.; Hazai, L.; Kalaus, Gy.; Szántay, Cs. Cyclopropanation of some alkaloids. *Periodica Politechnica Chem. Eng.* **2015**, *59*, 3–15. [CrossRef]
17. Beaulieu, L.-P.; Zimmer, L.E.; Charette, A.B. Enantio- and diastereoselective iodocyclopropanation of allylic alcohols by using a substituted zinc carbenoid. *Chem. Eur. J.* **2009**, *15*, 11829–11832. [CrossRef] [PubMed]
18. Gorka-Kereskényi, Á.; Szabó, L.; Hazai, L.; Lengyel, M.; Szántay, Cs., Jr.; Sánta, Zs.; Kalaus, Gy.; Szántay, Cs. Aromatic electrophilic substitutions on vindoline. *Heterocycles* **2007**, *71*, 1553–1563. [CrossRef]
19. Keglevich, Gy.; Keserű, Gy.M.; Forintos, H.; Szöllősy, Á.; Ludányi, K.; Tőke, L. The effect of a sterically demanding *P*-substituent on the reactivity of *P*-heterocycles: Selective transformations during the ring enlargement of a 1-(2,4,6-triisopropylphenyl)-2,5-dihydro-1*H*-phosphole 1-oxide. *J. Chem. Soc. Perkin Trans. 1* **1999**, 1801–1805. [CrossRef]
20. Fahy, J.; du Boullay, V.T.; Bigg, D.C.H. New method of synthesis of *Vinca* alkaloid derivatives. *Bioorg. Med. Chem. Lett.* **2002**, *12*, 505–507. [CrossRef]
21. Johnson, P.D.; Sohn, J.-H.; Rawall, V.H. Synthesis of C-15 vindoline analogues by palladium-catalyzed cross-coupling reactions. *J. Org. Chem.* **2006**, *71*, 7899–7902. [CrossRef] [PubMed]
22. Sundberg, R.J.; Gadamasetti, K.G.; Hunt, P.J. Mechanistic aspects of the formation of anhydrovinblastine by Potier-Polonovski oxidative coupling of catharanthine and vindoline. Spectroscopic observation and chemical reactions of intermediates. *Tetrahedron* **1992**, *48*, 277–296. [CrossRef]
23. Kutney, J.P.; Bokelman, B.H.; Ichikawa, M.; Jahngen, E.; Joshua, A.V.; Liao, P.-H.; Worth, B.R. Studies on the synthesis of bisindole alkaloids. IV. Novel oxigenated catharanthine derivatives. *Heterocycles* **1976**, *4*, 1267–1273. [CrossRef]
24. Mewald, M.; Medley, J.W.; Movassaghi, M. Concise and enantioselective total synthesis of (−)-mehranine, (−)-methylenebismehranine, and related Aspidosperma alkaloids. *Angew. Chem. Int. Ed.* **2014**, *53*, 11634–11639. [CrossRef] [PubMed]
25. Éles, J.; Kalaus, Gy.; Greiner, I.; Kajtár-Peredy, M.; Szabó, P.; Keserű, Gy.M.; Szabó, L.; Szántay, Cs. Synthesis of Vinca alkaloids and related compounds. 100. Stereoselective oxidation reactions of compounds with the aspidospermane and quebrachamine ring system. First synthesis of some alkaloids containing the epoxy ring. *J. Org. Chem.* **2002**, *67*, 7255–7260. [CrossRef] [PubMed]

26. Mayer, Sz.; Keglevich, P.; Ábrányi-Balogh, P.; Szigetvári, Á.; Dékány, M.; Szántay, Cs., Jr.; Hazai, L. Attempted Diels-Alder Reactions on Vindoline Derivatives. *Peroid. Polytech. Chem. Eng.* **2017**, *64*, 258–263. [CrossRef]
27. Langlois, N.; Gueritte, F.; Langlois, Y.; Potier, P. Application of a modification of the Polonovski reaction to the synthesis of vinblastine-type alkaloids. *J. Am. Chem. Soc.* **1976**, *98*, 7017–7024. [CrossRef] [PubMed]
28. Langlois, Y.; Guéritte, F.; Andriamialisoa, R.Z.; Langlois, N.; Potier, P.; Chiaroni, A.; Riche, C. Rearrangement du squelette de la catharanthine. *Tetrahedron* **1976**, *32*, 945–949. [CrossRef]
29. Ferroud, C.; Rool, P. A singlet oxygen mediated new access to hydroxyindolenine-catharanthine derivatives by two sequential oxidations. *Heterocycles* **2001**, *55*, 545–555. [CrossRef]
30. Sharma, P.; Cordell, G.A. Heyneanine hydroxyindolenine, a new indole alkaloid from *Ervatamia coronaria* var. plena. *J. Nat. Prod.* **1988**, *51*, 528–531. [CrossRef] [PubMed]
31. Atta-ur-Rahman; Ali, I.; Bashir, M.; Choudhary, M.I. Isolation and structure of rosamine—A new pseudoindoxyl alkaloid from *Catharanthus roseus*. *Z. Naturforsch.* **1984**, *39b*, 1292–1293.

Sample Availability: Samples of the compounds are not available from the authors.

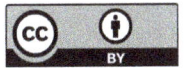

© 2018 by the authors. Licensee MDPI, Basel, Switzerland. This article is an open access article distributed under the terms and conditions of the Creative Commons Attribution (CC BY) license (http://creativecommons.org/licenses/by/4.0/).

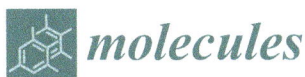

Article

Evaluation of Alkaloids Isolated from *Ruta graveolens* as Photosynthesis Inhibitors

Olívia Moreira Sampaio [1], Lucas Campos Curcino Vieira [2], Barbara Sayuri Bellete [3], Beatriz King-Diaz [4], Blas Lotina-Hennsen [4], Maria Fátima das Graças Fernandes da Silva [5] and Thiago André Moura Veiga [6],*

[1] Department of Chemistry, Federal University of Mato Grosso, Cuiabá-MT 78068-600, Brazil; olysampa@ufmt.br
[2] Engineering Institute, Federal University of Mato Grosso, Várzea Grande-MT 78060-900, Brazil; lucasccurcino@gmail.com
[3] Department of Chemistry, Federal University of Lavras, Minas Gerais-MG 37200-000, Brazil; barbarabellete@gmail.com
[4] Department of Biochemistry, University Nacional Autonoma de Mexico, Mexico City 04510, Mexico; kingbeat@unam.mx (B.K.-D.); blas@unam.mx (B.L.-H.)
[5] Department of Chemistry, Federal University of São Carlos, São Carlos-SP 13565-905, Brazil; dmfs@ufscar.br
[6] Department of Chemistry, Federal University of São Paulo, Diadema-SP 09972-270, Brazil
* Correspondence: tveiga@unifesp.br; Tel.: +55-11-4044-0500

Academic Editor: John C. D'Auria
Received: 12 September 2018; Accepted: 6 October 2018; Published: 19 October 2018

Abstract: Eight alkaloids (**1–8**) were isolated from *Ruta graveolens*, and their herbicide activities were evaluated through in vitro, semivivo, and in vivo assays. The most relevant results were observed for Compounds **5** and **6–8** at 150 µM, which decreased dry biomass by 20% and 23%, respectively. These are significant results since they presented similar values with the positive control, commercial herbicide 3-(3,4-dichlorophenyl)-1,1-dimethylurea (DCMU). Based on the performed assays, Compound **5** (graveoline) is classified as an electron-transport inhibitor during the light phase of photosynthesis, as well as a plant-growth regulator. On the other hand, Compounds **6–8** inhibited electron and energy transfers, and are also plant-growth inhibitors. These phytotoxic behaviors based on acridone and quinolone alkaloids may serve as a valuable tool in the further development of a new class of herbicides since natural products represent an interesting alternative to replace commercial herbicides, potentially due their low toxicity.

Keywords: *Ruta graveolens*; photosystem II; Chl *a* fluorescence; Hill reaction inhibitors; acridone alkaloids

1. Introduction

Ruta graveolens L. (Rutaceae) is a medicinal plant whose roots and aerial parts contain more than 120 special metabolites as coumarins, flavonoids, acridones, and furoquinoline alkaloids [1,2]. Many of these metabolites have attracted biological and pharmacological interest, demonstrating antifungal, phytotoxic, and antidotal activities [3–9]. In this context, the effect of the natural products as photosynthesis inhibitors has been efficiently evaluated [10–12]. The photosynthetic process is divided into three parts: the initial light-harvesting process and local charge separation, proton-coupled electron transfer, and multielectronic redox catalysis [13]. During the phenomenon, light absorption by antenna molecules is followed by efficient charge separation across the membrane via photosynthetic reaction centers [14]. The antenna system absorbs and converts light into chemical energy at P_{680}. Accordingly, charge recombination is prevented by the presence of an electron-transport chain driving electrons towards P_{700}; a second light-harvesting process occurs at photosystem I (PSI), providing additional energy to electrons for their final purpose: production of adenosine triphosphate (ATP) and dihydronicotinamide-adenine dinucleotide phosphate (NADPH), which are used for CO_2 fixation through the Calvin cycle (biochemistry phase) [13,14]. Therefore, we analyzed chlorophyll *a* fluorescence kinetic transients to verify the damage on photosynthetic apparatus, demonstrating the quantitative and qualitative effects of herbicides on both photosystems [15,16]. From this perspective, the main goal of this report was to investigate the effects of alkaloids (**1–8**) isolated from *Ruta graveolens* L. (Figure 1) on photosynthetic activities through polarography, chlorophyll (Chl) *a* fluorescence, and in vivo plant-growth experiments. Our results suggested that these techniques are powerful and sensitive enough to localize, in detail, the mechanisms of action related to such a complex target, photosynthesis.

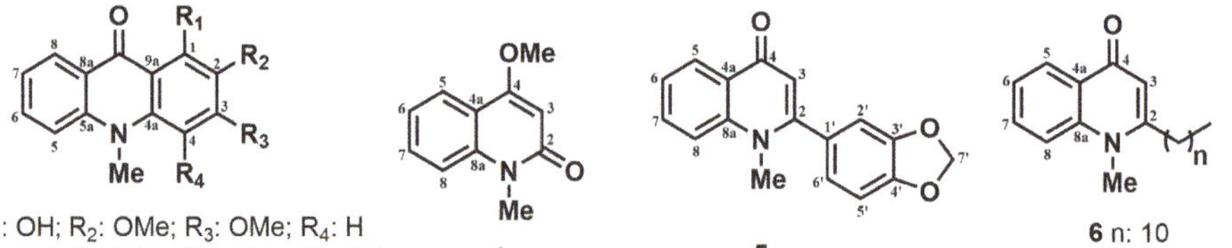

1 R_1: OH; R_2: OMe; R_3: OMe; R_4: H
2 R_1: OH; R_2: OMe; R_3: OMe; R_4: OH
3 R_1: OH; R_2: H; R_3: OMe; R_4: H

4

5

6 n: 10
7 n: 11
8 n: 12

Figure 1. Alkaloids isolated from *Ruta graveolens*.

2. Results and Discussion

2.1. *Effect of Alkaloids* **1–8** *on Noncyclic Electron Transport and* H^+*-ATPase Activity*

Compounds **2** and **3** did not present an effect on noncyclic electron transport in preliminary tests. On the other hand, the other alkaloids inhibited noncyclic electron transport from H_2O to methylviologen (MV) in chloroplasts isolated from *Spinacea oleracea* L. Arborinine (**1**) inhibited phosphorylating and uncoupled electron flow by 100% at 100 μM, which demonstrated that (**1**) behaves as a potent electron-transport inhibitor (Figure 2A). The basal electron flow was increased at low concentrations (around 15 μM), but electron flow at concentrations higher than 25 μM was decreased, inhibiting electron flow by 20% at 100 μM, which means that (**1**) binds to the CF_1CF_0-ATP*ase* complex, suggesting inhibitory activity on ATP synthesis. The results found, with regard to electron-transport reaction, a increment of the step as well as a decrease in the phosphorylating and uncoupled steps, indicating that (**1**) exhibited a dual effect by inhibiting both energy transfer and electron transport [17].

Compound **4** increased basal and phosphorylating electron transports by 80% and 40%, respectively, at the beginning of the illumination, and then decreased them, since the concentrations were higher than 80 μM (Figure 2B). As well as Compound (**1**), (**4**) decreased the uncoupled phase at concentrations close to 80 μM. Therefore, (**4**) did not demonstrate electron-transport inhibition, but rather acted as a decoupling agent. Graveoline (**5**) inhibited the basal, phosphorylating, and uncoupled electron transport by 40% at 300 μM, which suggested Hill reaction inhibitory behavior (Figure 2C).

Homolog mixture **6–8** inhibited energy transfer at 25 μM and showed slight inhibitory activity on electron-transport reactions at concentrations up to 100 μM (Figure 2D). Compounds **6–8** increased basal and phosphorylating electron transport by 230% and 140%, respectively. The uncoupled electron transport showed a small increase in concentrations below 100 μM. In this way, the mixture behaved mainly as an energy-transfer inhibitor and showed electron-transport inhibitory activity at higher concentrations.

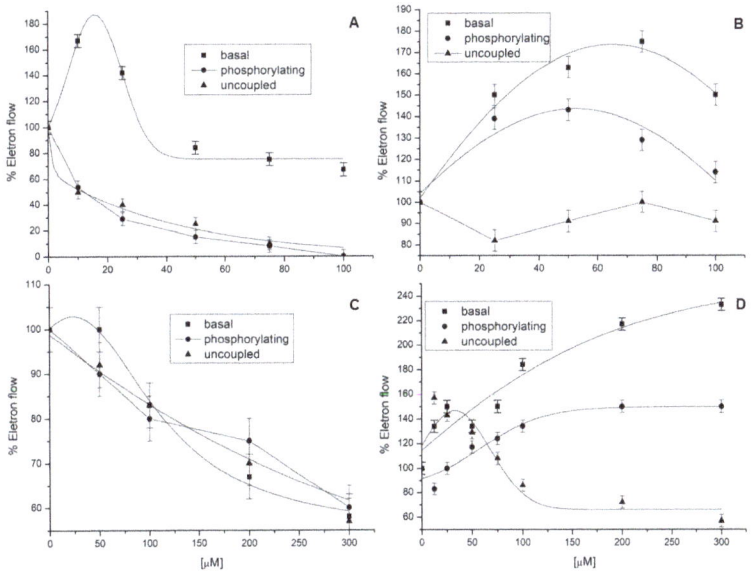

Figure 2. Effect of the alkaloids isolated from *R. graveolens* on electron flow. Control-rate values for electron transport from basal, phosphorylating, and uncoupled conditions were 450, 620, and 1200 µequiv e$^-$ h^{-1} mg^{-1} chlorophyll (Chl)$^{-1}$, respectively. Panel (**A**): Compound **1**; Panel (**B**): Compound **4**; Panel (**C**): Compound **5**; and Panel (**D**): Mixtures **6–8**.

When there is a significant increase on the basal electron-transport step, as observed for Compounds **1**, **4**, and **6–8**, this is an indication that the compounds are acting on the ATP–synthase complex [17]. Cyclic electron transport is happening normally, as can be observed in the basal reaction, due the behavior of the chloroplasts in the reaction medium. The percentage of the basal curve means that the effect is happening over the ATP–synthase complex once the basal reaction works harder to equilibrate this damage, thus increasing the speed of action.

Due to this, ATP*ase* analysis for Compounds **1**, **4**, and **6–8** was needed to confirm if they interfere on the CF$_1$CF$_0$-ATP*ase* complex, acting by direct inhibition of ATP synthesis. The experiments (Table 1) revealed that Compound **4** binds to CF$_1$CF$_0$-ATP*ase* complex exerting a direct inhibition of the H$^+$ gradient dissipation and the Compounds **1** and **6–8** act as energy transfer inhibitors (H$^+$-ATP*ase* inhibitor) [17].

The electron-transport increase on the basal reaction up to 100% indicates that the compounds acted on the ATP–synthase complex, blocking the energy transfer or acting as proton-transfer decoupling. This behavior was observed for Compounds **1** and **6–8** through the increase of the basal step for Compound **4** by the increment of the basal and phosphorylating reactions [18,19].

To confirm if Compounds **1** and **6–8** act as energy-transfer inhibitors, and if Compound **4** acts as a decoupling agent, we performed H$^+$-ATP*ase* assays to verify their effect on the catalytic unit of the H$^+$-ATP*ase* complex (CF$_0$-CF$_1$) [17]. Compounds **1** and **6–8** inhibited the energy transfer, as they decreased the inorganic phosphate (Pi) concentrations in the reaction medium by 25% at 100 µM and 300 µM, respectively. Corroborating the electron-transport data, both compounds are inhibitors of the CF$_0$-CF$_1$ enzymatic site of the ATPase complex (Table 1). In its turn, Compound **4** increased Pi concentration by 18% at 100 µM, which confirmed its proton-gradient uncoupling profile.

Table 1. Effect of Compounds **1**, **4**, and **6–8** on inorganic phospate (P*i*).

Compound	(µM)	P*i* (%)
Control	0	100
1	25	90
	50	78
	100	77
4	25	104
	50	108
	100	118
6–8	100	93
	200	88
	300	77

2.2. Uncoupled PSI and PSII Electron-Flow Determination

To localize the inhibition sites of the alkaloids on the thylakoid electron-transport chain, their effects on PSI and PSII (including partial reactions) were evaluated employing artificial donors and acceptors of electrons, as well as appropriate inhibitors [20]. Arborinine (**1**) inhibited uncoupled electron transport on PSII from water to DCBQ (from H_2O to Q_B) and the partial reactions from water to sodium silicomolybdate (SiMo) (from H_2O to Q_A) by 60% at 400 µM (Table 2). There were no significant results (<4%) for the reactions from DPC to 2,6-dichlorophenolindophenol (DCPIP) (from P_{680} to Q_B).

Table 2. Effects of arborinine (**1**) on photosynthetic electron transport on photosystem II (PSII). Note: DCPIP, 2,6-dichlorophenolindophenol.

(µM)	H$_2$O to DCBQ		H$_2$O to Sodium Silicomolybdate (SiMo)		DPC to DCPIP	
	a	*b*	*A*	*b*	*c*	*b*
0	547.5 ± 2.74	100	511.0 ± 2.56	100	256.0 ± 1.28	100
50	-	-	-	-	283.0 ± 1.42	110.6
100	401.5 ± 2.00	74	328.5 ± 1.64	65	268.0 ± 1.34	104.5
200	292.0 ± 1.46	54	255.5 ± 1.28	50	268.0 ± 1.34	104.5
300	255.5 ± 1.28	47	237.3 ± 1.19	47	-	-
400	219.0 ± 1.09	40	219.0 ± 1.09	43	-	-

a (µequiv e$^-$ h^{-1} mg^{-1} Chl^{-1}), *b* (%), *c* (µM DCPIP$_{red}$ mg^{-1} Chl^{-1}).

The polarographic measures indicated that **1** inhibited the passage from H_2O to Q_A, that is, on both sides of the electron transport on PSII. The first inhibition site (H_2O to SiMo) occurs in the enzyme where water photo-oxidation happens, and the other at DPC (donates electron at P680) to DCPIPox (accepts electrons at Q_B site), located at the water-splitting enzyme complex (OEC) and between the range of electron flow from P680 to Q_A. These results indicated that **1** inhibited PSII at the span of electron transport from H_2O to Q_A due the fact that SiMo accepts electrons exactly at the Q_A site. Table 2 shows that the span of electron transport from P680 to Q_B was not inhibited in all concentrations. Compound **1** inhibited the PSI uncoupled electron transport from reduced DCPIP to MV by 50% at 200 µM (Table 3). However, no changes were observed on inhibitory activity at higher concentrations.

Table 3. Effects of arborinine (**1**) on photosynthetic uncoupled electron transport at PSI.

(µM)	DCPIP$_{red}$ a Methylviologen (MV)	
	a	b
0	1467.4 ± 7.34	100
100	867.1 ± 4.34	59.1
200	733.7 ± 3.67	50
400	667.0 ± 3.34	46

a (µequiv e^{-} h^{-1} mg^{-1} Chl^{-1}) b (%).

2.3. Chl a Fluorescence Measurements in Spinach Leaf Discs

The Chl *a* fluorescence assay is a widely used tool to evaluate the photosynthetic apparatus in plants submitted to different stresses, as well as to provide detailed information about the structure and function of PSII [10,20]. For this experiment, all alkaloids were evaluated at 150 and 300 µM. Compounds **1–4** showed very low activity during the experiment, less than 20% compared to negative control (data not shown).

Compound **5** increased dV/dt$_0$ and decreased PI$_{abs}$, both parameters by 60% at 150 µM, which represents a stressful event occurring in the plant. The association of these parameters suggests that the natural redox process of photosynthesis was interfered with (Figure 3A). Parameters PSI$_0$, PHI(E$_0$), Sm, ET$_0$/CS$_0$, and ET$_0$/RC were reduced by 40%, which directly represents that electron transport on the redox process was interrupted, indicating damage to PSII. The decrease in Sm demonstrates that not all absorbed energy was used, and then it was eliminated from the process. Energy dissipation was confirmed through the increase of the nonphotochemical "de-excitation" constant (Kn) by 40% and the quantum yield (t = 0) of dissipation energy (PHI(Do)) by 20%. Thus, the energy contained in the system was released as heat or transferred to another molecule.

Compounds **6–8** were active at both concentrations during the leaf-disc fluorescence assay (Figure 3A,B). The PI$_{abs}$ parameter showed a decrease of 70% at 150 µM, indicating a nontraditional photosynthesis process. Parameters PSI$_0$, PHI(E$_0$), ET$_0$/CS$_0$ and ET$_0$/RC were reduced by 40, 40, 60 and 40%, respectively, at 150 µM. These decrements represent damage in electron transport on PSII, showing that the calculated quantum-yield values for the electron transport decreased in the process of the flux being inhibited. The reduction of ET$_0$/CS$_0$, ET$_0$/RC, and RC/CS$_0$ parameters by 30% indicated that the electron transport was being blocked, as well as a reduction in reaction centers participating in the process. Like Compound **5**, the increment was promoted by the mixture of analogs on the dV/dt$_0$, SmK, Kn, and PHI(D$_0$) parameters.

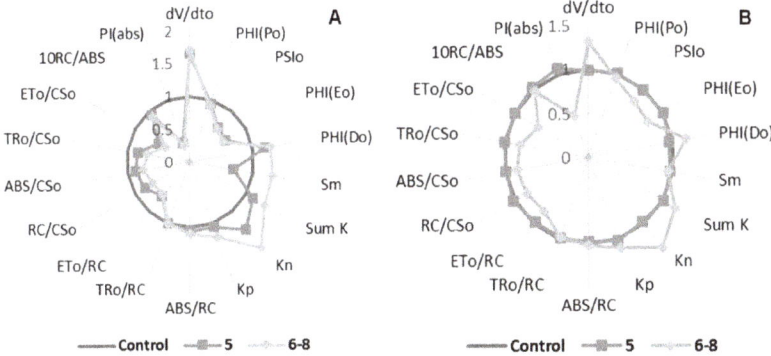

Figure 3. Radar plot of Compounds **5** and **6–8** effects on Chl *a* fluorescence parameters calculated from an OJIP transient curve. Panel (**A**) 150 µM, and Panel (**B**) 300 µM.

A *J* band (2 ms) was observed at the *OJIP* transient curve for Compound 5 (150 µM), which indicates inhibition at the quinone level, on the acceptor side of PSII (Figure 4A). An increase at *J* step can be understood as evidence for reduced-form QA accumulation (QA$^-$) due electron-transport deceleration beyond QA [21]. Since the PSII electron flux was inhibited, the maximum PSII microelectrons field carries less QA$^-$. This aspect corroborated the reduction of the PSI$_0$ and PHI(E$_0$) quantum parameters. The results of the fluorescence emission on spinach-leaf discs confirm the in vitro electron transport results, which revealed Compound 5 acting as a Hill reaction inhibitor.

The same *J* band was observed when the mixture of quinolone alkaloids was submitted to the assays (Figure 4B), which confirms that Compounds 6–8 also behave like 3-(3,4-dichlorophenyl)-1,1-dimethylurea (DCMU), inhibiting the acceptor side of the PSII [10]. The Chl *a* experiment also showed the appearance of the *I* band near 30 ms (Figure 4C), which exclusively refers to the efficiency of the quinone pool. This event indicates whether plastoquinones are active or not during the QA reduction process. When the *I* band is found in negative values (on the graph), it suggests that the QA pool is functioning excellently, and an increase in the *J* band is also observed, that is, this indicates that the interaction site is the reaction center (P680). The transient bands show exactly this effect (Figure 4A,B). Phase *I* appears when a dynamic equilibrium is reached between the reduction of the plastoquinone pool by the electron flow from the PSII and its oxidation due to PSI activity [22].

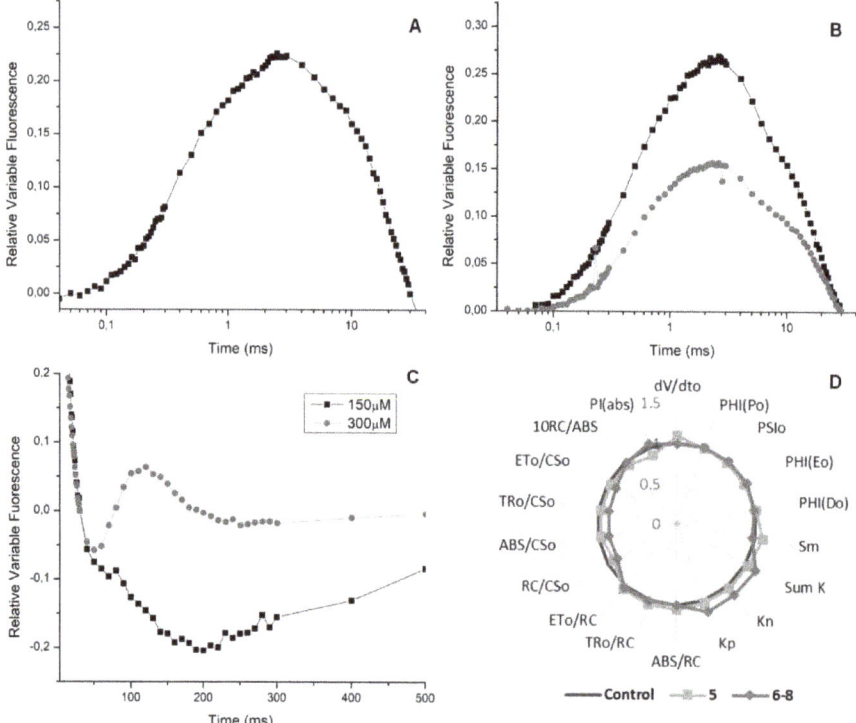

Figure 4. Panel (**A**) Appearance of the J-band in the presence of Compound 5 at 150 µM. Panel (**B**) Appearance of the J-band in the presence of Compounds 6–8 at 150 and 300 µM. Panel (**C**) Appearance of the I-band in the presence of 6–8 at 150 and 300 µM. Panel (**D**) Radar plot of Compounds 5 and 6–8 effects on Chl *a* fluorescence parameters calculated from OJIP curve of sprayed *Lolium perenne* plants after 72 h.

2.4. In Vivo Assays: Chl a Fluorescence Determination in Intact L. Perenne Leaves

The in vivo Chl *a* fluorescence experiment represents a powerful tool to evaluate the performance of the photosynthesis system in living plants without causing any damage to them [23]. To evaluate compound activity, solutions at 150 and 300 µM were sprayed on the leaves of *L. perenne* plants. However, only Compound **5** and the mixture **6–8** were tested because they presented the best results on a semivivo assay. After 24, 48, and 72 h of treatment, Chl *a* fluorescence transients were measured and the OJIP parameters were calculated employing Biolyser HP software.

Data showed that **5** and **6–8** on plants after 24 and 48 h were insignificant, but a small variation on photosynthetic parameters was observed after 72 h at 150 µM (Figure 4D). In short, the in vivo results are less significant than the results observed on the semivivo assay. We justify this because there are many natural obstacles that the compounds have to transcend to reach their target (the chloroplast), for example, cell walls and membranes [23].

2.5. Dry Biomass Determination

Dry biomass results were obtained using *L. perenne* plants 15 days after compound application. Compound **5** and the mixture **6–8** were evaluated at 150 and 300 µM. The other compounds were not tested, as they did not present any activity in the previously assays. DCMU, a herbicide, was used as positive control (Table 4). Fortunately, the best results were observed for the lowest concentration, 150 µM. Treatments **5** and **6–8** decreased dry biomass by 20% and 23%, respectively, compared to negative control. These are significant results since they behaved like DCMU, which reduced 23% of the biomass of the target plant.

Table 4. Dry biomass assay for Compounds **5** and **6–8**. Note: DCMU, 3-(3,4-dichlorophenyl)-1,1-dimethylurea.

Treatment	(µM)	Dry Biomass (mg)	Percentage (%)
Control	0	400.0 ± 2.00	100
DCMU	10	307.0 ± 1.54	77
5	150	320.0 ± 1.60	80
	300	327.0 ± 1.64	82
6–8	150	310.0 ± 1.55	77
	300	350.0 ± 1.75	87

Based on in vitro, semivivo, and in vivo approaches, Compound **5** acts as a photosynthetic electron-transport inhibitor and as a plant-growth regulator. Mixture **6–8**, on the other hand, acts as an electron-transport and energy-transfer inhibitor, as well as plant-growth regulator. Our results showed that almost all alkaloids behaved as photosynthesis inhibitors once some of them acted as Hill reaction inhibitors. Through fluorescence measurement, we could observe the presence of transient bands *J* and *I* (obtained from OJIP-test). These steps suggest that compounds isolated from *R. graveolens* inhibited electron flow on the acceptor side of PSII, exactly like DCMU does. Therefore, the aim of our work was to present that natural products still could be employed on programs to lead to new scaffold models for herbicides in the future, since natural products remains an interesting alternative to replace the commercial herbicides.

3. Materials and Methods

3.1. Alkaloid Isolation from Ruta Graveolens

The ethanolic extract (203.6 g) from *Ruta graveolens* leaves was solubilized in $CH_3OH:H_2O$ (1:3, v:v) and extracted by liquid–liquid partition with hexane and dichloromethane to obtain the partitioned extract fractions.

The dichloromethane fraction (14.6 g) from *Ruta graveolens* leaves was subjected to a chromatographic column using silica gel 60 (70–230 mesh), employing as a mobile phase increasing hexane, dichloromethane, acetone, and methanol concentrations to obtain 6 fractions (1–6). Fraction 5 (0.746 g) was subjected to a new chromatographic procedure using Sephadex LH-20 with isocratic elution formed by dichloromethane:methanol (1:1, v:v) to afford arborinine (**1**, 18.4 mg) and 1,4-dihydroxy-2,3-dimethoxy-*N*-methylacridone (**2**, 16.5 mg) [24].

1-hydroxy-3-methoxy-*N*-methylacridone (**3**, 17.9 mg) was obtained from the dichloromethane:hexane fraction of *Ruta graveolens* leaves using silica gel (70–230 mesh) and solvents of increasing polarity (hexane, dichloromethane, acetone, and methanol), followed by a second chromatographic purification over Sephadex LH-20 with isocratic elution dichloromethane: methanol (1:1, v:v) [25].

From the methanol fraction of *Ruta graveolens* leaves, the *N*-methyl-4-methoxy-2-quinolone (**4**, 19.3 mg) and graveoline (**5**, 14.1 mg) compounds were purified using a chromatographic column with silica gel as support, and hexane, dichloromethane, acetone, and methanol as the mobile phase [26].

The ethanolic extract (7.0 g) from the *Ruta graveolens* roots was solubilized with methanol:water (1:3 v:v), and subjected to liquid–liquid extraction with hexane to provide the respective fraction (1.53 g). The hexanic fraction was subjected to purification using silica gel (70–230 mesh). The mobile phase was composed of increasing portions of hexane, dichloromethane, acetone, and methanol to obtain 8 fractions (I–VIII). Fraction II (0.105 g) was subjected to new chromatographic purification by Sephadex LH-20 with isocratic elution dichloromethane:methanol (3:7, v:v) to obtain a homolog mixture of **6**, **7**, and **8**. The mixture was analyzed with GC-MS. The instrument was set to an initial temperature of 150 °C, and maintained at that temperature for 1 min. At the end of this period, the oven temperature was increased to 300 °C, at the rate of 10 °C/min, and maintained for 20 min. The chromatogram presented 3 peaks at retention times (t_R) 11.5 min (**6**, m/z 313), 12.0 min (**7**, m/z 327), and 13.0 min (**8**, m/z 341). Based on the GC-MS experiment, a ratio of 8:1:1 (based on the peak areas) was estimated for **6**, **7**, and **8** [27].

Compound 1. ^{1}H-NMR (200 MHz, CDCl$_3$) δ: 3.81 (s, 3H, *N*-Me), 3.92 (s, 3H, 3-OMe), 4.00 (s, 3H, 2-OMe), 6.23 (s, 1H, H-4), 7.23 (ddd, J = 8.0, 6.8 and 0.7 Hz, 1H, H-7), 7,50 (dl, J = 8.0 Hz, 1H, H-5), 7.73 (ddd, J = 8.0, 6.8 and 1.4 Hz, 1H, H-6), 8.42 (dd, J = 8.0 and 1.4 Hz, 1H, H-8), 14.75 (s, 1H, OH). ^{13}C-NMR (100 MHz, CDCl$_3$) δ: 34.1 (*N*-Me), 56.0 (C3-OMe), 60.8 (C2-OMe), 86.8 (C-4), 105.8 (C-9a), 114.5 (C-5), 120.8 (C-8a), 121.5 (C-7), 126.2 (C-8), 130.2 (C-2), 134.6 (C-6), 140.5 (C-4a), 142.0 (C-5a), 156.2 (C-1), 159.3 (C-3), 180.8 (C-9).

Compound 2. ^{1}H-NMR (200 MHz, CDCl$_3$) δ: 3.96 (s, 3H, *N*-Me), 3.99 (s, 3H, 2-OMe), 4.03 (s, 3H, 3-OMe), 7.32 (ddd, J = 8.0, 7.5 and 1.6 Hz, 1H, H-7), 7.48 (dl, J = 8.7 Hz, 1H, H-5), 7.76 (ddd, J = 8.7, 7.5 and 1.6 Hz, 1H, H-6), 8.36 (dd, J = 8.7 and 1,6 Hz, 1H, H-8), 14.69 (s, 1H, 1-OH). ^{13}C-NMR (50 MHz, CDCl$_3$) δ: 44.0 (*N*-Me), 61.0 (C2-OMe), 61.5 (C3-OMe), 109.4 (C-9a), 116.6 (C-5), 121.3 (C-8a), 122.1 (C-8), 126.2 (C-7), 134.6 (C-6), 134.7 (C-2), 140.0 (C-3), 146.1 (C-5a), 151.5 (C-4), 155.8 (C-1), 157.0 (C-4a), 182.3 (C-9).

Compound 3. ^{1}H-NMR (200 MHz, CDCl$_3$) δ: 3.77 (s, 3H, *N*-Me), 3.90 (s, 3H, OMe), 6.30 (s, 2H, H-2 and H-4), 7.30 (ddd, J = 8.0, 7.2 and 1.6 Hz, 1H, H-7), 7.40 (dl, J = 8.0 Hz, 1H, H-5), 7.73 (ddd, J = 8.0, 7.2 and 1.6 Hz, 1H, H-6), 8.44 (dd, J = 8.0 and 1.6 Hz, 1H, H-8), 14.75 (s, 1H, OH), ^{13}C-NMR (50 MHz, CDCl$_3$) δ: 33.3 (*N*-Me), 55.6 (OMe), 90.1 (C-4), 94.1 (C-2), 105.0 (C-9a), 114.4 (C-5), 121.0 (C-8a), 121.4 (C-7), 126.7 (C-8), 134.1 (C-6), 142.0 (C-5a), 144.0 (C-4a), 166.0 (C-1), 166.1 (C-3), 180.0 (C-9).

Compound 4. ^{1}H-NMR (200 MHz, CDCl$_3$) δ: 3.64 (s, 3H, N-Me), 3.92 (s, 3H, OMe), 6.23 (s, 1H, H-3), 7.96 (dd, J = 8.0 and 1.5 Hz, 1H, H-5), 7.21 (ddd, J = 8.0, 7.1 and 1.5 Hz, 1H, H-6), 7.34 (dl, J = 8.0 Hz, 1H, H-8), 7.58 (ddd, J = 8.0, 7.1 and 1.5 Hz, 1H, H-7). ^{13}C-NMR (50 MHz, CDCl$_3$) δ: 28.8 (N-Me), 55.3 (OMe), 96.1 (C-3), 113.8 (C-8), 116.2 (C-4a), 121.4 (C-6), 123.1 (C-5), 131.0 (C-7), 139.4 (C-8a), 162.4 (C-4), 163.6 (C-2).

Compound 5. ^{1}H-NMR (400 MHz, CDCl$_3$) δ: 3.59 (s, 3H, N-Me), 5.99 (s, 2H, H-7′), 6.26 (s 1H, H-3), 6.78 (dd, J = 1.6 and 0.4 Hz, 1H, H-2′), 6.81(dd, J = 8.0 and 1.6 Hz, 1H, H-6′), 6.84 (dd, J = 8.0 and 0.4 Hz, 1H, H5′), 7.34 (ddd, J = 8.0, 6.8 and 1.6 Hz, 1H, H-6), 7.49 (dl, J = 8.4 Hz, 1H, H-8), 7.64 (ddd, J = 8.4, 6.8 and 1.6 Hz, 1H, H-7), 8.37(dd, J = 8.0 and 1.6 Hz, 1H, H-5).

Compounds 6–8. ^{1}H-NMR (400 MHz, CDCl$_3$) δ: 0.87 (t, J = 8.0 Hz, 3H, CH$_3$-9′), 1.26–2.37 (2H-2′ to 2H-8′, overlapping with the signals of **7** and **8**), 3.05 (qt, J = 8.0 Hz, 2H, H-1′), 4.12 (s, 3H, N-Me), 6.70 (s, 1H, H-3), 7.54 (tl, J = 8.0 Hz, 1H, H-8), 7.77 (tl, J = 8 Hz, 1H, H-6), 8.19 (tl, J = 8.0 Hz, 1H, H-5), 8.19 (tl, J = 8.0 Hz, 1H, H-7).

3.2. Chloroplast Isolation and Chlorophyll Quantitative Determination

Intact chloroplasts were isolated from spinach leaves (*Spinacea oleracea* L.), as previously described [12,22,25]. Chlorophyll concentration was measured spectrophotometrically through a chloroplast suspension in a solution of 400 mM sucrose, 5 mM MgCl, 10 mM KCl, 30 mM tricine-KOH, and pH 8.0 [12].

3.3. Measurement of Noncyclic Electron Transport Rate

The light-induced noncyclic electron-transport activity from water to MV was determined polarographically employing a Clark-type electrode in the presence of 50 µM of MV [19]. Basal electron transport was quantified by illuminating a solution of chloroplasts (20 µg Chl/mL) in 3 mL of 100 mM sorbitol, 10 mM KCl, 5 mM MgCl$_2$, 0.5 mM KCN, 15 mM tricine-KOH, and 50 µM MV at pH 8.0 for 1 min. The phosphorylating electron-transport rate was estimated for the basal electron transport from water to MV, adding 1 mM of ADP and 3 mM KH$_2$PO$_4$. In turn, uncoupled electron transport was evaluated in the same solution used for basal step, with 6 mM NH$_4$Cl added as an uncoupler [12].

3.4. Uncoupled PSI and PSII Electron-Flow Determination

Electron-flow activities were monitored by an oxygen monitor yellow spring instrument model 5300A using a Clark-type electrode. All reaction mixtures were illuminated with filtered light (5 cm filter of 1% CuSO$_4$ solution) from a projector lamp (GAF 2660) at room temperature. For each reaction, a blank experiment was performed with chloroplasts in the reaction medium. Uncoupled PSII from H$_2$O to DCPIP was measured through the reduction of DCPIP-supported O$_2$ evolutions, monitored polarographically. The reaction medium for assaying PSII activity was composed by the same basal electron-transport medium, but in the presence of 1 µM 2,5-dibromo-3-methyl-6-isopropyl-1,4-p-benzoquinone (DBMIB), 100 µM DCPIP, and 300 µM K$_3$[Fe(CN)$_6$] and 6 mM NH$_4$Cl [28].

To determine the uncoupled partial reaction of PSII from water to SiMo, solutions of 200 µM of SiMo and 10 µM of DCMU were added to the solution used for the PSII reactions (3 mL), then chloroplasts (20 µg Chl/mL) were added and illuminated for 1 min [29].

Uncoupled PSI electron transport from the reduced DCPIP with sodium ascorbate to MV was determined in a similar form in a basal noncyclic electron-transport medium. However, the following reagents were added: 10 µM DCMU, 100 µM DCPIP, 50 µM MV, 300 µM sodium ascorbate, and 6 mM NH$_4$Cl [30]. All measurements were performed in triplicate and compared to negative control (solvent, dimethyl sulfoxide (DMSO)).

3.5. H^+-ATPase Activity Measurements

Intact chloroplasts isolated from *S. oleracea L.* were resuspended in a solution of 0.35 M sorbitol, 2 mM EDTA, 1 mM $MgCl_2 \cdot 6H_2O$, 1 mM $MnCl_2$, and 50 mM Hepes medium at pH 7.6. H^+-ATPase activity was measured as reported [24]. NH_4Cl and DMSO were employed as positive and negative controls, respectively. Pi was quantified using a UV spectrophotometer with measurements in $\lambda = 660$ nm.

3.6. Chlorophyll A Fluorescence Measurements in Spinach-Leaf Discs

Ten 7 mM leaf discs were placed in Petri dishes with 10 mL of a modified Krebs medium containing 115 mM NaCl, 5.9 mM KCl, 1.2 mM $MgCl_2$, 1.2 mM KH_2PO_4, 1.2 mM Na_2SO_4, 2.5 mM $CaCl_2$, and 25 mM $NaHCO_3$ (pH 7.4). The Petri dishes were maintained in orbital stirring for 12 h at room temperature. All alkaloids, **1–8**, were added to the system for a new period of stirring (12 h). The discs were dark-adapted for 30 min and chlorophyll *a* fluorescence was measured at room temperature through a Hansatech Fluorescence Handy PEA (Plant Efficiency Analyzer, King's Lynn, UK) [16,25].

3.7. Plant Material for In Vivo Assays

A suspension of *Lolium perenne* seeds prepared with 10% sodium hypochlorite solution was kept in an orbital shaker for 15 min. Then, the sodium hypochlorite solution was removed and the seeds were washed 3 times with distilled water; 100 seeds were placed in 12 cm diameter pots containing a mixture of 50:25:25 ($w/w/w$) soil/peat-moss/agrolite. All pots were watered daily and maintained in a greenhouse at 25–30 °C under normal day/night illumination (12/12 h). *L. perenne* plants were selected by uniformity after being 15 days old. The plants were separated in 3 groups: negative control (DMSO), positive control (50 µM of DCMU), and plants treated with each alkaloid at 150 and 300 µM [12] by being manually sprayed.

3.8. Chlorophyll a Fluorescence Determination in Intact L. Perenne Leaves and Dry Biomass Determination

Chl *a* fluorescence was measured in leaves from the control plants and those treated with alkaloids **1–8** at 150 and 300 µM. After 24, 48, and 72 h of spraying, the leaves that adapted to the dark for 15 min were excited by light from an array of 3 light-emitting diodes delivering 3000 µmol m^{-2} s^{-1} of red light (650 nm). The Chl *a* fluorescence induction curves were measured at room temperature with a portable Hansatech Fluorescence Handy PEA apparatus. Photosynthetic parameters like as PI_{abs}, dV/dt_0, Sm, ABS/RC, TR_0/RC, ET_0/RC, TR_0/ABS, ET_0/TR_0, ET_0/ABS, $PHI(D_0)$, ABS/CS_0, TR_0/CS_0, ET_0/CS_0, kp, kn, and Sum$k$ were represented in a radar plot [12]. For the dry-biomass experiment, 15 days old *L. perenne* plants treated with alkaloids **1–8** at 150 and 300 µM were dried in an oven at 65 °C to reach a constant weight. Then, the dry biomass was measured using analytical balance [12].

Author Contributions: Conceptualization, T.A.M.V., B.L.-H. and O.M.S.; Methodology, B.S.B., O.M.S. and B.K.-D.; Software, L.C.C.V.; Validation, O.M.S. and B.K.-D.; Formal Analysis, B.S.B., O.M.S., T.A.M.V. and B.K.-D.; Investigation, O.M.S.; Resources, M.F.d.G.F.d.S. and B.L.-H.; Data Curation, O.M.S., T.A.M.V., L.C.C.V. and B.K.-D.; Writing-Original Draft Preparation, O.M.S.; Writing-Review and Editing, O.M.S., T.A.M.V. and L.C.C.V.; Visualization, O.M.S., T.A.M.V. and L.C.C.V.; Supervision, T.A.M.V., B.L.-H. and M.F.d.G.F.d.S.; Project Administration, B.L.-H. and M.F.d.G.F.d.S.; Funding Acquisition, B.L.-H. and M.F.d.G.F.d.S.

Funding: The authors gratefully acknowledge financial support from Grants DGAPA-UNAM, IN 205806; CNPq, and CAPES—Finance Code 001.

Acknowledgments: Olívia Moreira Sampaio thanks FAPESP (Fundação de Amparo a Pesquisa do Estado de São Paulo-Brazil) for the scholarship support.

Conflicts of Interest: The authors declare no conflict of interest.

Abbreviations

ATP	adenosine triphosphate
Chl	chlorophyll
DBMIB	2,5-dibromo-3-methyl-6-isopropyl-1,4-p-benzoquinone
DCMU	3-(3,4-dichlorophenyl)-1,1-dimethylurea
DCPIP	2,6-dichlorophenolindophenol
DMSO	dimethyl sulfoxide
MV	methylviologen
NADPH	dihydronicotinamide-adenine dinucleotide phosphate
Pi	inorganic phospate
PSI	photosystem I
PSII	photosystem II
RC	reaction center
SiMo	sodium silicomolybdate

References

1. De Feo, V.; De Simone, F.; Senatore, F. Potential allelochemicals from the essential oil of *Ruta graveolens*. *Phytochemistry* **2002**, *61*, 573–578. [CrossRef]
2. Hale, A.L.; Meepagala, K.M.; Oliva, A.; Aliotta, G.; Duke, S.O. Phytotoxins from the leaves of Ruta graveolens. *J. Agric. Food Chem.* **2004**, *52*, 3345–3349. [CrossRef] [PubMed]
3. Kuzovkina, I.; Al'terman, I.; Schneider, B. Specific accumulation and revised structures of acridone alkaloid glucosides in the tips of transformed roots of Ruta graveolens. *Phytochemistry* **2004**, *65*, 1095–1100. [CrossRef] [PubMed]
4. Wansi, J.D.; Wandji, J.; Mbaze Meva'a, L.; Kamdem Waffo, A.F.; Ranjit, R.; Khan, S.N.; Asma, A.; Iqbal, C.M.; Lallemand, M.-C.; Tillequin, F.; Fomum-Tanee, Z. Alpha-glucosidase inhibitory and antioxidant acridone alkaloids from the stem bark of Oriciopsis glaberrima ENGL. (Rutaceae). *Chem. Pharm. Bull.* **2006**, *54*, 292–296. [CrossRef] [PubMed]
5. Michael, J.P. Quinoline, quinazoline and acridone alkaloids. *Nat. Prod. Rep.* **2007**, *24*, 223. [CrossRef] [PubMed]
6. Musiol, R.; Serda, M.; Hensel-Bielowka, S.; Polanski, J. Quinoline-Based Antifungals. *Curr. Med. Chem.* **2010**, *17*, 1960–1973. [CrossRef] [PubMed]
7. Lacroix, D.; Prado, S.; Kamoga, D.; Kasenene, J.; Bodo, B. Structure and in vitro antiparasitic activity of constituents of Citropsis articulata root bark. *J. Nat. Prod.* **2011**, *74*, 2286–2289. [CrossRef] [PubMed]
8. Torres-Romero, D.; King-Díaz, B.; Strasser, R.J.; Jiménez, I.A.; Lotina-Hennsen, B.; Bazz-Cchi, I.L. Friedelane triterpenes from celastrus vulcanicola as photosynthetic inhibitors. *J. Agric. Food Chem.* **2010**, *58*, 10847–10854. [CrossRef] [PubMed]
9. Menezes-De-Oliveira, D.; Aguilar, M.I.; King-Díaz, B.; Vieira-Filho, S.A.; Pains-Duarte, L.; De Fátima Silva, G.D.; Lotina-Hennsen, B. The triterpenes 3β-Lup-20(29)-en-3-ol and 3β-Lup-20(29)-en-3-yl acetate and the carbohydrate 1,2,3,4,5,6-hexa-O-acetyl-dulcitol as photosynthesis light reactions inhibitors. *Molecules* **2011**, *16*, 9939–9956. [CrossRef] [PubMed]
10. Sampaio, O.M.; de Castro Lima, M.M.; Veiga, T.A.M.; King-Díaz, B.; da Silva, M.F.d.G.F.; Lotina-Hennsen, B. Evaluation of antidesmone alkaloid as a photosynthesis inhibitor. *Pestic. Biochem. Phys.* **2016**, *134*, 55–62. [CrossRef] [PubMed]
11. Andreiadis, E.S.; Chavarot-Kerlidou, M.; Fontecave, M.; Artero, V. Artificial photosynthesis: From molecular catalysts for light-driven water splitting to photoelectrochemical cells. *Photochem. Photobiol.* **2011**, *87*, 946–964. [CrossRef] [PubMed]
12. McConnell, I.; Li, G.H.; Brudvig, G.W. Energy Conversion in Natural and Artificial Photosynthesis. *Chem. Biol.* **2010**, *17*, 434–447. [CrossRef] [PubMed]
13. Chen, S.; Zhou, F.; Yin, C.; Strasser, R.J.; Yang, C.; Qiang, S. Application of fast chlorophyll a fluorescence kinetics to probe action target of 3-acetyl-5-isopropyltetramic acid. *Environ. Exp. Bot.* **2011**, *73*, 31–41. [CrossRef]
14. Strasserf, R.J.; Srivastava, A. Govindjee polyphasic chlorophyll a fluorescence transient in plants and cyanobacteria. *Photochem. Photobiol.* **1995**, *61*, 32–42. [CrossRef]

15. Hasan, C.; Ahmed, N.; Haque, R.; Haque, M.; Begum, S.; Sohrab, M.; Ahsan, M. Secondary metabolites from the stem of Ravenia spectabilis Lindl. *Pharmacogn. Mag.* **2013**, *9*, 76. [CrossRef] [PubMed]
16. Spatafora, C.; Tringali, C. Bioactive metabolites from the bark of Fagara macrophylla. *Phytochem. Anal.* **1997**, *8*, 139–142. [CrossRef]
17. Macías-Rubalcava, M.L.; García-Méndez, M.C.; King-Díaz, B.; Macías-Ruvalcaba, N.A. Effect of phytotoxic secondary metabolites and semisynthetic compounds from endophytic fungus Xylaria feejeensis strain SM3e-1b on spinach chloroplast photosynthesis. *J. Photochem. Photobiol. B Biol.* **2017**, *166*, 35–43. [CrossRef] [PubMed]
18. Hernández-Terrones, M.G.; Aguilar, M.I.; King-Diaz, B.; Lotina-Hennsen, B. Interference of methyl trachyloban-19-oate ester with CF0of spinach chloroplast H+-ATPase. *Arch. Biochem. Biophys.* **2003**, *418*, 93–97. [CrossRef]
19. Xiang, M.; Chen, S.; Wang, L.; Dong, Z.; Huang, J.; Zhang, Y.; Strasser, R.J. Effect of vulculic acid produced by Nimbya alternantherae on the photosynthetic apparatus of Alternanthera philoxeroides. *Plant Physiol. Biochem.* **2013**, *65*, 81–88. [CrossRef] [PubMed]
20. Paunov, M.; Koleva, L.; Vassilev, A.; Vangronsveld, J.; Goltsev, V. Effects of different metals on photosynthesis: Cadmium and zinc affect chlorophyll fluorescence in durum wheat. *Int. J. Mol. Sci.* **2018**, *19*. [CrossRef] [PubMed]
21. Marchi, G.; Marchi, E.C.S.; Wang, G.; Mcgiffen, M. Effect of age of a sorghum-sudangrass hybrid on its allelopathic action. *Planta Daninha* **2008**, *26*, 707–716. [CrossRef]
22. King-Díaz, B.; Dos Santos, F.J.L.; Rubinger, M.M.M.; Piló-Veloso, D.; Lotina-Hennsen, B. A diterpene γ-lactone derivative from Pterodon polygalaeflorus Benth. as a photosystem II inhibitor and uncoupler of photosynthesis. *Z. Naturforsch. C* **2006**, *61*, 227–233. [CrossRef] [PubMed]
23. Castelo-Branco, P.; Santos, F.J.L.; Rubinger, M.; Ferreira-Alves, D.; Piló-Veloso, D.; King, B.; Lotina-Hennsen, B. Inhibition and uncoupling of photosynthetic electron transport by diterpene lactone amide derivatives. *Z. Naturforsch. C* **2008**, *63*. [CrossRef]
24. Min, Y.D.; Kwon, H.C.; Yang, M.C.; Lee, K.H.; Choi, S.U.; Lee, K.R. Isolation of limonoids and alkaloids from Phellodendron amurense and their multidrug resistance (MDR) reversal activity. *Arch. Pharm. Res.* **2007**, *30*, 58–63. [CrossRef] [PubMed]
25. Seya, K.; Furukawa, K.-I.; Chiyoya, M.; Yu, Z.; Kikuchi, H.; Daitoku, K.; Motomura, S.; Murakami, M.; Oshima, Y.; Fukuda, I. 1-Methyl-2-undecyl-4(1H)-quinolone, a derivative of quinolone alkaloid evocarpine, attenuates high phosphate-induced calcification of human aortic valve interstitial cells by inhibiting phosphate cotransporter PiT-1. *J. Pharmacol. Sci.* **2016**, *131*, 51–57. [CrossRef] [PubMed]
26. Yruela, I.; Montoya, G.; Alonso, P.; Picorel, R. Identification of the Pheophytin-QA-Fe domain of the reducing side of the photosystem II as the Cu(II)-inhibitory binding site. *J. Biol. Chem.* **1991**, *266*, 22847–22850. [PubMed]
27. Giaquinta, R.T.; Dilley, R.A. A partial reaction in Photosystem II: Reduction of silicomolybdate prior to the site of dichlorophenyldimethylurea inhibition. *Bioenergetics* **1975**, *387*, 288–305. [CrossRef]
28. Garza-Ortiz, A.; King-Díaz, B.; Sosa-Torres, M.E.; Lotina-Hennsen, B. Interference of ruthenium red analogues at photosystem II of spinach thylakoids. *J. Photochem. Photobiol. B Biol.* **2004**, *76*, 85–94. [CrossRef] [PubMed]
29. Mills, J.D.; Mitchell, P.; Schürmann, P. Modulation of coupling factor ATPase activity in intact chloroplasts: The role of the thioredoxin system. *FEBS Lett.* **1980**, *112*, 173–177. [CrossRef]
30. Aguilar, M.I.; Romero, M.G.; Chávez, M.I.; King-Díaz, B.; Lotina-Hennsen, B. Biflavonoids isolated from Selaginella lepidophylla inhibit photosynthesis in spinach chloroplasts. *J. Agric. Food Chem.* **2008**, *56*, 6994–7000. [CrossRef] [PubMed]

Sample Availability: Samples of the compounds are not available from the authors.

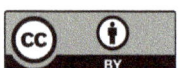 © 2018 by the authors. Licensee MDPI, Basel, Switzerland. This article is an open access article distributed under the terms and conditions of the Creative Commons Attribution (CC BY) license (http://creativecommons.org/licenses/by/4.0/).

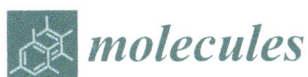

Article

8-Oxo-9-Dihydromakomakine Isolated from *Aristotelia chilensis* Induces Vasodilation in Rat Aorta: Role of the Extracellular Calcium Influx

Fredi Cifuentes [1], Javier Palacios [2,*], Adrián Paredes [3,4], Chukwuemeka R. Nwokocha [5] and Cristian Paz [6,*]

1. Laboratorio de Fisiología Experimental, Instituto Antofagasta, Universidad de Antofagasta, Antofagasta 1270300, Chile; fredi.cifuentes@uantof.cl
2. Facultad Ciencias de la Salud, Instituto de EtnoFarmacología (IDE), Universidad Arturo Prat, Iquique 1110939, Chile
3. Laboratorio de Química Biológica, Instituto Antofagasta, Universidad de Antofagasta, Antofagasta 1270300, Chile; adrian.paredes@uantof.cl
4. Departamento de Química, Facultad de Ciencias Básicas, Universidad de Antofagasta, Antofagasta 1270300, Chile
5. Department of Basic Medical Sciences Physiology Section, Faculty of Medical Sciences, The University of the West Indies, Mona, Kingston 7, KGN, Jamaica (W.I.); chukwuemeka.nwokocha@uwimona.edu.jm
6. Departamento de Ciencias Químicas y Recursos Naturales, Facultad de Ingeniería, Universidad de La Frontera, Temuco 4780000, Chile
* Correspondence: clpalaci@unap.cl (J.P.); cristian.paz@ufrontera.cl (C.P.); Tel.: +56-57-2526910 (J.P.); +56-45-2235424 (C.P.)

Academic Editor: John C. D'Auria
Received: 1 November 2018; Accepted: 17 November 2018; Published: 21 November 2018

Abstract: 8-Oxo-9-dihydromakomakine is a tetracyclic indole alkaloid extracted from leaves of the Chilean tree *Aristotelia chilensis*. The present study investigated the effects of this alkaloid on vascular response in tissues isolated from aortic segments obtained from normotensive rats. Our results showed that 8-oxo-9-dihydromakomakine induced a dose-dependent relaxation of aortic rings pre-contracted with phenylephrine (PE; 10^{-6} M). The vasorelaxation induced by 8-oxo-9-dihydromakomakine in rat aortic rings is independent of endothelium. The pre-incubation of aortic rings with 8-oxo-9-dehydromakomakine (10^{-4} M) significantly reduced the contractile response to KCl ($p < 0.001$) more than PE ($p < 0.05$). The highest dose of 8-oxo-9-dehydromakomakine (10^{-4} M) drastically reduced the contraction to KCl ($6 \cdot 10^{-2}$ M), but after that, PE (10^{-6} M) caused contraction ($p < 0.05$) in the same aortic rings. The addition of 8-oxo-9-dihydromakomakine (10^{-5} M) decreased the contractile response to tetraethylammonium (a voltage-dependent potassium channels blocker; TEA; 5×10^{-3} M; $p < 0.01$) and BaCl$_2$ (a non-selective inward rectifier potassium channel blocker; 5×10^{-3} M; $p < 0.001$) in rat aorta. 8-oxo-9-dihydromakomakine (10^{-5} M) decreased the contractile response to PE in rat aorta in the presence or absence of ouabain (an inhibitor of Na,K-ATPase; 10^{-3} M; $p < 0.05$). These results could indicate that 8-oxo-9-dihydromakomakine partially reduces plasma membrane depolarization-induced contraction. In aortic rings depolarized by PE, 8-oxo-9-dihydromakomakine inhibited the contraction induced by the influx of extracellular Ca^{2+} in a Ca^{2+} free solution ($p < 0.01$). 8-oxo-9-dihydromakomakine reduced the contractile response to agonists of voltage-dependent calcium channels type L (Bay K6844; 10^{-8} M; $p < 0.01$), likely decreasing the influx of extracellular Ca^{2+} through the voltage-dependent calcium channels. This study provides the first qualitative analysis indicating that traditional folk medicine *Aristotelia chilensis* may be protective in the treatment of cardiovascular pathologies.

Keywords: *Aristotelia chilensis* Molina Stuntz; vascular activity; endothelium-independent; indole alkaloid; 8-oxo-9-dihydromakomakine; voltage-dependent calcium channels

1. Introduction

Maqui (*Aristotelia chilensis* (Molina) Stuntz, *Elaeocarpaceae*) is a Chilean native tree sacred to the Araucanian people. Nowadays, maqui fruits have aroused special interest due to their beneficial properties for human health, such as antioxidant, cardioprotective, anti-inflammatory, and enzymatic activities [1–3]. These bioactivities could be useful for the treatment of vascular diseases such as hypertension, myocardial ischemia, and cerebral infarction, which have become worldwide epidemics in modern society [4].

Aristotelia chilensis produce various active components including a high concentration of flavonoids in fruits [1,2]. Chemical analysis have reported that maqui leaves consists of non-iridoid monoterpene indole alkaloids and polyphenolic compounds [5,6]. It is known that several pure compounds from plants may modulate the vascular response, and therefore act as antihypertensives. In fact, some flavonoids (quercetin or myricetin) cause vasoconstriction because they activate $Ca_v1.2$ channel, while flavonols (kaempferol and galangin), a flavone (chrysin), and an isoflavone (genistein) inhibit $Ca_v3.1$ channel by producing vasorelaxation [7]. In addition, galangin and chrysin can inhibit $Ca_v1.2$ channel [8].

However, there are a paucity of data and studies about the vascular response of alkaloids from *A. chilensis*. In order to have a more comprehensive idea of the pharmacological activity of alkaloids produced by *A. chilensis* on the cardiovascular system, the main component of leaves of maqui was purified and chemically characterized by NMR spectroscopy as 8-oxo-9-dihydromakomakine. Then, its activity was determined by the induction of tension change in vascular tissue isolated from aortic segments obtained from normotensive rats. The potential mechanisms were evaluated from the endothelium and nitric oxide (NO) production, together with the role of cytosolic calcium, and its modulation by calcium channels, potassium channels, and Na,K-ATPase.

2. Results

2.1. 8-Oxo-9-Dihydromakomakine Induced Vasodilation in Rat Aorta

8-Oxo-9-dehydromakomakine induced vascular relaxation on aortic rings pre-contracted with PE (10^{-6} M). In fact, 8-oxo-9-dehydromakomakine caused relaxation in intact aorta and endothelium-denuded aorta (Figure 1A). This result was confirmed because 8-oxo-9-dehydromakomakine also produced relaxation in aortic rings pre-incubated with 10^{-4} M N^ω-nitro-L-arginine methyl ester (L-NAME) (Figure 1B).

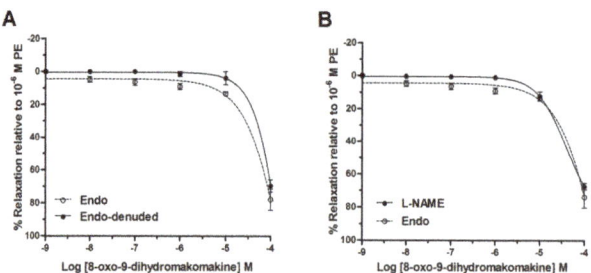

Figure 1. Vasorelaxation effect of 8-oxo-9-dihydromakomakine in intact (Endo) and denuded-endothelium (Endo-denuded) aortic rings (**A**), and in presence of 10^{-4} M L-NAME in the intact aorta (**B**). Values are mean ± standard error of the mean of 6 experiments. Two-way ANOVA followed by Bonferroni's post-hoc test.

2.2. 8-Oxo-9-Dihydromakomakine Reduced the Contractile Response to KCl and PE

The effect of 8-oxo-9-dihydromakomakine on contractile response induced by KCl and PE was studied in a new experiment (Figure 2).

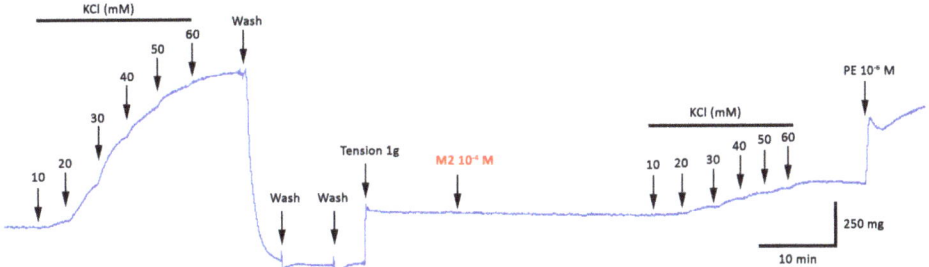

Figure 2. Original trace showing the time course of the concentration–response curves to KCl in intact aortic rings from male rats pre-incubated with M2 (8-oxo-9-dihydromakomakine; 10^{-4} M) for 20 min. Phenilephrine (PE; 10^{-6} M) increased drastically the contraction after the contractile response to 60 mM KCl.

Aortic rings were pre-incubated in absence and the presence of 8-oxo-9-dihydromakomakine (10^{-5} M and 10^{-4} M), before the addition of cumulative concentration of KCl (10 to 60 mM) and PE (10^{-10} to 10^{-5} M) (Figure 3). Results showed that the pre-incubation of aortic rings with 8-oxo-9-dihydromakomakine reduced the contractile response to KCl and PE. The pre-incubation with 8-oxo-9-dihydromakomakine decreased the maximal contraction (E_{max}) to 60 mM KCl (130 ± 3% control vs. 26 ± 1% with 10^{-4} M 8-oxo-9-dihydromakomakine; $p < 0.001$; Figure 3A). The maximal response to PE (10^{-5} M) decreased from 170 ± 7% for control to 137 ± 24% in rings pre-incubated with 8-oxo-9-dihydromakomakine (10^{-4} M, $p < 0.05$; Figure 3C).

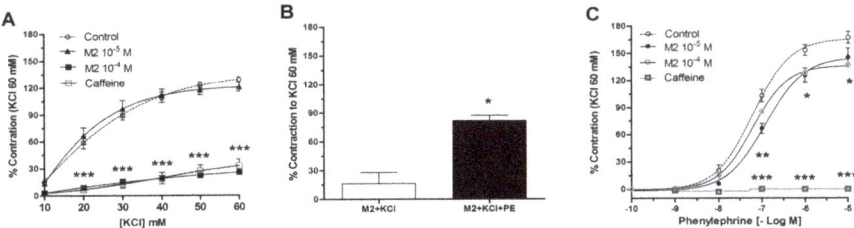

Figure 3. 8-Oxo-9-dihydromakomakine (M2) decreased the contraction induced with KCl and PE in aortic rings of rat. Contractile responses to KCl (**A**) and PE (**C**) are expressed in relation to the maximal response of 60 mM of KCl. 10^{-6} M PE induced a contraction after 60 mM KCl-induced contraction in aortic rings pre-incubated with 10^{-4} M 8-oxo-9-dehydromakomakine (**B**). The aortic rings were pre-incubated with 10^{-4} M 8-oxo-9-dehydromakomakine or 2×10^{-2} M caffeine for 20 min. Values are mean ± standard error of the mean of 5–10 experiments. Significant differences (SEM) are represented with * $p < 0.05$, ** $p < 0.01$, *** $p < 0.001$ versus the control. Two-way ANOVA followed by Bonferroni's post-hoc or test Student's t-test.

Interesting, we observed that the addition of 10^{-6} M PE significantly increased ($p < 0.05$) a 52 ± 11% contractile response in aortic rings pre-contracted with 60 mM KCl in presence of 10^{-4} M 8-oxo-9-dehydromakomakine (Figures 2 and 3). Also, caffeine (a methylxanthine alkaloid) significantly decreased the maximal contraction (E_{max}) to 60 mM KCl (33 ± 5 % with 2×10^{-2} M caffeine; $p < 0.001$; Figure 3A) and 10^{-5} M PE (1 ± 2 % with 2×10^{-2} M caffeine; $p < 0.001$; Figure 3C).

2.3. Role of Potassium Channels in the Vascular Response to 8-Oxo-9-Dihydromakomakine

To study the role of potassium channels on the depolarization-induced contraction to KCl, BaCl$_2$, and TEA, aortic rings of rat were pre-incubated with 8-oxo-9-dihydromakomakine. The contraction was induced by 30 mM KCl, 5×10^{-3} M BaCl$_2$, and 5×10^{-3} M TEA for 10 min. The aortic rings were pre-incubated with 8-oxo-9-dihydromakomakine (10^{-5} M) for 20 min, and showed a significantly lower contractile response to KCl ($p < 0.001$; Figure 4A), BaCl$_2$ ($p < 0.001$; Figure 4B), and TEA ($p < 0.01$; Figure 4C) than the control.

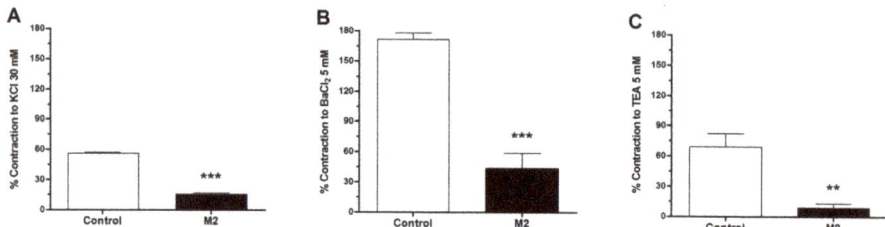

Figure 4. Effect of 8-oxo-9-dihydromakomakine on potassium channels. The pre-incubation of aortic rings with 10^{-5} M 8-oxo-9-dihydromakomakine significantly decreased the contractile response to 30 mM KCl (**A**), 5×10^{-3} M BaCl$_2$ (**B**), and 5×10^{-3} M TEA (**C**). Values are mean ± standard error of the mean of 6 experiments. Significant differences (SEM) are represented with ** $p < 0.01$, *** $p < 0.001$ versus the control. Student's t-test.

2.4. Role of Na,K-ATPase in the Vascular Response to 8-Oxo-9-Dihydromakomakine

To evaluate the role of the plasma membrane depolarization caused by the inhibition of Na,K-ATPase on the contractile response to PE, aortic rings were pre-incubated with ouabain (Figure 5). Cumulative doses of 8-oxo-9-dihydromakomakine (10^{-9} M to 10^{-4} M) were added to intact aortic rings pre-contracted with 10^{-6} M PE in the presence or absence of ouabain 10^{-3} M (Figure 5B). The pre-incubation of aortic rings with 10^{-3} M ouabain (an inhibitor of Na,K-ATPase) did not reduce the relaxation of 10^{-4} M 8-oxo-9-dihydromakomakine in aortic rings pre-contracted with 10^{-6} M PE.

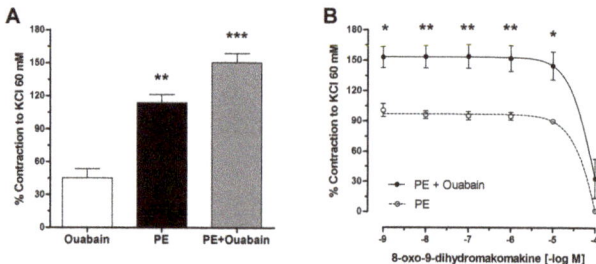

Figure 5. Effect of 8-oxo-9-dihydromakomakine on Na,K-ATPase function. Contractile response to Ouabain, PE and PE+Ouabain before adding 8-oxo-9-dihydromakomakine (**A**). The aortic rings were pre-incubated with 10^{-3} M ouabain for 20 min, and 8-oxo-9-dihydromakomakine was added in cumulative doses on aortic rings pre-contracted with 10^{-6} M PE (**B**). Values are mean ± standard error of the mean of 4 experiments. Significant differences (SEM) are represented with * $p < 0.05$, ** $p < 0.01$, *** $p < 0.001$ versus Ouabain or PE.

2.5. Role of Extracellular Calcium in the Vascular Response to 8-Oxo-9-Dihydromakomakine

We studied calcium fluxes to determine if the contractions induced by PE in the presence of 8-oxo-9-dihydromakomakine could be modulated by calcium inflow from the extracellular space. Thus, we added increasing concentrations of CaCl$_2$ to a calcium-free medium (Figure 6).

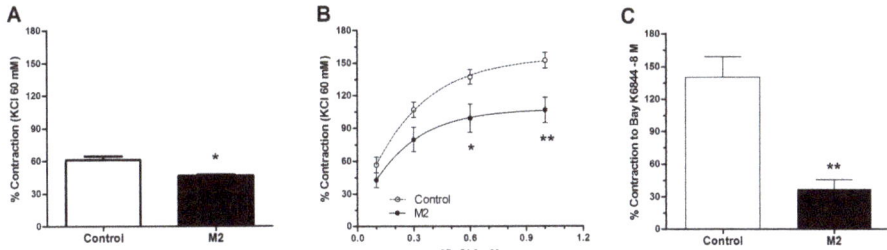

Figure 6. Effect of 8-oxo-9-dihydromakomakine (M2) on the calcium current blockage in calcium-free medium. The aortic rings were pre-incubated in a free calcium buffer for 10 min before PE was added (**A**), and then, the CaCl$_2$ (0.1, 0.3, 0.6, and 1.0 × 10^{-3} M) was added to the bath (**B**). Vasoconstriction occurred just when the agonist calcium channel (10^{-8} M Bay K6844) was added with 15 × 10^{-3} M KCl to the bath (**C**). Values are mean ± standard error of the mean of 6 experiments. Significant differences (SEM) are represented with * $p < 0.05$, ** $p < 0.01$. Student's t-test or two-way ANOVA followed by Bonferroni's post-hoc test.

Figure 6 shows that aortic rings pre-incubated with 10^{-5} M of 8-oxo-9-dihydromakomakine decreased contractile response to PE (10^{-6} M) in free calcium medium with values of 61 ± 3% control vs. 46 ± 1% ($p < 0.05$; Figure 6A) and presence of CaCl$_2$ in cumulative dose (0.1 to 1.0 × 10^{-3} M) with maximum values of 152 ± 21% control vs. 107 ± 14% with 1.0 × 10^{-3} M CaCl$_2$ (** $p < 0.01$; Figure 6B). To study the participation of calcium channels, an agonist of voltage-dependent calcium channels type L (Bay K6844) was used. As shown in Figure 6C, we confirmed that 10^{-5} M 8-oxo-9-dihydromakomakine significantly reduced the contractile response to 10^{-8} M Bay K6844 (140 ± 19% control vs. 37 ± 9% with 10^{-5} M M2; $p < 0.01$).

2.6. Chemical Characterization of 8-Oxo-9-Dihydromakomakine

The compound was formed by four fused rings, with a planar region composed by an indole moiety, and linked to two aliphatic rings by a ketone. The ^{1}H-NMR (Figure S1) and ^{13}C-NMR (Figure S2) results are in excellent agreement with previous data obtained by X-ray studies [6].

8-oxo-9-dihydromakomakine formula; $C_{20}H_{22}N_2O$, yellow crystals, mp 259–260 °C, $[\alpha]_D^{25}$ + 16.8 (CHCl$_3$, c 0.24), IR (cm^{-1}): 3248, 2970, 2938, 2431, 1589, 1504: ESIMS (M + 1) 307.1654.

3. Discussion

Aristotelia chilensis or Maqui is used in Chilean traditional medicine and nowadays its fruits are considered as "superfruit", due to the high concentration of polyphenols that display antioxidant and cardioprotective bioactivities bringing benefits to human health [1,2]. Earlier studies from Mexican plants have shown that triterpenes and polyphenolic compounds have vasodilator effects [7], which could explain or suggest vasodilatory activity by the fruits of *A. chilensis*. However, there is no information about the cardiovascular activity of the metabolites isolated from the leaves of this plant. In the present study, we evaluated the vasodilatory activity of 8-oxo-9-dihydromakomakine, a natural tetracyclic indole alkaloid isolated from the leaves of *A. chilensis*, in search of natural compounds that could be used to develop new therapeutic agents to treat cardiovascular diseases.

Results showed than 8-oxo-9-dihydromakomakine induced relaxation in aortic rings pre contracted with PE. The rings were obtained from normotensive rats and the relaxation was evidenced in a dose-dependent manner. The vasodilator activity of endothelium and the endothelial nitric oxide synthase (eNOS) were studied in two experiments. First, 8-oxo-9-dihydromakomakine caused vasodilation in intact and endothelium-denuded aortic rings when they were exposed to a cumulative concentrations of this one. Second, the inhition of the enzyme eNOS by pre-incubation of aortic rings with L-NAME did not alter the vasodilation caused by 8-oxo-9-dehydromakomakine.

These results suggest that the vasodilation mechanism is independent of endothelium [8]. Thus, 8-oxo-9-dihydromakomakine goes through the endothelium and evoke a vascular response in the smooth muscle.

In agreement with above relaxation data, the pre-incubation of aortic rings with 8-oxo-9-dehydromakomakine significantly reduced the KCl-induced contractions more than PE-induced contractions. The pre-incubation with 8-oxo-9-dihydromakomakine significantly decreased the contractile response to KCl, $BaCl_2$, and TEA in rat aorta. The KCl-induced contraction was caused by an increase of extracellular potassium, leading to membrane depolarization, which increases calcium influx from extracellular sources, involving voltage-dependent calcium channels [9]. $BaCl_2$ and TEA block inward rectifying potassium channels [10], or potassium channels activated by calcium [11], respectively, thus depolarizing the plasma membrane and vasoconstriction. Similar results were obtained with the inhibition of Na,K-ATPase, which causes depolarization of plasma membrane and induced vasoconstriction [12]. 8-oxo-9-dihydromakomakine significantly decreased the contractile responses to PE in rat aorta in the presence or absence of ouabain. Therefore, these results could indicate that 8-oxo-9-dihydromakomakine partially reduces plasma membrane depolarization-induced contraction.

To assess the effect of 8-oxo-9-dihydromakomakine on the calcium current blockage, aortic rings of rat were pre-incubated with or without 8-oxo-9-dihydromakomakine, and kept on calcium-free medium. Contractions to PE were reduced in aortic rings pre-incubated with 8-oxo-9-dihydromakomakine in a free calcium medium, and by extracellular Ca^{2+} addition. Since PE stimulates inositol 1,4,5-trisphosphate receptor via protein kinase C [13] and releases calcium from intracellular store, which opens the store-operated calcium channels [14], our result analysis will suggest that the reduction of contractile response is mediated via a reduction of the influx of extracellular Ca^{2+} [15].

Recently, some studies showed that secondary compounds from medicinal plants can modulate voltage-dependent calcium channels, and thus, the vascular response. The pre-incubation with caffeine (a methylxanthine alkaloid) blunted contractile response to both, KCl and PE. The vasodilation mechanism of caffeine involves activation of the ryanodine channels [16], inhibition of the IP3 receptor [17], and voltage-dependent calcium channels [18,19]. Dicentrine (an aporphine alkaloid), dihydrocorynantheine, and tetrandrine (a bisbenzyl isoquinoline) cause inhibition of α_1-adrenergic receptor and blocks calcium influx [20–22]. While, nantenine (an aporphine alkaloid) produces relaxation in aortic rings pre-contracted with noradrenaline or KCl [13]. We observed that 8-oxo-9-dihydromakomakine significantly reduced the contractile response to agonists of voltage-dependent calcium channels type L (Bay K6844), through a decrease of the calcium influx from extracellular sources [23]. In this way, it was confirmed that some alkaloid derivates may act as antihypertensives.

Since the aortic rings pre-incubated with the highest doses of 8-oxo-9-dehydromakomakine drastically reduced the contraction to KCl, and after responded to vasoactives substances, such as PE, it is possible to think that the high dose did not cause toxicity on vascular tissue [24]. Moreover, the effect induced by a toxic dose should be similar in vascular tissue pre-contracted with KCl or PE [25]; however, this was not observed in our study. Our use of aortic rings from rats to validate these findings are predicted on the observations that rat aorta assay provides a useful pharmacological tool for in vitro analysis, due to the low number of animals, good reproducibility of the experiments, and because the results are easily extrapolated to the in vivo models [26].

This study indicated that 8-oxo-9-dihydromakomakine reduces vascular tension endothelium-independently, and that the underlying mechanisms may involve decreases in the concentration of cytosolic Ca^{2+}, likely through the blocking of voltage-dependent calcium channels.

4. Materials and Methods

4.1. Reagents and Chemicals

Silica gel GF254 analytical chromatoplates, Silica gel grade 60 A for column chromatography were purchased from Merck Co., Santiago, Chile. Precoated thin-layer chromatography TLC plates SIL G-100 UV254, 1.0 mm, preparative were purchased from Machery–Nagel (GmbH&Co, KG), Dueren, Germany. 8-oxo-9-dihydromakomakine was 99% purified through recrystallization.

The drugs used were L-phenylephrine hydrochloride (PE), N^{ω}-nitro-L-arginine methyl ester (L-NAME), ouabain, and Bay K8644 (Sigma-Aldrich, St Luis, MO, USA). Caffeine, Tetraethylammonium (TEA), and Barium chloride dihydrate ($BaCl_2$) were obtained from Merck (Darmstadt, Germany). The drugs were dissolved in distilled deionized water (deionized water Millipore) and kept at 4 °C. The stock solution of 8-oxo-9-dihydromakomakine was dissolved in DMSO (Merck, Germany). Final DMSO concentration in the organ bath was lower than 0.1%. The Krebs-Ringer bicarbonate (KRB) solutions were freshly prepared before each experiment.

4.2. Plant Material

Leaves of *A. chilensis* were collected on S 36°50′01.51″ W 73°01′53.75″, Concepción, Chile, during the end of the winter season. A voucher specimen was deposited at the herbal collection of the Laboratory of Natural Products (C. Paz), Universidad de La Frontera, Chile.

4.3. Apparatus

Optical rotations were recorded on a JASCO P-200 polarimeter (JASCO, Tokyo, Japan). Fourier-transform infrared (FTIR) spectra were measured on a Nicolet 6700 from Thermo Electron Corporation, (Madison, WI, USA) with the Attenuated Total Reflectance (ATR)-unit Smart Performer. Melting points were determined on a Melting Point SMP10 (Stuart, Staffordshire, UK) uncorrected. The ^{1}H- and ^{13}C-NMR spectra were recorded in $CDCl_3$ solution in 5-mm tubes at room temperature (RT) on a Bruker Avance III spectrometer (Bruker Biospin GmbH, Rheinstetten, Germany) at 600.13 (^{1}H) and 150.61 (^{13}C) MHz, with the deuterium signal of the solvent as the lock and Tetramethylsilane (TMS; for ^{1}H) or the solvent (for ^{13}C) as internal standard. All spectra [^{1}H, ^{13}C, gradient-selected COrrelated SpectroscopY (gs-H,H-COSY), edited Heteronuclear Single Quantum Correlation (HSQC), and gradient-selected Heteronuclear Multiple Bond Correlation (gs-HMBC)] were acquired and processed with the standard Bruker software (Bruker, Rheinstetten, Germany). Tension changes in aortic rings were recorded with an Isometric force transducer (Radnoti, Monrovia, CA, USA), connected to a PowerLab 8/35 (ADInstruments, Bella Vista, Australia) for continuous recording of vascular tension using the LabChart Pro 8.1.2 computer program (ADInstruments, Bella Vista, Australia).

4.4. Isolation of 8-Oxo-9-Dihydromakomakine from Aristotelia chilensis

Fresh leaves of *A. chilensis* (7 kg) were crushed and extracted in acid water (pH 3, HCl) in the course of three days at room temperature. The aqueous layer was alkalinized to pH 11 with NaOH and subsequently extracted with EtOAc (3 × 1 L). The organic layer was evaporated at 45 °C and 200 mmHg to afford a gummy red residue. This total OH^- extract was chromatographed using a silica gel column (200–300 mesh) and increased solvent polarity (from hexane 100% to EtOAc 100%). The preparative chromatography was monitored by thin-layer chromatography (TLC; silica gel) and revealed using UV light, and later, Dragendorff's reagent; those fractions showing similar TLC patterns were pooled and concentrated in vacuo. With the mixture of eluents hex/EtOAc (1:1) appeared a clear spot in TLC, then this fraction was purified by Sephadex LH-20 column (MeOH) and further recrystallization from EtOAc, giving 8-oxo-9-dihydromakomakine (85 mg, 0.0012% yield, yellow crystals).

4.5. Animals

For vascular reactivity experiments, Male Sprague-Dawley rats (6–8 weeks of age, 150–180 g) from the breeding colony at the Universidad de Antofagasta were used. All animals were housed in a temperature-controlled (21 ± 1 °C), light-cycled (08:00–20:00 h) room with *ad libitum* access to drinking water and standard rat chow (Champion, Santiago, Chile). In this study, 12 rats were randomly allocated. The investigation was conformed to the Guide for the Care and Use of Laboratory Animals published by the U.S. National Institute of Health (NIH Publication revised 2013), and the local animal research committee approved the experimental procedure used in the present study (number CEIC REV/2013).

4.6. Isolation of Aortic Rings

Rats were sacrificed through cervical dislocation. The thoracic aorta was quickly excised and placed in physiological KRB at room temperature containing ($\times\ 10^{-3}$ M): 4.2 KCl, 1.19 KH_2PO_4, 120 NaCl, 25 Na_2HCO_3, 1.2 $MgSO_4$, 1.3 $CaCl_2$, and 5 D-glucose (pH 7.4). Rings (3–5 mm and 2–4 mg) were prepared after connective tissue was cleaned out from the aorta, taking special care to avoid endothelial damage. Aortic rings were equilibrated for 40 min in KRB at 37 °C by constant bubbling with 95% O_2 and 5% CO_2.

4.7. Vascular Reactivity Experiments

Aortic rings from the same animal were studied in duplicate, using different vasoactive substances (PE, KCl). The rings were mounted on two 25-gauge stainless steel wires; the lower one was attached to a stationary glass rod and the upper one was attached to an isometric force transducer connected to a PowerLab 8/35. The vascular tension was recorded with LabChart Pro 8.1.2 computer program (ADInstruments, Bella Vista, Australia). After the equilibration period for 30 min, the aortic rings were stabilized by three successive near-maximum contractions with KCl (6×10^{-2} M) for 10 min. The passive tension on aorta was 1.0 g, which was determined to be the resting tension for obtaining maximum active tension induced by 6×10^{-2} M KCl [10].

4.8. Assessment of the Effects of 8-Oxo-9-Dihydromakomakine on the Vasodilation in Isolated Aortic Rings Pre-Contracted with PE, with and without Endothelium

Aortic rings were pre-contracted with 10^{-6} M PE, and then increasing concentrations 8-oxo-9-dihydromakomakine (10^{-9} to 10^{-4} M) were added to the bath. The endothelium removal was by gentle rubbing off the endothelium using a small piece of cotton. To evaluate the vascular function of the endothelium, the vasodilation to 10^{-5} M acetylcholine (ACh, muscarinic agonist) in pre-contracted aortic rings with 10^{-6} M PE was tested. According to the general use of rat aorta as a pharmacological tool for in vitro, the aortic rings were considered with a functional endothelial response if vasodilation was up to 70–80% [11].

After a steady contraction of the aortic rings with or without endothelium induced by PE (10^{-6} M) or KCl (6×10^{-2} M) was achieved, 8-oxo-9-dihydromakomakine (10^{-9} to 10^{-4} M), dissolved in DMSO (0.1% on the bath), was cumulatively added to the Krebs solution, and the results were used to generate a concentration-response curve. In other protocols, an inhibitor of Na,K-ATPase (ouabain) was used. The aortic rings were pre-incubated with ouabain (10^{-3} M) for 20 min.

4.9. Assessment of the Effects of 8-Oxo-9-Dihydromakomakine on Endothelial Nitric Oxide Synthase (eNOS)

The role of endothelial nitric oxide (NO) in the rat aorta was studied. An inhibitor of eNOS (L-NAME) was used. The aortic rings were pre-incubated with L-NAME (10^{-4} M) for 20 min before the experiment. Then, the aortic rings were pre-contracted with 10^{-6} M PE, and then increasing concentrations 8-oxo-9-dihydromakomakine (10^{-9} to 10^{-4} M) were added to the bath.

4.10. Effect Calcium Dependence Extracellular Calcium Ionic and Effect of Barium chloride, Tetraethylammonium (TEA), and Bay K6844

To study the role of extracellular calcium, experiments were performed with a calcium-free KRB containing ($\times 10^{-3}$ M) 4.2 KCl, 1.19 KH$_2$PO$_4$, 125 NaCl, 25 NaHCO$_3$, 1.2 MgSO$_4$, and 5 D-glucose (pH 7.4). The aortic rings were first pre-incubated in a normal KRB for 30 min; then the normal KRB was replaced with KRB calcium-free for 5 min before PE (10^{-6} M) was added. Five min after contraction with PE (10^{-6} M), cumulative concentrations of CaCl$_2$ (0.1 to 1.0×10^{-3} M) were added to the medium. In other experiments, the contraction was induced by 5×10^{-3} M BaCl$_2$ or 5×10^{-3} M TEA for 10 min. BaCl$_2$ and TEA are used because they increases vasoconstriction by blocking of potassium channels, thus depolarizing the plasma membrane. In other protocols, the contractile response was induced by an agonist of voltage-dependent calcium channels (10^{-8} M Bay K6844). The aortic rings were pre-incubated with 8-oxo-9-dihydromakomakine (10^{-5} M) for 20 min before the experiment.

4.11. Effect Accumulative KCl and Phenylephrine Modulated by 8-Oxo-9-Dihydromakomakine

In the first curve, the aortic rings were stimulated with accumulative KCl doses (10 mM to 60 mM) or PE (10^{-9} to 10^{-5} M). In the second curve, the aortic rings were pre-incubated with 8-oxo-9-dihydromakomakine (10^{-5} M or 10^{-4} M) for 20 min and then stimulated with accumulative KCl doses (10 mM to 60 mM) or PE (10^{-9} to 10^{-5} M).

4.12. Statistical Analysis

Data shown in figures and tables are expressed as average ± standard errors of the mean. Statistical analysis was performed by means of one-way and two-way analysis of variance (ANOVA) followed by Bonferroni's post-hoc test, and some cases Student's *t*-test. Results are given in the text as probability values, with $p < 0.05$ adopted as the criterion of significance. The graphics and linear regression were done by the least square method, using GraphPad Prism software, version 6.0 (GraphPad Software, Inc, La Jolla, CA, USA).

5. Conclusions

This study demonstrates that the natural alkaloid 8-oxo-9-dihydromakomakine obtained from leaves of *Aristotelia chilensis*, a medicinal tree widely employed in Chilean traditional medicine, is able to decrease the tone of arterial smooth muscle. The vasodilator effect of this alkaloid involves responses independent of endothelium, probably due to calcium channels blockage and/or activation of potassium channels, whose mechanism of action remains to be clarified. Our data suggest that Chilean medicinal plants constitute an important reservoir of bioactive compounds that deserves intensive scientific exploration.

Supplementary Materials: The following are available online, Figure S1. Numbered structure of 8-oxo-9-dihydromakomakine. Figure S2: 1H-NMR (600 MHz, CD$_3$OD) spectra of 8-oxo-9-dihydromakomakine. Figure S3. 13C-NMR (150 MHz, CD$_3$OD) spectra of 8-oxo-9-dihydromakomakine. Figure S4. gs-H,H-COSY (CD$_3$OD) spectra of 8-oxo-9-dihydromakomakine. Figure S5. edited HSQC (CD$_3$OD) spectra of 8-oxo-9-dihydromakomakine. Figure S6. gs-HMBC (CD$_3$OD) spectra of 8-oxo-9-dihydromakomakine.

Author Contributions: F.C and A.P. conducted the pharmacological assays. A.P., C.R.N., and J.P. contributed to the preparation and writing the manuscript. C.P. isolated the tested compound and prepared the manuscript.

Funding: This research was supported by the grant [DI17-0049] from the Universidad de La Frontera, Chile and Network for Extreme Environments Research project (NEXER; Project [ANT1756], Universidad de Antofagasta, Chile).

Acknowledgments: The authors wish to express their gratitude to the Universidad de La Frontera and the Rectoria y Vicerrectoria de Investigacion, Innovacion y Postgrado Universidad de Antofagasta for their financial and technical support.

Conflicts of Interest: The authors declare no conflict of interest.

References

1. Cespedes, C.L.; Balbontin, C.; Avila, J.G.; Dominguez, M.; Alarcon, J.; Paz, C.; Burgos, V.; Ortiz, L.; Penaloza-Castro, I.; Seigler, D.S.; et al. Inhibition on cholinesterase and tyrosinase by alkaloids and phenolics from Aristotelia chilensis leaves. *Food Chem. Toxicol.* **2017**, *109*, 984–995. [CrossRef] [PubMed]
2. Cespedes, C.L.; El-Hafidi, M.; Pavon, N.; Alarcon, J. Antioxidant and cardioprotective activities of phenolic extracts from fruits of Chilean blackberry Aristotelia chilensis (Elaeocarpaceae), Maqui. *Food Chem.* **2008**, *107*, 820–829. [CrossRef]
3. Fredes, C.; Becerra, C.; Parada, J.; Robert, P. The microencapsulation of Maqui (*Aristotelia chilensis* (Mol.) Stuntz) juice by spray-drying and freeze-drying produces powders with similar anthocyanin stability and bioaccessibility. *Molecules* **2018**, *23*, 15. [CrossRef] [PubMed]
4. Halcox, J.P.; Quyyumi, A.A. Coronary vascular endothelial function and myocardial ischemia: Why should we worry about endothelial dysfunction? *Coron. Artery Dis.* **2001**, *12*, 475–484. [CrossRef] [PubMed]
5. Paz, C.; Becerra, J.; Silva, M.; Cabrera-Pardo, J.; Burgos, V.; Heydenreich, M.; Schmidt, B. (-)-8-Oxohobartine a new indole alkaloid from Aristotelia chilensis (Mol.) Stuntz. *Rec. Nat. Prod.* **2016**, *10*, 68–73.
6. Paz, C.; Becerra, J.; Silva, M.; Freire, E.; Baggio, R. A polymorphic form of 4,4-dimethyl-8-methylene-3-azabicyclo 3.3.1 non-2-en-2-yl 3-indolyl ketone, an indole alkaloid extracted from Aristotelia chilensis (maqui). *Acta Crystallogr. C Struct. Chem.* **2013**, *69*, 1509. [CrossRef] [PubMed]
7. Fusi, F.; Spiga, O.; Trezza, A.; Sgaragli, G.; Saponara, S. The surge of flavonoids as novel, fine regulators of cardiovascular Ca. *Eur. J. Pharmacol.* **2017**, *796*, 158–174. [CrossRef] [PubMed]
8. Luna-Vazquez, F.J.; Ibarra-Alvarado, C.; Rojas-Molina, A.; Rojas-Molina, I.; Zavala-Sanchez, M.A. Vasodilator compounds derived from plants and their mechanisms of action. *Molecules* **2013**, *18*, 5814–5857. [CrossRef] [PubMed]
9. Godfraind, T.; Miller, R.; Wibo, M. Calcium antagonism and calcium entry blockade. *Pharmacol. Rev.* **1986**, *38*, 321–416. [PubMed]
10. Cifuentes, F.; Palacios, J.; Nwokocha, C.R. Synchronization in the Heart Rate and the Vasomotion in Rat Aorta: Effect of Arsenic Trioxide. *Cardiovasc. Toxicol.* **2016**, *16*, 79–88. [CrossRef] [PubMed]
11. Palacios, J.; Vega, J.L.; Paredes, A.; Cifuentes, F. Effect of phenylephrine and endothelium on vasomotion in rat aorta involves potassium uptake. *J. Physiol. Sci.* **2013**, *63*, 103–111. [CrossRef] [PubMed]
12. Palacios, J.; Marusic, E.T.; Lopez, N.C.; Gonzalez, M.; Michea, L. Estradiol-induced expression of N(+)-K(+)-ATPase catalytic isoforms in rat arteries: Gender differences in activity mediated by nitric oxide donors. *Am. J. Physiol. Heart Circ. Physiol.* **2004**, *286*, H1793–H1800. [CrossRef] [PubMed]
13. Cicala, C.; Morello, S.; Iorio, C.; Capasso, R.; Borrelli, F.; Mascolo, N. Vascular effects of caffeic acid phenethyl ester (CAPE) on isolated rat thoracic aorta. *Life Sci.* **2003**, *73*, 73–80. [CrossRef]
14. Karaki, H.; Weiss, G.B. Calcium release in smooth muscle. *Life Sci.* **1988**, *42*, 111–122. [CrossRef]
15. Lee, C.H.; Poburko, D.; Sahota, P.; Sandhu, J.; Ruehlmann, D.O.; van Breemen, C. The mechanism of phenylephrine-mediated $[Ca^{2+}]_i$ oscillations underlying tonic contraction in the rabbit inferior vena cava. *J. Physiol.* **2001**, *534*, 641–650. [CrossRef] [PubMed]
16. Missiaen, L.; Parys, J.B.; De Smedt, H.; Himpens, B.; Casteels, R. Inhibition of inositol trisphosphate-induced calcium release by caffeine is prevented by ATP. *Biochem. J.* **1994**, *300*, 81–84. [CrossRef] [PubMed]
17. Martin, C.; Dacquet, C.; Mironneau, C.; Mironneau, J. Caffeine-induced inhibition of calcium channel current in cultured smooth cells from pregnant rat myometrium. *Br. J. Pharmacol.* **1989**, *98*, 493–498. [CrossRef] [PubMed]
18. Echeverri, D.; Montes, F.R.; Cabrera, M.; Galán, A.; Prieto, A. Caffeine's vascular mechanisms of action. *Int. J. Vasc. Med.* **2010**, *2010*, 834060. [CrossRef] [PubMed]
19. Iturriaga-Vásquez, P.; Miquel, R.; Ivorra, M.D.; D'Ocon, M.P.; Cassels, B.K. Simplified tetrandrine congeners as possible antihypertensive agents with a dual mechanism of action. *J. Nat. Prod.* **2003**, *66*, 954–957. [CrossRef] [PubMed]
20. Mustafa, M.R.; Achike, F.I. Dicentrine is preferentially antagonistic to rat aortic than splenic alpha 1-adrenoceptor stimulation. *Acta Pharmacol. Sin.* **2000**, *21*, 1165–1168. [PubMed]
21. Wang, K.; Zhou, X.Y.; Wang, Y.Y.; Li, M.M.; Li, Y.S.; Peng, L.Y.; Cheng, X.; Li, Y.; Wang, Y.P.; Zhao, Q.S. Macrophyllionium and macrophyllines A. and B., oxindole alkaloids from Uncaria macrophylla. *J. Nat. Prod.* **2011**, *74*, 12–15. [CrossRef] [PubMed]

22. Orallo, F.; Alzueta, A.F. Preliminary study of the vasorelaxant effects of (+)-nantenine, an alkaloid isolated from *Platycapnos spicata*, in rat aorta. *Planta Med.* **2001**, *67*, 800–806. [CrossRef] [PubMed]
23. Kim, J.E.; Choi, B.K.; Choi, J.Y.; Ryu, T.; Roh, W.S.; Song, S.Y. Role of calcium channels responsible for phenylephrine-induced contraction in rat aorta 3 days after acute myocardial infarction. *Korean J. Anesthesiol.* **2014**, *66*, 143–152. [CrossRef] [PubMed]
24. Maione, F.; Cicala, C.; Musciacco, G.; De Feo, V.; Amat, A.G.; Ialenti, A.; Mascolo, N. Phenols, Alkaloids and terpenes from medicinal plants with antihypertensive and vasorelaxant activities. A review of natural products as leads to potential therapeutic agents. *Nat. Prod. Commun.* **2013**, *8*, 539–544. [PubMed]
25. Ok, S.H.; Byon, H.J.; Kwon, S.C.; Park, J.; Lee, Y.; Hwang, Y.; Baik, J.; Choi, M.J.; Sohn, J.T. Lipid emulsion inhibits vasodilation induced by a toxic dose of bupivacaine via attenuated dephosphorylation of myosin phosphatase target subunit 1 in isolated rat aorta. *Int. J. Med. Sci.* **2015**, *12*, 958–967. [CrossRef] [PubMed]
26. Rameshrad, M.; Babaei, H.; Azarmi, Y.; Fouladia, D.F. Rat aorta as a pharmacological tool for in vitro and in vivo studies. *Life Sci.* **2016**, *145*, 190–204. [CrossRef] [PubMed]

Sample Availability: Samples of 8-oxo-9-dihydromakomakine is available from the corresponding author.

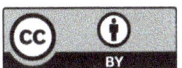

© 2018 by the authors. Licensee MDPI, Basel, Switzerland. This article is an open access article distributed under the terms and conditions of the Creative Commons Attribution (CC BY) license (http://creativecommons.org/licenses/by/4.0/).

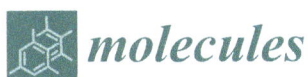

Article

Effect of *Aspergillus flavus* Fungal Elicitor on the Production of Terpenoid Indole Alkaloids in *Catharanthus roseus* Cambial Meristematic Cells

Chuxin Liang [1,†], Chang Chen [2,†], Pengfei Zhou [3,†], Lv Xu [1], Jianhua Zhu [1,2,*], Jincai Liang [2], Jiachen Zi [2] and Rongmin Yu [1,2,*]

1. Biotechnological Institute of Chinese Materia Medica, Jinan University, 601 Huangpu Avenue West, Guangzhou 510632, China; lcxliangcx@163.com (C.L.); xulv1818@163.com (L.X.)
2. Department of Natural Product Chemistry, College of Pharmacy, Jinan University, Guangzhou 510632, China; imchenchang@163.com (C.C.); yffsljc2006@sina.com (J.L.); jiachen_zi@163.com (J.Z.)
3. Department of Basic Medical Sciences, Xinxiang Medical University, Xinxiang 453003, China; zpf861223@163.com
* Correspondence: tzhujh@jnu.edu.cn (J.Z.); tyrm@jnu.edu.cn (R.Y.); Tel.: +86-20-85220386 (R.Y.); Fax: +86-20-85224766 (R.Y.)
† These authors contributed equally to this work.

Received: 22 October 2018; Accepted: 10 December 2018; Published: 11 December 2018

Abstract: This study reported the inducing effect of *Aspergillus flavus* fungal elicitor on biosynthesis of terpenoid indole alkaloids (TIAs) in *Catharanthus roseus* cambial meristematic cells (CMCs) and its inducing mechanism. According to the results determined by HPLC and HPLC-MS/MS, the optimal condition of the *A. flavus* elicitor was as follows: after suspension culture of *C. roseus* CMCs for 6 day, 25 mg/L *A. flavus* mycelium elicitor were added, and the CMC suspensions were further cultured for another 48 h. In this condition, the contents of vindoline, catharanthine, and ajmaline were 1.45-, 3.29-, and 2.14-times as high as those of the control group, respectively. Transcriptome analysis showed that *D4H*, *G10H*, *GES*, *IRS*, *LAMT*, *SGD*, *STR*, *TDC*, and *ORCA3* were involved in the regulation of this induction process. The results of qRT-PCR indicated that the increasing accumulations of vindoline, catharanthine, and ajmaline in *C. roseus* CMCs were correlated with the increasing expression of the above genes. Therefore, *A. flavus* fungal elicitor could enhance the TIA production of *C. roseus* CMCs, which might be used as an alternative biotechnological resource for obtaining bioactive alkaloids.

Keywords: *Catharanthus roseus*; cambial meristematic cells; *Aspergillus flavus*; terpenoid indole alkaloids; biosynthesis

1. Introduction

Catharanthus roseus (L.) Don is a perennial medicinal plant of the family Apocynaceae. At present, over 130 alkaloids have been isolated from *C. roseus*, most of which are terpenoid indole alkaloids (TIAs) [1]. Some TIAs such as vinblastine, vincristine, and ajmaline exhibit strong pharmacological activities, and some are widely used in the treatment of various diseases [2–5]. Ajmalicine is a potent antihypertensive reagent [5]. Vinblastine and vincristine, two bisindole alkaloids derived from coupling vindoline and catharanthine, are natural anticancer drugs and are still among the most valuable agents used to treat cancer [3,4].

These secondary metabolites are produced from the TIA biosynthetic pathway in *C. roseus*, which is complex and highly regulated (Figure 1) [2,6,7]. The TIA biosynthetic pathway consists of TIA feeder pathways and the downstream of the TIA biosynthetic pathway. The TIA feeder pathways are the monoterpenoid pathway and indole pathway [7]. The downstream of the TIA biosynthetic pathway in *C. roseus* starts with the formation of strictosidine from tryptamine and secologanin, which is catalyzed by strictosidine synthase (STR) [8]. Then, strictosidine is deglucosylated by strictosidine β-D-glucosidase (SGD) to form strictosidine aglycone. Further enzymatic steps result in the formation of numerous TIAs, and the TIA biosynthetic pathway is classified into several specific branches. One branch of the TIA biosynthetic pathway produces ajmalicine and serpentine, a second branch catharanthine, a third vindoline, and a fourth lochnericine and horhammericine [7]. Genes encoding enzymes catalyzing the production of vindoline from tabersonine, such as deacetoxyvindoline 4-hydroxylase (D4H) and deacetylvindoline O-acyltransferase (DAT), have now been identified [9–14]. The formation of α-3′,4′-anhydrovinblastine from vindoline and catharanthine is catalyzed by a major class III peroxidase (PRX1) [15]. Then, vinblastine and vincristine are formed through multiple enzymatic steps from α-3′,4′-anhydrovinblastine (Figure 1) [7]. The TIA biosynthetic pathway in *C. roseus* is highly regulated by enzymes and transcription factors (TFs). In 2000, Fits and Memelink discovered octadecanoid-derivative responsive *Catharanthus* A P2-domain protein 3 (ORCA3), a jasmonate-responsive AP2/ERF transcription factor, in *C. roseus* using the T-DNA activation tagging technology [16]. Since overexpression of *ORCA3* increases the expression of key genes in the TIA biosynthetic pathway, it is considered to be the core transcription factor in the TIA biosynthetic pathway in *C. roseus* [6]. In addition, *ORCA3* expression could be induced by jasmonates [17].

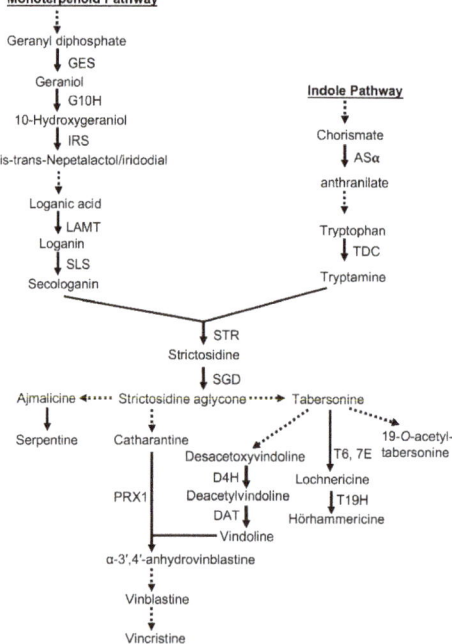

Figure 1. Terpenoid indole alkaloid (TIA) biosynthetic pathways of *C. roseus*. Enzyme abbreviations: GES: geranial synthase; G10H: geraniol 10-hydroxylase; IRS: iridoid synthase; LAMT: loganic acid methyltransferase; SLS: secologanin synthase; AS: anthranilate synthase; TDC: tryptophan decarboxylase; STR: strictosidine synthase; SGD: strictosidine β-D-glucosidase; D4H: deacetoxyvindoline 4-hydroxylase; DAT: deacetylvindoline 4-O-acetyltransferase; T6,7E: tabersonine 6,7-epoxidase; T19H: tabersonine/lochnericine 19-hydroxylase; PRX1: vacuolar class III peroxidase. Single arrows denote single steps, and dotted arrows denote multiple or unidentified steps.

However, the content of the pharmacological secondary metabolites in *C. roseus* is very low [18], and commercial production has used a semi-synthetic route to couple catharanthine and vindoline [3].

Therefore, developing methods to increase the yields of TIAs in *C. roseus* has become a focus for domestic and foreign scholars [19]. In recent years, an increasing number of studies has shown that fungal elicitors play an important role in regulating biological secondary metabolic pathways and intracellular information transmission [20,21]. The fungal elicitor is an active substance derived from fungus, which can rapidly and specifically induce the expression of specific plant genes, thereby activating specific secondary metabolic pathways and increasing the accumulation of interesting secondary metabolites [20]. The treatment of plant cell culture systems with fungal elicitors has become an effective method for rapidly increasing the yield of target product in plant cell culture [20,21]. Although fungal elicitors are known to regulate the production of secondary metabolites, the inducting effect varies depending on factors such as fungal species, elicitor components, dose, time of addition, and type of plant cell culture [22–24]. In 2016, Tonk reported that a low-dose *A. flavus* fungal elicitor effectively increased the growth rate of callus, embryo biomass, germination rate, and alkaloid content in the embryos of *C. roseus*, as well as increasing the shoot and root lengths of germinated somatic embryos. Further, antioxidant enzyme activity assays showed that a low-dose *A. flavus* elicitor caused an allergic reaction in the mature and germinating somatic embryos of *C. roseus*, resulting in an increase in alkaloid content [24]. Therefore, *A. flavus* may be a good elicitor for promoting the TIA production of *C. roseus* cell cultures.

More interestingly, our previous research showed that *C. roseus* cambial meristematic cells (CMCs) exhibit good characteristics when compared to *C. roseus* dedifferentiated plant cells (DDCs), such as faster growth, higher yields, diverse bioactive TIAs, lower variability, and high expression of TIA biosynthesis genes. In addition, after two years of being cultured, *C. roseus* CMCs remained stable in both genetic traits and alkaloid content; the production of vindoline, catharanthine, and ajmaline in *C. roseus* CMCs could be enhanced by β-cyclodextrin and methyl jasmonate (MeJA) [25]. Therefore, *C. roseus* CMCs may be a good system for the investigation of the biosynthesis and regulation of TIAs.

However, there is no report on the effect of the *A. flavus* fungal elicitor on the TIA production of *C. roseus* CMCs so far. In this research, we investigated the inducing effect of the *A. flavus* fungal elicitor on the biosynthesis of TIAs in *C. roseus* CMCs, and the inducing mechanism was explored by transcriptome analysis and determination of the expression of TIA biosynthesis-related genes via the quantitative real-time reverse transcription polymerase chain reaction (qRT-PCR) technique.

2. Results

2.1. Dry Cell Weight in Response to A. flavus Elicitation

Different concentrations of *A. flavus* medium elicitor were added to four-day-old or six-day-old suspensions of *C. roseus* CMCs. In the four-day-old suspensions of CMCs, we observed that the dry cell weight was slightly higher than that of the check group (CK) after *A. flavus* medium elicitor treatment for 24 h (Figure 2a). In the six-day-old suspensions of CMCs, we observed no significant difference in dry cell weight after the addition of the *A. flavus* medium elicitor (Figure 2b). Besides, the concentration of the *A. flavus* mycelium elicitor had no significant effect on the dry cell weight of *C. roseus* CMC suspension cultures (Figure 2c,d). For six-day-old suspensions of CMCs, the dry cell weight was slightly higher than that of the CK after 24-h treatment of 15 mg/L *A. flavus* mycelium elicitor (Figure 2d). Based on the results of Figure 2, the *A. flavus* elicitor (different concentrations: 5, 15, or 25 mg/L) had no negative effect on the growth of *C. roseus* CMCs in the selected concentration.

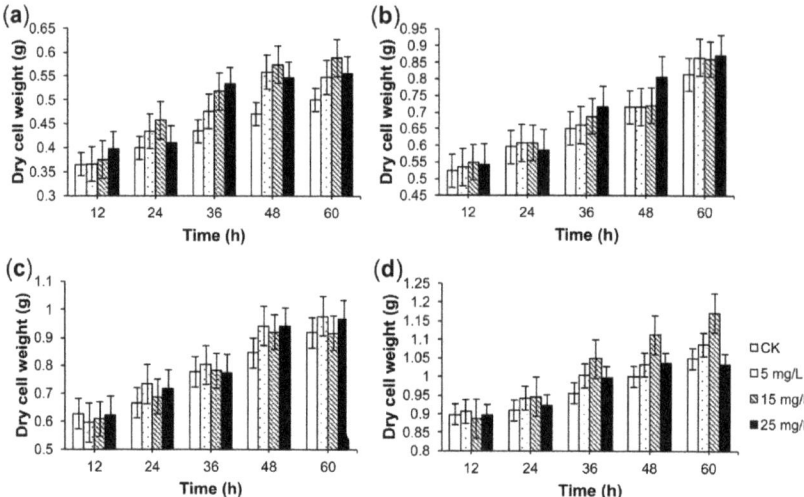

Figure 2. The effect of the *A. flavus* elicitor on the dry cell weight of *C. roseus* cambial meristematic cell (CMC) suspension cultures. The effect of the *A. flavus* medium elicitor on dry cell weight of four-day-old suspensions of *C. roseus* CMCs (**a**) or six-day-old suspensions of *C. roseus* CMCs (**b**). The effect of the *A. flavus* mycelium elicitor on the dry cell weight of four-day-old suspensions of *C. roseus* CMCs (**c**) or six-day-old suspensions of *C. roseus* CMCs (**d**). *C. roseus* CMC cultures treated by sterile water were labeled as the check group (CK). Data are given as the means ± SD (n = 3).

2.2. HPLC-MS/MS Analysis of Alkaloids

The *C. roseus* CMC cultures were harvested after suspension culture for six days. Then, the separation of the compounds of *C. roseus* CMCs was performed by reversed-phase high-performance liquid chromatography (RP-HPLC) with photodiode array detection, as well as by electrospray ionization tandem mass spectrometry (ESI-MS/MS) in positive mode (Figure S1). The MS spectra of the identified compounds are displayed in Figure S1c.

Compound **1**, identified by MS and chromatographic behavior comparison with that of the authentic standard, was ajmalicine (Rt 26.9 min. +MS: 353 [M + H]$^+$; +MS2: 353, 321, 284, 252, 222, 210, 178, 144, 143, 117) (Figure S1).

Compound **2**, equally identified by MS and chromatographic behavior comparison with that of the authentic standard, was catharanthine (Rt 31.3 min. +MS: 337 [M + H]$^+$; +MS2: 337, 248, 219, 204, 173, 165, 144, 143, 133, 128, 127, 93, 91, 77) (Figure S1).

Another compound (**3**) with [M + H]$^+$ at 457 putatively corresponded to vindoline. Compound **3** (Rt 37.1 min) with [M + H]$^+$ at 337 was noticed, and its UV spectrum (UV: 240, 294 nm) was similar to that of catharanthine; therefore, it was the catharanthine isomer. Further comparison showed that its MS spectrum (+MS: 457 [M + H]$^+$; +MS2: 457, 439, 397, 379, 347, 337, 295, 258, 232, 222, 188, 173, 162, 157, 145, 134, 122) (Figure S1c) was in line with that of the vindoline authentic standard.

2.3. TIA Content in Response to Elicitation

To obtain the optimal *A. flavus* elicitor treatment condition, different concentrations of the *A. flavus* medium elicitor and mycelium elicitor were tested for their inducing effects in *C. roseus* CMC suspension cultures.

The effect of the *A. flavus* elicitor on TIA content in *C. roseus* CMCs is shown in Figures 3 and 4. As shown in these figures, *A. flavus* increased the TIA content in *C. roseus* CMCs. For different alkaloids, the induction condition for the highest yield was different. The content of catharanthine reached its maximum (3.39 mg/L), which was 3.6-times as high as that of the CK, after 24-h treatment with

25 mg/L *A. flavus* medium elicitor in four-day-old suspensions of CMCs (Figure 3b). The content of vindoline reached as high as 8.79 mg/L, which was 1.45-times as high as that of the CK, after 48-h treatment with 25 mg/L *A. flavus* mycelium elicitor in six-day-old suspensions of CMCs (Figure 4a). As for ajmaline, the content reached 9.84 mg/L, which was 3.4-times as high as that of CK, after 24-h treatment with 25 mg/L *A. flavus* mycelium elicitor in six-day-old suspensions of CMCs (Figure 4c).

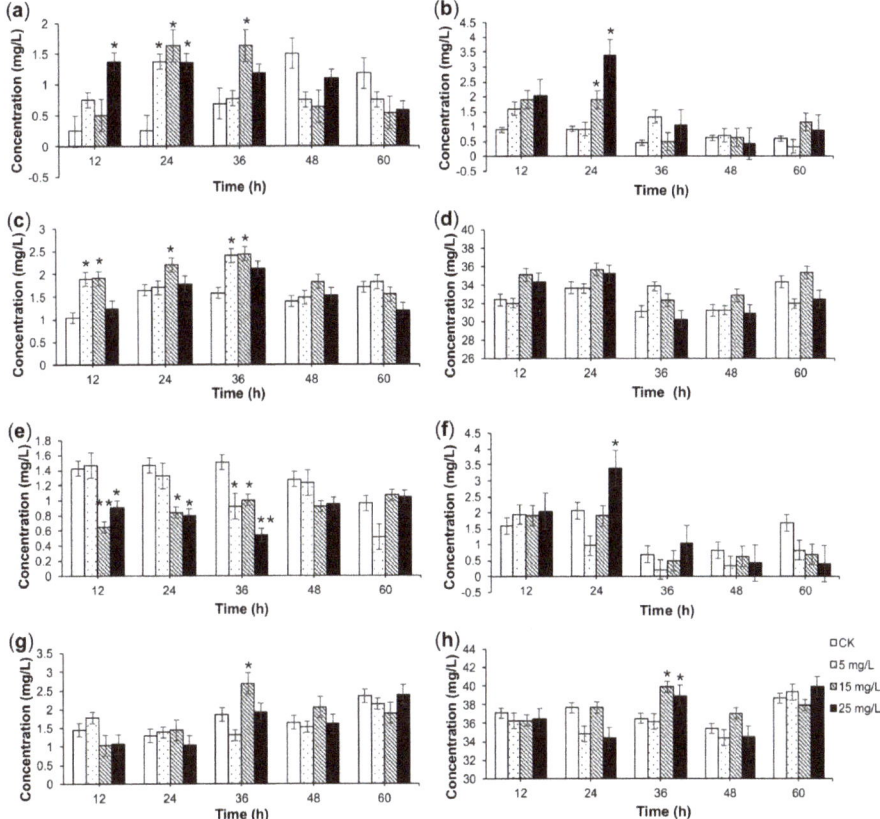

Figure 3. The effect of the *A. flavus* medium elicitor on the concentrations of TIAs. The effect of the *A. flavus* medium elicitor on the concentrations of vindoline (**a**), catharanthine (**b**), ajmaline (**c**), and total alkaloids (**d**) in four-day-old suspensions of *C. roseus* CMCs. The effect of *A. flavus* medium elicitor on the concentrations of vindoline (**e**), catharanthine (**f**), ajmaline (**g**), and total alkaloids (**h**) in six-day-old suspensions of *C. roseus* CMCs. *C. roseus* CMC cultures treated by sterile water were labeled as the check group (CK). Data are given as the means ± SD ($n = 3$). * $p < 0.05$, ** $p < 0.01$, compared to the CK group.

According to the timing when the contents of vindoline, catharanthine, and ajmaline were all relatively high (compared with those of the CK and other experimental groups), the optimal condition was confirmed. The optimal condition for the *A. flavus* elicitor treatment in *C. roseus* CMCs was as follows: after suspension culture of *C. roseus* CMCs for six days, 25 mg/L *A. flavus* mycelium elicitor were added, and the CMC suspensions were further cultured another 48 h. Although the content of total alkaloids was slightly lower than that of the CK under this condition, the contents of vindoline, catharanthine, and ajmaline reached 8.79, 2.81, and 8.95 mg/L, respectively, which were 1.45-, 3.29-, and 2.14-times as high as those of the CK, respectively (Figure 4e–g).

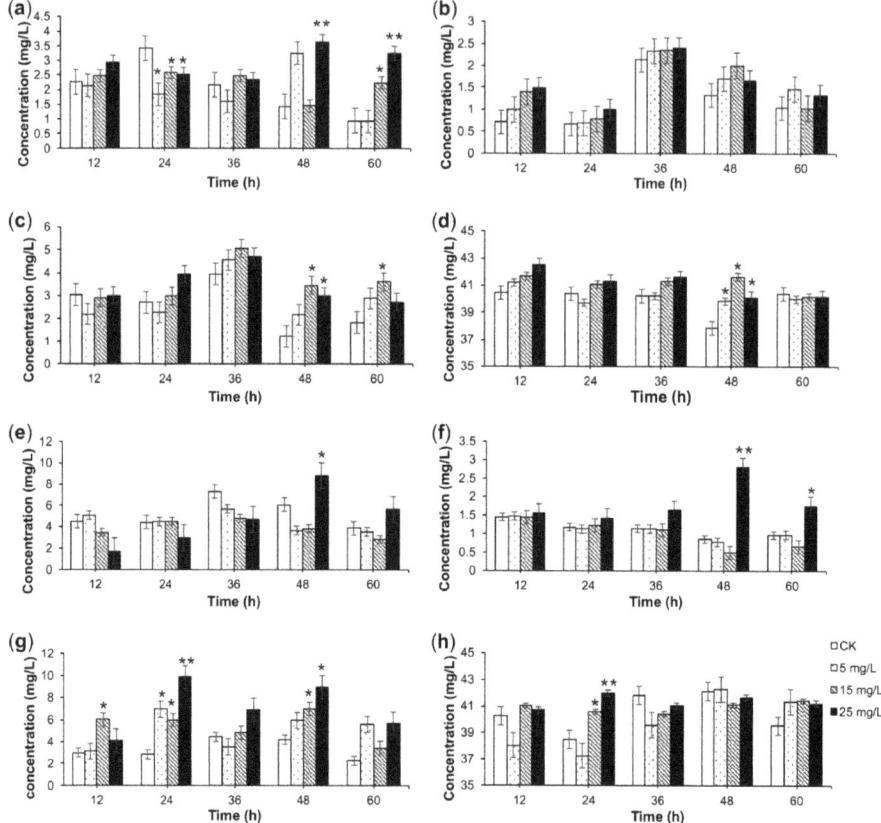

Figure 4. The effects of the *A. flavus* mycelium elicitor on the concentrations of TIAs. The effects of the *A. flavus* mycelium elicitor on the concentrations of vindoline (**a**), catharanthine (**b**), ajmaline (**c**), and total alkaloids (**d**) in four-day-old suspensions of *C. roseus* CMCs. The effect of the *A. flavus* mycelium elicitor on the concentrations of vindoline (**e**), catharanthine (**f**), ajmaline (**g**), and total alkaloids (**h**) in six-day-old suspensions of *C. roseus* CMCs. *C. roseus* CMCs treated by sterile water were labeled as the check group (CK). Data are given as the means ± SD (n = 3). * $p < 0.05$, ** $p < 0.01$, compared with the CK group.

2.4. Functional Annotation and Functional Classification of Unigenes

To identify the key genes in the TIA biosynthetic pathway in *C. roseus* CMCs, the transcriptomes of *C. roseus* DDCs (callus) treated with an equal amount of sterile water, *C. roseus* CMCs (the check treated with an equal amount of sterile water, CK), and *C. roseus* CMCs under optimal *A. flavus* elicitor treatment condition (the experimental group, EG) were determined.

In total, approximately 170.7 million Illumina raw data were generated from the three different samples (Table S1). After filtering the raw data, approximately 59.7, 50.7, and 57.8 million clean reads remained for the callus, CK, and EG transcriptomes, respectively (Table S1). All clean reads were subsequently subjected to de novo assembly with the Trinity program, producing 121,532 transcripts and 105,552 unigenes (Table S2).

Functional annotations of unigenes in the seven largest databases are shown in Table S3. A total of 83,742 unigenes (79.33%) were annotated based on the information available from seven public protein databases including the NCBI non-redundant protein sequences (NR), NCBI non-redundant nucleotide sequences (NT), Swiss-Prot, Protein family (Pfam), Gene Ontology (GO), euKaryotic Ortholog Groups

(KOG), and the Kyoto Encyclopedia of Genes and Genomes (KEGG) using the Basic Local Alignment Search Tool (BLAST) with an E-value cut-off of 1 e^{-10} (Table S3). A total of 79,711 unigenes (75.51% of the total assembled unigenes) had a match in the NR database, and 59,272 (56.15%), 63,496 (60.15%), 61,591 (58.35%), 61,829 (58.57%), 26,674 (25.27), and 34,367 (32.55%) unigenes showed significant similarity to sequences in the NT, Swiss-Prot, Pfam, GO, KOG, and KEGG databases, respectively (Table S3).

All unigenes were subjected to a search against the GO database to classify unigene functions based on the NR annotation. Of the 105,552 assembled unigenes, 61,829 unigenes were successfully assigned to one or more GO terms, and these unigenes were classified into three main GO categories and 56 groups (Figure S2). Within the "biological process" domain, the most evident matches were the terms "cellular process" (37,633), "metabolic process" (35,132), and "single-organism process" (28,250). In the "cellular component" domain, the terms "cell" (20,343) and "cell part" (20,343) were most frequently assigned. For the "molecular function" domain, the assignments were mostly enriched in the terms "binding" (37,680) and "catalytic activity" (31,249).

For further analysis, the unigenes were mapped onto the KEGG database for categorization of gene function and identification of biochemical pathways. A total of 34,367 unigenes were annotated and assigned to 5 main KEGG metabolic pathways, 19 sub-branches, and 300 KEGG pathways. Among them, the most common sub-branch was "carbohydrate metabolism" (2904), followed by "translation" (2711) and "folding, sorting and degradation" (2575) (Figure S3). In addition, there were seven unigene matches in "indole alkaloid biosynthesis" (ko00901), 43 in "monoterpenoid biosynthesis" (ko00902), and 314 in "terpenoid backbone biosynthesis" (ko00900) (Table S4).

As shown in Table S5, the detected unigenes contained transcription factors of the orphans, AP2-EREBP, and SET families.

2.5. High and Differential Expression Analysis of Unigenes

The correlation of gene transcription levels between samples could reflect differences in gene expression patterns. The closer the correlation coefficient is to one, the higher the degree of similarity of the gene expression pattern between samples. On the other hand, the closer the correlation coefficient is to zero, the bigger the difference in gene expression pattern between samples. As shown in Figure S4a, the square of the Pearson correlation coefficient (R^2) was 0.539, indicating that there was a significant difference between the callus and CK groups in the level of gene expression. Thus, the gene expression pattern of the *C. roseus* CMCs was very different from that of the *C. roseus* DDCs. Besides, R^2 was 0.86 between the EG and CK groups (Figure S4b), showing that *A. flavus* elicitor treatment could indeed cause differences in gene expression levels.

Differentially-expressed genes (DEGs) ($|\log_2$ (fold change)$| \geq 1$ and q-value ≤ 0.005) were defined as unigenes that were significantly enriched or depleted in one sample relative to the other. A volcano plot was constructed to illustrate the distribution of DEGs in the callus vs. CK and EG vs. CK groups (Figure S5). The results of the differential expression analysis indicated that the expression levels of some genes in the callus group were significantly up- or down-regulated when compared with the CK. Further, compared with the CK, the expression levels of a few genes in the EG group were significantly up- or down-regulated, but the significant degree was lower than that of the callus vs. CK. The number of common differential genes among the two comparative combinations was 133, while the number of unique differential genes was 4825 in callus vs. CK and 139 in EG vs. CK (Figure S6).

To further understand the biological functions of DEGs, they were annotated with the GO and KEGG pathways. Compared with the CK, there were 2035 up-regulated DEGs and 1859 down-regulated DEGs in the callus group and 232 up-regulated DEGs and 114 down-regulated DEGs in EG (Figure S7). Partial results of KEGG pathways analysis of DEGs, which were associated with TIA biosynthesis and induced by the *A. flavus* elicitor, are shown in Figure S8. Compared with the *C. roseus* DDCs (the callus group), some genes related to the biosynthesis of TIAs were up-regulated in the *C. roseus* CMCs (the CK group). Combining the results of differential expression analysis,

GO enrichment, and KEGG pathway analysis of DEGs in callus vs. CK and EG vs. CK, the DEGs associated with TIA biosynthesis and induced by the *A. flavus* elicitor were screened, and their sequences were aligned with the genes in the NCBI database via the BLAST tool. The genes identified were *D4H*, 10-hydroxylase geraniol (*G10H*), geraniol synthase (*GES*), iridoid synthase (*IRS*), loganic acid O-methyltransferase (*LAMT*), *SGD*, *STR*, tryptophan decarboxylase (*TDC*), and *ORCA3*, of which *ORCA3* was a transcription factor gene.

2.6. qRT-PCR

Under the optimal *A. flavus* elicitor treatment condition, the transcription levels of *D4H*, *G10H*, *GES*, *IRS*, *LAMT*, *SGD*, *STR*, *TDC*, and *ORCA3* were much higher in EG than in CK. Specifically, their expression were 4.49-, 1.75-, 1.71-, 1.42-, 3.12-, 2.33-, 2.87-, 2.51-, and 5.97-times as high as those of CK, respectively (Figure 5).

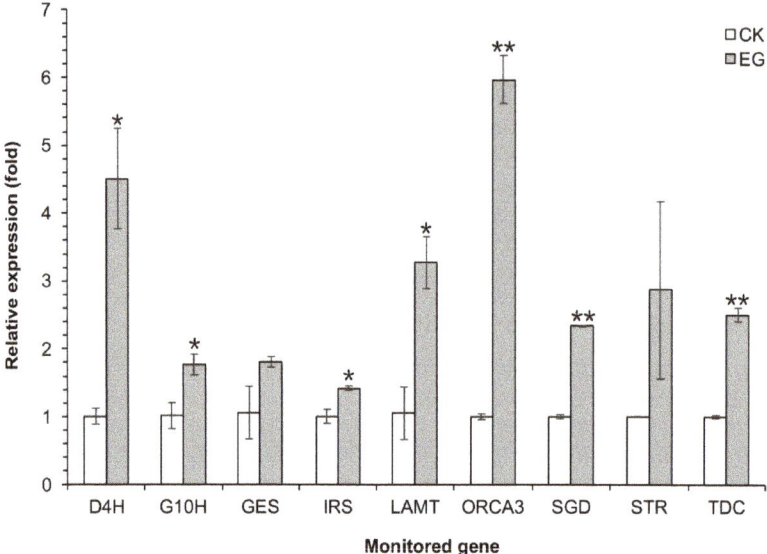

Figure 5. The effects of the *A. flavus* elicitor on the expression of TIA biosynthesis key genes in *C. roseus* CMCs under the optimal *A. flavus* elicitor treatment condition. *C. roseus* CMCs cultured under the optimal *A. flavus* elicitor treatment condition were labeled as the experimental group (EG). *C. roseus* CMCs treated by sterile water were labeled as the check group (CK). Data are given as the means ± SD (n = 3). * $p < 0.05$, ** $p < 0.01$, compared with the CK group.

3. Discussion

Since the low content of the pharmacological TIAs in *C. roseus* [18] and commercial production has used a semi-synthetic route to couple vindoline and catharanthine [3], developing methods to enhance the TIA production of *C. roseus* cell cultures has become a focus for domestic and foreign scholars [19]. According to our previous research, undifferentiated *C. roseus* CMCs were capable of maintaining not only good cellular morphology, but also stable and high production of alkaloid metabolites [25]. Therefore, *C. roseus* CMCs were used as plant cell materials for the investigation of the biosynthesis of TIAs.

In previous reports, fungal elicitors could increase the accumulation of secondary metabolites of interest by activating specific secondary metabolic pathways [20]. Tonk et al. showed that not only the callus growth rate, but also the alkaloid content in the embryos of *C. roseus* could be effectively increased after being treated with a low-dose *A. flavus* fungal elicitor [24]. However, there has been no research on the effect of *A. flavus* fungal elicitor on the yields of TIAs in *C. roseus* CMCs. Generally, the optimal time for adding the fungal elicitor to cell cultures is at the log phase of the culture cycle, when the cell cultures are most sensitive to elicitation. Our previous research showed that the log phase of the *C. roseus* CMC culture cycle lasts from 4–9 days [25]. Besides, the results of our preliminary experiment in this research showed that the *C. roseus* CMC cultures turned brown after three days of treatment or when the suspension cultures of *C. roseus* CMCs were treated with the fungal elicitor after a nine-day culture. Thus, we finally added three different concentrations of the *A. flavus* medium elicitor or the *A. flavus* mycelium elicitor to four-day-old or six-day-old suspensions of *C. roseus* CMCs. After inducing treatment, we found that the *A. flavus* mycelium elicitor could promote the TIA production without a negative effect on the growth of *C. roseus* CMCs in the selected concentration. According to the results determined by HPLC and HPLC-MS, the optimal condition of the *A. flavus* elicitor was as follows: after suspension culture of *C. roseus* CMCs for six days, 25 mg/L *A. flavus* mycelium elicitor were added, and the CMC suspensions were further cultured for another 48 h. Under this condition, the contents of vindoline, catharanthine, and ajmaline were 1.45-, 3.29-, and 2.14-times as high as those of the CK group, respectively (Figure 4e–g).

The TIA biosynthetic pathway in *C. roseus* is complex and highly regulated [2,6–8]. Hao et al. comprehensively analyzed the differential gene expression profiles of 24 h of continuous light, 24 h of dark treatment, 4 h of MeJA treatment under continuous light conditions, and 4 h of MeJA treatment under dark conditions in *Artemisia annua* seedlings using Illumina transcriptome sequencing. As a result, some TFs in the light signaling pathway were identified that can respond to MeJA [26]. Thus, transcriptome analysis is an effective method of investigating the inducing mechanism. To explore the inducing mechanism at the gene expression level, we analyzed the transcriptome data of *C. roseus* DDCs treated with sterile water, *C. roseus* CMCs treated with sterile water, and *C. roseus* CMCs under the optimal *A. flavus* elicitor treatment condition. This transcriptome analysis showed that *D4H*, *G10H*, *GES*, *IRS*, *LAMT*, *SGD*, *STR*, *TDC*, and *ORCA3* were involved in the regulation of this induction process. The functions of the above genes in the TIA biosynthetic pathway are shown in Figure 1. Among the above genes, *ORCA3* is the core transcription factor gene in the TIA biosynthetic pathway [6]. Then, we further analyzed the transcription levels of the above genes by qRT-PCR. The results of qRT-PCR showed that, under the optimal *A. flavus* elicitor treatment condition, the transcription levels of *D4H*, *G10H*, *GES*, *IRS*, *LAMT*, *SGD*, *STR*, *TDC*, and *ORCA3* were much higher in EG than in CK (Figure 5). These results indicated that the increasing accumulations of vindoline, catharanthine, and ajmaline in *C. roseus* CMCs were correlated with the increasing expression of the above genes. As previous reports showed, the expression of the transcription factor *ORCA3* gene could be induced by elicitors (such as MeJA and jasmonic acid), and elicitors could increase the expression of *D4H*, *G10H*, *STR*, *GES*, *SGD*, and *TDC* [6,17,25,27,28]. Since overexpression of *ORCA3* increases the expression of key genes such as *STR* in the TIA biosynthetic pathway [6], it is extremely meaningful to explore whether the up-regulation of TIA biosynthesis-related genes is related to the increasing transcription level of *ORCA3* under the *A. flavus* mycelium elicitor treatment.

In conclusion, the *A. flavus* mycelium elicitor could promote the TIA production of *C. roseus* CMCs. Under the optimal *A. flavus* elicitor treatment condition, the contents of vindoline, catharanthine, and ajmaline were 1.45-, 3.29-, and 2.14-times as high as those of the CK group, respectively. Transcriptome analysis and qRT-PCR experiment revealed that *D4H*, *G10H*, *GES*, *IRS*, *LAMT*, *SGD*, *STR*, *TDC*, and *ORCA3* were involved in the regulation of this induction process. Furthermore, the up-regulation of TIA biosynthesis-related genes was related to the inducting effect of the *A. flavus* mycelium elicitor, which in turn promoted the accumulation of vindoline, catharanthine, and ajmaline in *C. roseus* CMCs.

4. Materials and Methods

4.1. Plant Materials and Culture Conditions

C. roseus CMCs were established using the reported method [25], and *C. roseus* DDCs were established using the method of [29]. *C. roseus* CMCs were placed on pH-adjusted (5.75–5.80) Murashige and Skoog (MS) solid medium [30] supplemented with 2.0 mg/L α-naphthalene acetic acid (NAA), 10 g/L sucrose, and 4 g/L gellan gum, cultured at 25 °C in darkness, and maintained by serial subculturing every 12 days [25]. *C. roseus* DDCs were sub-cultured under the same condition as that of *C. roseus* CMCs.

Four or six days prior to the fungal elicitor experiments, CMCs were inoculated into 100 mL of MS liquid medium supplemented with 2.0 mg/L NAA and 20 g/L sucrose in a 250-mL Erlenmeyer flask at concentrations of 50.0 g fresh weight/L [25] and grown at 25 °C at 110 rpm with a 24-h light photoperiod. The suspension culture condition of *C. roseus* DDCs was the same as that of *C. roseus* CMCs.

4.2. Procurement, Fungal Culture, and Preparation of Elicitor

A. flavus elicitors were prepared using the methods of Tonk et al. [24] with slight modifications. The *A. flavus* strain (CGMCC No. 3.6434) was obtained from the China General Microbiological Culture Collection Center (CGMCC, Beijing, China). The fungus was grown at 28 °C in 100-mL Erlenmeyer flasks containing potato dextrose agar (BAM Media M127, Guangdong Huankai Microbial Sci.&Tech.Co., Ltd., Guangzhou, China) and maintained by serial subculture every 7 days. After 7 days of subculture, the mycelium was separated from the fungal mat with forceps.

The mycelium was washed several times with distilled water and homogenized with distilled water at 5.0, 15.0, and 25.0 g/L. Then, *A. flavus* mycelium elicitors were sterilized at 120 °C for 20 min and stored at 4 °C. At the same time, *A. flavus* medium elicitors were prepared from the fungal mat by the same method used to prepare *A. flavus* mycelium elicitors and stored at 4 °C.

4.3. Induction Treatment with Fungal Elicitor

The *A. flavus* fungal elicitor (0.1 mL) (*A. flavus* mycelium elicitor or *A. flavus* medium elicitor) was added to 4-day-old or 6-day-old suspensions of CMCs at final concentrations of 5, 15, and 25 mg/L. The check group (CK) was treated with 0.1 mL sterile distilled water. Then, the CMCs were further cultured at 25 °C at 110 rpm with a 24-h light photoperiod. After culturing for another 12, 24, 36, 48, and 60 h, the cultures and liquid media were harvested.

4.4. Measurement of Dry Cell Weight

The *C. roseus* CMCs were separated from the media by vacuum filtration and transferred to a Petri dish lined with a piece of filter paper. The cells were dried to constant weight at 50 °C and weighed on a ten-thousandth scale. All samples were measured in triplicate.

4.5. Alkaloid Extraction and Determination

4.5.1. Chemicals

Vindoline, catharanthine, and ajmalicine were HPLC grade and were purchased from Aladdin (Aladdin Reagents Co., Shanghai, China), and all other chemicals were of analytical grade.

4.5.2. HPLC-MS Analysis of Alkaloids

The alkaloid extraction from 6-day-old suspensions of *C. roseus* CMCs was performed according to the methods of Wang [31]. Alkaloid extracts were dissolved in 1.0 mL of methanol and analyzed by HPLC-MS/MS according to the methods of Ferreres et al. [32] with slight modifications.

The HPLC system was equipped with an Agilent 1260 series system (Agilent Technologies, Santa Clara, California, USA). Chromatographic separations were carried out on a 250 mm × 4.6 mm, 5 µm, Phenomenex Gemini C18 column (Phenomenex Inc., Torrance, CA, USA) at 25 °C. Elution was performed with a flow rate of 1 mL/min. Solvents used were acetonitrile (A) and acetic acid 1% (B). The gradient was as follows: 12% A at 0 min, 20% A at 30 min, 50% A at 40 min, 50% A at 45 min, 12% A at 47 min, 12% A at 55 min and the injection volume 10 µL. Spectroscopic data from all peaks were accumulated in the range 240–400 nm, and chromatograms were recorded at 255, 280, 290, 306, and 320 nm.

The mass detector was an X500R QTOF mass spectrometer (AB Sciex Pte. Ltd., Redwood City, CA, USA) equipped with an electrospray ionization (ESI) system and controlled by SCIEX OS 1.3.1 software (AB Sciex Pte. Ltd., Redwood City, CA, USA). The experimental parameters were as follows: curtain gas, 30 psi; ion source gas, GS1 60 psi and GS2 60 psi; temperature, 550 °C; ion spray voltage, 5.5 kV; collision gas, 7 psi. Other parameters were as follows: declustering potential (DP), 80 V; collision energy (collision energy spread), 10 V (0 V), and 35 V (15 V). The mass spectrometer was operated in the full-scan mode in the m/z range of 100–1500. The information-dependent acquisition spectra were automatically performed with helium as the collision gas in the m/z range of 50–1500. MS data were acquired in positive ionization mode. The isolation width of the parent ions for the following MS fragmentation events was set at ±50 mDa.

4.5.3. Quantitative Analysis of Alkaloids

Alkaloid extraction was performed according to the methods of Wang et al. [31]. Alkaloid extracts were dissolved in 1.0 mL of methanol and analyzed by HPLC and ion-pair extraction-spectrophotometry as described by Yang et al. [33].

The contents of vindoline, catharanthine, and ajmalicine were determined at 25 °C by HPLC analysis using an Agilent 1260 series system (Agilent Technologies, Santa Clara, CA, USA) and a Phenomenex Gemini C18 column (250 mm × 4.6 mm, 5 µm) (Phenomenex Inc., Torrance, CA, USA). The mobile phase consisted of methanol/acetonitrile/10 mM ammonium acetate (15:40:45, $v/v/v$) at a flow rate of 1.0 mL/min. The detection wavelength was 280 nm, and the injection volume was 10 µL. Before injection, all samples were filtered with 0.45-µm nylon membrane filters (Jinteng Corp., Tianjin, China). Alkaloids were identified and quantified by comparing retention time and UV absorbance spectra with the standards. In a citric acid-phosphate buffer of pH 3.0, an ion-pair complex was formed between all alkaloids in the sample and the color reagent bromophenol blue upon 5 min of reaction at 30 °C. The complex was extracted with $CHCl_3$ in which the absorbance of total alkaloids was measured at the wavelength of 413 nm. Vindoline was used as a reference standard in the preparation of the calibration curve. Each sample was analyzed in triplicate.

4.6. Transcriptome Determination and Analysis

4.6.1. Sample Preparation

After pre-culture of *C. roseus* CMC and DDC suspension cultures for 6 day, 25 mg/L *A. flavus* mycelium elicitor was added to the CMCs (the experimental group, EG), and the EG was further cultured for another 48 h. The CMC check (CK) group and DDC group (the callus group, callus) were treated with an equal amount of sterile water.

4.6.2. RNA Extraction, Library Preparation, and Transcriptome Sequencing

The cultures were frozen in liquid nitrogen and ground into powder with a mortar and pestle, and RNA extraction was performed as described by Liu et al. [34]. RNA purity was verified using the NanoPhotometer® spectrophotometer (IMPLEN, Los Angeles, CA, USA). The purity and concentration of the purified RNA were examined with a NanoPhotometer® spectrophotometer

(IMPLEN, Los Angeles, CA, USA) and a Qubit® RNA Assay Kit in a Qubit® 2.0 Fluorometer (Life Technologies, Los Angeles, CA, USA).

A total amount of 1.5 µg RNA per sample was used as input material for RNA sample preparation. Sequencing libraries were generated using the NEBNext® UltraTM RNA Library Prep Kit for Illumina® (NEB) following the manufacturer's recommendations, and index codes were added to attribute sequences in each sample. PCR products were purified (AMPure XP system, Beckman Coulter Inc., Brea, CA, USA), and library quality was assessed on the Agilent Bioanalyzer 2100 system (Genomics & Bioinformatics Core Facility, Fort Wayne, IN, USA).

The clustering of the index-coded samples was performed on a cBot Cluster Generation System using TruSeq PE Cluster Kit v3-cBot-HS (Illumina, Brea, CA, USA) according to the manufacturer's instructions. After cluster generation, the library preparations were sequenced on an Illumina Hiseq platform, and paired-end reads were generated.

4.6.3. De Novo Transcriptome Assembly and Gene Functional Annotation

Raw data (raw reads) in the FASTQ format were first processed through in-house Perl scripts. In this step, clean data (clean reads) were obtained by removing reads containing adapter and/or poly-N and low-quality reads from raw data.

Transcriptome assembly was accomplished based on the clean data using the Trinity de novo transcriptome assembly software (Trinity Technologies & software Solutions Pvt Ltd., Bengaluru, Karnataka, India) with min_kmer_cov set to 2 by default and all other parameters set to default in absence of a public reference genome for *C. roseus* [35].

All de novo-assembled unigenes were annotated based on the following databases: NCBI non-redundant protein sequences (NR, http://www.ncbi.nlm.nih.gov); NCBI non-redundant nucleotide sequences (NT, http://www.ncbi.nlm.nih.gov); Swiss-Prot (a manually-annotated and reviewed protein sequence database, http://www.expasy.ch/sprot); Protein family (Pfam, http://xfam.org/) [36]; Gene Ontology (GO, http://www.geneontology.org); euKaryotic Ortholog Groups (KOG, http://www.ncbi.nlm.nih.gov) [37], and the Kyoto Encyclopedia of Genes and Genomes (KEGG, http://www.genome.jp/l2eg) using BLASTX alignment with an E-value = 1e-10 [38,39].

The transcription factor families were identified and annotated using the iTAK software (IAITAM, Canton, OH, USA) [40,41].

4.6.4. Differential Expression Analysis of Unigenes

Gene expression levels were estimated by RSEM [42] for each sample. Clean data were mapped back onto the assembled transcriptome. The read count for each gene was obtained from the mapping results.

Prior to differential gene expression analysis, the read counts were adjusted for each sequenced library using the edgeR program package through one scaling/normalization factor. Differential expression analysis of two samples was performed using the DEGseq R package [43,44]. The p-value was adjusted using the q-value [45]. q-value < 0.005, and $|\log_2 (\text{fold change})| > 1$ was set as the threshold for significantly differential expression.

GO enrichment analysis of the differentially-expressed genes (DEGs) was implemented by the GOseq R package-based Wallenius non-central hyper-geometric distribution [46], which can adjust for gene length bias in DEGs.

KEGG is a database resource for understanding high-level functions and utilities of biological systems, such as the cell, the organism, and the ecosystem, from molecular-level information, especially large-scale molecular datasets generated by genome sequencing and other high-throughput experimental technologies [47]. KOBAS software (Peking University, Beijing, China) [48] was used to test the statistical enrichment of differential expression genes in KEGG pathways.

4.7. Gene Transcription Level Analysis by qRT-PCR

After a 6 days of pre-cultivation of the CMCs, the *A. flavus* mycelium elicitor was added at 25 mg/L. Then, the CMCs (experimental group, EG) and the sterile water-treated CMCs (the check group, CK) were cultured for another 48 h.

The cultures were frozen in liquid nitrogen and ground into a powder with a mortar and pestle, and RNA extraction was performed as described by Liu et al. [34]. The HiScript II 1st Strand cDNA Synthesis Kit (Vazyme, Nanjing, Jiangsu, China) was used to treat 1 µg of total RNA with DNase to remove genomic DNA, after which cDNA was synthesized according to manufacturer instructions.

Transcript levels of the genes encoding the 40S ribosomal protein S9 (*RPS9*, the housekeeping gene), *D4H*, *G10H*, *GES*, *IRS*, *LAMT*, *SGD*, *STR*, *TDC*, and the transcription factor *ORCA3* were monitored in CMC cultures. Primer sequences for *RPS9*, *IRS*, *LAMT* [49], *D4H*, *G10H*, *GES*, *STR*, *TDC*, *ORCA3* [50], *SGD* [27], and *GES* [25] are shown in Table S6.

The qRT-PCR mixture was prepared using ChamQ SYBR qPCR Master Mix (Q311-02) (Vazyme, Nanjing, Jiangsu, China), and reactions were performed using a LightCycler® 480 II System (Roche, Basel, Switzerland). Amplification included a holding stage of 30 s at 95 °C and 40 cycles, each consisting of 10 s at 95 °C followed by 30 s at 60 °C. Melt curve analysis at 95–60–95 °C was then used to verify the specificity of the amplicons. The expression stability of the qRT-PCR results was assayed using the LightCycler® 480 II Software (Roche, Basel, Switzerland). All samples were measured in triplicate.

Supplementary Materials: The following are available online. Figure S1: HPLC-MS/MS spectra of the alkaloids in six-day-old suspensions of *C. roseus* CMCs. (a) UV chromatogram at 280 nm; (1) ajmalicine; (2) catharanthine; (3) vindoline. (b) Total ion current (TIC) chromatogram. (c) MS spectra of the identified alkaloids. Figure S2: Gene Ontology (GO) functional classification of assembled unigenes. A total of 61,829 unigenes were assigned to at least one GO term and grouped into three main GO categories and 56 groups (26 groups in the "biological process" domain, 20 in the "cellular component" domain, and 10 in the "molecular function" domain). The y-axis indicates the number of genes in a sub-category. Figure S3: Functional classification and pathway assignment of assembled unigenes by the Kyoto Encyclopedia of Genes and Genomes (KEGG). A total of 34,367 unigenes were classified to the five main KEGG metabolic pathways: cellular processes (A), environmental information processing (B), genetic information processing (C), metabolism (D), and organismal systems (E). The y-axis represents the name of the KEGG metabolic pathway. The x-axis indicates the number of unigenes annotated to the KEGG metabolic pathway and the ratio of their number to the total number of annotated unigenes. Figure S4: Correlation coefficient between the callus vs. CK (a) and EG vs. CK (b) samples. The x-axis indicates the $\log_{10}$ (FPKM + 1) of Sample 1 and the y-axis the $\log_{10}$ (FPKM + 1) of Sample 2, and R^2 was the square of the Pearson correlation coefficient. Figure S5: Correlation coefficient between the callus vs. CK (a) and EG vs. CK (b) samples. The x-axis indicates the $\log_{10}$ (FPKM + 1) of Sample 1 and the y-axis the $\log_{10}$ (FPKM + 1) of Sample 2, and R^2 was the square of the Pearson correlation coefficient. Figure S6: Venn diagram of DEGs from callus vs. CK and EG vs. CK samples. Figure S7: GO enrichment analysis of DEGs in callus vs. CK and EG vs. CK samples. The x-axis indicates the comparative combination and the y-axis the number of DEGs. Figure S8: Partial results of KEGG pathway analysis of DEGs in callus vs. CK and EG vs. CK samples. The x-axis indicates the KEGG pathway and the y-axis the number of DEGs. Table S1: Summary of sequencing reads after filtering. Table S2: Summary of the sequence assembly results. Table S3: Summary of functional annotation for assembled unigenes. Table S4: Summary of KEGG pathways involved in the *Catharanthus roseus* transcriptome. Table S5: Gene transcription factor analysis of unigenes. Table S6: Sequences of primers for *Catharanthus roseus* genes used in the qRT-PCR assay.

Author Contributions: Methodology, J.Z. (Jianhua Zhu), J.Z. (Jiachen Zi) and C.L.; investigation, C.L., P.Z., L.X. and C.C..; formal analysis, J.Z. (Jianhua Zhu), J.L., C.L. and C.C.; resources, J.Z. (Jianhua Zhu), J.Z. (Jiachen Zi) and R.Y.; writing—original draft preparation, C.L., J.L., P.Z, L.X. and C.C.; writing—review and editing, J.Z. (Jianhua Zhu) and R.Y.; supervision, J.Z. (Jianhua Zhu) and R.Y.; project administration, J.Z. (Jianhua Zhu); funding acquisition, J.Z. (Jianhua Zhu) and R.Y.

Funding: This study was supported by the National Natural Science Foundation of China (Nos. 81573568 and 81673571), the Guangdong Province Natural Science Fund for Distinguished Young Scholars (No. 2016A030306009), and the Key Laboratory of Chemical Biology (Ministry of Education) Open Projects Fund (Project No. CB-201707).

Conflicts of Interest: The authors declare no conflict of interest.

References

1. Almagro, L.; Fernándezpérez, F.; Pedreño, M.A. Indole alkaloids from *Catharanthus roseus*: Bioproduction and their effect on human health. *Molecules* **2015**, *20*, 2973–3000. [CrossRef] [PubMed]
2. Verma, P.; Mathur, A.K.; Srivastava, A.; Mathur, A. Emerging trends in research on spatial and temporal organization of terpenoid indole alkaloid pathway in *Catharanthus roseus*: A literature update. *Protoplasma* **2012**, *249*, 255–268. [CrossRef] [PubMed]
3. Van Der Heijden, R.; Jacobs, D.I.; Snoeijer, W.; Hallard, D.; Verpoorte, R. The *Catharanthus* alkaloids: Pharmacognosy and biotechnology. *Curr. Med. Chem.* **2004**, *11*, 607–628. [CrossRef] [PubMed]
4. Guo, Z.G.; Liu, Y.; Xing, X.H. Enhanced catharanthine biosynthesis through regulation of cyclooxygenase in the cell suspension culture of *Catharanthus roseus* (L.) G. Don. *Prog. Biochem.* **2011**, *46*, 783–787. [CrossRef]
5. Liu, W.; Chen, R.; Chen, M.; Zhang, H.; Peng, M.; Yang, C.; Ming, X.; Lan, X.; Liao, Z. Tryptophan decarboxylase plays an important role in ajmalicine biosynthesis in *Rauvolfia verticillata*. *Planta* **2012**, *236*, 239–250. [CrossRef] [PubMed]
6. Peebles, C.A.; Hughes, E.H.; Shanks, J.V.; San, K.Y. Transcriptional response of the terpenoid indole alkaloid pathway to the overexpression of ORCA3 along with jasmonic acid elicitation of *Catharanthus roseus* hairy roots over time. *Metab. Eng.* **2009**, *11*, 76–86. [CrossRef] [PubMed]
7. Li, C.Y.; Leopold, A.L.; Sander, G.W.; Shanks, J.V.; Zhao, L.; Gibson, S.I. CrBPF1 overexpression alters transcript levels of terpenoid indole alkaloid biosynthetic and regulatory genes. *Front. Plant Sci.* **2015**, *6*, 818. [CrossRef]
8. McKnight, T.D.; Roessner, C.A.; Devagupta, R.; Scott, A.I.; Nessler, C.L. Nucleotide sequence of a cDNA encoding the vacuolar protein strictosidine synthase from *Catharanthus roseus*. *Nucleic Acids Res.* **1990**, *18*, 4939. [CrossRef]
9. Vazquez-Flota, F.; De Carolis, E.; Alarco, A.M.; De Luca, V. Molecular cloning and characterization of desacetoxyvindoline-4-hydroxylase, a 2-oxoglutarate dependent-dioxygenase involved in the biosynthesis of vindoline in *Catharanthus roseus* (L.) G. Don. *Plant Mol. Biol.* **1997**, *34*, 935–948. [CrossRef]
10. St-Pierre, B.; Laflamme, P.; Alarco, A.M.; De Luca, V. The terminal O-acetyltransferase involved in vindoline biosynthesis defines a new class of proteins responsible for coenzyme A-dependent acyl transfer. *Plant J.* **1998**, *14*, 703–713. [CrossRef]
11. Schröder, G.; Unterbusch, E.; Kaltenbach, M.; Schmidt, J.; Strack, D.; De Luca, V.; Schröder, J. Light-induced cytochrome P450-dependent enzyme in indole alkaloid biosynthesis: Tabersonine 16-hydroxylase. *FEBS Lett.* **1999**, *458*, 97–102. [CrossRef]
12. Levac, D.; Murata, J.; Kim, W.S.; De Luca, V. Application of carborundum abrasion for investigating the leaf epidermis: Molecular cloning of *Catharanthus roseus* 16-hydroxytabersonine-16-O-methyltransferase. *Plant J.* **2008**, *53*, 225–236. [CrossRef] [PubMed]
13. Liscombe, D.K.; Usera, A.R.; O'Connor, S.E. Homolog of tocopherol C methyltransferases catalyzes N methylation in anticancer alkaloid biosynthesis. *P. Natl Acad. Sci. USA* **2010**, *107*, 18793–18798. [CrossRef] [PubMed]
14. Qu, Y.; Easson, M.L.A.E.; Froese, J.; Simionescu, R.; Hudlicky, T.; De Luca, V. Completion of the seven-step pathway from tabersonine to the anticancer drug precursor vindoline and its assembly in yeast. *P. Natl Acad. Sci. USA* **2015**, *112*, 6224–6229. [CrossRef] [PubMed]
15. Costa, M.M.R.; Hilliou, F.; Duarte, P.; Pereira, L.G.; Almeida, I.; Leech, M.; Memelink, J.; Barceló, A.R.; Sottomayor, M. Molecular cloning and characterization of a vacuolar class III peroxidase involved in the metabolism of anticancer alkaloids in *Catharanthus roseus*. *Plant Physiol.* **2008**, *146*, 403–417. [CrossRef] [PubMed]
16. Van der Fits, L.; Memelink, J. ORCA3, a jasmonate-responsive transcriptional regulator of plant primary and secondary metabolism. *Science* **2000**, *289*, 295–297. [CrossRef] [PubMed]
17. Wei, S. Methyl jasmonic acid induced expression pattern of terpenoid indole alkaloid pathway genes in *Catharanthus roseus* seedlings. *J. Plant Growth Regul.* **2010**, *61*, 243–251. [CrossRef]
18. Noble, R.L. The discovery of the vinca alkaloids—chemotherapeutic agents against cancer. *Biochem. Cell Biol.* **1990**, *68*, 1344–1351. [CrossRef] [PubMed]

19. Pandey, S.S.; Singh, S.; Babu, C.S.V.; Shanker, K. Fungal endophytes of Catharanthus roseus enhance vindoline content by modulating structural and regulatory genes related to terpenoid indole alkaloid biosynthesis. *Sci. Rep. UK* **2016**, *6*, 26583. [CrossRef]
20. Hahn, M.G. Microbial elicitors and their receptors in plants. *Ann. Rev. Phytopathol.* **1996**, *34*, 387–412. [CrossRef]
21. Wang, J.W.; Wu, J.Y. Effective elicitors and process strategies for enhancement of secondary metabolite production in hairy root cultures. *Adv. Biochem. Eng. Biotech.* **2013**, *134*, 55–89.
22. Xu, M.J.; Dong, J.F. Elicitor-induced nitric oxide burst is essential for triggering catharanthine synthesis in Catharanthus roseus suspension cells. *Appl. Microbiol. Biotechnol.* **2005**, *67*, 40–44. [CrossRef] [PubMed]
23. Zhao, J.; Zhu, W.H.; Hu, Q. Selection of fungal elicitors to increase indole alkaloid accumulation in Catharanthus roseus suspension cell culture. *Enzyme Microb. Technol.* **2001**, *28*, 666–672. [CrossRef]
24. Tonk, D.; Mujib, A.; Maqsood, M.; Ali, M.; Zafar, N. Aspergillus flavus fungus elicitation improves vincristine and vinblastine yield by augmenting callus biomass growth in *Catharanthus roseus*. *Plant Cell Tiss. Organ Cult.* **2016**, *126*, 291–303. [CrossRef]
25. Zhou, P.; Yang, J.; Zhu, J.; He, S.J.; Zhang, W.J.; Yu, R.M.; Zi, J.C.; Song, L.Y.; Huang, X.S. Effects of β-cyclodextrin and methyl jasmonate on the production of vindoline, catharanthine, and ajmalicine in Catharanthus roseus cambial meristematic cell cultures. *Appl. Microbiol. Biotechnol.* **2015**, *99*, 7035–7045. [CrossRef] [PubMed]
26. Hao, X.; Zhong, Y.; Fu, X.; Lv, Z.; Shen, Q.; Yan, T.; Shi, P.; Ma, Y.; Chen, M.; Lv, X. Transcriptome analysis of genes associated with the artemisinin biosynthesis by jasmonic acid treatment under the light in *Artemisia annua*. *Front. Plant Sci.* **2017**, *8*, 971. [CrossRef] [PubMed]
27. Goklany, S.; Loring, R.H.; Glick, J.; Lee-Parsons, C.W. Assessing the limitations to terpenoid indole alkaloid biosynthesis in Catharanthus roseus hairy root cultures through gene expression profiling and precursor feeding. *Biotechnol. Progr.* **2009**, *25*, 1289–1296. [CrossRef] [PubMed]
28. Simkin, A.J.; Miettinen, K.; Claudel, P.; Burlat, V.; Guirimand, G.; Courdavault, V.; Papon, N.; Meyer, S.; Godet, S.; St-Pierre, B.; et al. Characterization of the plastidial geraniol synthase from Madagascar periwinkle which initiates the monoterpenoid branch of the alkaloid pathway in internal phloem associated parenchyma. *Phytochemistry* **2013**, *85*, 36–43. [CrossRef] [PubMed]
29. Guo, S.J.; Yang, C.Y.; Feng, L.L.; Zhang, G.B.; Fan, M.H.; Zhang, Z.H.; Liu, S.N.; Zhou, J.Y. Effects on induction and proliferation of *Catharanthus roseus* (L.) G.Don callus. *J. Central China Normal Univ. (Natl. Sci.)* **2004**, *38*, 228–230.
30. Murashige, T.; Skoog, F. A Revised medium for rapid growth and bio assays with tobacco tissue cultures. *Physiol. Plant.* **1962**, *15*, 473–497. [CrossRef]
31. Wang, M.; Zi, J.; Zhu, J.; Chen, S.; Wang, P.; Song, L.; Yu, R. Artemisinic acid serves as a novel ORCA3 inducer to enhance biosynthesis of terpenoid indole alkaloids in *Catharanthus roseus* cambial meristematic cells. *Nat. Prod. Commun.* **2016**, *11*, 715–717. [PubMed]
32. Ferreres, F.; Pereira, D.M.; Valentão, P.; Oliveira, J.M.A.; Faria, J.; Gaspar, L.; Sottomayor, M.; Andrade, P.B. Simple and reproducible HPLC-DAD-ESI-MS/MS analysis of alkaloids in *Catharanthus roseus* roots. *J. Pharm. Biomed. Anal.* **2010**, *51*, 65–69. [CrossRef] [PubMed]
33. Yang, L.; Liu, Y.; Zhang, L.; Zu, Y.G. Ion-pair extraction-spectrophotometric determination of total alkaloids in *Catharanthus roseus* with bromophenol blue as color reagent. *Phys. Test. Chem. Anal. Part B Chem. Anal.* **2008**, *44*, 427–432.
34. Liu, J.; Zhu, J.; Tang, L.; Wen, W.; Lv, S.; Yu, R. Enhancement of vindoline and vinblastine production in suspension-cultured cells of *Catharanthus roseus* by artemisinic acid elicitation. *World J. Microb. Biot.* **2014**, *30*, 175–180. [CrossRef] [PubMed]
35. Grabherr, M.G.; Haas, B.J.; Yassour, M.; Levin, J.Z.; Thompson, D.A.; Amit, I.; Adiconis, X.; Fan, L.; Raychowdhury, R.; Zeng, Q.; et al. Full-length transcriptome assembly from RNA-Seq data without a reference genome. *Nat. Biotechnol.* **2011**, *29*, 644–652. [CrossRef]
36. Finn, R.D.; Coggill, P.; Eberhardt, R.Y.; Eddy, S.R.; Mistry, J.; Mitchell, A.L.; Potter, S.C.; Punta, M.; Qureshi, M.; Sangrador-Vegas, A.; et al. The Pfam protein families database: Towards a more sustainable future. *Nucleic Acids Res.* **2016**, *44*, 279–285. [CrossRef]

37. Conesa, A.; Gotz, S.; Garcia-Gomez, J.M.; Terol, J.; Talon, M.; Robles, M. Blast2GO: A universal tool for annotation, visualization and analysis in functional genomics research. *Bioinformatics* **2005**, *21*, 3674–3676. [CrossRef]
38. Altschul, S.F.; Madden, T.L.; Schäffer, A.A.; Zhang, J.; Zhang, Z.; Miller, W.; Lipman, D.J. Gapped BLAST and PSI-BLAST: A new generation of protein database search programs. *Nucleic Acids Res.* **1997**, *25*, 3389–3402. [CrossRef]
39. Camacho, C.; Coulouris, G.; Avagyan, V.; Ma, N.; Papadopoulos, J.; Bealer, K.; Madden, T.L. BLAST+: Architecture and applications. *BMC Bioinforma.* **2009**, *10*, 421. [CrossRef]
40. Perez-Rodriguez, P.; Riano-Pachon, D.M.; Correa, L.G.; Rensing, S.A.; Kersten, B.; Mueller-Roeber, B. PlnTFDB: Updated content and new features of the plant transcription factor database. *Nucleic Acids Res.* **2010**, *38*, 822–827. [CrossRef]
41. Jin, J.; Zhang, H.; Kong, L.; Gao, G.; Luo, J. PlantTFDB 3.0: A portal for the functional and evolutionary study of plant transcription factors. *Nucleic Acids Res.* **2014**, *42*, 1182–1187. [CrossRef] [PubMed]
42. Li, B.; Dewey, C.N. RSEM: Accurate transcript quantification from RNA-Seq data with or without a reference genome. *BMC Bioinform.* **2011**, *12*, 323. [CrossRef] [PubMed]
43. Anders, S.; Huber, W. Differential expression analysis for sequence count data. *Genome Biol.* **2010**, *11*, R106. [CrossRef] [PubMed]
44. Wang, L.; Feng, Z.; Wang, X.; Wang, X.; Zhang, X. DEGseq: An R package for identifying differentially expressed genes from RNA-seq data. *Bioinformatics* **2010**, *26*, 136–138. [CrossRef] [PubMed]
45. Storey, J.D.; Tibshirani, R. Statistical significance for genomewide studies. *P Natl Acad Sci USA* **2003**, *100*, 9440–9445. [CrossRef]
46. Young, M.D.; Wakefield, M.J.; Smyth, G.K.; Oshlack, A. Gene ontology analysis for RNA-seq: Accounting for selection bias. *Genome Biol.* **2010**, *11*, R14. [CrossRef]
47. Kanehisa, M.; Araki, M.; Goto, S.; Hattori, M.; Hirakawa, M.; Itoh, M.; Katayama, T.; Kawashima, S.; Okuda, S.; Tokimatsu, T. KEGG for linking genomes to life and the environment. *Nucleic Acids Res.* **2008**, *36*, 480–484. [CrossRef]
48. Mao, X.; Cai, T.; Olyarchuk, J.G.; Wei, L. Automated genome annotation and pathway identification using the KEGG Orthology (KO) as a controlled vocabulary. *Bioinformatics* **2005**, *21*, 3787–3793. [CrossRef]
49. Geu-Flores, F.; Sherden, N.H.; Courdavault, V.; Burlat, V.; Glenn, W.S.; Wu, C.; Nims, E.; Cui, Y.; O'Connor, S.E. An alternative route to cyclic terpenes by reductive cyclization in iridoid biosynthesis. *Nature* **2012**, *492*, 138–142. [CrossRef]
50. William Sander, G. Quantitative Analysis of Metabolic Pathways in *Catharanthus roseus* Hairy Roots Metabolically Engineered for Terpenoid indole Alkaloid Overproduction. Ph.D. Thesis, Iowa State University, Ames, IA, USA, 2009.

Sample Availability: *Catharanthus roseus* plant materials are available from the authors.

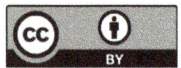

© 2018 by the authors. Licensee MDPI, Basel, Switzerland. This article is an open access article distributed under the terms and conditions of the Creative Commons Attribution (CC BY) license (http://creativecommons.org/licenses/by/4.0/).

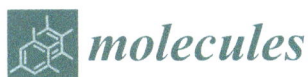

Article

Two New Cytotoxic Steroidal Alkaloids from *Sarcococca Hookeriana*

Shaojie Huo [1], Jichun Wu [1], Xicheng He [1], Lutai Pan [2] and Jiang Du [1,2,*]

[1] Guiyang College of Traditional Chinese Medicine, Guiyang 550025, China; 15038115764@163.com (S.H.); wujichun2018@sina.com (J.W.); hexicheng53@126.com (X.H.)
[2] Guizhou Provincial Key Laboratory of Miao Medicine, Guiyang 550025, China; ltpan@sina.cn
* Correspondence: dujang.gz@163.com; Tel.: +86-871-8830-8060

Academic Editor: John C. D'Auria
Received: 1 December 2018; Accepted: 19 December 2018; Published: 20 December 2018

Abstract: Two new steroidal alkaloids, named hookerianine A (**1**) and hookerianine B (**2**) were isolated from the stems and roots of *Sarcococca hookeriana* Baill., along with two known compounds, sarcorucinine G (**3**) and epipachysamine D (**4**). On the basis of spectroscopic methods and by comparison with literature data, their structures were determined. As well as X-ray crystallography was performed to confirm compound **4**. To identify novel antitumor inhibitors, all compounds were performed a CCK-8 assay against five human cancer cell lines SW480, SMMC-7721, PC3, MCF-7 and K562 in vitro. Compound **2** exhibited moderate cytotoxic activities to all cell lines with IC_{50} values in the range of 5.97–19.44 µM. Compound **3** was the most effective one against SW480 and K562 cell lines with IC_{50} values of 5.77 and 6.29 µM, respectively.

Keywords: Buxaceae; *Sarcococca hookeriana*; steroidal alkaloid; cytotoxicity

1. Introduction

The *Sarcococca* genus (Buxaceae) consists of about 20 species, widely distributed in the southwestern region of China and other south Asian countries [1]. The members of *Sarcococca* plants are used as TCM and traditional folk medicine for the treatment of stomach pain, rheumatism, swollen sore throat and traumatic injury [2–4]. Previous investigations on several species of this genus indicated that steroidal alkaloids are the major chemical components with a broad spectrum of biological activities, such as cholinesterase inhibition [5–7], antitumor [8], antibacterial [9], antileishamanial [10], antidiabetic [11] and estrogen biosynthesis-promoting [12].

Sarcococca hookeriana, one of *Sarcococca* plants, is usually confusedly used by ethnic minorities in China. Although dozens of steroidal alkaloids have been discovered from *S. hookeriana* of Nepal [13–17], there were few phytochemical or biological studies on this species which grows in China. Enlightened by the diverse bioactivities of steroidal alkaloids and the use of *Sarcococca* plants as folk medicine, *S. hookeriana* was chosen for searching antitumor agent by our research group and several cytotoxic steroidal alkaloids have been reported [18]. In continuation of our ongoing study on this plant, two new steroidal alkaloids, named hookerianine A (**1**) and hookerianine B (**2**), together with two known ones, sarcorucinine G (**3**) [19] and epipachysamine D (**4**) [20] (Figure 1), were characterized and their cytotoxicity were evaluated in vitro with a CCK-8 assay. Herein, we describe the isolation, structure elucidation and cytotoxicity of the isolates.

2. Results and Discussion

2.1. Elucidation of the Chemical Structure of Compounds

Hookerianine A (**1**) was obtained as white amorphous powder, positive to Dragendorff's reagent. The molecular formula of $C_{31}H_{48}N_2O$ was determined by HR-ESI-MS (m/z 465.3833, [M + H]$^+$). The IR absorption at 3294, 1637, 1539, 1496 and 760 cm^{-1} indicated the presence of a secondary amine, amide carbonyl and aromatic ring, respectively. The ^{1}H-NMR spectra (Table 1) exhibited signals of five aromatic protons (δ_H 7.37, 7.33 and 7.28) and five methyls (δ_H 2.17, 0.87, 0.74 and 0.63). The ^{13}C-NMR (Table 1) signals at (δ_C 135.5, 129.4, 129.1 and 127.4) were characteristic for a monosubstituted aromatic ring, whereas the signal at δ_C 170.1 was due to the carbonyl carbon. The NMR data of compound **1** was similar to epipachysamine D (**4**), having one more methylene. HMBCs (Figure 2) from H-C(2′) to C(1′), C(3′) and C(4′) indicated that the additional methylene was placed between C(1′) and C(3′). Thus, compound **1** possessed a novel phenylacetyl group instead of benzoyl group located at C(3). The relative configuration of C(3) was assigned as α-orientation by correlations of N-H with Hα-C(1), Hα-C(5), and Hβ-C(1) with H-C(19) in ROESY (Figure 2). Therefore, compound **1** was characterized as (20S)-20-(N,N-dimethylamino)-3α-phenylacetylamino -5α-pregnane, to which we give the trivial name hookerianine A.

Table 1. ^{1}H- (500 MHz) and ^{13}C- (125 MHz) NMR data of compounds **1–2** in CDCl$_3$.

Position	1		2	
	δ_H (J in Hz)	δ_C	δ_H (J in Hz)	δ_C
1	1.45 (m), 0.65 (m)	33.2 (t)	1.72 (m), 1.10 (m)	37.2 (t)
2	1.63 (m), 1.52 (m)	25.9 (t)	1.93 (d, J = 14.8), 1.38 (m)	28.8 (t)
3	4.06 (m)	44.8 (d)	3.96 (m)	49.3 (d)
4	1.45 (m), 1.28 (m)	32.7 (t)	1.70 (m), 1.24 (m)	35.4 (t)
5	0.79 (m)	41.0 (d)	1.24 (m)	45.4 (d)
6	1.12 (m)	28.5 (t)	1.32 (m), 1.24 (m)	28.4 (t)
7	1.64 (m), 0.77 (m)	32.1 (t)	1.62 (m), 0.95 (m)	31.6 (t)
8	1.31 (m)	35.4 (d)	1.62 (m)	33.8 (d)
9	0.46 (d, J = 11.8, 3.9)	54.7 (d)	0.73 (m)	54.5 (d)
10		36.0 (s)		35.6 (s)
11	1.42 (m), 1.18 (m)	20.8 (t)	1.62 (m), 1.29 (m)	20.8 (t)
12	1.87 (m), 1.08 (m)	39.8 (t)	1.62 (m), 1.47 (m)	32.8 (t)
13		41.7 (s)		42.2 (s)
14	1.01 (m)	56.8 (d)	1.24 (m)	45.1 (d)
15	1.58 (m), 1.02 (m)	24.0 (t)	1.84 (dd, J = 12.0, 4.8), 1.20 (m)	27.2 (t)
16	1.85 (m), 1.44 (m)	27.7 (t)	3.55 (s)	60.9 (d)
17	1.36 (d, J = 9.9)	54.9 (d)		73.6 (s)

Table 1. Cont.

Position	1		2	
	δ_H (J in Hz)	δ_C	δ_H (J in Hz)	δ_C
18	0.63 (s)	12.4 (q)	0.87 (s)	15.8 (q)
19	0.74 (s)	11.5 (q)	0.83 (s)	12.2 (q)
20	2.41 (dq, J = 10.2, 6.4)	61.2 (d)	2.84 (q, J = 6.6)	55.7 (d)
21	0.87 (s)	10.0 (q)	1.14 (s)	13.6 (q)
N(Me)2	2.17 (s)	39.9 (q)	2.24 (s)	43.1 (q)
1'		170.1 (s)		166.7 (s)
2'	3.57 (dt, J = 6.8, 1.2)	44.2 (t)		135.0 (s)
3'		135.5 (s)	7.74 (dt, J = 6.8, 1.2)	126.8 (d)
4'	7.28 (m)	129.4 (d)	7.41 (m)	128.5 (d)
5	7.37 (m)	129.1 (d)	7.47 (m)	131.2 (d)
6'	7.33 (m)	127.4 (d)	7.41 (m)	128.5 (d)
7'	7.37 (m)	129.1 (d)	7.47 (m)	126.8 (d)
8'	7.28 (m)	129.4 (d)		
NH	5.66 (d, J = 8.0)		5.98 (d, J = 8.0)	

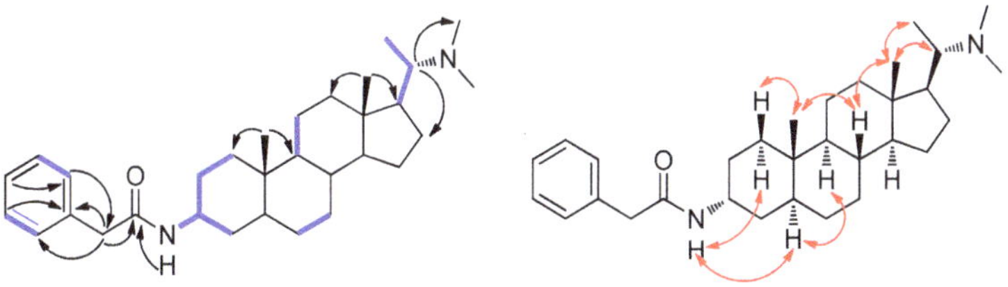

Figure 2. Key ^{1}H,^{1}H-COSY (━), HMBC (H→C), and ROESY (↔) correlations of compound **1**.

Hookerianine B (**2**) was obtained as white amorphous powder also reacts positively with Dragendorff's reagent. The molecular formula of $C_{30}H_{44}N_2O_2$ was determined by HR-ESI-MS (m/z 465.3471, [M + H]$^+$). The IR absorption at 3402, 1644, 1603, 1521, 1488 and 718 cm^{-1} indicated the presence of a secondary amine, amide carbonyl and aromatic ring, respectively. The ^{1}H-NMR spectra (Table 1) exhibited signals of five aromatic protons (δ_H 7.74, 7.47 and 7.41) and five methyls (δ_H 2.24, 1.14, 0.87 and 0.83). The ^{13}C-NMR spectra (Table 1) displayed 30 carbon signals including one carbonyl carbon at (δ_C 166.7) and six carbons of an aromatic ring (δ_C 135.0, 131.2, 128.5 and 126.8), respectively. whereas the signals at (δ_C 73.6 and 60.9) were due to two oxygenated carbons. The NMR data of compound **2** was similar to epipachysamine D (**4**), and the difference was the downfield chemical shift of C(16) and C(17) at δ(C) 73.6 and 60.9, which suggested that compound **2** possessed an epoxy group at C(16) and C(17), confirmed by HMBCs (Figure 3) from H-C(16) to C(14) and C(15), from H-C(18) and H-C(21) to C(15). The ROESY correlations (Figure 3) of N-H with Hα-C(5), and Hβ-C(16) with N-Me suggested that the substituent at C(3) and the epoxy group at C(16) and C(17) all had α-orientations. Thus, compound **2** was characterized as (20S)-20-(N,N-dimethylamino)-16α,17α-epoxy-3α-benzoylamino-5α-pregnane, to which we give the trivial name hookerianine B.

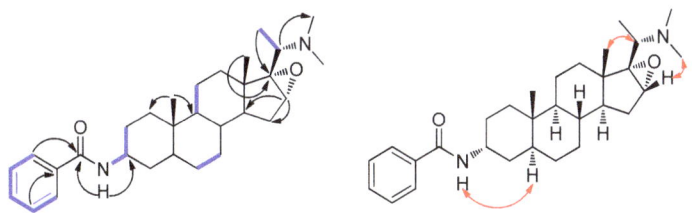

Figure 3. Key ^{1}H,^{1}H-COSY (━), HMBC (H→C), and ROESY (↔) correlations of compound **2**.

The structures of known compounds **3–4** were determined by comparing their spectral data with literature data. To further confirm the chemical structure of compound **4**, a colorless crystal was obtained from CH$_2$Cl$_2$, and X-ray crystallography analysis with Mo Kα radiation was performed. Through structural refinement by direct method SHELX-2014 [21,22], the chemical structure of **4** was identified as shown in Figure 4.

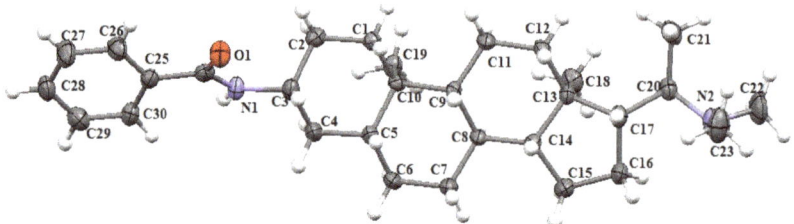

Figure 4. ORTEP drawing of compound **4**.

2.2. Results of the Cytotoxicity Test

The IC$_{50}$ values of four compounds against five human cancer cell lines: SW480, SMMC-7721, PC3, MCF-7 and K562 are summarized in Table 2 (DDP and 5-FU was used as the positive control). The compound **2**, a new steroidal alkaloid, exhibited moderate cytotoxic activities to all cell lines with IC$_{50}$ values in the range of 5.97–19.44 µM. Compared to the positive control 5-FU with IC$_{50}$ values of 7.65 and 4.78 µM against SW480 and K562 cell lines, the compound **3** was the most effective one against these cell lines with IC$_{50}$ values of 5.77 and 6.29 µM, respectively. The structure-activity relationships of compound **1** and **4** showed that steroidal alkaloids possessed a novel phenylacetyl group instead of benzoyl group located at C-3 can increase the cytotoxicity to human cancer cell lines: SW480, SMMC-7721, PC3 and K562. Interestingly, the cytotoxicity of compound **3** is stronger than compound **4**, which indicated that the presence of double bond between C-16 and C-17 can increase the cytotoxicity. Meanwhile, compared to compound **4**, compound **2** possessed an epoxy group at C-16 and C-17 also showed better cytotoxicity. The results suggested that C-16 and C-17 of steroidal alkaloids play an important role in anticancer potential.

Table 2. Cytotoxicity of compounds **1–4** against SW480, SMMC-7721, PC3, MCF-7 and K562 cells in vitro.

Compounds	IC$_{50}$ (µM) [a] (n = 3)				
	SW480	SMMC-7721	PC3	MCF-7	K562
1	10.97 ± 1.36	41.31 ± 3.02	32.97 ± 3.78	37.30 ± 0.99	11.86 ± 0.82
2	5.97 ± 0.13	16.19 ± 0.56	11.57 ± 0.86	19.44 ± 1.70	7.95 ± 0.02
3	5.77 ± 0.29	10.84 ± 1.19	11.79 ± 2.96	44.97 ± 4.73	6.29 ± 0.53
4	45.92 ± 1.56	71.13 ± 5.37	>100	28.92 ± 1.22	85.48 ± 6.77
DDP [b]	4.71 ± 0.20	4.03 ± 0.62	6.50 ± 0.44	6.86 ± 0.42	5.49 ± 0.83
5-FU [c]	7.65 ± 0.26	7.86 ± 0.38	8.18 ± 0.73	6.74 ± 0.89	4.78 ± 0.27

[a] Values of IC$_{50}$ expressed as mean ± SD, n = 3 for all groups. [b] DDP, the abbreviation of cisplatin, used as reference drug. [c] 5-FU, the abbreviation of 5-fluorouracil, used as reference drug.

3. Materials and Methods

3.1. General Experimental Procedures

Optical rotations were measured with a Rudolph Autopol I automatic polarimeter (Rudolph, Hackettstown, NJ, USA). UV spectra were obtained on a Shimadzu UV-2401PC spectrophotometer (Shimadzu, Kyoto, Japan). IR spectra were measured with a Bruker TENSOR-27 spectrophotometer

(Bruker, Bremerhaven, Germany) using KBr pellets. The 1D and 2D NMR spectra were recorded on JEOL ECX 500 MHz spectrometers (JEOL Ltd, Kyoto, Japan) with TMS as an internal standard. Chemical shifts (δ) were expressed in ppm with reference to solvent signals. High-Resolution Electrospray Ionization Mass Spectrometry (HR-ESI-MS) was recorded on a Bruker Daltonics micrOTOF-Q II spectrometer (Bruker, Bremerhaven, Germany). Column chromatography (CC) was performed on Silica gel (200–300 and 300–400 mesh, Qingdao Marine Chemical Ltd., Qingdao, China). Fractions were monitored by TLC (GF 254, Qingdao Haiyang Chemical Co., Ltd., Qingdao, China), and spots were visualized by Dragendorff's reagent. Solvents were distilled prior to use for extraction and isolation.

3.2. Plant Material

The plants of *S. hookeriana* were collected from Hezhang Country, Guizhou Province of China, in July 2015 and identified by Prof. JunHua Zhao, Guiyang College of Traditional Chinese Medicine. A voucher specimen (No. 150708) was deposited at College of Pharmacy, Guiyang College of Traditional Chinese Medicine.

3.3. Extraction and Isolation

The powdered stems and roots of *S. hookeriana* (14.5 Kg) were extracted ultrasonically with MeOH for three times. The combined extracts were concentrated and then partitioned between EtOAc and 1% aq. H_2SO_4. The acid-soluble fraction was alkalinized with aq. Na_2CO_3 to pH 9 and followed by exhaustive extraction with CH_2Cl_2 to afford crude alkaloids (156 g). The crude alkaloids were roughly separated by CC (SiO_2; CH_2Cl_2/MeOH/Et_2NH, 100:0:0→10:1:0→5:1:1) to give five fractions: *Frs. A-E*. *Fr. A* (32 g) was passed through CC [SiO_2; petroleum ether (PE)/CH_2Cl_2/Et_2NH 50:1:1→10:1:1, then cyclohexane/acetone/Et_2NH 20:1:1] to afford **3** (150 mg), **4** (800 mg). *Fr. B* (24 g) was subjected to CC (PE/CH_2Cl_2/ Et_2NH, 50:1:1→20:1:1, then CH_2Cl_2/MeOH 20:1) to yield **1** (60 mg) and **2** (40 mg).

3.3.1. Compound **1**

The Hookerianine A (**1**): White amorphous powder. $[\alpha]_D^{14}$ = +21.2 (c = 0.565, CH_2Cl_2). UV ($CHCl_3$) λ_{max} (log ε) 242.0 (0.25) nm. IR (KBr) v_{max}: 3294, 3029, 2929, 2865, 2761, 1637, 1539, 1496, 760 cm^{-1}. ^{1}H- and ^{13}C-NMR data are shown in Table 1. HR-ESI-MS m/z 465.3833 ([M + H]$^+$, $C_{31}H_{49}N_2O^+$; calc. 465.3839).

3.3.2. Compound **2**

Hookerianine B (**2**): White amorphous powder. $[\alpha]_D^{14}$ = +21.2 = +3.7 (c = 0.092, CH_2Cl_2). UV ($CHCl_3$) λ_{max} (log ε) 244.5 (1.53). IR (KBr) v_{max}: 3402, 3032, 2930, 2853, 2767, 1644, 1603, 1521, 1488, 718, 694 cm^{-1}. ^{1}H- and ^{13}C-NMR data are shown in Table 1. HR-ESI-MS m/z 465.3471 ([M + H] $^+$, $C_{30}H_{45}N_2O_2^+$; calc. 465.3476).

3.4. Single Crystal X-Ray Data of Compound **4**

Crystal data of **4** (from CH_2Cl_2): $C_{30}H_{46}N_2O$, M = 450.69, space group $P2_1$ (No. 4), monoclinic, Z = 2, a = 5.895(14) Å, b = 9.983(2) Å, c = 22.033(5) Å, α = 90°, β = 95.971(6)°, γ = 90°, V = 1289.4(5)Å^3, T = 173 K, μ (Mo Kα) = 0.71073 mm^{-1}. A crystal of dimensions of 0.18 × 0.08 × 0.05 mm^3 was measured on a Bruker APEX-II CCD diffractometer with a graphite monochromator (φ-ω scans, 2θ$_{max}$ = 55.18°), Mo Kα radiation. 9787 reflections were measured, 5785 independent reflections were observed (R_{int} = 0.0530). The final R_1 values were 0.0625 (I >= 2σ (I)). The final wR_2 values were 0.1278 (I >= 2σ (I)). The final R_1 values were 0.1008 (all data). The final wR_2 values were 0.1449 (all data). The goodness of fit on F^2 was 0.971. CCDC 1875789 for compound **4** contains the supplementary crystallographic data for this paper. These data can be obtained free of charge via https://www.ccdc.cam.ac.uk/.

3.5. Cytotoxicity Assay

To identify novel antitumor inhibitors, compounds **1–4** were tested on five human cancer cell lines SW480, SMMC-7721, PC3, MCF-7 and K562 by using a CCK-8 assay. All cells were obtained from Centre of Drug Safety Evaluation and Research of Hunan Province. Those cells were cultured in a DMEM medium (high glucose) (Hyclone, Logan, UT, USA), which was supplemented with 10% fetal bovine serum (Sciencell, San Diego, CA, USA) in a humidified 5% CO_2 atmosphere at 37 °C. CCK-8 was purchased from American Bimake Company (Bimake, Houston, TE, USA).

The cytotoxicity assay was performed according to the Cell Counting Kit-8 assay methods as described by elsewhere [23]. Briefly, all cells were seeded into 96-well plates at 3×10^3 cells per well and allowed to culture for 12 h before the addition of the drug. Then, each tumor cell line was exposed to the tested compounds at different concentrations (100–0 µM) for 72 h. DDP (Tokyo Chemical Industry, Tokyo, Japan) and 5-FU (Amresco, Portland, ME, USA) was used as positive control. After treatment, 10 µL of CCK-8 was added to each well, and the plates were incubated for an additional 12 h. OD_{450} absorbance was determined using a Spectramax-i3x (Molecular Devices, Sunnyvale, CA, USA). The experiments were performed in triplicate to obtained IC_{50} values.

4. Conclusions

In this study, two new steroidal alkaloids, hookerianine A (**1**) and hookerianine B (**2**), together with two known ones, scorucinine G (**3**) and epipachysamine D (**4**), were isolated from the stems and roots of *S. hookeriana*. To the best of our knowledge, four compounds were isolated from this plant for the first time. Two new compounds were shown to possess a 3α substituent, which were rarely reported. In addition, compound **1** represents the first example of pregnane-type steroidal alkaloid possessed a novel phenylacetyl group at C-3. Based on the preliminary structure-activity relationships study, we found that the different substituents at C-3 and the presence of double bond and epoxy group between C-16 and C-17 have an important effect on the cytotoxicity of steroidal alkaloids. Inspired by this, it deserves further structural modification and in-depth mechanism research on steroid alkaloids with those characteristics. The results suggested that these types of steroidal alkaloids may have the potential to be anticancer agents.

All of the ^{1}H-NMR, ^{13}C-NMR, 2D-NMR and HR-ESI-MS spectra of compound **1** and **2** are available in Supplementary Material.

Supplementary Materials: The following ^{1}H-NMR, ^{13}C-NMR, 2D-NMR, and HR-ESI-MS spectra are available as supporting data. Supplementary materials are available online.

Author Contributions: J.D. and J.W. designed the experiments and revised the paper; S.H. and J.W. performed the experiments, analyzed the data, and wrote the paper; S.H. and X.H. contributed to bioassay reagents and materials and analyzed the data; L.P. and J.D. revised the paper. All authors read and approved the final manuscript.

Acknowledgments: This research was supported by the National Natural Science Foundation of China [No. 30960529] and the Science and Technology Project of Guizhou Province [No. 2016-1015]. We are grateful to the Centre of Drug Safety Evaluation and Research of Hunan Province for measuring cytotoxicity.

Conflicts of Interest: The authors declare no conflict of interest.

References

1. Editorial Committee of Flora of China. *Flora Reipublicae Popularis Sinicae*; Science Press: Beijing, China, 2004; Volume 45, pp. 41–56.
2. Yu, S.S.; Zou, Z.M.; Zen, J.; Yu, D.Q.; Cong, P.Z. Four new steroidal alkaloids from the roots of *Sarcococca vagans*. *Chin. Chem. Lett.* **1997**, *8*, 511–514.
3. He, K.; Du, J. Two New steroidal alkaloids from the roots of *Sarcococca ruscifolia*. *J. Asian Nat. Prod. Res.* **2010**, *12*, 233–238. [CrossRef] [PubMed]
4. Ghayur, M.N.; Gilani, A.H. Studies on cardio-suppressant, vasodilator and tracheal relaxant effects of *Sarcococca saligna*. *Arch. Pharm. Res.* **2006**, *29*, 990–997. [CrossRef] [PubMed]

5. Devkota, K.P.; Lenta, B.N.; Fokou, P.A.; Sewald, N. Terpenoid alkaloids of the Buxaceae family with potential biological importance. *Nat. Prod. Rep.* **2008**, *25*, 612–630. [CrossRef] [PubMed]
6. Rahman, A.; Feroz, F.; Naeem, I.; Haq, Z.; Nawaz, S.A.; Khan, N.; Khan, M.R.; Choudhary, M.I. New pregnane-type steroidal alkaloids from *Sarcococca saligna* and their cholinesterase inhibitory activity. *Steroids* **2004**, *69*, 735–741. [CrossRef]
7. Rahman, A.; Haq, Z.; Fareeda, F.; Khalid, A.; Nawaz, S.A.; Khan, M.R.; Choudhary, M. New cholinesterase-inhibiting steroidal alkaloids from *Sarcococca saligna*. *Helv. Chim. Acta* **2004**, *87*, 439–448. [CrossRef]
8. Yan, Y.X.; Sun, Y.; Chen, J.C.; Wang, Y.Y.; Li, Y.; Qiu, M.H. Cytotoxic steroids from *Sarcococca saligna*. *Planta Med.* **2011**, *77*, 1725–1729. [CrossRef]
9. Rahman, A.; Anjum, S.; Farooq, A.; Khan, M.R.; Choudhary, M. Two new pregnane-type steroidal alkaloids from *Sarcococca saligna*. *Phytochemistry* **1997**, *46*, 771–775. [CrossRef]
10. Devkota, K.P.; Choudhary, M.I.; Ranjit, R.; Samreen; Sewald, N. Structure activity relationship studies on antileishmanial steroidal alkaloids from *Sarcococca hookeriana*. *Nat. Prod. Res.* **2007**, *21*, 292–297. [CrossRef]
11. Ullah Jan, N.; Ali, A.; Ahmad, B.; Iqbal, N.; Adhikari, A.; Inayat Ur, R.; Musharraf, S.G. Evaluation of antidiabetic potential of steroidal alkaloid of *Sarcococca saligna*. *Biomed. Pharm.* **2018**, *100*, 461–466. [CrossRef]
12. Zhang, P.Z.; Wang, F.; Yang, L.J.; Zhang, G.L. Pregnane alkaloids from *Sarcococca hookeriana* var. digyna. *Fitoterapia* **2013**, *89*, 143–148. [CrossRef] [PubMed]
13. Choudhary, M.I.; Devkota, K.P.; Nawaz, S.A.; Shaheen, F.; Rahman, A. Cholinesterase-inhibiting new steroidal alkaloids from *Sarcococca hookeriana* of nepalese origin. *Helv. Chim. Acta* **2004**, *87*, 1099–1108. [CrossRef]
14. Choudhary, M.I.; Devkota, K.P.; Nawaz, S.A.; Ranjit, R.; Rahman, A. Cholinesterase inhibitory pregnane-type steroidal alkaloids from *Sarcococca hookeriana*. *Steroids* **2005**, *70*, 295–303. [CrossRef] [PubMed]
15. Devkota, K.P.; Lenta, B.N.; Choudhary, M.I.; Naz, Q.; Fekam, F.B.; Rosenthal, P.J. Cholinesterase inhibiting and antiplasmodial steroidal alkaloids from *Sarcococca hookeriana*. *Chem. Pharm. Bull.* **2007**, *55*, 1397–1401. [CrossRef] [PubMed]
16. Devkota, K.P.; Lenta, B.N.; Wansi, J.D.; Choudhary, M.I.; Kisangau, D.P.; Naz, Q.; Samreen; Sewald, N. Bioactive 5α-pregnane-type steroidal alkaloids from *Sarcococca hookeriana*. *J. Nat. Prod.* **2008**, *71*, 1481–1484. [CrossRef] [PubMed]
17. Devkota, K.P.; Wansi, J.D.; Lenta, B.N.; Khan, S.; Choudhary, M.I.; Sewald, N. Bioactive steroidal alkaloids from *Sarcococca hookeriana*. *Planta Med.* **2010**, *76*, 1022–1025. [CrossRef] [PubMed]
18. He, K.; Wang, J.X.; Zou, J.; Wu, J.C.; Huo, S.J.; Du, J. Three new cytotoxic steroidal alkaloids from *Sarcococca hookeriana*. *Molecules* **2018**, *23*, 1181. [CrossRef] [PubMed]
19. Zhang, P.; Shao, L.; Shi, Z.; Zhang, Y.; Du, J.; Cheng, K.J. Pregnane alkaloids from *Sarcococca ruscifolia* and their cytotoxic activity. *Phytochem. Lett.* **2015**, *14*, 31–34. [CrossRef]
20. Rahman, A.; Anjum, S.; Farooq, A.; Khan, M.R.; Parveen, Z.; Choudhary, M.I. Antibacterial steroidal alkaloids from *Sarcococca saligna*. *J. Nat. Prod.* **1998**, *61*, 202–206. [CrossRef]
21. Sheldrick, G.M. SHELXT-integrated space-group and crystal-structure determination. *Acta. Cryst. Sect. A* **2015**, *71*, 3–8. [CrossRef]
22. Sheldrick, G.M. Crystal structure refinement with SHELXL. *Acta. Cryst. Sect. C* **2015**, *71*, 3–8. [CrossRef] [PubMed]
23. Kageyama, M.; Li, K.J.; Sun, S.; Xing, G.Q.; Gaoe, R.; Leia, Z.F. Anti-tumor and anti-metastasis activities of honey bee larvae powder by suppressing the expression of EZH2. *Biomed. Pharma.* **2018**, *105*, 690–696. [CrossRef] [PubMed]

Sample Availability: Samples of the compounds **1**–**4** are available from the authors.

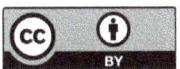

© 2018 by the authors. Licensee MDPI, Basel, Switzerland. This article is an open access article distributed under the terms and conditions of the Creative Commons Attribution (CC BY) license (http://creativecommons.org/licenses/by/4.0/).

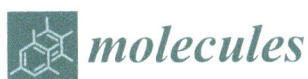

Article
Reaction of Papaverine with Baran Diversinates™

Folake A. Egbewande, Mark J. Coster, Ian D. Jenkins and Rohan A. Davis *

Griffith Institute for Drug Discovery, Griffith University, Brisbane, QLD 4111, Australia;
f.egbewande@griffith.edu.au (F.A.E.); m.coster@griffith.edu.au (M.J.C.); i.jenkins@griffith.edu.au (I.D.J.)
* Correspondence: r.davis@griffith.edu.au; Tel: +61-7-3735-6043; Fax: +61-7-3735-6001

Academic Editor: John C. D'Auria
Received: 30 September 2019; Accepted: 28 October 2019; Published: 31 October 2019

Abstract: The reaction of papaverine with a series of Baran Diversinates™ is reported. Although the yields were low, it was possible to synthesize a small biodiscovery library using this plant alkaloid as a scaffold for late-stage C–H functionalization. Ten papaverine analogues (**2–11**), including seven new compounds, were synthesized. An unexpected radical-induced exchange reaction is reported where the dimethoxybenzyl group of papaverine was replaced by an alkyl group. This side reaction enabled the synthesis of additional novel fragments based on the isoquinoline scaffold, which is present in numerous natural products. Possible reasons for the poor yields in the Diversinate™ reactions with this particular scaffold are discussed.

Keywords: late-stage functionalization; sulfinate; Diversinate™; natural product; medicinal chemistry; papaverine; scaffold; library; biodiscovery

1. Introduction

Late-stage functionalization of organic molecules has emerged as an important strategy in modern drug discovery programs as it allows for direct derivatization without the need for pre-functionalized synthetic handles [1]. This strategy, which involves the direct substitution of a C–H bond with a new functionality, is currently under-utilized in the field of natural products where the generation of analogues provides structure–activity relationships (SAR), a critical component often missing in current biodiscovery programs. The ability to make unusual derivatives of a bioactive scaffold via a simple one-step procedure is of particular relevance in the field of natural products where typically, only small amounts of material or analogues are available. Nitrogen-rich heterocyclic compounds sourced from nature have played a profound role in human health and these motifs are found in many of the current drugs that are used to treat various diseases [2]. Transition-metal-mediated cross-coupling reactions that require pre-functionalized starting materials have been used extensively in the synthesis of such molecules [3–5]; however, the direct C–H functionalization of biologically active heterocycles is still underdeveloped and worthy of further investigations [6–14].

Recent developments in radical-mediated C–H functionalization of heterocycles, including Minisci [15], borono-Minisci [7], and reactions with sulfinate reagents [2], have led to a resurgence in the use of radical-based methods, due primarily to improvements in substrate scope and mild reaction conditions.

In 1971, Minisci et al. reported the addition of carbon-centered radicals to heteroaromatic bases through the silver-mediated decarboxylation of carboxylic acids in the presence of persulfate [15]. One feature that makes this form of innate C–H functionalization appealing for pharmaceutical applications is that protection and deprotection protocols are rarely needed [6]. While these conditions are compatible with alkyl and acyl radicals (derived from alkyl halides, carboxylic acids, and related derivatives), limitations in functional group compatibility, high reaction temperatures (>70 °C), and the requirement of transition-metal additives and strongly oxidizing conditions [6] make them unsuitable for more complex chemical structures. Since this initial publication, numerous methods of C–H functionalization have been reported by Baran [2,7,9,14], Molander [8], and others [16,17], which have significantly increased the scope and generality of this strategy. With the goal of the direct transformation of C–H bonds into C–C bonds in a more practical manner, Baran et al. have developed a radical-based functionalization strategy that involves the use of zinc bis(alkanesulfinate) reagents [12,14]. The most notable features of C–C bond formation using this sulfinate chemistry are that it involves a one-pot reaction, occurs under mild conditions with no need for pre-functionalized starting materials, and the reactions can be conducted in open flasks as they do not require the exclusion of air or moisture [2]. This approach has the advantage of rapidly accelerating drug discovery timelines regardless of whether the compounds of interest are natural or synthetic.

With the intent of identifying hit or lead compounds that are based on bioactive natural products, our research focuses on the semi-synthesis of biodiscovery libraries using unique natural product scaffolds that have been isolated from sources such as fungi, plants and marine invertebrates [18–24]. Herein, we report late-stage functionalization studies on papaverine, a nitrogen-containing heterocyclic natural product, using the commercially available sulfinate reagents known as Diversinates™. Some unexpected chemistry was identified during these studies.

2. Results and Discussion

Commercially available papaverine hydrochloride (**1a**) [25] was chosen as a model compound for our initial foray into C–H functionalization studies utilizing the sulfinate chemistry that has been described by Baran and other research groups [2,9,14]. Fluoroalkyl substituents have become increasingly valuable in modern drug discovery due to their resistance toward oxidation by cytochrome P450 oxidases. Also, incorporation of halogen atoms on hit/lead compounds has been performed in order to exploit their steric effects through the ability of these atoms to occupy the active site of molecular targets [26–28], and establish intermolecular bonds in a manner that resembles H-bonding [29–31].

Baran et al. have published a number of sulfinate reaction conditions, where the Diversinate™ reagents are compatible with different organic solvents (e.g., DMSO, CH_2Cl_2, $ClCH_2CH_2Cl$, perfluorotoluene, perfluorohexane, and anisole). Furthermore, it has been determined that fluoroalkyl zinc sulfinate reagents react best in halogenated solvents, such as CH_2Cl_2, alkyl zinc sulfinate salts react more favorably in DMSO [2], and stoichiometric conditions for the peroxide and Diversinate™ reagents, as well as reaction temperatures and times, vary greatly in the literature. Before synthesizing the targeted papaverine library, we initially conducted several experiments that tested the effect of solvents (e.g., DMSO/CH_2Cl_2/H_2O), reagent stoichiometry, and additives [e.g., trifluoroacetic acid (TFA)] with papaverine HCl (**1a**) and the commonly used Diversinate™, zinc trifluoromethanesulfinate [$(CF_3SO_2)_2Zn$] (Table S71). From this data, it was clear that the best yield for the major mono-CF_3 analogue (**2**) was obtained using 6 mol eq. of $(CF_3SO_2)_2Zn$ and 6 mol eq. of *tert*-butyl hydroperoxide (TBHP) in CH_2Cl_2 for 16 h. In order to ascertain whether the presence of HCl was affecting the yields (the chloride ion could be competitively oxidized by TBHP), we generated the free base of papaverine (**1b**) and repeated the test reactions. Surprisingly, the reaction on the free base gave a lower yield of **2** (15%) compared to the papaverine HCl reaction (compound **2**, 24%). Subsequently, the effect of the addition of TFA was investigated using both the free base and HCl salt of papaverine and a mixture of products was produced, with the free base (**1b**) affording the best yield (10%) with the solvent conditions CH_2Cl_2/TFA/H_2O (1 mol eq. TFA). Based on these data (Table S71), all subsequent reactions were performed using the HCl salt of papaverine and 6 mol eq. of the Diversinate™ reagent in CH_2Cl_2/H_2O (2.5:1) for the fluorinated Diversinates™, while DMSO/H_2O (2.5:1) was chosen for use with the non-fluorinated Diversinates™.

For example, scaffold **1a** (0.1 mmol of the HCl salt) was treated with $(CF_3SO_2)_2Zn$ (0.6 mmol) in a mixture of CH_2Cl_2 (100 μL) and H_2O (40 μL) at 0 °C. The mixture was stirred at 0 °C and TBHP (0.6 mmol) was slowly added, followed by stirring for 20 min. The mixture was then allowed to warm to room temperature over 16 h [2], before evaporation under a stream of nitrogen and chromatography

(HPLC on NH$_2$-bonded silica) was undertaken in order to give the major products, substituted papaverines **2** (24%) and **3** (4%), and the recovered starting material (7%) (Scheme 1). HPLC showed a multitude of UV-active peaks. This, and the recovery of only 7% of the starting material, suggested that the reaction of trifluoromethyl radicals with papaverine was very unselective and/or the products were unstable under the reaction conditions. The preferred attack on the electron-rich 3,4-dimethoxybenzyl ring was not surprising as the trifluoromethyl radical is electrophilic.

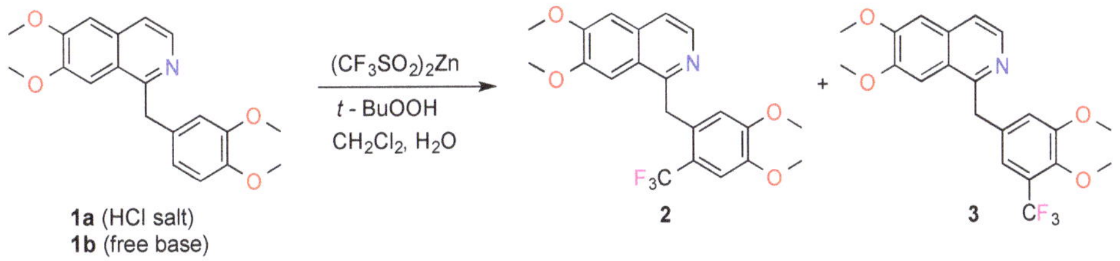

Scheme 1. Reaction of papaverine HCl (**1a**) and free base (**1b**) with zinc trifluoromethanesulfinate [(CF$_3$SO$_2$)$_2$Zn] and *tert*-butyl hydroperoxide (TBHP) in CH$_2$Cl$_2$/H$_2$O.

Interestingly, when the reaction was repeated with the less electrophilic reagent sodium 1,1-difluoroethanesulfinate, the products obtained were those involving substitution on the isoquinoline ring, rather than substitution on the dimethoxybenzyl ring. The products obtained were **4** (7%) and **5** (3%), as well as the recovered starting material (8%) (Figure 1). In all of these reactions, a significant amount (generally between 7 and 14%) of starting material was recovered even though a six-fold excess of reagents was employed.

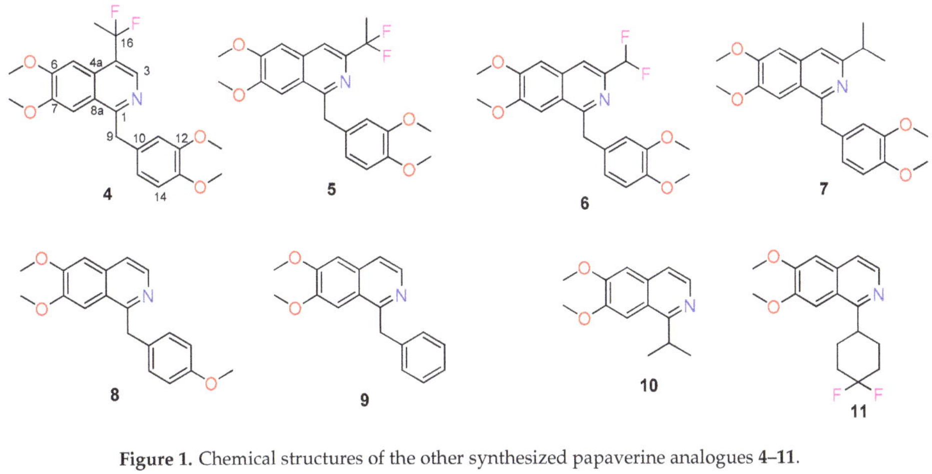

Figure 1. Chemical structures of the other synthesized papaverine analogues **4–11**.

The closely related zinc difluoromethanesulfinate gave a low yield of **6** (3%) analogous to **5**, but only when the reaction was carried out in the presence of TFA (0.1 mmol). No products were detected in the absence of TFA. Although the reaction employed the HCl salt of papaverine under the reaction conditions of excess (CF$_2$HSO$_2$)$_2$Zn and *t*-BuOOH, the HCl would be neutralized by the zinc hydroxide formed. Presumably, the addition of TFA ensured at least partial protonation of the isoquinoline nitrogen, rendering the papaverine more electrophilic and therefore more reactive toward radicals that had some nucleophilic character. Baran et al. found that the difluoromethyl radical had nucleophilic properties, preferring to attack *N*-heterocyclic compounds at electron-deficient centers [12].

Use of the nucleophilic radical precursor zinc isopropylsulfinate gave the papaverine derivative **7** (4%), analogous to **5** and **6**. Once again, TFA was required for the formation of **7**. Surprisingly, the major product was **10** (19%), formed by an apparent radical substitution reaction. Analogous reactions were observed with the nucleophilic radical precursors zinc 4-methoxybenzylsulfinate, zinc benzylsulfinate, and 4,4-difluorocyclohexylsulfinate to give **8** (4%), **9** (14%), and **11** (4%), respectively. A suggested mechanism for these radical substitution reactions is outlined in Scheme 2.

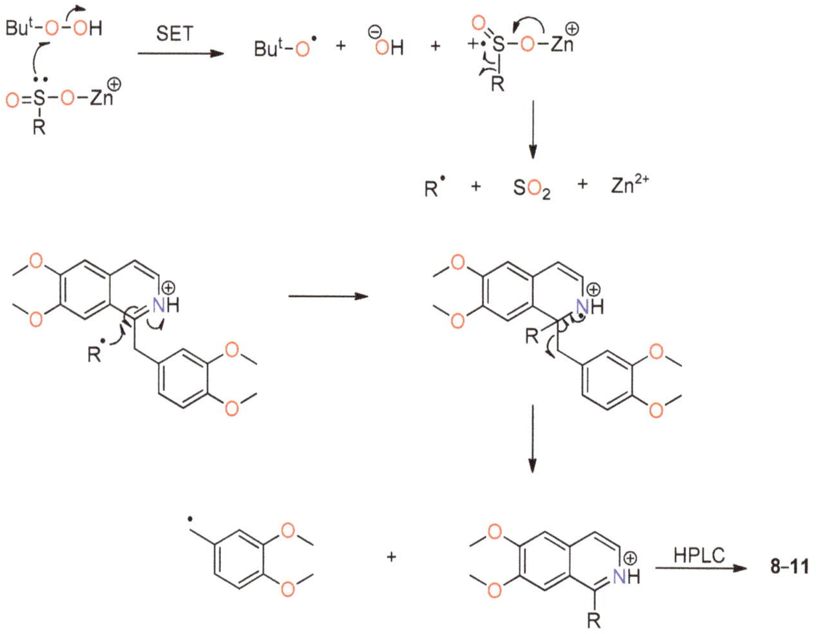

Scheme 2. Proposed single-electron transfer (SET) mechanism for the formation of the side-products **8–11**.

The isolated yields in these reactions were generally low. This was partly due to the large number of minor products formed with this particular scaffold (as evidenced by the HPLC data) and partly due to losses during HPLC purification. Some of these minor products may be due to the attack by trifluoromethyl radicals on the dimethoxyisoquinoline ring and/or bis-trifluoromethylation (which could yield 21 different compounds). In addition, the papaverine scaffold contains four methoxyl groups and a benzylic methylene group, all of which could undergo hydrogen atom abstraction by *tert*-butoxyl radicals leading to a plethora of minor products. Interestingly, Kuttruff et al. [32] have recently reported rather low yields (3–30%) and sometimes extensive decomposition with these reactions. They employed a range of scaffolds incorporating benzene, pyridine, pyrimidine, imidazole, pyrazole and thiazole rings. They also explored different reaction conditions and were able to achieve modest increases in yields in some cases via the addition of Fe(acac)$_3$. However, in other cases, the presence of Fe(acac)$_3$ led to rapid decomposition. Baran et al. [9] have also noted that one of the limitations of the method is that some substrates deliver only moderate amounts of product.

We suggest that the main reason for the poor reactivity of **1a** toward difluoromethyl radicals is the presence of the dimethoxybenzyl group at position 1. Difluoromethyl radicals react readily with isoquinoline and with 3-methylisoquinoline at position 1 (the most electrophilic position), but they do not react with 1-methylisoquinoline [33]. It is interesting to note that the more nucleophilic isopropyl radicals attack at position 1 of the papaverine despite the significant steric hindrance to attack at this position. This is followed by loss of the (more stable) 3,4-dimethoxybenzyl radical to give **10** in moderate (19%) yield.

Compounds **2**, **8**, and **9** have previously been synthesized via multi-step syntheses; **2** was generated using the copper-mediated trifluoromethylation-allylation of arynes [34]; **8** was produced from a reaction of Raney nickel with N-benzylsulfonamide [35], and via the desulfonylation of N-sulfonyl tetrahydroisoquinolines with KF/Al$_2$O$_3$ [36]; and **9** was synthesized using a ruthenium-mediated dual catalytic reaction, and oxidative cross-dehydrogenative coupling with methyl arenes [37,38]. However, this is the first report of the synthesis of **2**, **8**, and **9** using sulfinate chemistry. Furthermore, these three compounds were only partially characterized and none of them had their ^{1}H and ^{13}C chemical shifts assigned to specific positions within the alkaloidal skeleton. We report here the first synthesis of several other papaverine analogues as their free base; full characterization using 1D/2D NMR, UV, IR, and MS data was performed during these studies.

The first products to be fully characterized were compounds **2** and **3**. The ^{1}H NMR spectra (Table 1) of these two mono-CF$_3$ derivatives enabled the definitive positioning of the CF$_3$. Careful comparison of the natural product scaffold (**1b**) NMR data in CD$_3$OD with the fluorinated analogue **2** indicated that this molecule had a CF$_3$ group attached to C-15, since the ^{1}H NMR chemical shifts and multiplicities associated with the pendant benzyl moiety of the starting material had changed from a classic 1,3,4-trisubstituted benzene system (δ_H 7.03, d, J = 2.1 Hz, H-11, 6.92, d, J = 8.4 Hz, H-14 and 6.82, dd, J = 8.4, 2.1 Hz, H-15) to a 1,3,4,6-tetrasubstituted benzene system (δ_H 6.41, s, H-11 and 7.26, s, H-14) (Table 1). Furthermore, a heteronuclear multiple bond correlation (HMBC) (Figure 2) from H-14 (δ_H 7.26) to CF$_3$ (δ_C 126.4) provided further proof of the structural assignment. In a similar fashion to **2**, NMR data analysis of **3** also showed that the CF$_3$ was attached to the pendant aromatic ring of papaverine; however, in this case, the fluorinated moiety was attached to C-14, as indicated once again by the ^{1}H NMR chemical shifts and multiplicities associated with the pendant benzyl moiety of papaverine that had changed from the 1,3,4-trisubstituted benzene system to a 1,3,4,5-tetrasubstituted benzene system (δ_H 7.22, d, J = 2.2 Hz, H-11 and 7.11, d, J = 2.2 Hz, H-15) (Table 1). The HMBC spectrum analysis of **3** was also critical in confirming the CF$_3$ positioning; key HMBC correlations for **3** are shown in Figure 2.

Detailed 2D NMR data analyses were also performed on all other analogues generated during these studies (see Supplementary Materials).

Surprisingly, the reactions that used other commercially available Diversinates™, such as zinc chloromethanesulfinate, zinc chloroethanesulfinate, sodium (2,4-dichlorophenyl)methanesulfinate, sodium 1-(trifluoromethyl)cyclopropanesulfinate, and sodium tert-butylsulfinate were not successful using our methodology (with or without TFA), as determined by LCMS analysis of the crude reaction mixtures after 16 h. The lack of reaction with sodium tert-butylsulfinate and sodium 1-(trifluoromethyl)cyclopropanesulfinate was possibly due to steric hindrance, but it is unclear why the other Diversinate™ reactions were unsuccessful.

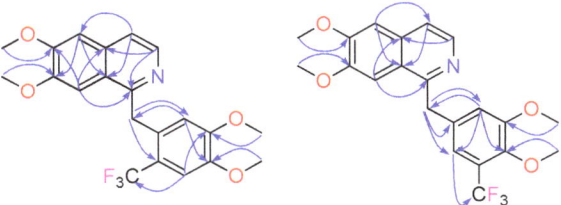

Figure 2. Key HMBC (⟶) correlations for **2** and **3**.

Table 1. ^{1}H (800 MHz) and ^{13}C (200 MHz) NMR data for the mono-CF$_3$ papaverine analogues 2 and 3 in CD$_3$OD at 25 °C.

Position	Mono-CF$_3$ Analogue 2		Mono-CF$_3$ Analogue 3	
	δ_C, type, (J in Hz)	δ_H, mult. (J in Hz)	δ_C, type, (J in Hz)	δ_H, mult. (J in Hz)
1	157.6, C		158.2, C	
3	140.7, CH	8.25, d (5.7)	140.7, CH	8.23, d (5.7)
4	120.9, CH	7.65, d (5.7)	120.8, CH	7.62, d (5.7)
4a	135.4, C		135.6, C	
5	106.7, CH	7.30, s	106.7, CH	7.30, s
6	154.7, C		154.7, C	
7	152.1, C		152.0, C	
8	104.5, CH	7.19, s	105.1, CH	7.46, s
8a	124.3, C		124.2, C	
9	38.4, CH$_2$	4.67, s	41.7, CH$_2$	4.60, s
6-OMe	56.8, CH$_3$	3.98, s	56.51, CH$_3$	3.98, s
7-OMe	56.5, CH$_3$	3.78, s	56.4, CH$_3$	3.91, s
12-OMe	56.1, CH$_3$	3.49, s	56.54, CH$_3$	3.81, s
13-OMe	56.2, CH$_3$	3.85, s	61.7, CH$_3$	3.80, s
10	132.3, C, q, (2.1)		137.1, C	
11	114.5, CH	6.41, s	117.9, CH	7.22, d (2.2)
12	153.1, C		154.9, C	
13	148.8, C		147.3, C, q, (2.3)	
14	110.7, CH, q, (5.9)	7.26, s	120.8, C, q, (39.2)	
15	121.2, C, q, (30.3)		118.6, CH, q, (5.2)	7.11, d (2.2)
CF$_3$	126.4, C, q, (272.1)		124.8, C, q, (269.4)	

In Scheme 2, we propose that the zinc bis(alkanesulfinate) underwent oxidation by TBHP via a single-electron transfer (SET) process to give a *tert*-butoxyl radical, hydroxide ion, and the radical cation of the zinc sulfinate, which then underwent fragmentation to give the alkyl radical and sulfur dioxide. The nucleophilic alkyl radical then underwent addition at position 1 of papaverine followed by elimination of the dimethoxybenzyl radical. This addition–elimination mechanism is analogous to that proposed for the reaction of carbon-centered radicals with β-bromostyrene [39]. The *tert*-butoxyl radical generated in the first step could oxidize a second molecule of sulfinate to give the *tert*-butoxide anion and the radical cation of the zinc sulfinate. A similar mechanism has been proposed by Baran et al. [9] where the presence of a trace metal initiates *tert*-butoxyl radical formation, compared to our proposed mechanism that involves SET. The dimethoxybenzyl radical could also be oxidized by TBHP to give the corresponding dimethoxybenzyl alcohol and a *tert*-butoxyl radical.

Again, it is interesting that the more nucleophilic radicals attack position 1 of the isoquinoline ring, while the 1,1-difluoroethyl and difluoromethyl radicals, which appear to have both nucleophilic and electrophilic properties, prefer to attack at the 3- or 4-position.

In a final attempt to improve the yields and/or the selectivity of these reactions, we decided to modify the reactivity of the papaverine scaffold. It was envisaged that converting papaverine to its N-oxide might increase reactivity, particularly toward electrophilic trifluoromethyl radicals. The free base of papaverine was readily converted to the corresponding N-oxide derivative 12 in moderate yield (58%) using *meta*-chloroperbenzoic acid (MCPBA) in CHCl$_3$ without the need for chromatography, using a method previously described by Bremner et al. [40] (Scheme 3). Unfortunately, treatment of 12 with (CF$_3$SO$_2$)$_2$Zn and TBHP under the same conditions as that used for 1a did not result in an improvement in the yield of the desired Diversinate^{TM} product. After work-up and C$_{18}$ HPLC purification of the reaction mixture, ^{1}H NMR and LCMS analysis indicated that the major product formed was compound 13, albeit with a low yield (<12%) and purity (<80%). Significant amounts of starting material (12, 26%) were isolated, indicating that papaverine N-oxide was less reactive than papaverine toward zinc trifluoromethanesulfinate. As the yield of the desired product had not improved, the reaction of papaverine N-oxide with other Diversinate^{TM} reagents was not investigated.

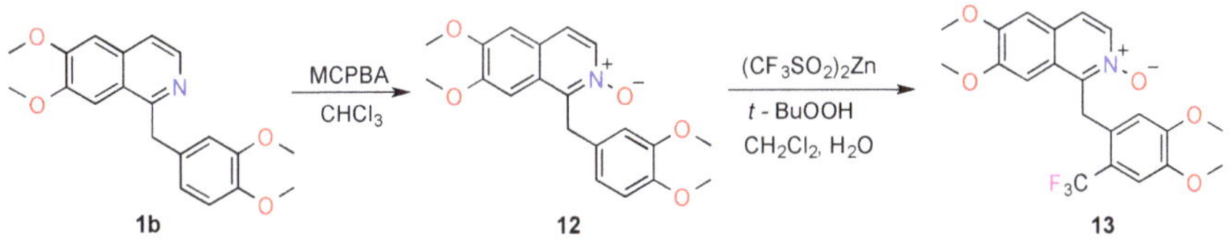

Scheme 3. Conversion of papaverine free base (**1b**) to papaverine *N*-oxide (**12**) using *meta*-chloroperbenzoic acid (MCPBA) in CHCl$_3$ and the subsequent reaction of **12** with zinc trifluoromethanesulfinate [(CF$_3$SO$_2$)$_2$Zn] and *tert*-butyl hydroperoxide (TBHP) in CH$_2$Cl$_2$/H$_2$O to form compound **13**.

3. Materials and Methods

3.1. General Experimental Procedures

NMR spectra were recorded at 25 °C on a Bruker AVANCE HDX 800 MHz spectrometer (Fällanden, Zürich, Switzerland) equipped with a TCI cryoprobe. The ^{1}H and ^{13}C NMR chemical shifts were referenced to the solvent peak for CD$_3$OD (δ_H 3.31 and δ_C 49.00) and CDCl$_3$ (δ_H 7.26 and δ_C 77.16). UV spectra were recorded using a JASCO V-650 UV/vis spectrophotometer (Tokyo, Japan). IR data were acquired using an attached Universal Attenuated Total Reflectance (UATR) Two module on a PerkinElmer spectrophotometer (Waltham, MA, USA). LRESIMS data were recorded on a Thermo Fisher MSQ Plus single quadrupole mass spectrometer (Waltham, MA, USA). HRESIMS data were recorded on a Bruker maXis II ETD ESI-qTOF (Bremen, Germany). A Thermo Scientific Dionex Ultimate 3000 HPLC (Waltham, MA, USA) was used for semi-preparative HPLC separations. An Alltech stainless steel guard cartridge (10 mm × 30 mm) (Sydney, NSW, Australia) was used for loading pre-adsorbed synthetic reaction products onto the semi-preparative HPLC columns. Alltech Davisil NH$_2$-bonded silica (35–75 µm, 150 Å) (Sydney, NSW, Australia) and C$_{18}$-bonded silica (35–75 µm, 150 Å) (Sydney, NSW, Australia) were used for pre-adsorption work before HPLC separations. TLC was carried out on Merck gel F$_{254s}$ pre-coated NH$_2$ glass plates (Darmstadt, Germany) and was observed using UV light. A YMC NH$_2$-bonded silica column (5 µm, 120 Å, 20 mm × 150 mm) (Kyoto, Japan) and a ThermoElectron Betasil C$_{18}$-bonded silica column (5 µm, 143 Å, 21.2 × 150 mm) (Waltham, MA, USA) were used for semi-preparative HPLC separations. All solvents used for chromatography, UV and MS were Honeywell Burdick & Jackson HPLC grade (Muskegon, MI, USA), and the H$_2$O was Sartorius arium proVF (Göttingen, Germany) filtered. All synthetic reagents (including papaverine HCl) were purchased from Sigma-Aldrich (St. Louis, MO, USA) and used without further purification. NMR spectra were processed using MestReNova version 11.0 (Santiago de Compostela, Spain).

3.2. Generation of the Papaverine Library (TFA-Free Method): Compounds 2–5, 9, and 11

Papaverine hydrochloride (**1a**, 37.5 mg, 0.1 mmol) was dissolved in CH$_2$Cl$_2$/H$_2$O or DMSO/H$_2$O (2.5:1, 100 µL:40 µL) before the addition of the sulfinate reagent (85.6–198.9 mg, 0.6 mmol) at room temperature. The mixture was cooled to 0 °C before TBHP (40 µL, 0.6 mmol) was slowly added, after which time the stirred mixture slowly warmed to room temperature over 16 h. Crude reaction products were dried under N$_2$ and pre-adsorbed to NH$_2$-bonded silica (≈1 g) overnight with the dry material packed into a stainless steel guard cartridge, which was subsequently attached to a NH$_2$ semi-preparative HPLC column. Isocratic conditions of 100% *n*-hexane for 10 min, followed by a linear gradient to 20% *i*-PrOH/*n*-hexane over 50 min, then isocratic conditions of 20% *i*-PrOH/*n*-hexane for 10 min all at a flow rate of 9 mL/min was used for each HPLC separation. Sixty fractions (60 × 1 min) were collected from the start of the HPLC run. Fractions containing UV-active material from each HPLC run were analyzed using ^{1}H NMR spectroscopy and LCMS, and relevant fractions with a purity >90% were combined to produce the desired products. Compounds **2–5** and **11** were synthesized using the CH$_2$Cl$_2$/H$_2$O solvent system, while compound **9** was generated using the DMSO/H$_2$O mixture.

3.2.1. Compound **2**

Colorless gum (6.0 mg, 15%); UV (MeOH) λ_{max} (log ε) 241 (4.20), 279 (3.30), 327 (3.19) nm; IR (UATR) ν_{max} 3440, 2981, 1747, 1709, 1279, 1199, 1167, 1078, 1026, 976, 712 cm^{-1}; For NMR data see Table 1; (+)-LRESIMS m/z (rel. int.) 408 (100) [M + H]$^+$; (+)-HRESIMS m/z 408.1425 [M + H]$^+$ (calcd for $C_{21}H_{21}F_3NO_4$, 408.1417).

3.2.2. Compound **3**

Colorless gum (1.9 mg, 4%); UV (MeOH) λ_{max} (log ε) 240 (4.24), 283 (3.47), 324 (3.20) nm; IR (UATR) ν_{max} 3440, 2982, 1746, 1709, 1278, 1199, 1168, 1078, 1026, 975, 712 cm^{-1}; For NMR data see Table 1; (+)-LRESIMS m/z (rel. int.) 408 (100) [M + H]$^+$; (+)-HRESIMS m/z 408.1422 [M + H]$^+$ (calcd for $C_{21}H_{21}F_3NO_4$, 408.1417).

3.2.3. Compound **4**

Colorless gum (2.7 mg, 7%); UV (MeOH) λ_{max} (log ε) 240 (4.08), 276 (3.35), 327 (3.17) nm; IR (UATR) ν_{max} 3400, 2981, 1747, 1705, 1278, 1200, 1164, 1078, 975, 712 cm^{-1}; ^{1}H NMR (800 MHz, CD$_3$OD) δ_H 2.17 (3H, t, J = 18.8 Hz, H-17), 3.74 (3H, s, 12-OMe), 3.75 (3H, s, 13-OMe), 3.87 (3H, s, 7-OMe), 3.97 (3H, s, 6-OMe), 4.56 (2H, s, H-9), 6.77 (1H, dd, J = 8.2, 2.0 Hz, H-15), 6.83 (1H, d, J = 8.2 Hz, H-14), 6.92 (1H, d, J = 2.0 Hz, H-11), 7.51 (1H, s, H-5), 7.53 (1H, s, H-8), 8.42 (1H, s, H-3); ^{13}C NMR (200 MHz, CD$_3$OD) δ_C 25.5 (t, $^2J_{CF}$ = 28.6 Hz, C-17), 42.4 (C-9), 56.36 (12-OMe), 56.38 (13-OMe), 56.41 (7-OMe), 56.5 (6-OMe), 104.4 (C-5), 106.4 (C-8), 113.2 (C-14), 113.6 (C-11), 122.0 (C-15), 124.0 (t, $^1J_{CF}$ = 238.3 Hz, C-16), 124.6 (C-8a), 126.8 (t, $^2J_{CF}$ = 25.3 Hz, C-4), 131.2 (C-4a), 133.1 (C-10), 138.1 (t, $^3J_{CF}$ = 9.3 Hz, C-3), 149.3 (C-13), 150.6 (C-12), 151.6 (C-7), 154.8 (C-6), 162.1 (C-1); (+)-LRESIMS m/z (rel. int.) 404 (100) [M + H]$^+$; (+)-HRESIMS m/z 426.1481 [M + Na]$^+$ (calcd for $C_{22}H_{23}F_2NO_4Na$, 426.1487).

3.2.4. Compound **5**

Colorless gum (1.3 mg, 3%); UV (MeOH) λ_{max} (log ε) 243 (3.95), 283 (3.19), 328 (3.08) nm; IR (UATR) ν_{max} 3400, 2972, 1747, 1705, 1279, 1199, 1165, 1078, 976, 712 cm^{-1}; ^{1}H NMR (800 MHz, CD$_3$OD) δ_H 2.08 (3H, t, J = 18.4 Hz, H-17), 3.73 (3H, s, 12-OMe), 3.75 (3H, s, 13-OMe), 3.88 (3H, s, 7-OMe), 3.97 (3H, s, 6-OMe), 4.56 (2H, s, H-9), 6.80 (1H, dd, J = 8.3, 2.0 Hz, H-15), 6.83 (1H, d, J = 8.3 Hz, H-14), 6.95 (1H, d, J = 2.0 Hz, H-11), 7.34 (1H, s, H-5), 7.46 (1H, s, H-8), 7.86 (1H, s, H-4); ^{13}C NMR (200 MHz, CD$_3$OD) δ_C 24.4 (t, $^2J_{CF}$ = 28.7 Hz, C-17), 41.9 (C-9), 56.3 (12-OMe), 56.39 (13-OMe), 56.41 (7-OMe), 56.5 (6-OMe), 107.4 (C-5), 105.5 (C-8), 113.0 (C-14), 113.4 (C-11), 115.7 (t, $^3J_{CF}$ = 5.3 Hz, C-4), 121.8 (C-15), 122.5 (t, $^1J_{CF}$ = 237.4 Hz, C-16), 124.3 (C-8a), 133.5 (C-10), 135.0 (C-4a), 147.6 (t, $^2J_{CF}$ = 28.3 Hz, C-3), 149.0 (C-13), 150.4 (C-12), 152.3 (C-7), 154.7 (C-6), 159.8 (C-1); (+)-LRESIMS m/z (rel. int.) 404 (100) [M + H]$^+$; (+)-HRESIMS m/z 426.1478 [M + Na]$^+$ (calcd for $C_{22}H_{23}F_2NO_4Na$, 426.1487).

3.2.5. Compound **9**

Colorless gum (4.0 mg, 14%); UV (MeOH) λ_{max} (log ε) 241 (3.90), 326 (2.94) nm; IR (UATR) ν_{max} 3458, 2981, 1747, 1705, 1278, 1199, 1165, 1078, 1026, 975, 712 cm^{-1}; ^{1}H NMR (800 MHz, CD$_3$OD) δ_H 3.83 (3H, s, 7-OMe), 3.97 (3H, s, 6-OMe), 4.60 (2H, s, H-9), 7.16 (1H, m, H-13), 7.24 (2H, m, H-11, H-15), 7.27 (1H, s, H-5), 7.38 (1H, s, H-8), 7.40 (2H, m, H-12, H-14), 7.61 (1H, d, J = 5.7 Hz, H-4), 8.22 (1H, d, J = 5.7 Hz, H-3); ^{13}C NMR (200 MHz, CD$_3$OD) δ_C 42.5 (C-9), 56.3 (7-OMe), 56.5 (6-OMe), 105.5 (C-8), 106.5 (C-5), 120.6 (C-4), 124.3 (C-8a), 127.4 (C-13), 129.6 (2C, C-11, C-15), 129.5 (2C, C-12, C-14), 135.5 (C-4a), 140.5 (C-10), 140.8 (C-3), 151.7 (C-7), 154.6 (C-6), 158.9 (C-1); (+)-LRESIMS m/z (rel. int.) 280 (100) [M + H]$^+$; (+)-HRESIMS m/z 280.1327 [M + H]$^+$ (calcd for $C_{18}H_{18}NO_2$, 280.1332).

3.2.6. Compound **11**

Colorless gum (1.2 mg, 4%); UV (MeOH) λ_{max} (log ε) 237 (3.94), 327 (2.96) nm; IR (UATR) ν_{max} 3436, 2986, 1747, 1705, 1280, 1199, 1166, 1078, 1026, 975, 712 cm^{-1}; ^{1}H NMR (800 MHz, CD$_3$OD) δ_H

2.00–2.11 (4H, m, H-10, H-14), 2.12–2.21 (4H, m, H-11, H-13), 3.71 (1H, m, H-9), 3.99 (3H, s, 6-OMe), 4.03 (3H, s, 7-OMe), 7.28 (1H, s, H-5), 7.52 (1H, d, J = 5.7 Hz, H-4), 7.54 (1H, s, H-8), 8.19 (1H, d, J = 5.7 Hz, H-3); ^{13}C NMR (200 MHz, CD$_3$OD) δ_C 29.6 (2C, d, $^3J_{CF}$ = 10.3 Hz, C-10, C-14), 34.8 (2C, dd, $^2J_{CF}$ = 25.5, 22.6 Hz, C-11, C-13), 40.2 (C-9), 56.46 (6-OMe), 56.54 (7-OMe), 104.2 (C-8), 106.9 (C-5), 119.9 (C-4), 123.3 (C-8a), 124.5 (dd, $^1J_{CF}$ = 242.0, 239.2 Hz, C-12), 135.2 (C-4a), 140.9 (C-3), 152.0 (C-7), 154.5 (C-6), 162.3 (C-1); (+)-LRESIMS m/z (rel. int.) 308 (100) [M + H]$^+$; (+)-HRESIMS m/z 308.1454 [M + H]$^+$ (calcd for C$_{17}$H$_{20}$F$_2$NO$_2$, 308.1457).

3.3. Generation of the Papaverine Library (TFA-Addition Method): Compounds 6–8 and 10

Papaverine hydrochloride (**1a**, 37.5 mg, 0.1 mmol) was dissolved in CH$_2$Cl$_2$/H$_2$O or DMSO/H$_2$O (2.5:1, 100 µL:40 µL) before the addition of the sulfinate reagent (85.6–198.9 mg, 0.6 mmol) and TFA (7.7 µL, 0.1 mmol) at room temperature. The mixture was cooled to 0 °C before TBHP (40 µL, 0.6 mmol) was slowly added, after which time, the stirred mixture slowly warmed to room temperature over 16 h. Crude reaction products was dried under N$_2$ and pre-adsorbed to NH$_2$-bonded silica (≈1 g) overnight before being subjected to identical NH$_2$ semi-preparative HPLC conditions, which are described above. This method generated compound **6** using the CH$_2$Cl$_2$/H$_2$O solvent system, while compounds **7**, **8**, and **10** were generated using the DMSO/H$_2$O mixture.

3.3.1. Compound **6**

Colorless gum (1.0 mg, 3%); UV (MeOH) λ$_{max}$ (log ε) 240 (4.15), 273 (3.36), 327 (3.08) nm; IR (UATR) ν$_{max}$ 3458, 2981, 1747, 1705, 1278, 1199, 1165, 1078, 1026, 975, 712 cm^{-1}; ^{1}H NMR (800 MHz, CD$_3$OD) δ_H 3.72 (3H, s, 12-OMe), 3.76 (3H, s, 13-OMe), 3.87 (3H, s, 7-OMe), 3.98 (3H, s, 6-OMe), 4.57 (2H, s, H-9), 6.78 (1H, dd, J = 8.3, 2.0 Hz, H-15), 6.83 (1H, d, J = 8.3 Hz, H-14), 6.84 (1H, t, J = 55.7 Hz, H-16), 6.93 (1H, d, J = 2.0 Hz, H-11), 7.37 (1H, s, H-5), 7.48 (1H, s, H-8), 7.88 (1H, s, H-4); ^{13}C NMR (200 MHz, CD$_3$OD) δ_C 42.0 (C-9), 56.4 (12-OMe), 56.45 (13-OMe), 56.49 (7-OMe), 56.6 (6-OMe), 107.4 (C-5), 105.8 (C-8), 113.2 (C-14), 113.6 (C-11), 115.6 (t, $^1J_{CF}$ = 238.0 Hz, C-16), 117.4 (t, $^3J_{CF}$ = 4.8 Hz, C-4), 121.9 (C-15), 125.0 (C-8a), 133.4 (C-10), 135.0 (C-4a), 144.9 (t, $^2J_{CF}$ = 24.3 Hz, C-3), 149.2 (C-13), 150.6 (C-12), 152.6 (C-7), 154.9 (C-6), 160.1 (C-1); (+)-LRESIMS m/z (rel. int.) 390 (100) [M + H]$^+$; (+)-HRESIMS m/z 390.1506 [M + H]$^+$ (calcd for C$_{21}$H$_{22}$F$_2$NO$_4$, 390.1511).

3.3.2. Compound **7**

Colorless gum (1.5 mg, 4%); UV (MeOH) λ$_{max}$ (log ε) 239 (3.72), 276 (3.00), 328 (2.83) nm; IR (UATR) ν$_{max}$ 3413, 2986, 1756, 1718, 1279, 1198, 1170, 1078, 1025, 973, 712 cm^{-1}; δ_H 1.40 (6H, d, J = 6.9 Hz, H-17), 3.22 (1H, sept, J = 6.9 Hz, H-16), 3.72 (3H, s, 12-OMe), 3.76 (3H, s, 13-OMe), 3.84 (1H, s, 7-OMe), 3.96 (3H, s, 6-OMe), 4.53 (1H, s, H-9), 6.78 (1H, dd, J = 8.5, 2.2 Hz, H-15), 6.83 (1H, d, J = 8.5 Hz, H-14), 6.91 (1H, d, J = 2.2 Hz, H-11), 7.21 (1H, s, H-5), 7.44 (1H, s, H-4), 7.37 (1H, s, H-8); ^{13}C NMR (200 MHz, CD$_3$OD) δ_C 23.2 (2C, C-17), 36.6 (C-16), 41.7 (C-9), 56.31 (6-OMe), 56.33 (7-OMe), 56.4 (12-OMe), 56.5 (13-OMe), 105.4 (C-8), 106.5 (C-5), 113.1 (C-14), 113.4 (C-11), 115.3 (C-4), 121.8 (C-15), 123.0 (C-8a), 133.7 (C-10), 136.2 (C-4a), 149.0 (C-13), 159.3 (C-3), 151.0 (C-12), 151.8 (C-7), 154.4 (C-6), 158.7 (C-1); (+)-LRESIMS m/z (rel. int.) 382 (100) [M + H]$^+$; (+)-HRESIMS m/z 382.2024 [M + H]$^+$ (calcd for C$_{23}$H$_{28}$NO$_4$, 382.2013).

3.3.3. Compound **8**

Colorless gum (1.3 mg, 4%); UV (MeOH) λ$_{max}$ (log ε) 241 (3.90), 326 (2.94) nm; IR (UATR) ν$_{max}$ 3456, 2981, 1745, 1705, 1279, 1199, 1167, 1079, 1026, 978, 712 cm^{-1}; ^{1}H NMR (800 MHz, CD$_3$OD) δ_H 3.72 (3H, s, 13-OMe), 3.84 (3H, s, 7-OMe), 3.96 (3H, s, 6-OMe), 4.52 (2H, s, H-9), 7.15 (2H, m, H-11, H-15), 7.26 (1H, s, H-5), 7.39 (1H, s, H-8), 6.81 (2H, m, H-12, H-14), 7.58 (1H, d, J = 5.7 Hz, H-4), 8.20 (1H, d, J = 5.7 Hz, H-3); ^{13}C NMR (200 MHz, CD$_3$OD) δ_C 41.6 (C-9), 55.6 (13-OMe), 56.3 (7-OMe), 56.5 (6-OMe), 105.6 (C-8), 106.6 (C-5), 120.5 (C-4), 124.2 (C-8a), 130.4 (2C, C-11, C-15), 115.0 (2C, C-12, C-14), 135.5 (C-4a), 132.7 (C-10), 140.5 (C-3), 151.7 (C-7), 154.6 (C-6), 159.7 (C-1), 159.3 (C-13); (+)-LRESIMS m/z (rel. int.) 310 (100) [M + H]$^+$; (+)-HRESIMS m/z 310.1436 [M + H]$^+$ (calcd for C$_{19}$H$_{20}$NO$_3$, 310.1438).

3.3.4. Compound 10

Colorless gum (4.5 mg, 19%); UV (MeOH) λ_{max} (log ε) 237 (3.91), 324 (2.83) nm; IR (UATR) ν_{max} 3413, 2986, 1747, 1709, 1281, 1198, 1169, 1078, 1026, 973, 712 cm^{-1}; ^{1}H NMR (800 MHz, CD$_3$OD) δ_H 1.40 (6H, d, J = 6.8 Hz, H-10), 3.91 (1H, sept, J = 6.8 Hz, H-9), 3.97 (1H, s, 6-OMe), 3.98 (3H, s, 7-OMe), 7.23 (1H, s, H-5), 7.47 (1H, d, J = 5.6 Hz, H-4), 7.51 (1H, s, H-8), 8.17 (1H, d, J = 5.6 Hz, H-3); ^{13}C NMR (200 MHz, CD$_3$OD) δ_C 22.4 (2C, C-10, C-11), 31.9 (C-9), 56.4 (2C, 6-OMe, 7-OMe), 104.4 (C-8), 106.8 (C-5), 119.6 (C-4), 123.3 (C-8a), 135.1 (C-4a), 140.8 (C-3), 151.8 (C-7), 154.4 (C-6), 165.1 (C-1); (+)-LRESIMS m/z (rel. int.) 232 (100) [M + H]$^+$; (+)-HRESIMS m/z 232.1333 (calcd for C$_{14}$H$_{18}$NO$_2$, 232.1332).

3.4. Synthesis of Papaverine N-oxide (12)

Using a method previously reported by Bremner et al. [40], the free base of papaverine (**1b**, 0.50 g, 1.5 mmol) was dissolved in CHCl$_3$ (10 mL) and treated portion wise with MCPBA (0.35 g, 2.4 mmol) over 5 min. After completion of the addition, the solution was stirred at room temperature for 19 h. The colorless precipitate that formed was filtered and the filtrate was extracted with 5% NaOH (3 × 25 mL). The CHCl$_3$-soluble material was dried down then recrystallized from acetone to yield pure papaverine N-oxide (**12**, 310 mg, 58%).

Comparison of the ^{1}H NMR and LRMS data of product **12** with literature values confirmed the compound [40], although the ^{1}H NMR chemical shifts for two methoxyl signals had been incorrectly assigned to δ_H 6.14 and 6.15; this being a typographical error. The ^{1}H NMR data for papaverine N-oxide was initially reported in CDCl$_3$ at 60 MHz; no ^{13}C NMR data was reported in the original article [40], hence we recorded 1D and 2D NMR data for **12** in both CDCl$_3$ and CD$_3$OD, and report the full NMR assignments here for completeness.

Compound **12**

White amorphous solid (310 mg, 58%); ^{1}H NMR (800 MHz, CDCl$_3$) δ_H 3.800^a (3H, s, 12-OMe), 3.803^a (3H, s, 13-OMe), 3.94 (3H, s, 7-OMe), 3.99 (3H, s, 6-OMe), 4.73 (2H, s, H-9), 6.73 (1H, d, J = 8.3 Hz, H-14), 6.80 (1H, dd, J = 8.3, 2.1 Hz, H-15), 7.01 (1H, d, J = 2.1 Hz, H-11), 7.03 (1H, s, H-5), 7.21 (1H, s, H-8), 7.42 (1H, d, J = 7.0 Hz, H-4), 8.16 (1H, d, J = 7.0 Hz, H-3); ^{13}C NMR (200 MHz, CDCl$_3$) δ_C 31.8 (C-9), 56.00^b (12-OMe), 56.01^b (13-OMe), 56.2 (7-OMe), 56.3 (6-OMe), 103.1 (C-8), 106.1 (C-5), 111.4 (C-14), 112.3 (C-11), 120.4 (C-15), 121.1 (C-4), 124.9 (C-8a), 125.7 (C-4a), 130.1 (C-10), 135.3 (C-3), 145.8 (C-1), 147.9 (C-13), 149.3 (C-12), 151.3 (C-6), 151.8 (C-7); ^{1}H NMR (800 MHz, CD$_3$OD) δ_H 3.747^b (3H, s, 12-OMe), 3.748^b (3H, s, 13-OMe), 3.91 (3H, s, 6-OMe), 3.96 (3H, s, 7-OMe), 4.79 (2H, s, H-9), 6.79 (1H, dd, J = 8.3, 1.8 Hz, H-15), 6.82 (1H, d, J = 8.3 Hz, H-14), 7.01 (1H, d, J = 1.8 Hz, H-11), 7.33 (1H, s, H-5), 7.38 (1H, s, H-8), 7.72 (1H, d, J = 7.0 Hz, H-4), 8.14 (1H, d, J = 7.0 Hz, H-3); ^{13}C NMR (200 MHz, CD$_3$OD) δ_C 32.2 (C-9), 56.44^c (12-OMe), 56.47^c (13-OMe), 56.63^d (7-OMe), 56.66^d (6-OMe), 104.8 (C-8), 107.3 (C-5), 113.2 (C-14), 113.8 (C-11), 121.9 (C-15), 123.2 (C-4), 125.6 (C-8a), 129.1 (C-4a), 131.3 (C-10), 134.8 (C-3), 148.4 (C-1), 149.4 (C-13), 150.7 (C-12), 153.6 (C-7), 154.1 (C-6); (+)-LRESIMS m/z (rel. int.) 356 (100) [M + H]$^+$. ^{a,b,c,d} Interchangeable signals.

3.5. Synthesis of Papaverine N-oxide Diversinate^{TM} Analogue (13)

Papaverine N-oxide (**12**, 35.5 mg, 0.1 mmol) was dissolved in CH$_2$Cl$_2$/H$_2$O (2.5:1, 100 µL:40 µL) before the addition of (CF$_3$SO$_2$)$_2$Zn (198.9 mg, 0.6 mmol) at room temperature. The mixture was cooled to 0 °C before TBHP (40 µL, 0.6 mmol) was slowly added, after which time, the stirred mixture slowly warmed to room temperature over 16 h. The crude reaction product was dried under N$_2$ and pre-adsorbed to C$_{18}$-bonded silica (≈1 g) overnight with the dry material packed into a stainless-steel guard cartridge, which was subsequently attached to a C$_{18}$ semi-preparative HPLC column. Isocratic conditions of H$_2$O/MeOH/TFA (90:10:0.1) were run for the first 10 min, followed by a linear gradient of MeOH/TFA (100:0.1) over 40 min, then isocratic conditions of MeOH/TFA (100:0.1) for a further 10 min, all at a flow rate of 9 mL/min. Sixty fractions (60 × 1 min) were collected from the start of the HPLC run. Fractions containing UV-active material were analyzed using ^{1}H NMR spectroscopy and LCMS in order to identify products of interest. The starting material (**12**, 9.3 mg, 26%) eluted in fraction 39, while a mixture (<80% pure) containing predominantly the mono-CF$_3$ papaverine N-oxide analogue (**13**, 5.1 mg, <12%) eluted in fraction 43. While ^{1}H NMR and LCMS analysis of the fraction 43 mixture indicated product **13** had been made, the paucity of material and low yield, meant no further purification or characterization was undertaken.

*3.6. Generation of the Free Base of Papaverine (**1b**)*

Papaverine hydrochloride (**1a**, 200 mg) was dissolved in a mixture of ammoniated H$_2$O (9:1, H$_2$O:28% aq. NH$_3$, 20 mL) and then extracted with CH$_2$Cl$_2$ (3 × 20 mL). The free base of papaverine (**1b**) was soluble in the CH$_2$Cl$_2$ layer, and following evaporation, yielded the desired product with a high purity and yield (174 mg, 93%).

*3.7. Generation of Compounds **2** and **3** Using the Free Base of Papaverine (**1b**)*

The free base of papaverine (**1b**, 33.9 mg, 0.1 mmol) was dissolved in CH$_2$Cl$_2$/H$_2$O or DMSO/H$_2$O (2.5:1, 100 µL:40 µL) before the addition of the (CF$_3$SO$_2$)$_2$Zn (198.9 mg, 0.6 mmol) at room temperature. Where TFA was used, 7.7 µL (0.1 mmol) was added to the reaction while stirring. The mixture was cooled to 0 °C before TBHP (40 µL, 0.6 mmol) was added, after which time, the stirred mixture was slowly warmed to room temperature over 16 h. The crude reaction product was dried under N$_2$ and pre-adsorbed to NH$_2$-bonded silica (≈1 g) overnight before being subjected to identical NH$_2$ semi-preparative HPLC conditions, which are described above. Reaction conditions and yields for these free base reactions can be found in Table S71.

4. Conclusions

The papaverine scaffold reacted with (CF$_3$SO$_2$)$_2$Zn and TBHP to give dimethoxybenzyl ring-substituted products. With other sulfinates, however, the products featured substitution on the isoquinoline ring. The use of nucleophilic radical precursors, such as zinc isopropylsulfinate, resulted in the replacement of the 3,4-dimethoxybenzyl substituent as the major reaction. A mechanism was suggested for this unusual radical replacement reaction. Despite the fact that the papaverine scaffold was a poor substrate for Diversinate^{TM} chemistry resulting in low yields, we were able to prepare a small library of ten papaverine derivatives (including seven new compounds), some of which would be difficult to prepare by other means. Oxidizing the scaffold to papaverine N-oxide had no significant impact on the Diversinate^{TM} yield or selectivity. To the best of our knowledge, these are the first examples of the derivatization of a benzylisoquinoline using Diversinate^{TM} C–H functionalization chemistry. This unique library has been added to the Davis open-access natural product-based library for future drug discovery and chemical biology evaluations [41].

Supplementary Materials: The following are available online: 1D/2D NMR spectra for compounds **1–12** and Diversinate^{TM} optimization conditions on papaverine HCl salt and papaverine free base.

Author Contributions: R.A.D. and F.A.E. conceived, designed, and conceptualized the study. F.A.E. collected the data and literature for the manuscript and performed the experiments. R.A.D. and M.J.C. supervised the study. R.A.D., M.J.C., I.D.J. and F.A.E. wrote the manuscript and all authors reviewed the manuscript. All authors have read and approved the final version of the manuscript.

Funding: The authors acknowledge the National Health and Medical Research Council (grant APP1024314 to R.A.D.), the Australian Research Council for support towards NMR and MS equipment (grants LE0668477, LE140100119, and LE0237908), and financial support (grant LP120200339 to R.A.D.).

Acknowledgments: F.A.E. thanks Griffith University for two Ph.D. scholarships, the Griffith University Postgraduate Research Scholarship and the Griffith University International Postgraduate Research Scholarship.

Conflicts of Interest: The authors declare no conflict of interest.

References

1. Wencel-Delord, J.; Glorius, F. C–H bond activation enables the rapid construction and late-stage diversification of functional molecules. *Nat. Chem.* **2013**, *5*, 369–375. [CrossRef] [PubMed]
2. Fujiwara, Y.; Dixon, J.A.; O'Hara, F.; Funder, E.D.; Dixon, D.D.; Rodriguez, R.A.; Baxter, R.D.; Herle, B.; Sach, N.; Collins, M.R.; et al. Practical and innate carbon–hydrogen functionalization of heterocycles. *Nature* **2012**, *492*, 95–99. [CrossRef] [PubMed]
3. Miyaura, N.; Yamada, K.; Suzuki, A. A new stereospecific cross-coupling by the palladium-catalyzed reaction of 1-alkenylboranes with 1-alkenyl or 1-alkynyl halides. *Tetrahedron Lett.* **1979**, *20*, 3437–3440. [CrossRef]
4. Kalyani, D.; Deprez, N.R.; Desai, L.V.; Sanford, M.S. Oxidative C–H activation/C–C bond forming reactions: Synthetic scope and mechanistic insights. *J. Am. Chem. Soc.* **2005**, *127*, 7330–7331. [CrossRef]
5. Boorman, T.C.; Larrosa, I. Gold-mediated C–H bond functionalisation. *Chem. Soc. Rev.* **2011**, *40*, 1910–1925. [CrossRef]
6. Duncton, M.A. Minisci reactions: Versatile CH-functionalizations for medicinal chemists. *MedChemComm* **2011**, *2*, 1135–1161. [CrossRef]
7. Seiple, I.B.; Su, S.; Rodriguez, R.A.; Gianatassio, R.; Fujiwara, Y.; Sobel, A.L.; Baran, P.S. Direct C–H arylation of electron-deficient heterocycles with arylboronic acids. *J. Am. Chem. Soc.* **2010**, *132*, 13194–13196. [CrossRef]
8. Molander, G.A.; Colombel, V.; Braz, V.A. Direct alkylation of heteroaryls using potassium alkyl-and alkoxymethyltrifluoroborates. *Org. Lett.* **2011**, *13*, 1852–1855. [CrossRef]
9. Ji, Y.; Brueckl, T.; Baxter, R.D.; Fujiwara, Y.; Seiple, I.B.; Su, S.; Blackmond, D.G.; Baran, P.S. Innate CH trifluoromethylation of heterocycles. *Proc. Natl. Acad. Sci.* **2011**, *108*, 14411–14415. [CrossRef]
10. Langlois, B.R.; Laurent, E.; Roidot, N. Trifluoromethylation of aromatic compounds with sodium trifluoromethanesulfinate under oxidative conditions. *Tetrahedron Lett.* **1991**, *32*, 7525–7528. [CrossRef]
11. Minisci, F.; Vismara, E.; Fontana, F. Recent developments of free-radical substitutions of heteroaromatic bases. *Heterocycles* **1989**, *28*, 489–519. [CrossRef]
12. Brückl, T.; Baxter, R.D.; Ishihara, Y.; Baran, P.S. Innate and guided C–H functionalization logic. *Acc. Chem. Res.* **2012**, *45*, 826–839. [CrossRef] [PubMed]
13. Fujiwara, Y.; Domingo, V.; Seiple, I.B.; Gianatassio, R.; Del Bel, M.; Baran, P.S. Practical C–H Functionalization of Quinones with Boronic Acids. *J. Am. Chem. Soc* **2011**, *133*, 3292–3295. [CrossRef] [PubMed]
14. Fujiwara, Y.; Dixon, J.A.; Rodriguez, R.A.; Baxter, R.D.; Dixon, D.D.; Collins, M.R.; Blackmond, D.G.; Baran, P.S. A new reagent for direct difluoromethylation. *J. Am. Chem. Soc.* **2012**, *134*, 1494–1497. [CrossRef] [PubMed]
15. Minisci, F.; Bernardi, R.; Bertini, F.; Galli, R.; Perchinummo, M. Nucleophilic character of alkyl radicals—VI: A new convenient selective alkylation of heteroaromatic bases. *Tetrahedron* **1971**, *27*, 3575–3579. [CrossRef]
16. Punta, C.; Minisci, F. Minisci Reaction: A Friedel-Crafts Type Process with Opposite Reactivity and Selectivity. Selective Homolytic Alkylation, Acylation, Carboxylation and Carbamoylation of Heterocyclic Aromatic Bases. *Trends Heterocycl. Chem.* **2008**, *13*, 1–68. [CrossRef]
17. Stout, E.P.; Choi, M.Y.; Castro, J.E.; Molinski, T.F. Potent fluorinated agelastatin analogues for chronic lymphocytic leukemia: Design, synthesis, and pharmacokinetic studies. *J. Med. Chem.* **2014**, *57*, 5085–5093. [CrossRef]
18. Barnes, E.C.; Choomuenwai, V.; Andrews, K.T.; Quinn, R.J.; Davis, R.A. Design and synthesis of screening libraries based on the muurolane natural product scaffold. *Org. Biomol. Chem.* **2012**, *10*, 4015–4023. [CrossRef]
19. Choomuenwai, V.; Andrews, K.T.; Davis, R.A. Synthesis and antimalarial evaluation of a screening library based on a tetrahydroanthraquinone natural product scaffold. *Bioorg. Med. Chem.* **2012**, *20*, 7167–7174. [CrossRef]
20. Davis, R.A.; Carroll, A.R.; Quinn, R.J. The synthesis of a combinatorial library using a tambjamine natural product template. *Aust. J. Chem.* **2001**, *54*, 355–359. [CrossRef]
21. Kumar, R.; Sadowski, M.C.; Levrier, C.; Nelson, C.C.; Jones, A.J.; Holleran, J.P.; Avery, V.M.; Healy, P.C.; Davis, R.A. Design and synthesis of a screening library using the natural product scaffold 3-chloro-4-hydroxyphenylacetic acid. *J. Nat. Prod.* **2015**, *78*, 914–918. [CrossRef] [PubMed]
22. Davis, R.A.; Pierens, G.K.; Parsons, P.G. Synthesis and spectroscopic characterisation of a combinatorial library based on the fungal natural product 3-chloro-4-hydroxyphenylacetamide. *Magn. Reson. Chem.* **2007**, *45*, 442–445. [CrossRef] [PubMed]

23. Egbewande, F.A.; Nilsson, N.; White, J.M.; Coster, M.J.; Davis, R.A. The design, synthesis, and anti-inflammatory evaluation of a drug-like library based on the natural product valerenic acid. *Bioorg. Med. Chem. Lett.* **2017**, *27*, 3185–3189. [CrossRef] [PubMed]
24. Egbewande, F.A.; Sadowski, M.C.; Levrier, C.; Tousignant, K.D.; White, J.M.; Coster, M.J.; Nelson, C.C.; Davis, R.A. Identification of Gibberellic Acid Derivatives that Deregulate Cholesterol Metabolism in Prostate Cancer Cells. *J. Nat. Prod.* **2018**, *81*, 838–845. [CrossRef]
25. Aboutabl, E.A.; El-Azzouny, A.A.; Afifi, M.S. ^{1}H-NMR assay of papaverine hydrochloride and formulations. *Phytochem. Anal.* **2002**, *13*, 301–304. [CrossRef]
26. Geronikaki, A.A.; Lagunin, A.A.; Hadjipavlou-Litina, D.I.; Eleftheriou, P.T.; Filimonov, D.A.; Poroikov, V.V.; Alam, I.; Saxena, A.K. Computer-aided discovery of anti-inflammatory thiazolidinones with dual cyclooxygenase/lipoxygenase inhibition. *J. Med. Chem.* **2008**, *51*, 1601–1609. [CrossRef]
27. La Motta, C.; Sartini, S.; Mugnaini, L.; Salerno, S.; Simorini, F.; Taliani, S.; Marini, A.M.; Da Settimo, F.; Lavecchia, A.; Novellino, E. Exploiting the pyrazolo [3, 4-d] pyrimidin-4-one ring system as a useful template to obtain potent adenosine deaminase inhibitors. *J. Med. Chem.* **2009**, *52*, 1681–1692. [CrossRef]
28. Monforte, A.-M.; Logoteta, P.; Ferro, S.; De Luca, L.; Iraci, N.; Maga, G.; De Clercq, E.; Pannecouque, C.; Chimirri, A. Design, synthesis, and structure–activity relationships of 1, 3-dihydrobenzimidazol-2-one analogues as anti-HIV agents. *Bioorg. Med. Chem.* **2009**, *17*, 5962–5967. [CrossRef]
29. Metrangolo, P.; Neukirch, H.; Pilati, T.; Resnati, G. Halogen bonding based recognition processes: A world parallel to hydrogen bonding. *Acc. Chem. Res.* **2005**, *38*, 386–395. [CrossRef]
30. Metrangolo, P.; Resnati, G. Halogen Versus Hydrogen. *Science* **2008**, *321*, 918–919. [CrossRef]
31. Müller, K.; Faeh, C.; Diederich, F. Fluorine in pharmaceuticals: Looking beyond intuition. *Science* **2007**, *317*, 1881–1886. [CrossRef] [PubMed]
32. Kuttruff, C.A.; Haile, M.; Kraml, J.; Tautermann, C.S. Late-Stage Functionalization of Drug-Like Molecules Using Diversinates. *ChemMedChem* **2018**, *13*, 983–987. [CrossRef] [PubMed]
33. Tung, T.T.; Christensen, S.B.; Nielsen, J. Difluoroacetic Acid as a New Reagent for Direct C–H Difluoromethylation of Heteroaromatic Compounds. *Chem. Eur. J.* **2017**, *23*, 18125–18128. [CrossRef] [PubMed]
34. Yang, X.; Tsui, G.C. Copper-Mediated Trifluoromethylation–Allylation of Arynes. *Org. Lett.* **2018**, *20*, 1179–1182. [CrossRef]
35. Larghi, E.L.; Kaufman, T.S. Preparation of N-benzylsulfonamido-1, 2-dihydroisoquinolines and their reaction with Raney nickel. A mild, new synthesis of isoquinolines. *Tetrahedron Lett.* **1997**, *38*, 3159–3162. [CrossRef]
36. Silveira, C.C.; Bernardi, C.R.; Braga, A.L.; Kaufman, T.S. Desulfonylation of N-sulfonyl tetrahydroisoquinoline derivatives by potassium fluoride on alumina under microwave irradiation: Selective synthesis of 3, 4-dihydroisoquinolines and isoquinolines. *Synlett* **2002**, *6*, 0907–0910. [CrossRef]
37. Wang, T.-H.; Lee, W.-C.; Ong, T.-G. Ruthenium-Mediated Dual Catalytic Reactions of Isoquinoline via C–H Activation and Dearomatization for Isoquinolone. *Adv. Synth. Catal.* **2016**, *358*, 2751–2758. [CrossRef]
38. Wan, M.; Lou, H.; Liu, L. C$_1$-Benzyl and benzoyl isoquinoline synthesis through direct oxidative cross-dehydrogenative coupling with methyl arenes. *Chem. Commun.* **2015**, *51*, 13953–13956. [CrossRef]
39. Sølvhøj, A.; Ahlburg, A.; Madsen, R. Dimethylzinc-Initiated Radical Coupling of β-Bromostyrenes with Ethers and Amines. *Chem. Eur. J.* **2015**, *21*, 16272–16279. [CrossRef]
40. Bremner, J.; Wiriyachitra, P. The photochemistry of papaverine N-oxide. *Aust. J. Chem.* **1973**, *26*, 437–442. [CrossRef]
41. Askin, S.; Bond, T.E.; Sorenson, A.E.; Moreau, M.J.; Antony, H.; Davis, R.A.; Schaeffer, P.M. Selective protein unfolding: A universal mechanism of action for the development of irreversible inhibitors. *Chem. Commun.* **2018**, *54*, 1738–1741. [CrossRef] [PubMed]

Sample Availability: Samples of all compounds are available from the corresponding author, R.A.D.

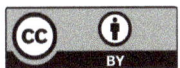 © 2019 by the authors. Licensee MDPI, Basel, Switzerland. This article is an open access article distributed under the terms and conditions of the Creative Commons Attribution (CC BY) license (http://creativecommons.org/licenses/by/4.0/).

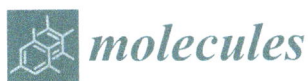

Article

Integrated Analytical Tools for Accessing Acridones and Unrelated Phenylacrylamides from *Swinglea glutinosa*

Ana Calheiros de Carvalho [1], Luiza De Camillis Rodrigues [2], Alany Ingrid Ribeiro [3], Maria Fátima das Graças Fernandes da Silva [3], Lívia Soman de Medeiros [2] and Thiago André Moura Veiga [2,*]

[1] Programa de Pós-Graduação em Biologia Química, Department of Chemistry, Federal University of São Paulo, Diadema-SP 09972-270, Brazil; carvalho.ac08@gmail.com
[2] Department of Chemistry, Federal University of São Paulo, Diadema-SP 09972-270, Brazil; decamillisluiza@gmail.com (L.D.C.R.); livia.soman@unifesp.br (L.S.d.M.)
[3] Department of Chemistry, Federal University of São Carlos, São Carlos-SP 13565-905, Brazil; alanyiribeiro@gmail.com (A.I.R.); dmfs@ufscar.br (M.F.d.G.F.d.S.)
* Correspondence: tveiga@unifesp.br; Tel.: +55-11-4044-0500

Academic Editor: Derek J. McPhee
Received: 16 November 2019; Accepted: 24 December 2019; Published: 30 December 2019

Abstract: In natural product studies, the purification of metabolites is an important challenge. To accelerate this step, alternatives such as integrated analytical tools should be employed. Based on this, the chemical study of *Swinglea glutinosa* (Rutaceae) was performed using two rapid dereplication strategies: *Target Analysis* (Bruker Daltonics®, Bremen, Germany) MS data analysis combined with MS/MS data obtained from the GNPS platform. Through UHPLC-HRMS data, the first approach allowed, from crude fractions, a quick and visual identification of compounds already reported in the *Swinglea* genus. Aside from this, by grouping compounds according to their fragmentation patterns, the second approach enabled the detection of eight molecular families, which presented matches for acridonic alkaloids, phenylacrylamides, and flavonoids. Unrelated compounds for *S. glutinosa* have been isolated and characterized by NMR experiments, Lansamide I, Lansiumamide B, Lansiumamide C, and *N*-(2-phenylethyl)cinnamamide.

Keywords: *Swinglea glutinosa*; dereplication; acridones; phenylacrylamides

1. Introduction

Currently, a combination of hyphenated techniques (i.e., two or more analytical techniques) may increase the efficiency and speed of analysis, being useful tools to determine unknown natural products. Recent methodologies developed to discover new metabolites include molecular dereplication, which is defined as the analysis of a natural product, fraction, or crude extract without previous purification steps. Usually, this is done based on spectroscopic, structural, or biological activity, using data comparisons obtained from "in-house" and/or commercial databases [1].

In this sense, one of the most employed approaches is the Global Natural Products Social Molecular Networking (GNPS), which consists of a database that analyzes mass spectrometry data and compares it with previously registered data to establish the molecular networking maps. GNPS has been created to improve and accelerate the discovery of natural products, allowing the identification of substances not yet reported [2].

Another tool recently developed to distinguish known and unknown secondary metabolites is HRMS data processing through Target Analysis software (Bruker Daltonics®) [3]. This screening method interacts with previously known compound databases by an internal application (Excel spreadsheet) that generates searching lists, which indicate reported detected compounds. This enables accelerated and efficient identification of known compounds, saving time for isolating unknown compounds or bioactive substances. This strategy was developed by Klitgaard et al. (2013) [3].

Based on the advantages of the application of modern strategies, this work aims to explore the chemical profile of *Swinglea glutinosa*, a species from the Rutaceae family, which belongs to a monotypic genus, according to Engler (1931) [4]. It is a plant from the Philippines, but is already widespread throughout the world including Latin America, especially Colombia and Brazil. Biosynthetically, it is characterized by the presence of alkaloids, especially acridones [5] and benzoyltyramines [6].

Some reports have shown that acridones present antiparasitic activity against *Plasmodium falciparum* and *Trypanosoma brucei rhodesiense*, which are responsible for transmitting malaria and sleeping sickness, respectively. Acridone 5-hydroxynoracronycine (**6**), among those tested, was the most active against *T. b. rhodesiense* (IC^T_{50} 1.0 µM). On the other hand, glycocitrine-IV (**5**), was more active (IC^P_{50} 0.3 µM) against *P. falciparum* [7]. The acridones also presented an effect on cathepsin V, an enzyme that degrades random proteins in the lysosome, which is associated with some diseases, the progression of tumors, muscular dystrophy, Alzheimer's disease, rheumatoid arthritis, and osteoporosis. Among the tested compounds, citibrasine (**4**) was the most potent inhibitor, with an IC_{50} value of 1.2 µM [8].

Beyond these effects, we can find reports on the potential of this class of compounds on photosynthesis inhibition. Citrusinine-I (**1**), glycocitrine-IV (**5**), 1,3,5-trihydroxy-10-methyl-2,8-bis(3-methylbut-2-en-1-yl)-9(10*H*)-acridinone, (2*R*)-2-*tert*-butyl-3,10-dihydro-4,9-dihydroxy-11-methoxy-10-methylfuro-[3,2-b]acridin-5(2*H*)-one, and (3*R*)-2,3,4,7-tetrahydro-3,5,8-trihydroxy-6-methoxy-2,2,7-trimethyl-12*H*-pyrano [2,3-a]acridin-12-one affect photosynthesis through different mechanisms of action [5]. We also can find reports on anticancer activity, for instance, compound 1,3-dimethoxy-10-methylacridone, which presented cytotoxic effects with IC_{50} values from 3.38 µM (toward MDA-MB-231-BCRP cells) to 58.10 µM (toward leukemia CEM/ADR5000 cells) [9].

Given the reports and the biological activities associated with compounds isolated from *Swinglea glutinosa*, we have decided to continue [5] our search for compounds still undiscovered in the plant. Thus, the selected modern analytical tools have been very useful for conducting this work, which led us to isolate and characterize substances of interest, in this case, unrelated phenylacrylamides to the *Swinglea* genus.

2. Results and Discussion

Before starting the chemical fractionation of *S. glutinosa* extracts, to detail the chemical profile of the plant, a literature review (including the use of the Dictionary of Natural Products) of all compounds previously reported for the *Swinglea* genus was performed. Thus, an "in-house" database was created by feeding an Excel spreadsheet containing the molecular formula and the name of all cataloged compounds. In total, 27 compounds were cataloged, belonging to the acridone and benzoyltyramine classes.

Among the fractions obtained from the ethanolic extract fractionation of *S. glutinosa*, the hexane stem and hexane leaf fractions were analyzed through the dereplication approaches. Thus, it was possible to observe on the chromatogram of the hexane stem fraction that many detected compounds corresponded to compounds listed in the "in-house" database, most of them belonging to the acridonic alkaloid, benzoyltyramine, and phenylacrylamide classes (Figures 1A and 2; Table 1). The numbers indicated on the chromatograms (Figure 1A,B) correspond to the molecular formulas for the compounds present in the "in-house" database. These compounds are shown in Figure 2 and Table 1.

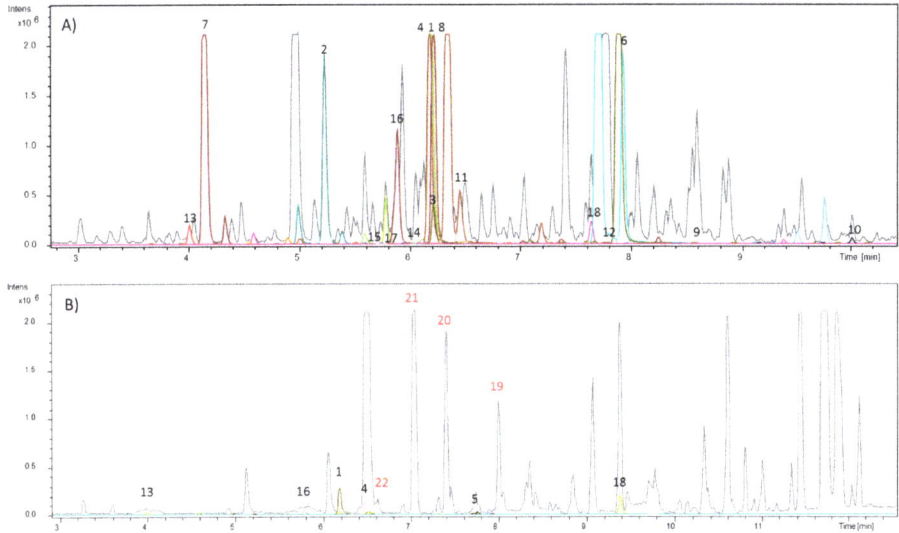

Figure 1. (**A**) Base peak chromatogram (BPC) of *S. glutinosa* hexane stem fractions. (**B**) BPC of *S. glutinosa* hexane leaf fraction. The chromatogram is overlaid with the extracted-ion chromatogram from detected compounds. The colored peaks represent compounds listed in the "in-house" database, some of them identified in Table 1 and Figure 2. The peaks numbered in red correspond to the isolated amides in this work, not yet reported for the genus.

Table 1. Identified compounds from the hexane stem and hexane leaf fractions of *Swinglea glutinosa* through UHPLC-HRMS (using Target Analysis), their molecular formulas, exact masses, and accurate masses.

Compound Name (Code)	Molecular Formula	Exact Mass	Accurate Mass [M + H]$^+$
citrusinine-I (1)	$C_{16}H_{15}NO_5$	301.0950	302.1018
citrusinine-II (2)	$C_{15}H_{13}NO_5$	287.0794	288.0862
pyranofoline (3)	$C_{20}H_{19}NO_5$	353.1263	354.1334
citibrasine (4)	$C_{17}H_{17}NO_6$	331.1056	332.1131
glycotrycine IV (5)	$C_{20}H_{21}NO_5$	355.1420	356.1488
5-hydroxynoracronycine (6)	$C_{19}H_{17}NO_4$	323.1158	324.1230
2,3-dihydro-4,9-dihydroxy-2-(2-hydroxypropan-2-yl)-11-methoxy-10-methylfuro[3,2-b]acridin-5(10H)-oneI (7)	$C_{20}H_{21}NO_6$	371.1369	372.1439
3,4-dihydro-3,5,8-trihydroxy-6-methoxy-2,2,7-trimethyl-2H-pyrano[2,3-a]acridin-12(7H)-one (8)	$C_{20}H_{21}NO_6$	371.1369	372.1452
des-N-methylnoracronycine (9)	$C_{19}H_{17}NO_3$	307.1208	308.1250
5-hydroxy-N-methylseverifoline (10)	$C_{24}H_{25}NO_4$	391.1784	392.1842
glyfoline (11)	$C_{18}H_{19}NO_7$	361.1162	362.1272
atalaphyllinine (12)	$C_{23}H_{23}NO$	377.1627	378.1446
(E)-N-methylcinnamamide [(E)-N-methylphenylacrylamide] (13)	$C_{10}H_{11}NO$	161.0841	162.0912
N-benzoyl-O-(4-acetoxyl-6,7-dihydroxy)geranylthiramine (14)	$C_{27}H_{35}NO_6$	469.2464	470.2522
N-benzoyl-O-(6-acetoxyl-4,7-dihydroxy)geranylthiramine (15)	$C_{27}H_{35}NO_6$	469.2464	470.2522
N-{2-[4-(butoxy-3-one) phenyl]ethyl}benzamide (16)	$C_{19}H_{21}NO_3$	311.1521	312.1591
N-{2 [4-(2,3-dihydroxy-2-methylbutoxyethyl)phenyl] ethyl}benzamide (17)	$C_{20}H_{23}NO_6$	373.1525	374.1573
N-benzoyltyramine (18)	$C_{15}H_{15}NO_2$	241.1103	242.1175
lansamide I (19)	$C_{18}H_{17}NO$	263.131	264.1379
lansiumamide B (20)	$C_{18}H_{17}NO$	263.131	264.1381
lansiumamide C (21)	$C_{18}H_{19}NO$	265.147	266.1554
N-(2-phenylethyl)cinnamamide (22)	$C_{17}H_{17}NO$	251.131	252.1397

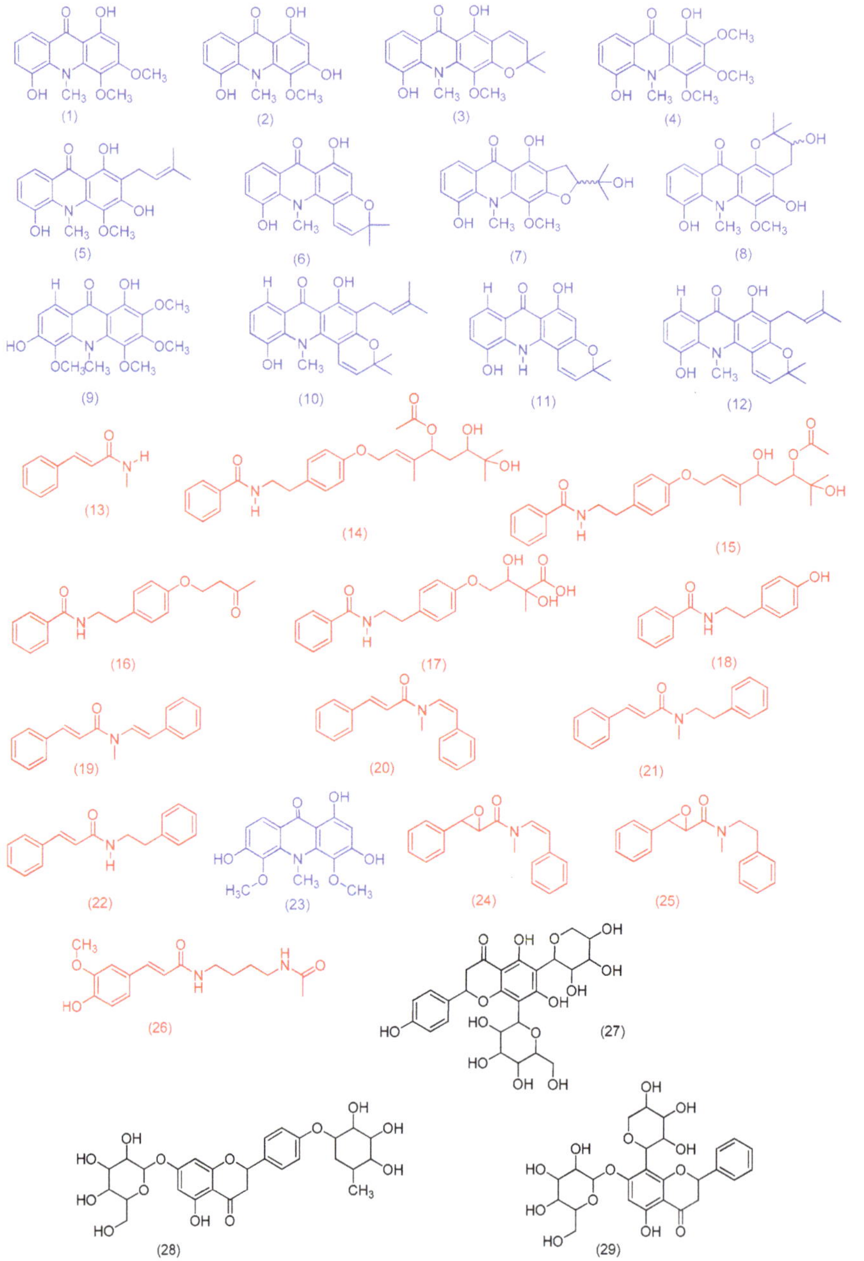

Figure 2. Identified compounds from *Swinglea glutinosa* through UHPLC-HRMS (compounds **1–22**, using Target Analysis; compounds **23–29** using GNPS). The compounds indicated in red correspond to the phenylacrylamide class; the compounds in blue belong to the acridonic alkaloid class and in black are compounds belonging to the flavonoid class.

On the other hand, from the analysis of the hexane leaf fraction (Figure 1B), we observed that its major compounds did not correspond to the cataloged metabolites in our database. To find out which classes of compounds were present in the fraction as well as in the other fractionated amounts, we decided to use a complementary dereplication strategy: the free website GNPS.

Currently, the use of molecular networking is a powerful analytical tool for metabolic mapping by molecular fragmentation data through tandem mass spectrometry [2]. This makes it possible to represent and to group a set of spectral data based on the fragmentation similarity (MS/MS spectra) of compounds present in one or more target samples. Directly, such grouping suggests a structural similarity between compounds, thus facilitating the detection of biosynthetic analogues [10]. Therefore, through the analysis of the obtained molecular families from the extracts of *S. glutinosa* (Figure 3 and Figure S1), it was possible to visualize the establishment of eight predominant clusters.

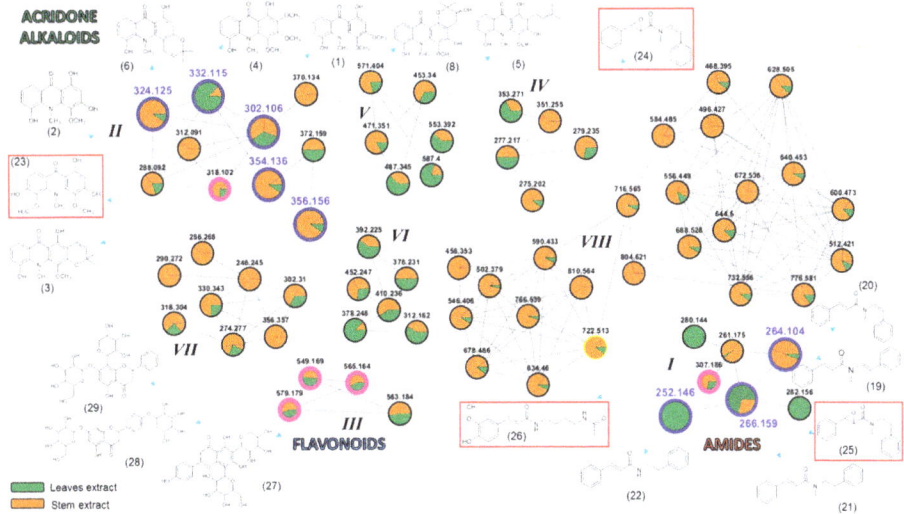

Figure 3. Molecular families for *S. glutinosa* extracts. Nodes outlined in blue represent isolated and identified compounds in this work. The nodes outlined in pink represent dereplicated compounds, which had the chemical structure suggested by the GNPS platform. Compounds indicated from non-prominent nodes suggest substances compatible with metabolites already described for *S. glutinosa*. Structures highlighted in the red frame indicate compounds not related to the *Swinglea* genus and that were identified by our "in-house" database. Different portions visualized at nodes are not quantitatively representative.

The orange and green colors represented in the nodes (Figure 3) illustrate the presence of the described precursor ions found in the extracts from the stems and leaves of the plant, respectively. It is important to highlight that the indicated proportions should not be associated with the amounts of metabolite detected in each extract. The observed differences correspond to the number of spectral counts recorded for each ion, according to the program processing standardization.

The molecular family I indicates the detection of seven metabolites belonging to the N-benzoyltyramine class, a known group of compounds found in the *Swinglea* genus [6]. However, all seven biosynthetic congeners have not been described for *S. glutinosa* yet. Given this, we decided to isolate the compounds represented by *m/z* 264.104, 252.146, and 266.159 through the use of preparative HPLC. NMR data allowed for the identification of the metabolites as: Lansamide I (**19**) [11], Lansiumamide B (**20**) [12], Lansiumamide C (**21**) [12], and N-(2-phenylethyl)cinnamamide (**22**) [13] (Figure 2). In the chromatogram shown in Figure 1B, the characteristic peaks of these compounds are highlighted in red. Noteworthy, compounds (**19**) and (**20**) are configurational isomers, whose *m/z* is 264.104. Furthermore, compounds represented by *m/z* 280.144 and 282.156 (Figure 3) are correlated with metabolites found in another Rutaceae plant, *Clausena lansium* [14] as well as the isolated and identified compounds.

The GNPS platform was important to identify compound (**26**), whose m/z is 307.186, as (*E*)-*N*-(4-acetamidobutyl)-3-(4-hydroxy-3-methoxyphenyl)prop-2-enamide. These data confirm the consistent result for grouping the compounds in cluster I, which is also highlighted by the obtained cosine values (higher than 0.7), pointing to significant fragmentation similarities among the clustered compounds. The comparison between the experimental and registered (GNPS database) spectra (Figure 4) also demonstrates the resemblances around the fragmentation pattern, which was important for compound identification.

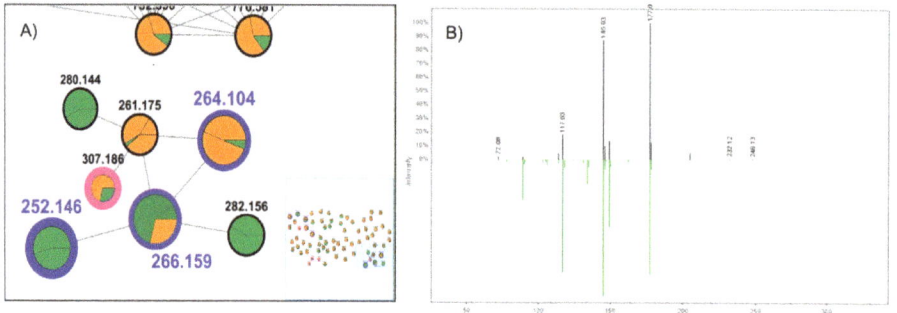

Figure 4. (**A**) Part of molecular family I, corresponding to amide detection, with highlighted cosine values. (**B**) MS/MS spectrum acquired (black) vs. registered spectrum on the GNPS platform (green), for the ion m/z 307.186. The pseudomolecular ion was not detected in both cases.

Molecular family II is basically formed by acridones, a class of natural products quite characteristic in *Swinglea glutinosa* [4,5,15]. In this work, some of them were isolated and identified: citrusinine-I (**1**) [16], citrusinine (**2**) [17], glycotrycine IV (**5**) [18], and 5-hydroxynoracronycine (**6**) [19]. In addition, the presence of cluster II also suggests the likely production of other alkaloids that have not been reported for *S. glutinosa* yet. The nodes represented by m/z 312.091, m/z 370.134, and m/z 318.102 did not show any correlation with our "in-house" database. The last one was identified using MS/MS spectra comparison at the GNPS platform as 1,3,6-trihydroxy-4,5-dimethoxy-10-methylacridin-9-one (**23**) [20]. Therefore, our approach revealed the potential of finding untapped acridones in *S. glutinosa*.

In its turn, for molecular family III, it was observed as a flavonoid cluster, some of whose compounds were identified according to MS/MS spectra matches through the GNPS database [2]. The candidates suggested for m/z 565.164, m/z 579.179, and m/z 549.169 were 5,7-dihydroxy-2-(4-hydroxyphenyl)-8-[3,4,5-trihydroxy-6-(hydroxymethyl)oxanitrile)-2-yl]-6-(3,4,5-trihydroxyoxan-2-yl)chromen-4-one (**27**), 5-hydroxy-7-[3,4,5-trihydroxy-6-(hydroxymethyl)oxan-2-yl]-oxy-2-[4-(3,4,5-trihydroxy-6-methoxan-2-yl)oxiphenyl]chromen-4-one (**28**), and 5,7-dihydroxy-2-phenyl-6-[3,4,5-trihydroxy-6-(hydroxymethyl)oxan-2-yl]-8-(3,4,5-trihydroxyoxan-2-yl)chromen-4-one (**29**), respectively. Furthermore, clusters IV–VIII were also observed, but any corresponding metabolite was identified using the described analytical tools.

Employing the two mentioned dereplication strategies, it was possible to identify 29 compounds, 11 of them not described for the *Swinglea* genus. These methodologies guided the isolation of four phenylacrylamides, alkaloid-based compounds that were also first shown in the plant genus.

In a nutshell, the use of the combined approaches has been useful for exploring the chemical profile of the *Swinglea* genus, in particular regarding the detection of alkaloid-based compounds produced by the plant. Altogether, the results point toward still hidden specialized metabolites from *Swinglea glutinosa* to be revealed in the ongoing work.

3. Materials and Methods

3.1. Target Analysis and Molecular MS/MS Networking-Based Dereplication

A list creation for target candidates in the Target Analysis 1.3 (Bruker Daltonics®, Bremen, Germany) program processing was performed through the Microsoft Excel interface, with the compound name and the molecular formula, according to the literature information. Considered processing parameters were SigmaFit at 1000 (broad, isotope-free), 60 (medium), 20 (low), mass accuracy accessed lower than 5 ppm, and mSigma lower than 50. Area cut-off was set to 2000 counts as the default and DataAnalysis 4.2 software (Bruker Daltonics®) was used for manual comparison of extracted-ion chromatograms (EIC) generated by Target Analysis.

For MS/MS dereplication via molecular networking analysis (GNPS), MS/MS data were acquired using AutoMS mode and converted to .mzXML format using MS-Convert software, which is part of ProteoWizard (Palo Alto, CA, USA). The networks were generated using the online platform (https://gnps.ucsd.edu/ProteoSAFe/static/gnps-splash.jsp) [2]. All MS/MS peaks within ±17 Da deviations from the precursor ions were filtered out. MS/MS spectra were selected from only the six best peaks, considering a range of ±50 Da across the spectrum. The data were grouped with a tolerance of 0.02 Da for precursor ions and 0.02 Da for fragment ions in the construction of "consensus" spectra (identical spectra for each precursor, which are combined to create the node to be visualized). Consensus spectra with less than two spectra were not considered. Connections between nodes were filtered to values greater than 0.7 of the cosine parameter, with compatibility for more than six peaks. For the dereplication of compounds, the generated network spectra were consulted at the GNPS libraries, using the same selection criteria for the analyzed samples. GNPS data were analyzed and viewed using Cytoscape 3.7.0 software (U.S. National Institute of General Medical Sciences, Bethesda, MD, USA).

3.2. Acridone Alkaloids and Phenylacrylamides Isolation and Identification

The plant material was divided into two parts, stem and leaves, followed by drying in an air circulation oven at 40 °C. After grinding, materials were submitted to extraction by maceration in ethanol for three days. After three days, the ethanol was filtered off and evaporated. The procedure was repeated until the third extraction to obtain the extracts from the stems and leaves of *S. glutinosa*. In sequence, from the ethanolic crude extracts, the liquid–liquid extraction procedure was employed to prepare hexane, ethyl acetate, and butanol fractions.

The stems hexane fraction (0.93 g) was subjected to silica column chromatography (diameter: 4.0 cm; height: 1 cm) using hexane, ethyl acetate, and methanol as the gradient mode eluent yielding 16 subfractions (A1 to A16). Fractions A6 and A7 were submitted to preparative HPLC (C12—Synergi Max column—150 mm × 4.60 mm, 4 µ), allowing the isolation of one substance from A6 (6) and three substances from A7 (1, 2, and 5). The employed mobile phase was formed by acetonitrile (ACN) and H_2O (both with the addition of 0.1% formic acid) and the method used for all these substances was: 0.01–2.5 min—15% ACN; 2.5–12 min—15–95% ACN; 12–20 min—95% ACN; 20–23 min—95–15% ACN; 23–27 min—15% ACN; this procedure allowed us to obtain citrusinine-I (1) (5.0 mg) [16], citibrasine (2) (11.7 mg) [17], glycotrycine IV (5) (21.2 mg) [18], and 5-hydroxynoracronycine (6) (2.0 mg) [19].

The hexane fraction from the leaves (8.0 g) of *S. glutinosa* was fractionated using a silica chromatography column (diameter: 5.7 cm; height: 30 cm); hexane, ethyl acetate, and methanol were used as gradient mode eluents yielding 10 fractions (B1–B10). Fractions B5 and B7 were submitted to preparative HPLC (column C18—250 mm × 4.6 mm—Luna 5 µ). The mobile phase used was ACN and H_2O (both with addition of 0.1% formic acid) and the method used for isolation was: 0.01–2.5 min—60% ACN; 2.5–12 min—60–95% ACN; 12–20 min—95% ACN; 20–23 min—95–60% ACN; 23–27 min—60% ACN; this procedure allowed us to obtain Lansamide I (19) (8.1 mg) [11], Lansiumamide B (20) (3.8 mg) [12], Lansiumamide C (21) (20.6 mg) [12], and *N*-(2-phenylethyl)cinnamamide (22) (18.0 mg) [13]. The NMR spectra were recorded on a Bruker spectrometer (Bruker Daltonics®)

Ultrashield 300—Advance III operating at 300 MHz (^{1}H) and 75 MHz (^{13}C). The spectra are presented in the Supplementary Materials (Figures S2–S14).

Lansamide I (**19**): ^{1}H NMR (CDCl$_3$, δ (J/Hz)): 7.77 (d, 16.4); 7.32 (d, 14,0); 7.20–7.59 (m); 7.02 (d, 15.4); 6.07 (d, 14.3); 3.37 (s); ^{13}C NMR (CDCl$_3$): 135.2; 130.2; 129.1; 128.2; 128.9; 126.8; 125.8; 117.3; 29.8. HRMS. m/z 264.1379 [M + H]$^+$ (calcd for C$_{18}$H$_{17}$NO, Δ3.4 ppm).

Lansiumamide B (**20**): ^{1}H NMR (CDCl$_3$, δ (J/Hz)): 7.55 (d, 15.0); 7.20–7.34 (m); 6.93 (d, 15.0); 6.50 (d, 8.6); 6.24 (d, 8.7); 3.09 (s). ^{13}C NMR (CDCl$_3$): 141.4; 135.4; 124.1; 127.5–129.5; 118.9; 33.6. HRMS. m/z 264.1381 [M + H]$^+$ (calcd for C$_{18}$H$_{17}$NO, Δ2.6 ppm).

Lansiumamide C (**21**): ^{1}H NMR (CDCl$_3$, δ (J/Hz)): 7.72 (d, 15.4); 7.20–7.41 (m); 6.58 (d, 15.4); 3.71 (q, 7.2); 3.07 (s); 2.94 (t, 7.4). ^{13}C NMR (CDCl$_3$): 166.5; 142.2; 140.6–127.0; 119.5; 51.9; 36.1; 34.3. HRMS. m/z 266.1554 [M + H]$^+$ (calcd for C$_{18}$H$_{19}$NO, Δ3.3 ppm).

N-(2-phenylethyl)cinnamamide (**22**): ^{1}H NMR (CDCl$_3$): 7.54 (d, 15.5); 7.22–7.50 (m); 6.31 (d, 15.6); 5.60 (s); 3.67 (q, 6.5); 2.89 (t, 7.0). ^{13}C NMR (CDCl$_3$): 140.5; 130.2–127.0; 123.0; 41.6; 36.5. HRMS. m/z 252.1397 [M + H]$^+$ (calcd for C$_{17}$H$_{17}$NO, Δ3.5 ppm).

Supplementary Materials: The following are available online, Figure S1: Molecular families obtained from *Swinglea glutinosa* extracts, Figures S2–S14: NMR (^{1}H and ^{13}C) spectra of the compounds (**19–22**), Figures S15–S18: Fragmentation schemes for the compounds (**19–22**).

Author Contributions: Conceptualization, T.A.M.V.; methodology, A.I.R. and L.S.d.M.; software, L.S.d.M.; formal analysis, A.I.R.; investigation, A.C.d.C. and L.D.C.R.; data curation, L.S.d.M. and M.F.d.G.F.d.S.; writing—original draft preparation, A.C.d.C. and L.D.C.R.; writing—review and editing, L.S.d.M. and T.A.M.V.; supervision, L.S.d.M. and T.A.M.V.; project administration, T.A.M.V.; funding acquisition, T.A.M.V. All authors have read and agreed to the published version of the manuscript.

Funding: This research was funded by the Fundação de Amparo á Pesquisa do Estado de São Paulo, grant number 2018/04095-0, and ACC was funded by a PhD scholarship from Coordenação de Aperfeiçoamento de Pessoal de Nível Superior.

Acknowledgments: The authors thank the "*Programa de Pós-Graduação em Biologia Química*" for all their support and the "Central de Equipamentos e Serviços Multiusuários (CESM-UNIFESP)" for technical support.

Conflicts of Interest: The authors declare no conflict of interest.

References

1. Dinan, L. Dereplication and partial identification of compounds. In *Natural Products Isolation*, 2nd ed.; Sarker, S.D., Latif, Z., Gray, A.I., Eds.; Humana Press Inc.: Totowa, NJ, USA, 2005.
2. Wang, M.; Carver, J.J.; Phelan, V.V.; Sanchez, L.M.; Garg, N.; Peng, Y.; Nguyen, D.D.; Watrous, J.; Kapono, C.A.; Luzzatto-Knaan, T.; et al. Sharing and community curation of mass spectrometry data with GNPS. *Nat. Biotechnol.* **2016**, *34*, 828–837. [CrossRef] [PubMed]
3. Klitgaard, A.; Iversen, A.; Andersen, M.R.; Larsen, T.O.; Frisvad, J.C.; Nielsen, K.F. Aggressive dereplication using UHPLC-DAD-QTOF: Screening extracts for up to 3000 fungal secondary metabolites. *Anal. Bioanal. Chem.* **2014**, *406*, 1933–1943. [CrossRef] [PubMed]
4. Engler, A.; Prantl, K. *Die Naturlichen Pflanzenfamilien*; Engler, A., Prantl, K., Eds.; Wilhelm Engelmann: Leipzig, Germany, 1931; Volume 19, pp. 187–359.
5. Arato Ferreira, P.H.; Dos Santos, D.A.; Da Silva, M.F.; Vieira, P.C.; King-diaz, B.; Lotina-Hennsen, B.; Veiga, T.A. Acridone Alkaloids from *Swinglea glutinosa* (Rutaceae) and Their Effects on Photosynthesis. *Chem. Biodivers.* **2016**, *13*, 100–106. [CrossRef] [PubMed]
6. Do Nascimento Cerqueira, C.; Cerqueira, N.C.; Dos Santos, D.A.P.; Malaquias, K.S.; Lima, M.M.C.; Da Silva, M.F.G.; Fernandes, F.; Vieira, P.C. Novas n-benzoiltiraminas de *Swinglea Glutinosa* (rutaceae). *Quim. Nova* **2012**, *35*, 2181–2185. [CrossRef]
7. Santos, D.A.P.; Vieira, P.C.; Silva, M.F.G.F.; Fernandes, J.B.; Rattray, L.; Crof, S.L. Antiparasitic Activities of Acridone Alkaloids from *Swinglea glutinosa* (Bl.) Merr. *J. Braz. Chem. Soc.* **2009**, *20*, 644–651. [CrossRef]
8. Marques, E.F.; Vieira, P.C.; Severino, R.P. Acridone alkaloids as Inhibitors of Cathepsin L and V. *Quím. Nova* **2016**, *39*, 58–62. [CrossRef]

9. Kuete, V.; Fouotsa, H.; Mbaveng, A.T.; Wiench, B.; Nkengfack, A.E.; Efferth, T. Cytotoxicity of a naturally occurring furoquinoline alkaloid and four acridone alkaloids towards multi-factorial drug-resistant cancer cells. *Phytomedicine* **2015**, *22*, 946–951. [CrossRef]
10. Winnikoff, J.R.; Glukhov, E.; Watrous, J.; Dorrestein, P.C.; Gerwick, W.H. Quantitative molecular networking to profile marine cyanobacterial metabolomes. *J. Antibiot.* **2014**, *67*, 105–112. [CrossRef]
11. Goossen, L.J.; Gooben, L.; Blanchot, M.; Arndt, M.; Salih, K.S.M. Synthesis of botryllamides and lansiumamides via ruthenium-catalyzed hydroamidation of alkynes. *Synlett* **2010**, 1685–1687. [CrossRef]
12. Lin, J.H. Cinnamamide derivatives from *Clausena Lansium*. *Phitochemistry* **1989**, *28*, 621–622. [CrossRef]
13. Yamazaki, Y.; Kawano, Y.; Uebayasi, M. Induction of adiponectin by natural and synthetic phenolamides in mouse and human preadipocytes and its enhancement by docosahexaenoic acid. *Life Sci.* **2008**, *82*, 290–300. [CrossRef] [PubMed]
14. Matsui, T.; Ito, C.; Furukawa, H. Lansiumamide B and SB-204900 isolated from *Clausena lansium* inhibit histamine and TNF-a release from RBL-2H3 cells. *Inflamm. Res.* **2013**, *62*, 333–341. [CrossRef] [PubMed]
15. Weniger, B.; Um, B.-H.; Valentin, A.; Estrada, A.; Lobstein, A.; Anton, R.; Maille, M.; Sauvain, M. Bioactive acridone alkaloids from *Swinglea glutinosa*. *J. Nat. Prod.* **2001**, *64*, 1221–1223. [CrossRef] [PubMed]
16. Furukawa, H.; Yogo, M.; Wu, T.-S. Acridone Alkaloids. X. ^{13}C-Nuclear Magnetic Resonance Spectra of Acridone Alkaloids. *Chem. Pharm. Bull.* **1983**, *31*, 3084–3090. [CrossRef]
17. Wu, T.-S.; Furukawa, H. Acridone alkaloids. VII. Constituents of Citrus sinensis OSBECK var. brasiliensis TANAKA. Isolation and characterization of three new acridone alkaloids, and a new coumarin. *Chem. Pharm. Bull.* **1983**, *31*, 901–906. [CrossRef]
18. Ito, C.; Kondo, Y.; Wu, T.-S.; Furukawa, H. Chemical Constituents of *Glycosmis citrifolia* (Willd.) Lindl. Structures of four New Acridones and Three New Quinolone Alkaloids. *Chem. Pharm. Bull.* **2000**, *48*, 65–70. [CrossRef] [PubMed]
19. Wu, T.-S.; Kuoh, C.-S.; Furukawa, H. Acridone Alkaloids. VI, The constituents of *Citrus depressa*. Isolation and Structure Elucidation of New Acridone Alkaloids from *Citrus* genus. *Chem. Pharm. Bull.* **1983**, *31*, 895–900. [CrossRef]
20. Wu, T.-S.; Chen, C.-M. Acridone Alkaloids from the Root Bark of *Severinia buxifolia* in Hainan. *Chem. Pharm. Bull.* **2000**, *48*, 85–90. [CrossRef] [PubMed]

Sample Availability: Samples of the compounds are not available from the authors.

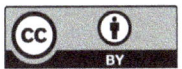

© 2019 by the authors. Licensee MDPI, Basel, Switzerland. This article is an open access article distributed under the terms and conditions of the Creative Commons Attribution (CC BY) license (http://creativecommons.org/licenses/by/4.0/).

MDPI
St. Alban-Anlage 66
4052 Basel
Switzerland
Tel. +41 61 683 77 34
Fax +41 61 302 89 18
www.mdpi.com

Molecules Editorial Office
E-mail: molecules@mdpi.com
www.mdpi.com/journal/molecules